2016

The Year Book of SURGERY®

Editor-in-Chief

Kevin E. Behrns, MD

Chairman, Edward R. Woodward Professor, Department of Surgery, University of Florida, Gainesville, Florida

ELSEVIER
MOSBY

ELSEVIER
MOSBY

Acquisitions Editor: John Vassallo
Developmental Editor: Alison Swety

2016 EDITION

Composition by TNQ Books and Journals Pvt Ltd, India

Editorial Office:
Elsevier
1600 John F. Kennedy Blvd.
Suite 1800
Philadelphia, PA 19103-2899

International Standard Serial Number: 0090-3671
International Standard Book Number: 978-0-323-44696-9

Editorial Board

Table of Contents

Journals Represented

Journals represented in this YEAR BOOK are listed below.

American Journal of Clinical Nutrition
American Journal of Surgery
American Journal of Transplantation
American Surgeon
Annals of Diagnostic Pathology
Annals of Plastic Surgery
Annals of Surgery
Annals of Surgical Oncology
Annals of the American Thoracic Society
Annals of the Rheumatic Diseases
Annals of Thoracic Surgery
Biochimica et Biophysica Acta
Biomaterials
British Journal of Surgery
Burns
Cancer
Chest
Clinical Endocrinology (Oxford)
Cochrane Database of Systematic Reviews
Critical Care Medicine
Digestive Diseases and Sciences
Diseases of the Colon and Rectum
Epidemiology and Infection
European Journal of Clinical Microbiology & Infectious Diseases
European Journal of Radiology
European Journal of Vascular and Endovascular Surgery
Gastroenterology
Hepatology
Injury
International Journal of Pediatric Ortorhinolaryngology
International Journal of Radiation Oncology *Biology* Physics
Journal of Burn Care & Research
Journal of Clinical Oncology
Journal of Heart and Lung Transplantation
Journal of Orthopaedic Trauma
Journal of Pediatric Gastroenterology and Nutrition
Journal of Pediatrics
Journal of Surgical Oncology
Journal of Surgical Research
Journal of the American College of Surgeons
Journal of the American Geriatrics Society
Journal of the American Medical Association
Journal of the American Medical Association dermatology
Journal of the American Medical Association surgery
Journal of Thoracic and Cardiovascular Surgery
Journal of Vascular Surgery
JPEN Journal of Parenteral and Enteral Nutrition

Kidney International
Lancet
Medicine (Baltimore)
Neurosurgery
New England Journal of Medicine
Proceedings of the National Academy of Sciences of the United States of America
Public Library of Science One
Surgery
Surgical Endoscopy
The Journal of Clinical Endocrinology and Metabolism
Thyroid
Transplantation
Wound Repair and Regeneration

Standard Abbreviations

The following terms are abbreviated in this edition: acquired immunodeficiency syndrome (AIDS), cardiopulmonary resuscitation (CPR), central nervous system (CNS), cerebrospinal fluid (CSF), computed tomography (CT), deoxyribonucleic acid (DNA), electrocardiography (ECG), health maintenance organization (HMO), human immunodeficiency virus (HIV), intensive care unit (ICU), intramuscular (IM), intravenous (IV), magnetic resonance (MR) imaging (MRI), ribonucleic acid (RNA), and ultrasound (US).

Note

The Year Book of Surgery is a literature survey service providing abstracts of articles published in the professional literature. Every effort is made to assure the accuracy of the information presented in these pages. Neither the editors nor the publisher of the Year Book of Surgery can be responsible for errors in the original materials. The editors' comments are their own opinions. Mention of specific products within this publication does not constitute endorsement.

To facilitate the use of the Year Book of Surgery as a reference tool, all illustrations and tables included in this publication are now identified as they appear in the original article. This change is meant to help the reader recognize that any illustration or table appearing in the Year Book of Surgery may be only one of many in the original article. For this reason, figure and table numbers appear to be out of sequence within the Year Book of Surgery.

1 General Considerations

National Cluster-Randomized Trial of Duty-Hour Flexibility in Surgical Training

Bilimoria KY, Chung JW, Hedges LV, et al (Northwestern Univ, Chicago, IL; Northwestern Univ, Evanston, IL; et al)

N Engl J Med 374:713-727, 2016

Background.—Concerns persist regarding the effect of current surgical resident duty-hour policies on patient outcomes, resident education, and resident well-being.

Methods.—We conducted a national, cluster-randomized, pragmatic, noninferiority trial involving 117 general surgery residency programs in the United States (2014–2015 academic year). Programs were randomly assigned to current Accreditation Council for Graduate Medical Education (ACGME) duty-hour policies (standard-policy group) or more flexible policies that waived rules on maximum shift lengths and time off between shifts (flexible-policy group). Outcomes included the 30-day rate of postoperative death or serious complications (primary outcome), other postoperative complications, and resident perceptions and satisfaction regarding their well-being, education, and patient care.

Results.—In an analysis of data from 138,691 patients, flexible, less-restrictive duty-hour policies were not associated with an increased rate of death or serious complications (9.1% in the flexible-policy group and 9.0% in the standard-policy group, $P = 0.92$; unadjusted odds ratio for the flexible-policy group, 0.96; 92% confidence interval, 0.87 to 1.06; $P = 0.44$; noninferiority criteria satisfied) or of any secondary postoperative outcomes studied. Among 4330 residents, those in programs assigned to flexible policies did not report significantly greater dissatisfaction with overall education quality (11.0% in the flexible-policy group and 10.7% in the standard-policy group, $P = 0.86$) or well-being (14.9% and 12.0%, respectively; $P = 0.10$). Residents under flexible policies were less likely than those under standard policies to perceive negative effects of duty-hour policies on multiple aspects of patient safety, continuity of care, professionalism, and resident education but were more likely to perceive negative effects on personal activities. There were no significant differences between study groups in resident-reported perception of the effect of fatigue on personal or patient safety. Residents in the flexible-policy group were less likely than those in the standard-policy group to report leaving during an operation (7.0% vs. 13.2%, $P < 0.001$) or handing off active patient issues (32.0% vs. 46.3%, $P < 0.001$).

Conclusions.—As compared with standard duty-hour policies, flexible, less-restrictive duty-hour policies for surgical residents were associated with noninferior patient outcomes and no significant difference in residents' satisfaction with overall well-being and education quality. (FIRST ClinicalTrials.gov number, NCT02050789.)

▶ Perhaps no topic in surgery has generated more discussion than duty-hour regulations, which were introduced by the Accreditation Council for Graduate Medical Education (ACGME) in 2003. The topic has been debated vigorously because of a lack of evidence about the risks and benefits of duty-hour regulations on patient safety and outcomes and resident well-being. Bilimoria et al addressed this important question by conducting a randomized, noninferiority trial of general surgery training programs and residents by comparing standard versus flexible duty hour regulations on outcomes measured by ACS NSQIP (American College of Surgeons National Surgical Quality Improvement Program) and ABSITE (American Board of Surgery In-Training Examination) results and surveys. The results showed no significant differences in patient safety or outcomes when training programs were randomized to standard versus flexible duty hours. Furthermore, residents in the flexible duty-hour group did not express significant differences in overall education quality or well-being. Residents in the flexible duty-hour group did express dissatisfaction with time for personal activities, however. Overall, flexibility in duty-hour regulations for surgical residents did not affect surgical outcomes, resident education, and trainee well-being. This obviously raises the question of what's next. These data suggest that ACGME duty-hour regulations that applied broadly across all disciplines of medicine may not have achieved the intended goals. Thus, a well-thought-out plan that addresses duty-hour regulations applied to specific disciplines or to groups of disciplines, all surgical disciplines for instance, may be more appropriate. In addition, a plan of duty-hour modifications must clearly describe the intended goals of duty-hour restrictions. Collectively, we need to strike a balance between optimal patient outcomes and outstanding resident education that is characterized by progressive acquisition of responsibility and autonomy. These parameters are difficult to reconcile for a large group of trainees and, thus we may be served by considering competency-based surgical education. Clearly, we are at a critical juncture in surgical education, and thoughtful approaches and leadership from multiple stakeholders is necessary to train the next generation of surgeons.

K. E. Behrns, MD

Investigating the Impact of the 2011 ACGME Resident Duty Hour Regulations on Surgical Residency Programs: The Program Director Perspective

Scally CP, Sandhu G, Magas C, et al (Univ of Michigan, Ann Arbor)

J Am Coll Surg 221:883-889.e1, 2015

Background.—The 2011 ACGME regulations required substantial changes to the structure of general surgery residency programs, due primarily to the 16-hour in-house rule for PGY1 residents. However, the scope of changes that programs have undertaken to meet these requirements, and the educational impact of those changes, are poorly understood.

Study Design.—We performed in-depth qualitative interviews with general surgery program directors. Twenty program directors participated in the study; interviews were conducted until adequate thematic saturation was achieved. Participants were recruited from a stratified random sampling of residency programs in the United States to ensure a representative cohort. Interviews focused on changes in call schedule, interns' educational requirements, development, and satisfaction.

Results.—Most programs used a month-long night float (NF) rotation (14 of 20 [75%]). A minority of programs (5 of 20 [25%]) used a weekly rotating schedule, in which interns worked 5 to 6 nights in a month. Multiple programs (65%) had an NF in place before 2011; these programs made changes to and expanded their existing schedule to accommodate the new regulations. Commonly cited challenges to instituting NF included weekend coverage (60%) and providing adequate days off during day-to-night transition. Interns spent as much as 3 months of the year on NF. Only 5 programs made explicit changes to teaching schedules or developed a curriculum for residents on NF. Seventy-five percent of programs excused interns, explicitly or implicitly, from didactic teaching when on NF. Common themes noted by program directors included delayed maturation of trainees, interns being isolated from the team culture, and a conflict between the professional behaviors of "following the rules" and "doing what is right."

▶ The 2011 ACGME duty-hour regulations specified that interns could work shifts no longer than 16 hours in duration. For some general surgery training programs, this regulation required a major schedule modification, whereas other programs made relatively minor changes to trainees' shifts. Most programs, however, implemented night float rotations to address the 2011 regulations. Although duty-hour changes incite many negative impressions, the 2011 regulations were implemented relatively quietly. The impact of these duty-hour changes has not been quantitatively or qualitatively documented until now. Scally et al used a semistructured interview of 20 general surgery program directors to assess the consequences of the 2011 duty-hour regulations. Their work showed nicely that many of the program directors recognized major limitations to increasing night float rotations for trainees. First, the education of trainees on night float rotations is essentially nonexistent. Second, because the trainees often worked 2 to 3 months of night float in a year, many of the potential daytime learning experiences were eliminated. These changes led to delayed development of the interns. In addition, surgical interns are a proud group, and being told that they can only work 16-hour shifts resulted in animosity and resentment from being told when to end a shift. The faculty, too, were not immune to feeling the effects of the duty-hour changes. Faculty expressed the need to more frequently attend to details, especially at night, and these behaviors created a sense of mistrust. In summary, it appears that the 2011 duty-hour changes created a training environment that reduced resident education, delayed maturation, and created a less than desirable work environment. For these reasons, we eagerly await the results of the FIRST (Flexibility in Duty Hour Requirements for Surgical Trainees Trial), which we hope will demonstrate equivalency, as judged by patient outcomes, between the 2003 and 2011 duty-hour regulations. If equivalency is established, perhaps we can revert to the 2003 duty-hour regulations, which despite several shortcomings, may allow more educational opportunities.

K. E. Behrns, MD

Using Patient Outcomes to Evaluate General Surgery Residency Program Performance

Bansal N, Simmons KD, Epstein AJ, et al (Perelman School of Medicine at the Univ of Pennsylvania, Philadelphia; Univ of Pennsylvania Health System, Philadelphia; et al)

JAMA Surg 151:111-119, 2016

Importance.—To evaluate and financially reward general surgery residency programs based on performance, performance must first be defined and measureable.

Objective.—To assess general surgery residency program performance using the objective clinical outcomes of patients operated on by program graduates.

Design, Setting, and Participants.—A retrospective cohort study was conducted of discharge records from 349 New York and Florida hospitals between January 1, 2008, and December 31, 2011. The records comprised 230 769 patients undergoing 1 of 24 general surgical procedures performed by 454 surgeons from 73 general surgery residency programs. Analysis was conducted from June 4, 2014, to June 16, 2015.

Main Outcomes and Measures.—In-hospital death; development of 1 or more postoperative complications before discharge; prolonged length of stay, defined as length of stay greater than the 75th percentile when compared with patients undergoing the same procedure type at the same hospital; and failure to rescue, defined as in-hospital death after the development of 1 or more postoperative complications.

Results.—Patients operated on by surgeons trained in residency programs that were ranked in the top tertile were significantly less likely to experience an adverse event than were patients operated on by surgeons trained in residency programs that were ranked in the bottom tertile. Adjusted adverse event rates for patients operated on by surgeons trained in programs that were ranked in the top tertile and those who were operated on by surgeons trained in programs that were ranked in the bottom tertile were, respectively, 0.483% vs 0.476% for death, 9.68% vs 10.79% for complications, 16.76% vs 17.60% for prolonged length of stay, and 2.68% vs 2.98% for failure to rescue (all $P < .001$). The differences remained significant in procedure-specific subset analyses. The rankings were significantly correlated among some but not all outcome measures. The magnitude of the effect of the residency program on the outcomes achieved by the graduates decreased with increasing years of practice. Within the analyses of surgeons within 20, 10, and 5 years of practice, the relative difference in adjusted adverse event rates across the individual models between the top and bottom tertiles ranged from 1.5% to 12.3% (20 years), 9.1% to 33.8% (10 years), and 8.0% to 44.4% (5 years).

Conclusions and Relevance.—Objective data were successfully used to rank the clinical outcomes achieved by graduates of general surgery residency programs. Program rankings differed by the outcome measured. The magnitude of differences across programs was small. Careful consideration must be used when identifying potential targets for payment-for-performance initiatives in graduate medical education.

▶ The recommendations from the 2014 Institute of Medicine (IOM) report on Graduate Medical Education (GME) include examining alternative methods of funding resident education. One suggestion was to reward those programs that are superior. An issue with this approach, however, is how to determine the programs that consistently train surgeons who perform better than their peers. In this report, Bansal et al offer an intriguing approach to measure general surgery resident program performance. As detailed in the article, this group cleverly used databases from Florida and New York to measure patient outcomes for up to 20 years to determine whether the outcomes correlated with training in specific programs. Impressively, those residents who trained in a top tertile program had significantly better patient outcomes as an independent surgeon than did those who did not train in a program with improved outcomes (Table 3 in the original article). The closer the surgeon was to residency training, the bigger the difference in outcomes, suggesting that the training program markedly influenced patient outcomes. This ingenious study is the first to demonstrate a linkage between outcomes at a training program and outcomes of graduates of training programs. This strong work clearly suggests that we must teach our trainees how to assess and measure quality outcomes, and, importantly, how to deliver care that results in excellent patient outcomes. I applaud the authors for fine work but am anxious to know the characteristics of the training programs that scored in the top tertile. Our real task is to model these programs as best practices and to disseminate their approach to patient care such that we can raise the level of performance of all groups. I trust the authors will publish a follow-up article that provides information about the characteristics of these top-tier programs.

K. E. Behrns, MD

Morbidity and Mortality Conference 2.0

Sacks GD, Lawson EH, Tillou A, et al (David Geffen School of Medicine at Univ of California–Los Angeles)
Ann Surg 262:228-229, 2015

Background.—The weekly Morbidity and Mortality (M&M) conference has been the means by which residents are exposed to safety and quality improvement (QI) issues. However, recent changes dictate that all graduating residents be trained in the science of patient safety and QI, and M&M conferences in the past have not accomplished this goal. Designing the M&M conference to educate residents as required and develop various QI initiatives involves a comprehensive identification of complications, a standardized case presentation that seeks care improvement and communication of clinical learning points, and a focus on translating what is discussed into meaningful QI projects.

Case Identification.—With the limited time in an M&M conference, planners must carefully select the most appropriate cases for presentation. Data sources from which to populate the conference are now abundant, providing data for evaluating hospital care as well as identifying complications from patient charts. Existing internal quality assurance initiatives can also be used as a referral base. Simple complications are visible on automatically generated electronic health record dashboards.

Once complications are identified, a senior resident and faculty member can review the list of complications and collate and categorize cases that meet the criteria for presentation. Cases can be presented by surgical service, operation type, complication type, or educational value.

Case Presentation.—Standardizing the format for case presentation helps presenters concentrate on the vital details and not irrelevant items. A useful framework is the Situation, Background, Assessment, Recommendations (SBAR) system. SBAR facilitates clear, consistent communication, producing a higher quality of presentation and improved educational value.

Assessment is the focus of the framework and is designed to identify individual and systemic factors that may contribute to the adverse outcome. A root-cause analysis framework considers the entire care pathway for environmental, team-related, and care process factors that may have contributed to the adverse event. This shifts the focus from individual blame to system-wide improvement. By recognizing the role of systemic factors, care path weaknesses can be addressed and similar complications avoided.

QI Initiatives.—The M&M conference can inform QI efforts in several ways. With the participation of residents, faculty, and quality officers, it is possible to brainstorm solutions, evaluate them from all sides, and implement changes to correct deficiencies. In addition, the results of the M&M conference can be directly communicated to existing QI teams, including surgery residents. This approach facilitates the successful crafting and implementation of a new QI strategy. In addition, less urgent QI issues can be tabled for future consideration and resident projects. The collective wisdom of all attendees of the M&M conference can inform refinements of the assessment process and identify targets for QI projects. Once these projects are undertaken and progress has been made, an update of the status is useful to underscore the importance of attending and participating in the M&M conference process.

Conclusions.—The M&M conference should be updated to use modern data analysis tools, standardize case presentation by using the root-cause analysis method, and effectively tailor the discussion to inform and complement ongoing QI efforts.

▶ Morbidity and mortality (M&M) conference is a long-held tradition in surgery. Traditionally, M&M was viewed as a mechanism to hold resident and faculty surgeons accountable, to educate trainees and surgeons alike, and to serve as a barometer for complications on a service. Over time, the M&M conference has served us well, but as pointed out in this article and many others, the capture rate of complications for M&M was low and personnel dependent. Furthermore, the conference was often geared toward accountability of an individual rather than looking at individual decision making in the context of a system. Sacks et al, appropriately highlight the need to change M&M conference. In a "just culture" with team-delivered care, M&M should focus on case identification, data reporting, establishment of processes to address the pertinent issues, and feedback to the larger audience. Teams that consist of faculty, residents, students, staff, and quality office personnel should conduct most of the work of establishing and implementing processes, as a strategy to mitigate complications. The teams should have short-term goals only, with rapid introduction of processes and outcomes assessment. The teams should not meet repetitively to establish an elaborate plan but address the most pertinent issues in the care pathway. This approach to M&M conference would be evidence-based, data-driven, and orientated at process improvement that leads to better outcomes. After all, the goal of M&M should be improved care for our patients, and, likely, future patients if we educate our trainees through this process.

K. E. Behrns, MD

Outcomes of Daytime Procedures Performed by Attending Surgeons after Night Work

Govindarajan A, Urbach DR, Kumar M, et al (Mount Sinai Hosp, NY; et al)
N Engl J Med 373:845-853, 2015

Background.—Sleep loss in attending physicians has an unclear effect on patient outcomes. In this study, we examined the effect of medical care provided by physicians after midnight on the outcomes of their scheduled elective procedures performed during the day.

Methods.—We conducted a population-based, retrospective, matched-cohort study in Ontario, Canada. Patients undergoing 1 of 12 elective daytime procedures performed by a physician who had treated patients from midnight to 7 a.m. were matched in a 1:1 ratio to patients undergoing the same procedure by the same physician on a day when the physician had not treated patients after midnight. Outcomes included death, readmission, complications, length of stay, and procedure duration. We used generalized estimating equations to compare outcomes between patient groups.

Results.—We included 38,978 patients, treated by 1448 physicians, in the study, of whom 40.6% were treated at an academic center. We found no significant difference in the primary outcome (death, readmission, or complication) between patients who underwent a daytime procedure performed by a physician who had provided patient care after midnight and those who underwent a procedure performed by a physician who had not treated patients after midnight (22.2% and 22.4%, respectively; $P = 0.66$; adjusted odds ratio, 0.99; 95% confidence interval, 0.95 to 1.03). We also found no significant difference in outcomes after stratification for academic versus nonacademic center, physician's age, or type of procedure. Secondary analyses revealed no significant difference between patient groups in length of stay or procedure duration.

Conclusions.—Overall, the risks of adverse outcomes of elective daytime procedures were similar whether or not the physician had provided medical services the previous night. (Funded by the University of Toronto Dean's Fund and others.)

▶ The introduction of resident duty hour regulations in 2003 has had a profound impact on patient care models, resident education, and regulation of residency training programs. Despite these weighty responses, the implementation of duty hour regulations and subsequent modified duty hour requirements has not improved definitively the quality and outcomes of patient care, which was the original premise for the creation and implementation of duty hours. Noticeably, little has been written about the effect of sleep deprivation of attending surgeons on the quality of care. Govindarajan et al, however, have closed the knowledge gap with this publication that examines surgical outcomes in nearly 40 000 patients cared for by 1448 surgeons who worked after midnight the night before performing daytime operations. Death, readmission, or complications were similar between groups that worked after midnight and those that did not, and these data were also similar in academic and nonacademic settings. The authors conclude that outcomes were similar between those that provided care the night before scheduled operation and those that did not. So where does this leave us? Are resident surgeons different from attending surgeons, who after years of nighttime work have acclimated appropriately to apparent sleep deprivation? It may be that residents and attendings are different, but likely, this is not the primary reason for the findings. It is more likely that nighttime work did not affect residents differently, and, thus, patient outcomes did not change for residents either. This publication should give us pause and make us reflect on our goals for duty hour restrictions. Have we achieved our goals? Did we have appropriate expectations? I doubt we strived to decrease the autonomy of residents or to increase the failure rate of general surgery certifying examination. As we are poised to reconsider our model of surgical training, we must first outline our goals for the delivery of high-quality surgical care that the public deserves.

K. E. Behrns, MD

Assessing Technical Competence in Surgical Trainees: A Systematic Review

Szasz P, Louridas M, Harris KA, et al (Univ of Toronto, Ontario, Canada; Royal College of Physicians and Surgeons of Canada, Ottawa, Ontario; et al)
Ann Surg 261:1046-1055, 2015

Objective.—To systematically examine the literature describing the methods by which *technical competence* is assessed in surgical trainees.

Background.—The last decade has witnessed an evolution away from time-based surgical education. In response, governing bodies worldwide have implemented competency-based education paradigms. The definition of *competence*, however, remains elusive, and the impact of these education initiatives in terms of assessment methods remains unclear.

Methods.—A systematic review examining the methods by which *technical competence* is assessed was conducted by searching MEDLINE, EMBASE, PsychINFO, and the Cochrane database of systematic reviews. Abstracts of retrieved studies were reviewed and those meeting inclusion criteria were selected for full review. Data were retrieved in a systematic manner, the validity and reliability of the assessment methods was evaluated, and quality was assessed using the Grading of Recommendations Assessment, Development and Evaluation classification.

Results.—Of the 6814 studies identified, 85 studies involving 2369 surgical residents were included in this review. The methods used to assess *technical competence* were categorized into 5 groups; Likert scales (37), benchmarks (31), binary outcomes (11), novel tools (4), and surrogate outcomes (2). Their validity and reliability were mostly previously established. The overall Grading of Recommendations Assessment, Development and Evaluation for randomized controlled trials was high and low for the observational studies.

Conclusions.—The definition of *technical competence* continues to be debated within the medical literature. The methods used to evaluate *technical competence* predominantly include instruments that were originally created to assess technical skill. Very few studies identify standard setting approaches that differentiate competent versus noncompetent performers; subsequently, this has been identified as an area with great research potential.

▶ In recent years, surgery program directors and leaders in surgical education have received feedback that some of our graduating surgical trainees are not ready for independent practice. The reasons for additional training have been enumerated previously in multiple publications, but a component of additional training is the need to attain technical competence. Clearly, our trainees spend less time in the operating room and have less independence, and, therefore, we need better tools to assess trainees' technical competence or readiness to conduct an operation independently. In this *Annals of Surgery* article, Szasz et al performed a systematic review to obtain an overview of assessment tools that allow measurement of technical competence. Their systematic review defined technical competence as "a minimum standard to safely perform a procedure or task independently." This definition appears appropriate, but can we truly assess this definition of technical competence with a Likert scale, benchmarks, binary outcomes, novel tools, or surrogate outcomes? I doubt these measurement tools are satisfactory and agree completely with the authors that this definition of technical competence requires substantial research to arrive at an appropriate assessment tool. Importantly, this definition of technical competence cannot be determined by an intraoperative assessment alone. Safety of an operation can only be determined after a patient recovers for an extended period of time, likely at least 90 days. Therefore, as we move forward with the goal of training technically competent surgeons, we need substantial education research to determine the type of assessment tools that will assist in the measurement of technical competence. I encourage all surgeons with interest in surgical training to participate in the development of these outcome tools.

K. E. Behrns, MD

Observations on Surgeons' Case Selection, Morbidity, and Mortality Following Board Certification

Guidry CA, Newhook TE, Turrentine FE, et al (Dept of Surgery, Charlottesville, VA; et al)
Ann Surg 263:487-492, 2016

Objective.—The purpose of this study is to determine if patient selection varies based on years of surgical practice.

Background.—The impact of hospital and surgeon volume as a marker of experience has demonstrated an inverse association with surgical outcomes. However, temporal measures of experience often demonstrate no effect. Additionally, a self-reporting survey demonstrated decreasing case complexity over time, suggesting that changes in patient selection may account for some of these observed discrepancies.

Methods.—General surgery cases at a single tertiary care center reported to the American College of Surgeons National Surgical Quality Improvement Program over a 10-year period were identified. Additionally general surgery cases from the ACS NSQIP 2008 PUF data were used to create risk models for any complications, 30-day mortality, or a composite complication or mortality outcome. These models then estimated risk for our local data. Years of experience after American Board of Surgery certification were calculated for each surgeon for each case. Multivariate linear regression, controlling for surgeon clustering, was used to determine the association between years of surgical experience and preoperative risk of complications and mortality.

Results.—Eighteen thousand six hundred and eighty eight cases were identified from our institution. Surgeons selected patients of increasing operative risk until 15 years of practice before selecting lower risk patients throughout the rest of their career. After adjusting for risk, no association was observed between years from board certification and mortality. However, there was a trend toward decreasing complication rates with increasing experience.

Conclusions.—Surgical experience significantly impacts patient selection. Surgeons with over 25 years of experience had lower complication rates. Experience had no impact on mortality (Fig 2).

▶ Providing high-value surgical care is dependent on numerous surgeon-specific and institution-centered factors. For the busy practicing clinical surgeon, delivery of high-value care can be broken down into the phases of care, including preoperative assessment, intraoperative management, and postoperative care including intensive care unit management, postoperative floor care, and discharge care. Furthermore, when assessing care, one should consider (1) the appropriateness of care—the correct operation at the right time; (2) conducting evidenced-based care assessment processes before an operation, that is, appropriate laboratory and imaging evaluations; (3) measuring "hard" outcomes such as mortality, morbidity, and length of stay; and (4) patient satisfaction. To date, too little emphasis has been placed on the appropriateness of surgical care. We should continually ask the question of whether this patient will reap significant benefits from an operation. Therefore, case selection is a primary driver of delivery of high-value surgical care. In this study, Guidry et al nicely studied the role of surgeon experience in case selection and outcomes. They used the National Surgical Quality Improvement Program Database to determine outcomes of board-certified surgeons as a function of time after certification. They applied sophisticated analyses and found that surgical experience significantly affects patient selection and that surgeons with more than 25 years of experience had fewer complications (Fig 2). These data suggest that accumulated surgeon experience may affect the appropriateness of care.

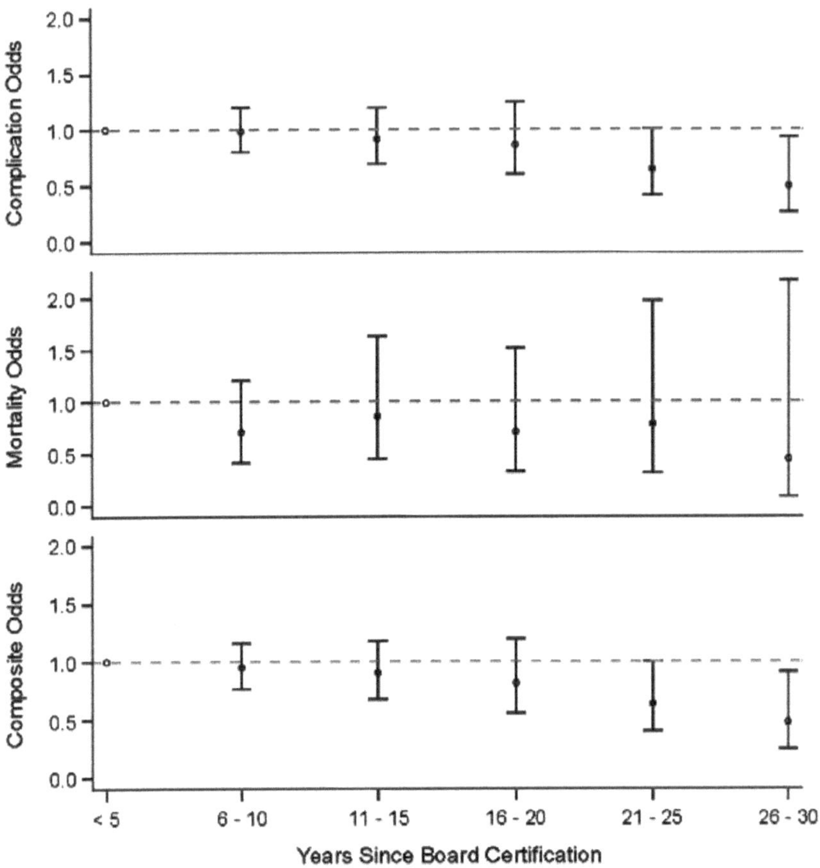

FIGURE 2.—Adjusted odds ratios for outcomes based on years of experience. OR indicates odds ratio. Values represent odds ratios listed with 99% confidence interval. (Reprinted from Guidry CA, Newhook TE, Turrentine FE, et al. Observations on surgeons' case selection, morbidity, and mortality following board certification. *Ann Surg*. 2016;263:487-492, with permission from Wolters Kluwer Health, Inc.)

What does this mean for us? These findings suggest that the practice of having 2 surgeons, 1 of which is preferable a senior colleague, see high-risk surgical patients and render an opinion on the advisability of performing an operation before committing to it is likely a valuable exercise that can reduce harm to a patient. The data also suggest that the surgeon should continue to use methods to determine the appropriateness of care by using patient-specific physiologic information and performing risk calculator analysis. Gone are the days of "eyeballing" a patient to determine the readiness for surgery: appropriate application of surgical care requires a disciplined and thorough approach.

K. E. Behrns, MD

"And I Think That We Can Fix It": Mental Models Used in High-risk Surgical Decision Making

Kruser JM, Pecanac KE, Brasel KJ, et al (Univ of Wisconsin, Madison; Med College of Wisconsin, Milwaukee; et al)

Ann Surg 261:678-684, 2015

Objective.—To examine how surgeons use the "fix-it" model to communicate with patients before high-risk operations.

Background.—The "fix-it" model characterizes disease as an isolated abnormality that can be restored to normal form and function through medical intervention. This mental model is familiar to patients and physicians, but it is ineffective for chronic conditions and treatments that cannot achieve normalcy. Overuse may lead to permissive decision making favoring intervention. Efforts to improve surgical decision making will need to consider how mental models function in clinical practice, including "fix-it."

Methods.—We observed surgeons who routinely perform high-risk surgery during preoperative discussions with patients. We used qualitative content analysis to explore the use of "fix-it" in 48 audio-recorded conversations.

Results.—Surgeons used the "fix-it" model for 2 separate purposes during preoperative conversations: (1) as an explanatory tool to facilitate patient understanding of disease and surgery, and (2) as a deliberation framework to assist in decision making. Although surgeons commonly used "fix-it" as an explanatory model, surgeons explicitly discussed limitations of the "fix-it" model as an independent rationale for operating as they deliberated about the value of surgery.

Conclusions.—Although the use of "fix-it" is familiar for explaining medical information to patients, surgeons recognize that the model can be problematic for determining the value of an operation. Whether patients can transition between understanding *how* their disease is fixed with surgery to a subsequent deliberation about *whether* they should have surgery is unclear and may have broader implications for surgical decision making.

► The conceptual framework used by surgeons to guide conversations with patients and families in surgical decision-making processes often use metaphors that familiarize the patient with concepts of an operation. One such frequently used metaphor is the "fix-it" model. Surgical operations are often likened to domestic activities, such as relieving a clogged household pipe as plumber would undertake. In this article, Kruser et al carefully articulated the advantages and disadvantages of the use of metaphors such as "fix it." Although phraseology like "fix it" may assist in establishing rapport with the patient and family, the notion that an operation will "fix" an underlying pathophysiologic defect may limit significantly the patient's and family's understanding of the complexities of an operation, and, importantly, may shortchange the risk of adverse events. As the authors correctly describe, the "fix-it" approach is no substitute for clearly delineating the substantial operative risk and potential long-term consequences of complicated operations. In today's environment, informed consent goes well beyond building rapport with a patient. Precise conversations, risk calculator demonstrations, and well-constructed consent forms that articulate likely patient outcomes in both the short-term and the foreseeable future are the currency of current informed consent, and "fix-it" conversations are no substitute for a conversation that may lead to a life-altering operation. We owe our patients these detailed discussions in the shared decision-making process.

K. E. Behrns, MD

Precision Medicine—Personalized, Problematic, and Promising

Jameson JL, Longo DL (Univ of Pennsylvania Perelman School of Medicine, Philadelphia)

N Engl J Med 372:2229-2234, 2015

Background.—Precision medicine refers to treatment targeted to the individual's specific needs based on genetic, biomarker, phenotypic, or psychosocial characteristics that distinguish him or her from other patients with similar clinical presentations. The goal is to improve the individual's clinical outcome while minimizing unneeded side effects for those who will likely not respond to treatment. Although the principles of precision medicine reflect the basis for medical practice throughout history, the pace of advances in diagnostic and treatment options has increased exponentially and will alter the applications of precision medicine.

Technology.—The convergence of many technologies has allowed the refinement of disease classifications, with implications for prognosis and treatment. Among these technologies are those in genetics, informatics, and imaging. Genetics and next-generation DNA sequencing methods appear to be the most influential changes currently. Clinical implications will balloon once the results of genetic testing become actionable, informing prognostic and treatment decisions. Imaging has supported the diagnosis of conditions with reasonable confidence, sparing patients from more invasive testing or unneeded surgery. Electronic health records are expected to eventually help in developing algorithms to identify patients with disease risk factors, individuals who require guideline-based screening, or tailored drug selection and administration methods. When genetic testing costs decrease, relevant genetic or pharmacogenomic data may be included and inform clinicians' decisions. Even the eligibility for clinical trials may be determined, with appropriate privacy controls and provider input.

Disruptions and Challenges.—The multitude of stakeholders involved in precision medicine makes for difficulty in aligning all interests. Patients want to understand their disease and receive the most effective treatment. Physicians and health care systems seek these goals as well as balance between individual patient needs and the management of overall health care utilization. Payers are concerned about rising health care expenditures and the actual usefulness of advances. Pharmaceutical companies seek opportunities for new drugs without losing previous lucrative drug uses.

With the advances in genetics and biomarkers, more precise definitions and more discrete disease entities will be identified. As a result, decision algorithms and treatment options may be expanded. However, disorders of some pathways can signal many diseases. Physicians, especially primary care providers, will have to navigate this complex system and will likely require informatics for assistance. Referral pathways will be needed to help connect patients with appropriate experts. In addition, better biomarkers are required to better detect disease and guide treatment, especially for common acquired conditions with no strong genetic predisposition. Developing new diagnostic tests tends to be less financially rewarding than creating new drugs, however.

Future Advances.—Among the areas where advances are expected are medications that target altered genetic pathways in cancer and targeted immunotherapies for cancer. Diagnostics and therapeutics will be combined in novel immunotherapeutic approaches. DNA sequencing has led to study of the microbiome, a large ecosystem embedded on the surface of the skin and mucosal tracts. Microbiome composition reflects innate immunity, the introduction of organisms early in life, diet, and exposure to environmental factors, including antibiotics. Study of the role of the microbiome in various disorders is underway. Finally, technology will be used to help with acute interventions in specific patients. With the use of mobile technology to monitor health and its integration into the health record, it may become a way to practice precision medicine as well.

Conclusions.—Various technologic advances are accelerating the practice of precision medicine. Whether the changes are helpful or disruptive remains to be seen, but changes are on the horizon. In response to these advances in technology, alterations will be required for payers, medical school curricula, physicians' use of informatics and algorithms, health systems, and regulatory agencies.

▶ The Human Genome Project was a daunting scientific endeavor of great magnitude and hope. With the majority of the human genome sequenced, the available genetic information can be mined to develop a personal gene signature for each patient. Although the project was a large undertaking with substantial expense, we now live in the era when an individual's genome can be sequenced at the relatively low price of approximately $1000. The information provided for this relatively inexpensive price is vast and may help predict responsiveness to medications or other treatments. In this *New England Journal of Medicine* Sounding Board article, Jameson and Longo detail the possibilities of precision medicine. How does this relate to surgery? What would precision surgery (is there another kind of surgery?) look like? As a surgical community, we should focus on how precision medicine or a gene signature may predict response to common surgical problems. For example, what if the genetic profile of an individual or group of individuals prognosticated a high likelihood of wound infection because a panel of immunoregulatory genes forecasted susceptibility to bacterial infection? Could we alter the treatment of such a patient to prevent infection and have a better patient outcome at lower costs? The changes in surgical management that may arise from precision medicine represent significant opportunities for surgeons to conduct groundbreaking, clinically relevant research that could have a marked impact on the care of our patients. I encourage you to read this article with an open mind and contemplate the possibilities to improve the care of our patients.

K. E. Behrns, MD

Profiling Individual Surgeon Performance Using Information from a High-Quality Clinical Registry: Opportunities and Limitations

Hall BL, Huffman KM, Hamilton BH, et al (Washington Univ in St Louis, MO; American College of Surgeons, Chicago, IL; et al)

J Am Coll Surg 221:901-913, 2015

Background.—There is increasing interest in profiling the quality of individual medical providers. Valid assessment of individuals should highlight improvement opportunities, but must be considered in the context of limitations.

Study Design.—High quality clinical data from the American College of Surgeons NSQIP, gathered in accordance with strict policies and specifications, was used to construct individual surgeon-level assessments. There were 39,976 cases evaluated, performed by 197 surgeons across 9 hospitals. Both 2-level (cases by surgeon) and 3-level (cases by surgeon by hospital) risk-adjusted, hierarchical regression analyses were performed. Outcomes were 30-day postoperative morbidity, surgical site infection, and mortality. Surgeon performance was compared in both absolute and relative terms. "Signal-to-noise" reliability was calculated for surgeons and models. Projected case requirements for reliability levels were generated.

Results.—Surgeon performances could be distinguished to different degrees: morbidity distinguished best, mortality least. Outliers could be identified for morbidity and infection, but not mortality. Reliability was also highest for morbidity and lowest for mortality. Even models with high overall reliability did not assess all providers reliably. Incorporating institutional effects had predictable effects: penalizing providers at "good" institutions, benefiting providers at "poor" institutions.

Conclusions.—Individual surgeon profiles can, at times, be distinguished with moderate or good reliability, but to different degrees in different models. Absolute and relative comparisons are feasible. Incorporating institutional level effects in individual provider modeling presents an interesting policy dilemma, appearing to benefit providers at "poor-performing" institutions, but penalizing those at "high-performing" ones. No portrayal of individual medical provider quality should be accepted without consideration of modeling rationale and, critically, reliability.

▶ Health care delivery is intently focused on quality outcomes, especially at the institutional level. Surgical outcomes, however, lend themselves to analyses of the individual performer—that is, the surgeon. The assessment of individual surgeon outcomes has proven difficult because the collection of data has not been consistent and reliable and comparative efforts are plagued by low sample size in some instances. In this article, Hall et al addressed some of these issues in a sophisticated analysis of individual surgeon data collected through the National Quality Surgical Improvement Project, a data set collected with meticulous methods. The results of this study showed that surgeon outcomes for morbidity and surgical site infection could differentiate performance, whereas the assessment of mortality did not distinguish surgeon performance. In addition, and somewhat surprisingly, surgeons at institutions that have inferior quality tended to fare better than surgeons at high-performing institutions. Most important, the overall message of the article is that comparing surgeon outcomes requires complicated analyses that have numerous assumptions. This work, although methodologically advanced, is important because it shows the extent to which analyses must be conducted to differentiate surgeon performance. Clearly, we are some distance from reliably assessing and comparing and fairly reporting surgeon performance. We should continue to seek sensible methods to assess surgeon outcomes.

K. E. Behrns, MD

Understanding Variation in 30-Day Surgical Readmission in the Era of Accountable Care: Effect of the Patient, Surgeon, and Surgical Subspecialties

Gani F, Lucas DJ, Kim Y, et al (Johns Hopkins Univ School of Medicine, Baltimore, MD; Walter Reed Natl Military Med, Ctr, Bethesda, MD)

JAMA Surg 150:1042-1049, 2015

Importance.—Readmission is a target area of quality improvement in surgery. While variation in readmission is common, to our knowledge, no study has specifically examined the underlying etiology of this variation among a variety of surgical procedures performed in a large academic medical center.

Objective.—To quantify the variability in 30-day readmission attributable to patient, surgeon, and surgical subspecialty levels in patients undergoing a major surgical procedure.

Design, Setting, and Participants.—Retrospective analysis of administrative claims data of patients discharged following a major surgical procedure at a tertiary care center between January 1, 2009, and, December 31, 2013. A total of 22 559 patients were included in this study and underwent a major surgical procedure performed by 56 surgeons practicing in 8 surgical subspecialties.

Main Outcomes and Measures.—In-hospital morbidity, 30-day readmission, and proportional variation in 30-day readmission at patient, surgeon, and surgical subspecialty levels.

Results.—Among the 22 559 patients in this study, patient age, race/ethnicity, and payer type differed across surgical subspecialties. Preoperative comorbidity was common and noted in 65.1% of patients.

Postoperative complications were noted in 21.6% of patients varying from 2.1% following breast, melanoma or endocrine surgery to 37.0% following cardiac surgery. The overall 30-day readmission was 13.2% (n = 2975). Readmission varied considerably across the 8 different surgical subspecialties, ranging from 24.8% following transplant surgery (n = 557) to 2.1% following breast, melanoma, or endocrine surgery (n = 32). After adjusting for patient- and surgeon-level variables, factors associated with readmission included African American race/ethnicity (odds ratio, 1.23; 95% CI, 1.11-1.36; $P < .001$), increasing comorbidity (Charlson Comorbidity Index score of 1: odds ratio, 1.16; 95% CI, 1.02-1.32; $P = .02$; and a Charlson Comorbidity Index score of ≥2: odds ratio, 1.38; 95% CI, 1.24-1.53; $P < .001$), postoperative complication (odds ratio, 1.19; 95% CI, 1.08-1.32; $P = .001$), and an extended length of stay (odds ratio, 1.78; 95% CI, 1.61-1.96; $P < .001$). The majority of the variation in readmission was attributable to patient-related factors (82.8%) while surgical subspecialty accounted for 14.5% of the variability, and individual surgeon-level factors accounted for 2.8%.

Conclusions and Relevance.—Readmission occurred in more than 1 in 10 patients, with considerable variation across surgical subspecialties. Variation in readmission was overwhelmingly owing to patient-level factors while only a minority of the variation was attributable to factors at the surgical subspecialty and individual surgeon levels.

▶ Health care delivery is undergoing significant evolution, and numerous outcome measures are now scrutinized heavily. One of these measures is the rate of hospital readmission. In fact, the Centers for Medicare and Medicaid Services introduced the Hospital Readmission Reductions Program (HRRP), which focused initially on financial penalties related to readmission for myocardial infarction, pneumonia, and heart failure. HRRP also introduced recently penalties for readmission for total hip and knee arthroplasty. In addition, surgical patients across several disciplines will be increasingly evaluated for readmission. Therefore, an improved understanding of structure and process issues that contribute to surgical readmission will be helpful. The work by Gani et al is a major contribution to our understanding of surgical readmissions. They used an administrative database to study more than 22 000 patients to determine patient-, surgical service-, and surgeon-related factors that influence readmission. The data across 8 surgical services are typical of other publications in that patients undergoing surgery for breast, melanoma, or endocrine conditions have a low readmission rate, whereas patients who had cardiac, transplant, and hepatopancreatobiliary procedures had significantly higher readmission rates. Importantly, this study attributed 83% of variation in readmission to patient-related factors and 14.5% to surgical service—related factors. Less than 3% of the variation in readmission was attributable to surgeon-related factors. This work is important because it shows us where to direct our efforts in terms of decreasing readmissions. A word of caution, however, is that patient-related factors become surgeon-related factors in decision making for an operation. For example, just under 50% of the patients in this study had a Charlson Co-Morbidity score of 2 or greater. Certainly, some of these patients may have been marginal candidates for an operation and, thus, surgical decision making rests, in part, on patient-related factors. This is an interesting era in surgical decision making, so stay tuned for further developments.

K. E. Behrns, MD

Wrong-Site Surgery, Retained Surgical Items, and Surgical Fires: A Systematic Review of Surgical Never Events

Hempel S, Maggard-Gibbons M, Nguyen DK, et al (Southern California Evidence-Based Practice Ctr, Santa Monica; Veterans Affairs Greater Los Angeles Healthcare System, CA; Univ of California, Los Angeles; et al)

JAMA Surg 150:796-805, 2015

Importance.—Serious, preventable surgical events, termed *never events*, continue to occur despite considerable patient safety efforts.

Objective.—To examine the incidence and root causes of and interventions to prevent wrong-site surgery, retained surgical items, and surgical fires in the era after the implementation of the Universal Protocol in 2004.

Data Sources.—We searched 9 electronic databases for entries from 2004 through June 30, 2014, screened references, and consulted experts.

Study Selection.—Two independent reviewers identified relevant publications in June 2014.

Data Extraction and Synthesis.—One reviewer used a standardized form to extract data and a second reviewer checked the data. Strength of evidence was established by the review team. Data extraction was completed in January 2015.

Main Outcomes and Measures.—Incidence of wrong-site surgery, retained surgical items, and surgical fires.

Results.—We found 138 empirical studies that met our inclusion criteria. Incidence estimates for wrong-site surgery in US settings varied by data source and procedure (median estimate, 0.09 events per 10 000 surgical procedures). The median estimate for retained surgical items was 1.32 events per 10 000 procedures, but estimates varied by item and procedure. The per-procedure surgical fire incidence is unknown. A frequently reported root cause was inadequate communication. Methodologic challenges associated with investigating changes in rare events limit the conclusions of 78 intervention evaluations. Limited evidence supported the Universal Protocol (5 studies), education (4 studies), and team training (4 studies) interventions to prevent wrong-site surgery. Limited evidence exists to prevent retained surgical items by using data-matrix–coded sponge-counting systems (5 pertinent studies). Evidence for preventing surgical fires was insufficient, and intervention effects were not estimable.

Conclusions and Relevance.—Current estimates for wrong-site surgery and retained surgical items are 1 event per 100 000 and 1 event per 10 000 procedures, respectively, but the precision is uncertain, and the per-procedure prevalence of surgical fires is not known. Root-cause analyses suggest the need for improved communication. Despite promising approaches and global Universal Protocol evaluations, empirical evidence for interventions is limited.

▶ In 2004, The Joint Commission issued the Universal Protocol as a measure to decrease the incidence of surgical safety issues. Since that time, numerous studies have assessed surgical safety, but the overall incidence of safety issues such as wrong-site surgery, retained surgical items, and operating room fires has not decreased significantly despite these measures. To document the incidence of these surgical safety measures, Hempel et al conducted a systematic review of these surgical never events. Their research identified an incidence of wrong-site surgery of 1 in 100 000 procedures and retained surgical items in 1 in 10 000 procedures (Fig 1 in the original article). The incidence of fires in the operating room could not be determined. Why do these surgical never events continue to occur despite interventions designed to eliminate these mishaps? Not surprisingly, lapses in communication, either written or verbal, are the major reason for continued wrong-site surgery and retained surgical items. Curiously, persons in the operating room identify risks but do not articulate these risks to the surgeon or team. In addition, over the past decade numerous advances have been implemented to reduce these surgical never events, but team-training and improved technology to detect retained items have not had a positive impact on the rate of these events. So how can we decrease the incidence of surgical never events, as the airline industry continues to decrease serious events? We must implement and adhere rigidly to high-reliability processes. High-reliability processes have 2 essential features; first, systematic processes that are designed to produce reliable outcomes are implemented; second, a high degree of professional accountability results in adherence to these processes. Leadership in the operating room must ensure that these high-reliability processes are in place and that the environment in the operating room is conducive to open communication so that we can ensure the safety of our patients and significantly reduce these surgical never events.

K. E. Behrns, MD

Escalation of Care in Surgery: A Systematic Risk Assessment to Prevent Avoidable Harm in Hospitalized Patients

Johnston M, Arora S, Anderson O, et al (Imperial College London, United Kingdom; et al)

Ann Surg 261:831-838, 2015

Objective.—To systematically risk assess and analyze the escalation of care process in surgery so as to identify problems and provide recommendations for intervention.

Background.—The ability to escalate care appropriately when managing deteriorating patients is a hallmark of surgical competence and safe postoperative care. Healthcare-Failure-Mode-Effects-Analysis (HFMEA) is a methodology adapted from safety-critical industries, which allows for hazardous process failures to be prospectively identified and solutions to be recommended.

Methods.—Forty-two hours of ethnographic observations on surgical wards in 3 London hospitals (phase 1) formed the basis of an escalation process diagram. A risk-assessment survey identified failures associated with process steps and attributed hazard scores (phase 2). Patient safety and clinical risk experts validated hazard scores through a group consensus meeting (phase 3). Hazardous failures were taken forward to multidisciplinary HFMEA where cause analysis was applied and interventions were recommended (phase 4).

Results.—Observations identified 33 steps in the escalation process. The risk assessment survey (30 surgical staff members, 100% response) and expert consensus group identified 18 hazardous failures associated with these steps. The HFMEA team identified 3 adequately controlled failures; therefore, 15 were subjected to cause analysis. Outdated communication technology, understaffing, and hierarchical barriers were identified as root causes of failure. Participants recommended interventions based on these findings including defined escalation protocols, human factors education, enhanced communication technology, and improved clinical supervision.

Conclusions.—Failures in the escalation process amenable to intervention were systematically identified. This mapping of the escalation process will allow tailored interventions to enhance surgical training and patient safety (Fig 1).

▶ One of the tenets of surgical care is to minimize complications, but although surgeons have long been in tune with the avoidance of complications,

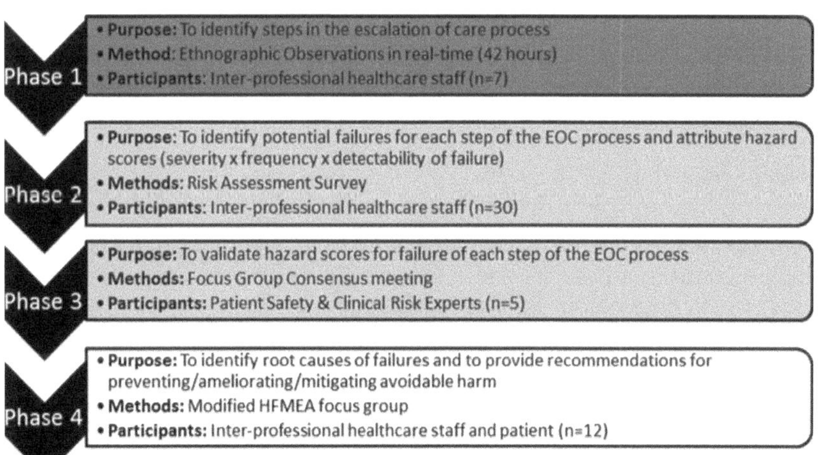

FIGURE 1.—A diagram showing the steps in the method for modified HFMEA. (Reprinted from Johnston M, Arora S, Anderson O, et al. Escalation of care in surgery: a systematic risk assessment to prevent avoidable harm in hospitalized patients. *Ann Surg*. 2015;261:831-838, with permission from Wolters Kluwer Health, Inc.)

complications persist despite our efforts. More recently, we routinely receive data that demonstrate our "failure to rescue" patients from serious complications. Indeed, while preventing complications may prove difficult, our ability to demonstrate early recognition and prompt action may limit the consequences of a complication. In the work by Johnston et al, prospective systematic approaches to process steps that may be involved in failure to rescue are outlined through an assessment termed HFMEA (Healthcare Failure mode and Effects Analysis; Fig 1). This logical and stepwise assessment of patient-caregiver and caregiver-caregiver interactions and decision making provides an in-depth view of how our care systems function (or do not function). Not surprisingly, failure in our care systems is related to errors in recognition, communication, response, and recovery. Mishaps in recognition may be related to failure of a patient to communicate a change in status or a nurse or junior surgeon not realizing a potentially dangerous clinical situation. Perhaps most disturbing are the errors in communication in which we fail to move a problem up the chain of command or do not adequately describe the clinical picture. Hopefully, it is rare that an experienced surgeon does not respond appropriately with action to a patient with deterioration. The HFMEA process is an excellent assessment tool to diminish the likelihood of failure to rescue, but as pointed out in the accompanying editorial by Ghaferi and Dimick,[1] a culture of safety must be present throughout the institution. This manuscript and the editorial are essential reading for surgical leaders, who strive for quality and safety in their surgical practice.

K. E. Behrns, MD

Reference

1. Ghaferi AA, Dimick JB. Understanding failure to rescue and improving safety culture. *Ann Surg*. 2015;261:839-840.

Effect of Hospital Safety-Net Burden on Cost and Outcomes After Surgery

Hoehn RS, Wima K, Vestal MA, et al (Univ of Cincinnati School of Medicine, OH; Sg2 Health Care and Hosp System Consultancy, Chicago, IL; et al)
JAMA Surg 151:120-128, 2016

Importance.—Safety-net hospitals provide broad services for a vulnerable population of patients and are financially at risk owing to impending reimbursement penalties and policy changes.

Objective.—To determine the effect of patient and hospital factors on surgical outcomes and cost at safety-net hospitals.

Design, Setting, and Participants.—Hospitals in the University HealthSystem Consortium database from January 1, 2009, through December 31, 2012 (n = 231), were grouped according to their safety-net burden, defined as the proportion of Medicaid and uninsured patient charges for all hospitalizations during that time (n = 12 638 166). Nine cohorts, based on a variety of surgical procedures, were created and examined with regard to preoperative characteristics, postoperative outcomes, and resource utilization. Multiple logistic regression was performed to analyze the effect of patient and center factors on outcomes. Hospital Compare data from the Centers for Medicare & Medicaid Services were linked and used to characterize and compare the groups of hospitals.

Main Outcomes and Measures.—Postoperative mortality, 30-day readmissions, and total direct cost.

Results.—For all 9 procedures examined in 231 hospitals comprising 12 638 166 patient encounters, patients at hospitals with high safety-net burden (HBHs) (vs hospitals with low and medium safety-net burdens) were most likely to be young, to be black, to be of the lowest socioeconomic status, and to have the highest severity of illness and the highest cost for surgical care ($P < .01$ for all). For 7 of 9 procedures, HBHs had the highest proportion of emergent cases and longest length of stay ($P < .01$ for all). After adjusting for patient characteristics and center volume, HBHs still had higher odds of mortality for 3 procedures (odds ratios [ORs], 1.81-2.08; $P < .05$), readmission for 2 procedures (ORs, 1.19-1.30; $P < .05$), and the highest cost of care associated with 7 of 9 procedures (risk ratios, 1.23-1.35; $P < .05$). Analysis of Hospital Compare data found that HBHs had inferior performance on Surgical Care Improvement Project measures, higher rates of surgical complications, and inferior markers of emergency department timeliness and efficiency (all $P < .05$).

Conclusions and Relevance.—These data suggest that intrinsic qualities of safety-net hospitals lead to inferior surgical outcomes and increased cost across 9 elective surgical procedures. These outcomes are likely owing to hospital resources and not necessarily patient factors. In addition, impending changes to reimbursement may have a negative effect on the surgical care at these centers.

▶ The Patient Protection and Affordable Care Act (PPACA) was designed to provide health care access and coverage to some of the most vulnerable patients, many of whom are cared for at safety-net hospitals. In this article, Hoehn et al examined the outcomes for 9 surgical procedures performed at safety-net hospitals in the academic community. The hospitals were stratified in 3 tiers (low, medium, and high) by the safety-net burden, or the percent of patients with Medicaid or no insurance. The results demonstrated that patients in high safety-net burden hospitals (HBH) might experience higher mortality, readmission rates, and costs even after adjusting for center volume and patient characteristics. Furthermore, performance on Surgical Care Improvement Project measures was poorer, surgical complications greater, and emergency department efficiency lower in HBH compared with low-burden hospitals (Table 3 in the original article). Thus, HBH are at high risk for receiving penalties for quality or value measures, and the very hospitals the PPACA was designed to help may receive crippling financial penalties. How can we combat this scenario? First, we must realize that patients' socioeconomic status reflects social determinants of health care and outcomes. Basic needs such as food, water, shelter, and sleep all affect surgical outcomes. Second, HBH need an incentive system that addresses the basic needs of patients such that HBH can work with community or public health departments to identify at-risk patients undergoing surgical care and monitor them throughout the entire episode of care. Too frequently, we perform operations and discharge patients to environments that are not suitable for a successful recovery from an operation. We need to work closely in multidisciplinary teams to provide a path for successful surgical recovery for our most vulnerable patients.

K. E. Behrns, MD

Understanding the determinants of patient satisfaction with surgical care using the Consumer Assessment of Healthcare Providers and Systems surgical care survey (S-CAHPS)

Schmocker RK, Cherney Stafford LM, Siy AB, et al (Univ of Wisconsin, Madison)

Surgery 158:1724-1733, 2015

Background.—Patient satisfaction has been emphasized increasingly in all aspects of medicine, including the imposition of financial penalties for underperformance. Current measures of patient satisfaction, however, do not address aspects specific to the care of operative patients. Therefore, our aim was to examine the recently validated Consumer Assessment of Healthcare Providers and Systems (S-CAHPS) to determine which aspects of perioperative care are predictive of satisfaction with the surgeon.

Methods.—All patients undergoing a general surgery operation at our institution during a 5-month period were sent a modified S-CAHPS within 3 days of discharge. Patients were then divided into 2 groups: those who rated their surgeon as the best possible and those giving a lower rating. Univariate and multivariate analyses were used to determine predictors of satisfaction with operative care. S-CAHPS results were then compared with other satisfaction measures in a subset of patients.

Results.—The response rate was 45.3% (456/1,007). The average age was 59 ± 16 years, duration of stay was 4.1 ± 6.6 days, and 23% underwent unscheduled operations. A total of 72% of patients rated their surgeon as the best surgeon possible. On multivariate analysis, preoperative communication and attentiveness on the day of operation were the most important determinants of overall surgeon rating. S-CAHPS scores correlated with other standard measures of satisfaction (HCAHPS scores).

Conclusion.—S-CAHPS is a novel operative satisfaction tool and is feasible to administer to patients undergoing general operative procedures. Surgeon characteristics most predictive of high patient satisfaction are effective preoperative communication and attentiveness on the day of operation.

▶ Patient satisfaction is a central theme in the measurement of health care delivery. Over the past decade, several validated surveys have been developed to assess patient satisfaction in various patient care venues. In this article,

Schmocker et al examine a niche survey, the Consumer Assessment of Healthcare Providers and Systems, which was designed to specifically address surgical care and the performance of the surgeon. In this study, the authors gathered 435 responses from patients who underwent operations performed by general surgeons. The responses were overwhelmingly favorable to the surgeons, and, not surprisingly, communication, preoperative preparation, and attentiveness on the day of surgery were highly valued by patients. Interestingly, the patients expressed relatively low satisfaction with shared decision making regarding the treatment options. These results suggest that although surgeons are compassionate and attentive, we still have work to do listening to patients. Frequently, the competency of communication is stressed, but we are guilty of assuming that this competency deals with the delivery of our message or perhaps the lack of delivering any message at all. In this important article, a message is that we need to become better listeners. The time pressures often seemingly compel us to give our spiel about an operation without truly listening to the patients concerns or desires. We should step back and engage our patients through attentive listening.

K. E. Behrns, MD

Readmissions, Observation, and the Hospital Readmissions Reduction Program

Zuckerman RB, Sheingold SH, Orav EJ, et al (Dept of Health and Human Services, Washington, DC)

N Engl J Med 2016 [Epub ahead of print]

Background.—The Hospital Readmissions Reduction Program, which is included in the Affordable Care Act (ACA), applies financial penalties to hospitals that have higher-than-expected readmission rates for targeted conditions. Some policy analysts worry that reductions in readmissions are being achieved by keeping returning patients in observation units instead of formally readmitting them to the hospital. We examined the changes in readmission rates and stays in observation units over time for targeted and nontargeted conditions and assessed whether hospitals that had greater increases in observation-service use had greater reductions in readmissions.

Methods.—We compared monthly, hospital-level rates of readmission and observation-service use within 30 days after hospital discharge among Medicare elderly beneficiaries from October 2007 through May 2015. We used an interrupted time-series model to determine when trends changed and whether changes differed between targeted and nontargeted conditions. We assessed the correlation between changes in readmission rates and use of observation services after adoption of the ACA in March 2010.

Results.—We analyzed data from 3387 hospitals. From 2007 to 2015, readmission rates for targeted conditions declined from 21.5% to 17.8%, and rates for nontargeted conditions declined from 15.3% to 13.1%. Shortly after passage of the ACA, the readmission rate declined quickly, especially for targeted conditions, and then continued to fall at a slower rate after October 2012 for both targeted and nontargeted conditions. Stays in observation units for targeted conditions increased from 2.6% in 2007 to 4.7% in 2015, and rates for nontargeted conditions increased from 2.5% to 4.2%. Within hospitals, there was no significant association between changes in observation-unit stays and readmissions after implementation of the ACA.

Conclusions.—Readmission trends are consistent with hospitals' responding to incentives to reduce readmissions, including the financial penalties for readmissions under the ACA. We did not find evidence that changes in observation-unit stays accounted for the decrease in readmissions.

▶ The Affordable Care Act (ACA) addressed many access-related issues in health care, but importantly, it also undertook reduction of hospital readmission for targeted conditions, which included acute myocardial infarction, heart failure, and pneumonia during the initial study period. Subsequently, total hip or knee arthroplasty and chronic obstructive pulmonary disease were added, and it is assumed that many other conditions will be phased in the assessment of readmission in the coming years. Since the implementation of the Hospital Readmissions Reduction Program (HRRP), few data have demonstrated its effect. Zuckerman et al studied the reduction in hospital readmissions to determine whether readmissions decreased for targeted and nontargeted conditions and to determine whether a reduction in readmissions was associated with an increase in observation cases. The results demonstrated a reduction in readmissions for both targeted and nontargeted conditions, but no relationship between readmissions and observation cases was evident. Why are these data important for surgeons? First, as already mentioned, the HRRP will soon be applied to surgical diagnoses, and the implementation of the program will be associated with financial penalties. Second, and more important, developing care processes that will permit efficient use of our resources will have a substantial impact on optimal care for our patients and resource conservation. As pressure grows to reduce the costs of health care, surgeons and other physicians must look for ways to decrease costs and efficiently use our resources such that the value of our care is increased.

K. E. Behrns, MD

Using Time-Limited Trials to Improve Surgical Care for Frail Older Adults

Neuman MD, Allen S, Schwarze ML, et al (Perelman School of Medicine at the Univ of Pennsylvania, Philadelphia; Univ of Wisconsin—Madison; et al)

Ann Surg 261:639-641, 2015

Background.—Surgical decision making can be challenging when the patient is an older adult with cognitive impairment, advanced frailty, or severe comorbidity. For younger adults or healthier older adults, treatment decisions are relatively straightforward, with surgery done as an isolated intervention to resolve a discrete issue. For impaired and older adults, the surgeon must also consider postoperative care and possible additional interventions. To address this situation, the perspectives of geriatrics and palliative care have coalesced to create a "time-limited trial." In this approach, the physician, patient, and patient's family agree that an intervention will be done to meet the immediate goal and the patient's status will be re-evaluated periodically thereafter.

Process.—Time-limited trials begin with a meeting between the care team and the patient and family to define the patient's acute problem and overall prognosis; to clarify the patient's goals and priorities; to identify objective markers for improvement or deterioration; to set a time frame, whether a few days or a month or longer, for re-assessment of the patient's status; and to define the potential actions possibly needed at the end of the trial or during the trial should complications arise. The process is designed to help facilitate value-based, goal-oriented medical decisions that fit logically within the broader context of the patient's prognosis and priorities for health care. It recognizes that the person's prognosis and goals of care change over time. For patients near the end of life, a time-limited trial offers an alternative to absolute commitment to a course of treatment that may involve unwelcome and painful interventions that no longer align with the patient's priorities. Patients are offered the opportunity for a good outcome if all goes well but a change in course if the burdens of treatment become excessive or a complication negates the possibility of a positive long-term result.

Time-limited trials specific to surgery also help patients, families, and physicians make better decisions about how to proceed. They allow flexibility in handling unexpected outcomes, unpredictable complications, and treatment burdens. The decisions about surgery and postoperative care are made in the context of the patient's prognosis and preferences for care, which may change with time and the occurrence of untoward events. Thus a major operation is not viewed as an isolated intervention but as the beginning of an uncertain process that will require regular reevaluation.

For surgeons, using a time-limited trial will require a major paradigm shift about how surgical success and failure are defined. Surgical failure must be recognized when overly burdensome, non-beneficial therapy is continued even if the patient is still alive. Time-limited trials help all concerned acknowledge the limitations of medicine and avoid the sense of personal failure when a patient cannot be saved.

Provisions.—Use of time-limited trials can be facilitated by promoting the collection and reporting of data on surgical quality of care for frail older adults that de-emphasizes comparisons based on 30-day mortality and replaces them with rewards for high-quality palliative care and patient engagement. A reporting system is needed specifically for palliative surgery that measures how well the treatment represents purposeful care that is valued and desired by patient and family. Variances in patient preferences and changes in priorities of care over time must also be accommodated.

Conclusions.—By bringing together the perspectives of geriatrics and palliative care with surgical decision making processes, older patients may experience better surgical care even with limited prognoses. The use of time-limited trials offers a practical way to make it clear that the decisions about a person's care, no matter what the context is, are not set in stone but rather choices to be made by informed patients and families regardless of their stage of life (Table 1).

▶ The emphasis on the value of care rather than the quantity of care has sharpened the focus on offering surgical interventions in high-risk scenarios. This situation occurs with some regularity in elderly, frail patients who develop

TABLE 1.—Application of the Time-limited Trial Model to a Family Discussion Regarding Care for a Frail 85-Year-old Man With a High-grade Small Bowel Obstruction

Communication Goal	What We Would Say
1. Define acute problem and overall prognosis; define options for treatment of the acute problem. Characterize potential benefits and risks of treatment options.	You have a bowel obstruction and we need to discuss the best way to care for you. We have a choice between operating on your bowels and focusing primarily on your comfort. We can operate on your bowel obstruction and you might be able to get back to your life at the nursing home where you could live for several months or maybe even a year or two. Based on your age and because you are quite frail, there is a high potential for complications. For example, the bowel could leak after surgery, or you could develop an abdominal infection; if one of these complications occurs, you would need to go back to the operating room for another surgery or need invasive treatments in the ICU. If your wishes are to avoid surgery, we can focus our efforts on helping you be comfortable and allow nature to take its course.
2. Clarify expectations for surgery and recovery; reconcile goals and treatment options.	From your perspective, what is the best outcome that we could have for you in this situation? What do you think about that outcome?
3. Identify objective markers for improvement or deterioration with the selected course of treatment.	If you decide to go ahead with surgery, we are going to be following your recovery closely to look for signs that you are getting better. If you are able to eat, breathe comfortably, and have less pain after surgery that will indicate to us that you are getting better.
4. Identify a time at which the initial treatment choice can be reevaluated.	If you are still unable to eat 1 week after surgery, or if you are struggling to breathe and are very uncomfortable, we should sit down and talk about all our options at that point.
5. Define potential actions during the trial and ask for initial preferences regarding subsequent treatments.	If you were to develop a leak or get an abdominal infection after surgery, you could become much sicker very quickly and a second surgery would be needed. How would you feel about having more surgery or needing a breathing tube or other treatments in the ICU?

ICU indicates intensive care unit.

Reprinted from Neuman MD, Allen S, Schwarze ML, et al. Using time-limited trials to improve surgical care for frail older adults. *Ann Surg.* 2015;261:639-641, with permission from Wolters Kluwer Health, Inc.

life-threatening conditions for which surgery is indicated. At this crucial, sometimes unexpected time, the patient and/or family must make difficult decisions about undergoing an operation and potentially dealing with complications and reduced quality of life. In this outstanding piece of work, Neuman et al frame the issue nicely and provide a construct, a time-limited trial, for addressing these delicate situations (Table 1). The time-limited trial model is logical and raises most of the pertinent questions. Perhaps another goal that should be explicitly stated with this model is that a decision can be reversed. The authors certainly allude to the reversible nature of decisions, but too often once we embark on a treatment course, especially if an operation was performed, we are reluctant to accept an alternative. In addition, in this work, the time-limited trial is posed in the context of an elderly frail patient, but young, nonfrail patients may also face dire circumstances, and this model may be of value to those patients and their families. As a surgeon with a high-risk practice, I have been applying this principle, somewhat naively, for years. The concept provides the patient, family, and surgeon with an excellent construct that will help guide difficult care.

K. E. Behrns, MD

Impact of Surgical Quality Improvement on Payments in Medicare Patients

Scally CP, Thumma JR, Birkmeyer JD, et al (Univ of Michigan, Ann Arbor)

Ann Surg 262:249-252, 2015

Objective.—To examine the financial impact of quality improvement using Medicare payment data.

Background.—Demonstrating a business case for quality improvement—that is, that fewer complications translates into lower costs—is essential to justify investment in quality improvement. Prior research is limited to crosssectional studies showing that patients with complications have higher costs. We designed a study to better evaluate the relationship between payments and complications by using quality improvement itself as a measured outcome.

Methods.—We used national Medicare data for patients undergoing general (n = 1,485,667) and vascular (n = 531,951) procedures. We calculated hospitals' rates of serious complications in 2 time periods: 2003—2004 and 2009—2010. We sorted hospitals into quintiles by the change in complication rates across these time periods. Costs were assessed using price-standardized Medicare payments, and regression analyses used to determine the average change in payments over time.

Results.—There was significant change in serious complication rates across the 2 time periods. The top 20% of hospitals demonstrated a 38% decrease (14.3% vs 11.6%, $P < 0.001$) in complications; in contrast the bottom 20% demonstrated a 25% increase (11.1% vs 16.5%, $P<0.001$). There was a strong relationship between quality improvement and payments. The top hospitals reduced their payments by $1544 per patient (95% confidence interval: $1334—1755), whereas the bottom of hospitals had no significant change (average \$67 increase, 95% confidence interval: −\$123 to \$258).

Conclusions.—Hospitals that reduced their complications over time had significant reductions in Medicare payments. This demonstrates that payers are clearly incentivized to invest in quality improvement (Fig 1).

▶ For several years now, we have heard that improving quality will decrease costs. Likewise, surgeons hear repeatedly that we must provide high-value care. High-value care is characterized as high quality with low costs. To assess our outcomes and improve care delivery, quality programs that monitor outcomes and safety are increasingly operational. These programs are important but come at cost. Similarly, payers have made internal and external investments in the quality programs, in theory, to reduce their costs. To date, however, few data exist to support the postulate that improved quality reduces payer costs. Thus, the business proposition to payers has not been validated. In this article by Scally et al, however, Medicare data were used to prove that higher quality may result in decreased cost for payers. The authors compared general surgery and vascular surgery procedures across 2 time periods, 2003-2004 and 2009-2010, across quintiles of hospitals. The top 20% of hospitals demonstrated a 38% reduction in complications between the 2 time periods, whereas the bottom 20% of hospitals had a 25% increase in complications. The major finding, however, was that top hospitals had Medicare payments reduced by \$1544 per patient, but the bottom 20% of hospitals had no change

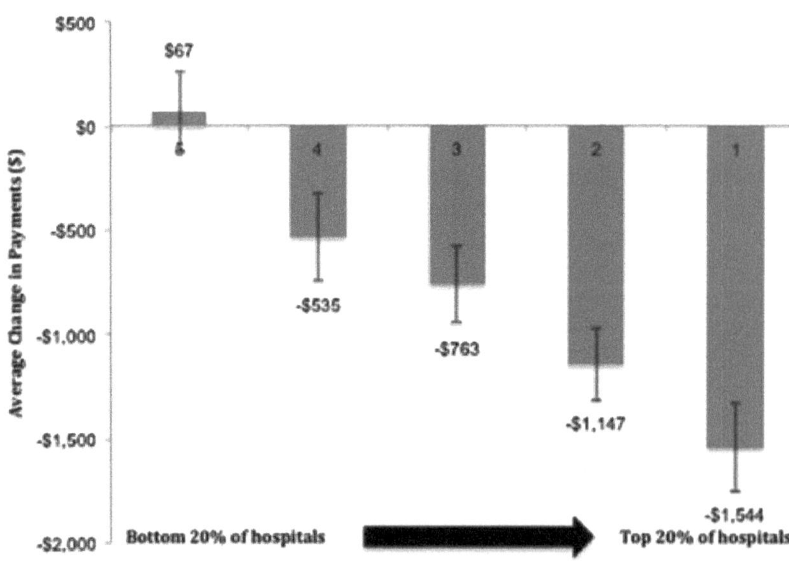

FIGURE 1.—Average change in Medicare payments for all procedure types between 2003–2004 and 2009–2010 for each Hospital Quintile of quality improvement. (Reprinted from Scally CP, Thumma JR, Birkmeyer JD, et al. Impact of surgical quality improvement on payments in medicare patients. *Ann Surg.* 2015;262:249-252, with permission from Wolters Kluwer Health, Inc.)

in payment (Fig 1). This work is noteworthy because moving forward providers will be sharing risk with payers and knowledge of the benefits and risks of this relationship will help guide discussions and lead to better quality programs. Our patients should be the ultimate beneficiaries of such collaboration.

K. E. Behrns, MD

2 Trauma

An evidence-based approach to patient selection for emergency department thoracotomy: A practice management guideline from the Eastern Association for the Surgery of Trauma

Seamon MJ, Haut ER, Van Arendonk K, et al (Hosp of the Univ of Pennsylvania, Philadelphia; the Johns Hopkins Hosp, Baltimore, MD; et al)

J Trauma Acute Care Surg 79:159-173, 2015

Background.—Within the GRADE (Grading of Recommendations Assessment, Development and Evaluation) framework, we performed a systematic review and developed evidence-based recommendations to answer the following PICO (Population, Intervention, Comparator, Outcomes) question: should patients who present pulseless after critical injuries (with and without signs of life after penetrating thoracic, extrathoracic, or blunt injuries) undergo emergency department thoracotomy (EDT) (vs. resuscitation without EDT) to improve survival and neurologically intact survival?

Methods.—All patients who underwent EDT were included while those involving either prehospital resuscitative thoracotomy or operating room thoracotomy were excluded. Quantitative synthesis via meta-analysis was not possible because no comparison or control group (i.e., survival or neurologically intact survival data for similar patients who did not undergo EDT) was available for the PICO questions of interest.

Results.—The 72 included studies provided 10,238 patients who underwent EDT. Patients presenting pulseless after penetrating thoracic injury had the most favorable EDT outcomes both with (survival, 182 [21.3%] of 853; neurologically intact survival, 53 [11.7%] of 454) and without (survival, 76 [8.3%] of 920; neurologically intact survival, 25 [3.9%] of 641) signs of life. In patients presenting pulseless after penetrating extrathoracic injury, EDT outcomes were more favorable with signs of life (survival, 25 [15.6%] of 160; neurologically intact survival, 14 [16.5%] of 85) than without (survival, 4 [2.9%] of 139; neurologically intact survival, 3 [5.0%] of 60). Outcomes after EDT in pulseless blunt injury patients were limited with signs of life (survival, 21 [4.6%] of 454; neurologically intact survival, 7 [2.4%] of 298) and dismal without signs of life (survival, 7 [0.7%] of 995; neurologically intact survival, 1 [0.1%] of 825).

Conclusion.—We strongly recommend that patients who present pulseless with signs of life after penetrating thoracic injury undergo EDT. We conditionally recommend EDT for patients who present pulseless and have absent signs of life after penetrating thoracic injury, present or absent signs of life after penetrating extrathoracic injury, or present signs of life after blunt injury. Lastly, we conditionally recommend against EDT for pulseless patients without signs of life after blunt injury.

Level of Evidence.—Systematic review/guideline, level III (Fig 7).

▶ Emergency department thoracotomy remains one of the most controversial procedures that physicians perform. When treating trauma victims presenting in extremis, clinicians are called on to make immediate life-or-death decisions. Such decisions consider the last chance of survival with the risk of salvaging patients with severe anoxic encephalopathy or exposing health care providers to bloodborne pathogens. The very low survival rates in conjunction with considerable potential risks, associated with emergency department thoracotomy, have continued to fuel this controversy. The publication of many outcome studies have led to a more discriminating focus on patients most likely to benefit from emergency department thoracotomy while limiting unnecessary risk. A selective approach to the performance of emergency department thoracotomy based on the presence or absence of several predictors of survival has thus emerged. The primary objective of this selection is to provide clear evidence-based recommendations for the physician facing the most common presenting clinical scenarios after critical injury. These recommendations are meant to provide an evidence-based framework from which clinicians can make rapid decisions regarding further resuscitation with emergency department thoracotomy or the determination of futile care. The expert committee provided 6 recommendations, based on an exhaustive systematic review of the existing literature, to guide the physician regarding emergency department thoracotomy. These recommendations are included as Fig 7. The conditional recommendations supporting emergency department thoracotomy all involve the most controversial indications that are still heavily debated. Despite assimilating and analyzing a

Question	Recommendation
PICO #1	In patients who present pulseless to the Emergency Department with signs of life after penetrating thoracic injury, we **strongly recommend** resuscitative Emergency Department thoracotomy. **Strong Recommendation**
PICO #2	In patients who present pulseless to the Emergency Department without signs of life after penetrating thoracic injury, we **conditionally recommend** resuscitative Emergency Department thoracotomy. **Conditional Recommendation**
PICO #3	In patients who present pulseless to the Emergency Department with signs of life after penetrating extra-thoracic injury, we **conditionally recommend** resuscitative Emergency Department thoracotomy. **Conditional Recommendation**
PICO #4	In patients who present pulseless to the Emergency Department without signs of life after penetrating extra-thoracic injury, we **conditionally recommend** resuscitative Emergency Department thoracotomy.[1] **Conditional Recommendation**
PICO #5	In patients who present pulseless to the Emergency Department with signs of life after blunt injury, we **conditionally recommend** resuscitative Emergency Department thoracotomy. **Conditional Recommendation**
PICO #6	In patients who present pulseless to the Emergency Department without signs of life after blunt injury, we **conditionally recommend against** resuscitative Emergency Department thoracotomy.[2] **Conditional Recommendation**

FIGURE 7.—Final recommendations. [1]Group voting for a recommendation was mixed. While all voted for a "conditional" recommendation, 11 members voted in favor of Emergency Department Thoracotomy and 4 voted against the procedure based on the PICO #4 Evidence Profile. [2]Group voting for a recommendation was mixed. While all voted against the performance of Emergency Department Thoracotomy based on the PICO #6 Evidence Profile, 10 members voted for a "strong" recommendation and 5 voted for a "conditional" recommendation. (Reprinted from Seamon MJ, Haut ER, Van Arendonk K, et al. An evidence-based approach to patient selection for emergency department thoracotomy: a practice management guideline from the Eastern Association for the Surgery of Trauma. *J Trauma Acute Care Surg.* 2015;79:159-173, with permission from Wolters Kluwer Health, Inc.)

vast amount of data, our knowledge of when to perform emergency department thoracotomy is largely unchanged.

D. W. Mozingo, MD

FAST Ultrasound Examination as a Predictor of Outcomes After Resuscitative Thoracotomy: A Prospective Evaluation

Inaba K, Chouliaras K, Zakaluzny S, et al (Univ of Southern California, Los Angeles)

Ann Surg 262:512-518, 2015

Objective.—The objective of this study was to examine the ability of Focused Assessment Using Sonography for Trauma (FAST) to discriminate between survivors and nonsurvivors undergoing resuscitative thoracotomy (RT).

Background.—RT is a high-risk, low-salvage procedure performed in arresting trauma patients with poorly defined indications.

Methods.—Patients undergoing RT from 10/2010 to 05/2014 were prospectively enrolled. A FAST examination including parasternal/subxiphoid cardiac views was performed before or concurrent with RT. The result was captured as adequate or inadequate with presence or absence of pericardial fluid and/or cardiac motion. A sensitivity analysis utilizing the primary outcome measure of survival to discharge or organ donation was performed.

Results.—Overall, 187 patients arrived in traumatic arrest and underwent FAST. Median age 31 (1–84), 84.5% male, 51.3% penetrating. Loss of vital signs occurred at the scene in 48.1%, en-route in 23.5%, and in the ED in 28.3%. Emergent left thoracotomy was performed in 77.5% and clamshell thoracotomy in 22.5%. Sustained cardiac activity was regained in 48.1%. However, overall survival was only 3.2%. An additional 1.6% progressed to organ donation. FAST was inadequate in 3.7%, 28.9% demonstrated cardiac motion and 8.6% pericardial fluid. Cardiac motion on FAST was 100% sensitive and 73.7% specific for the identification of survivors and organ donors.

Conclusions.—With a high degree of sensitivity for the detection of potential survivors after traumatic arrest, FAST represents an effective method of separating those that do not warrant the risk and resource burden of RT from those who may survive. The likelihood of survival if pericardial fluid and cardiac motion were both absent was zero (Fig 1).

► In comparison to the last selection, these authors describe the use of ultrasound examination of cardiac activity in the assessment of patients presenting in traumatic cardiac arrest. For patients presenting in traumatic cardiac arrest, an emergency department thoracotomy is often used as a final salvage maneuver. The quantitative yield on this procedure, however, is exceedingly low. Although proponents would argue that there is little to lose because not intervening would invariably end in death, there is an impact on society because of resource utilization and the potential risk of harm to the trauma care providers. The

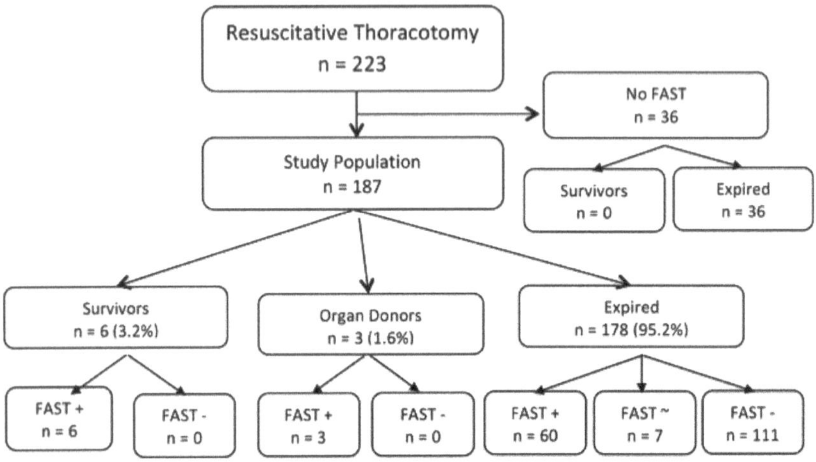

FIGURE 1.—Patient flow chart. FAST indicates Focused Assessment with Sonography for Trauma; FAST+, positive for cardiac motion or fluid; FAST−, negative for cardiac motion or fluid; FAST~, inadequate exam. (Reprinted from Inaba K, Chouliaras K, Zakaluzny S, et al. FAST ultrasound examination as a predictor of outcomes after resuscitative thoracotomy: a prospective evaluation. *Ann Surg.* 2015;262:512-518, with permission from Wolters Kluwer Health, Inc.)

recommendations discussed in the previous selection rely on the literature review of patients based on mechanism of injury and their probability of survival. This selection, however, offers new information and presents a specific tool that might better guide the selection of patients for emergency department thoracotomy. Fig 1 is included that demonstrates the ability of cardiac activity or pericardial fluid to predict outcomes in patients presenting with traumatic cardiac arrest. This is a single-center experience, so additional validation of the use of focused assessment using sonography for trauma for decision making regarding emergency department thoracotomy is necessary.

D. W. Mozingo, MD

Shock-induced systemic hyperfibrinolysis is attenuated by plasma-first resuscitation

Moore HB, Moore EE, Morton AP, et al (Univ of Colorado Denver; et al)
J Trauma Acute Care Surg 79:897-903, 2015

Background.—We developed a hemorrhagic shock animal model to replicate an urban prehospital setting where resuscitation fluids are limited to assess the effect of saline versus plasma in coagulopathic patients. An in vitro model of whole blood dilution with saline exacerbated tissue plasminogen activator (tPA)–mediated fibrinolysis, while plasma dilution did not change fibrinolysis. We hypothesize that shock-induced hyperfibrinolysis can be attenuated by resuscitation with plasma while exacerbated by saline.

Methods.—Sprague-Dawley rats were hemorrhaged to a mean arterial pressure of 25 mm Hg and maintained in shock for 30 minutes. Animals were resuscitated with either normal saline (NS) or platelet-free plasma (PFP) with a 10% total blood volume bolus, followed by an additional 5 minutes of resuscitation with NS to increase blood pressure to a mean arterial pressure of 30 mm Hg. Animals were observed for 15 minutes for the assessment of hemodynamic response and survival. Blood samples were analyzed with thrombelastography paired with protein analysis.

Results.—The median percentage of total blood volume shed per group were similar (NS, 52.5% vs. PFP, 55.7; $p = 0.065$). Survival was 50% in NS compared with 100% in PFP. The change in LY30 and tPA levels from baseline to shock was similar between groups (LY30 PFP, 10; interquartile range [IQR], 4.3–11.2; NS, 4.5; IQR, 4.1–14.2; $p = 1.00$; tPA PFP, 16.6 ng/mL; IQR, 13.7–27.8; NS, 22.4; IQR, 20.1–25.5; $p = 0.240$). After resuscitation, the median change in LY30 was greater in the NS group (13.5; IQR, 3.5–19.9) compared with PFP (−4.9%; IQR, −9.22 to 0.25 $p = 0.004$), but tPA levels did not significantly change (NS, 1.4; IQR, −6.2 to 7.1 vs. PFP, 1.7; IQR, −5.2 to 6.8; $p = 0.699$).

Conclusion.—Systemic hyperfibrinolysis is driven by hypoperfusion and associated with increased levels of tPA. Plasma is a superior resuscitation fluid to NS in a prehospital model of severe hemorrhagic shock as it attenuates hyperfibrinolysis and improves systemic perfusion (Fig 5).

▶ Prehospital volume restoration to correct shock in severely injured patients remains a challenge. Resuscitation with crystalloid has been associated with the development of hyperfibrinolysis; however, using plasma as the initial resuscitation agent in hyperfibrinolytic patients may be lifesaving because it provides substrate for controlling hemostasis in addition to being an effective volume expander. The authors of this selection undertook this study to better

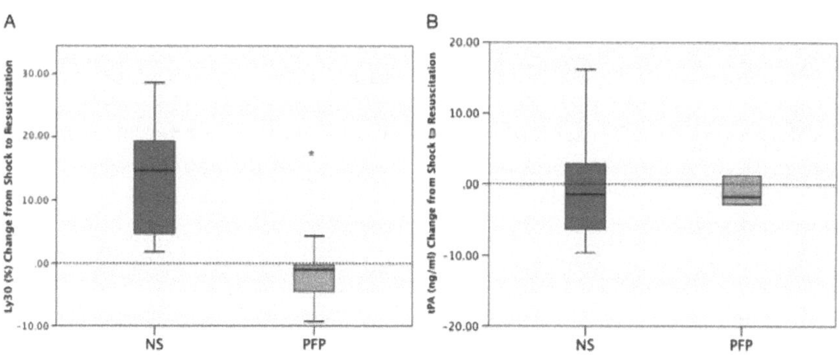

FIGURE 5.—*A*, LY30 after NS resuscitation and was attenuated with plasma. y-axis represents the change in LY30 from shock to partial resuscitation and 15 minutes of observation. NS resuscitation increased LY30, while plasma resuscitation tended to decrease LY30. *B*, tPA levels similar regardless of resuscitation. y-axis represents the change in tPA from shock to partial resuscitation and 15 minutes of observation. Both experimental groups showed a similar distribution of change in tPA. (Reprinted from Moore HB, Moore EE, Morton AP, et al. Shock-induced systemic hyperfibrinolysis is attenuated by plasma-first resuscitation. *J Trauma Acute Care Surg*. 2015;79:897-903, with permission from Wolters Kluwer Health, Inc.)

characterize these observations in an animal model of hemorrhagic shock and resuscitation. Fig 5 is included in this selection showing a dramatic continuation of the change in LY30, the percentage of clot that has lysed after 30 minutes by thromboelastography, with plasma resuscitation. This study adds additional evidence to support the use of plasma in severely injured patients in hemorrhagic shock. The ongoing randomized prehospital trials to evaluate the risk and benefit of treating trauma patients in the field with plasma are ongoing, and we look forward to seeing these results.

D. W. Mozingo, MD

Predicting progressive hemorrhagic injury from isolated traumatic brain injury and coagulation

Folkerson LE, Sloan D, Cotton BA, et al (Univ of Texas Health Science Ctr, Houston)

Surgery 158:655-661, 2015

Background.—Progressive hemorrhagic injury (PHI) in traumatic brain injury (TBI) patients is associated with poor outcomes. Early prediction of PHI is difficult yet vital. We hypothesize that TBI subtype and coagulation would be predictors of PHI.

Methods.—This was a retrospective analysis of highest level activation adult trauma patients with evidence of TBI (head Abbreviated Injury Scale ≥3). Coagulopathy was determined using rapid thrombelastography (r-TEG), complete blood counts, and conventional coagulation tests obtained on arrival. Patients were dichotomized into PHI and stable groups based on head computerized CT. Subtypes of TBI included subdural hematoma, intraparenchymal contusions (IPC), subarachnoid hemorrhage, epidural hematoma, and combined. Data are reported as median values with interquartile range (IQR). Multivariate logistic regression was used to assess the effect of subtype and coagulation on PHI.

Results.—We included 279 isolated TBI patients who met study criteria. There were 157 patients (56%) who experienced PHI; 122 (44%) were stable on repeat CT. Patients with PHI were older, had fewer hospital-free days, and higher mortality (all $P < .001$). No differences were noted in r-TEG parameters between groups; however, coagulopathy and age were independent predictors of progression in all subtypes (odds ratio [OR], 1.81; 95% CI, 1.09–3.01 [$P = .021$]; OR, 1.02, 95% CI, 1.01–1.04 [$P = .006$]). Controlling for age, Glasgow Coma Scale score, and coagulopathy, patients with IPC were more likely to experience PHI (OR, 4.49; 95% CI, 2.24–8.98; $P < .0001$).

Conclusion.—This study demonstrates that older patients with coagulation abnormalities and IPC on admission are more likely to experience PHI, identifying a target population for earlier therapies.

▶ The development of coagulopathy associated with trauma, coined the acute coagulopathy of trauma, has been associated with traumatic brain injury and is commonly observed in brain-injured patients with progressive hemorrhagic injury.

Progression of hemorrhagic injury is associated with a platelet count of <100 000/mL as well as an international normalized ratio >1.5. The authors of this selection noted there are no studies correlating coagulopathy with subtypes of isolated traumatic brain injury and clinical outcomes. Given the link between traumatic brain injury subtype, as well as coagulopathy, and progressive hemorrhagic injury, they hypothesized that a subtype of isolated brain injury and coagulation status would predict progressive hemorrhagic injury and allow targeting these patients for earlier interventions and therapies. Future prospective studies should be targeted at determining which admission laboratory values define coagulopathy more precisely in isolated traumatic brain injuries and finding individualized therapies aimed at correcting these derangements to diminish or prevent the frequency of progressive hemorrhagic injury.

D. W. Mozingo, MD

Pediatric solid organ injury operative interventions and outcomes at Harborview Medical Center, before and after introduction of a solid organ injury pathway for pediatrics

Dervan LA, King MA, Cuschieri J, et al (Seattle Children's Hosp, WA; Univ of Washington, Seattle)

J Trauma Acute Care Surg 79:215-220, 2015

Background.—Although nonoperative management has become the standard of care for solid organ injury, variability exists in the care patients receive, and there are limited data regarding nonoperative management in patients with high grades of organ injury and substantial overall injury. We aimed to evaluate operative intervention frequency, including splenectomy, and patient outcomes before and after institution of the pediatric solid organ injury pathway at Harborview Medical Center (HMC) in 2005.

Methods.—This is a retrospective cohort study conducted at HMC for all pediatric solid organ injury patients from 2001 to 2012. Patients were identified in the Harborview Trauma Registry via DRG International Classification of Diseases—9th Rev. (ICD-9) codes for the presence of liver and spleen injuries. Demographic information, clinical characteristics, and ICD-9 procedure codes were also obtained from the trauma registry. Outcomes including splenectomy, a related abdominal surgery (exploratory laparotomy, spleen or liver repair, or splenectomy), mortality, and length of stay were compared between periods before and after 2005, adjusted for Injury Severity Score (ISS).

Results.—The pediatric solid organ injury population at HMC ($n = 712$) has a high frequency of high-grade injury (35% Grade IV or V) and a high level of overall injury severity (median ISS, 21). Splenectomy was rare and remained stable over time despite an increase in severity of injury (from 2.4% to 0.8%, $p = 0.44$, among patients with isolated injury and from

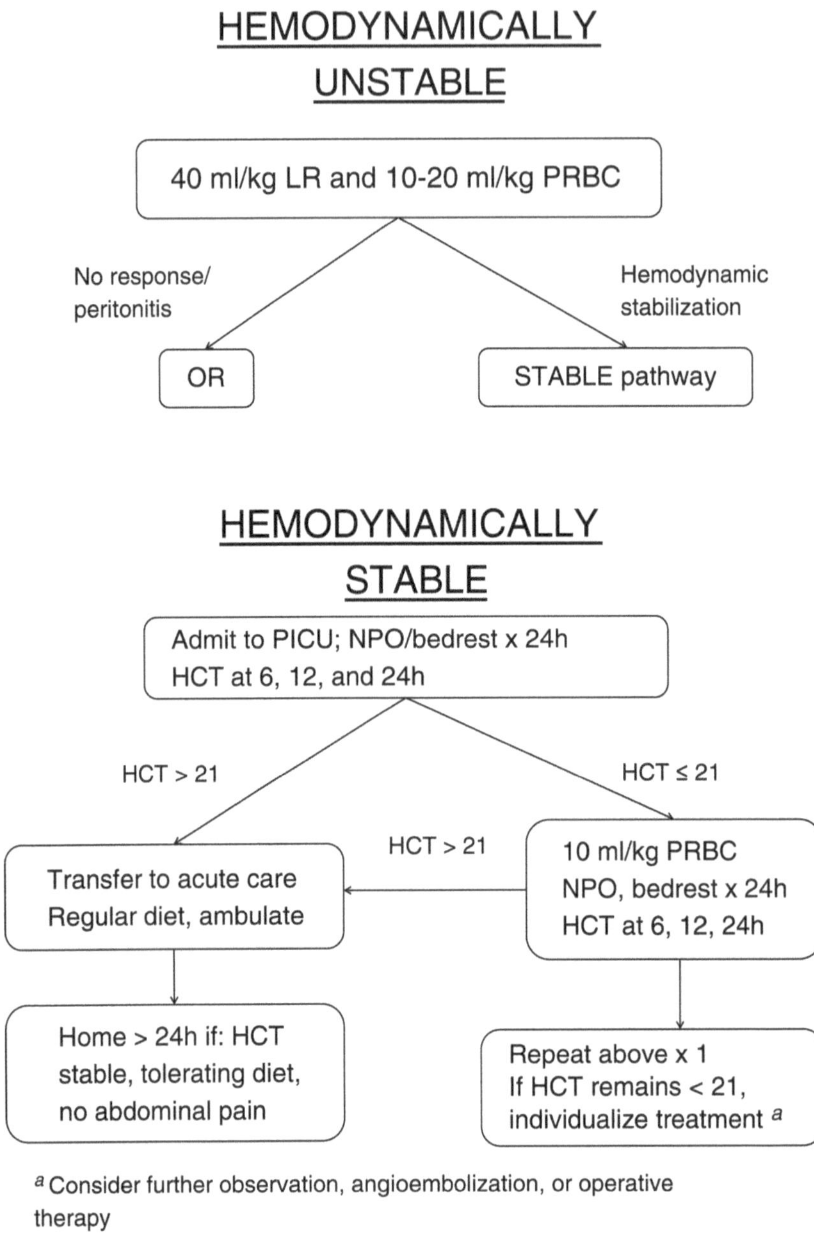

FIGURE 1.—HMC solid organ injury pathway for pediatrics. Hemodynamic status based on age-specific vital sign classification; see Table 1. *Editor's Note*: Please refer to original journal article for full references. (Reprinted from Dervan LA, King MA, Cuschieri J, et al. Pediatric solid organ injury operative interventions and outcomes at Harborview Medical Center, before and after introduction of a solid organ injury pathway for pediatrics. *J Trauma Acute Care Surg*. 2015;79:215-220, with permission from Wolters Kluwer Health, Inc.)

4.0% to 3.3%, $p = 0.78$, among patients with nonisolated injury). Other abdominal surgeries also remained stable over time. Mortality decreased among patients with nonisolated injury (from 11.2% to 4.8%, $p = 0.01$). Length of stay decreased among patients with isolated organ injury, from a median of 4 days (interquartile range, 3–5 days) to 2 days (interquartile range, 2–3 days) ($p < 0.0005$) as well as within the lower ISS strata among patients with nonisolated organ injury (from a median of 4 days to 2 days among ISS < 12, $p = 0.007$; from 5 days to 3 days among ISS of 12–20, $p = 0.0001$; and from 7 days to 4 days among ISS of 21–33, $p = 0.003$).

Conclusion.—Care in the recent period (2005–2012) was associated with a stable, low frequency of splenectomy; decreased mortality for patients with nonisolated injury; and decreased hospital length of stay among most subsets of patients, suggesting improved care despite an increase in patients' severity of injury.

Level of Evidence.—Therapeutic study, level IV; epidemiologic study, level III (Fig 1).

▶ Management algorithms and clinical practice guidelines are used increasingly to control for variability in clinical practice. There is, however, limited experience in the application of these guidelines to severely injured patients with high grades of solid organ injury. The authors of this selection developed a management algorithm and evaluated outcomes in all patients paying particular attention to those with high-grade injury. Their algorithm is included as Fig 1. A strength of this algorithm is that the pathway classifies the patients' hemodynamic status based on age-specific vital sign parameters to help guide resuscitation in operative decision making. The patients meeting the criteria for vital sign abnormalities tended to have serious injuries and poorer outcomes. The vital sign criteria may help alert providers to patients who are likely to be seriously ill; however, a portion of the pathway might be revised to improve its sensitivity for identifying patients who may benefit from more aggressive resuscitation. A major strength of this study is that it includes a large study population, including large numbers of severely injured patients and patients with Grade IV and V solid organ injury.

D. W. Mozingo, MD

The splenic injury outcomes trial: An American Association for the Surgery of Trauma multi-institutional study

Zarzaur BL, Kozar R, Myers JG, et al (Univ of Tennessee Health Science Ctr, Memphis; AAST Multi-Institutional Trials Committee; et al)

J Trauma Acute Care Surg 79:335-342, 2015

Background.—Delayed splenic hemorrhage after nonoperative management (NOM) of blunt splenic injury (BSI) is a feared complication, particularly in the outpatient setting. Significant resources, including angiography (ANGIO), are used in an effort to prevent delayed splenectomy (DS). No prospective, long-term data exist to determine the actual risk of splenectomy. The purposes of this trial were to ascertain the 180-day risk of splenectomy after 24 hours of NOM of BSI and to determine factors related to splenectomy.

Methods.—Eleven Level I trauma centers participated in this prospective observational study. Adult patients achieving 24 hours of NOM of their BSI were eligible. Patients were followed up for 180 days. Demographic, physiologic, radiographic, injury-related information, and spleen-related interventions were recorded. Bivariate and multivariable analyses were used to determine factors associated with DS.

Results.—A total of 383 patients were enrolled. Twelve patients (3.1%) underwent in-hospital splenectomy between 24 hours and 9 days after injury. Of 366 discharged with a spleen, 1 (0.27%) required readmission for DS on postinjury Day 12. No Grade I injuries experienced DS. The splenectomy rate after 24 hours of NOM was 1.5 per 1,000 patient-days. Only extravasation from the spleen at time of admission (ADMIT-BLUSH) was associated with splenectomy (odds ratio, 3.6; 95% confidence interval, 1.4–12.4). Of patients with ADMIT-BLUSH ($n = 49$), 17 (34.7%) did not have ANGIO with embolization (EMBO), and 2 of those (11.8%) underwent splenectomy; 32 (65.3%) underwent ANGIO with EMBO, and 2 of those (6.3%, $p = 0.6020$ compared with no ANGIO with EMBO) required splenectomy.

Conclusion.—Splenectomy after 24 hours of NOM is rare. After the initial 24 hours, no additional interventions are warranted for patients with Grade I injuries. For Grades II to V, close observation as an inpatient or outpatient is indicated for 10 days to 14 days. ADMIT-BLUSH is a strong predictor of DS and should lead to close observation or earlier surgical intervention.

Level of Evidence.—Prognostic/epidemiological study, level III; therapeutic study, level IV (Fig 1).

▶ There is significant debate in the literature regarding the optimal management for patients with blunt splenic injury who do not need urgent operative intervention. Most existing guidelines rely on retrospective studies and expert opinion. Recognizing this, a study group was formed by the American Association for the Surgery of Trauma including 11 level 1 trauma centers. Patients admitted with blunt splenic injury were followed for a total of 180 days. This study represents the first collection of multi-institutional, long-term prospective data for patients with blunt splenic injury. Fig 1 is included here, demonstrating the outcome of the 383 patients followed in the study. After the first 24 hours, the risk of splenectomy is rare, occurring in only 3.1% of patients. The risk is even lower in the outpatient setting over the 180 days of the study. A surprising finding in this study questions the benefits of angiography and embolization in patients with blunt splenic injury. There was relatively little difference in patients with an arterial blush on angiography with or without arterial

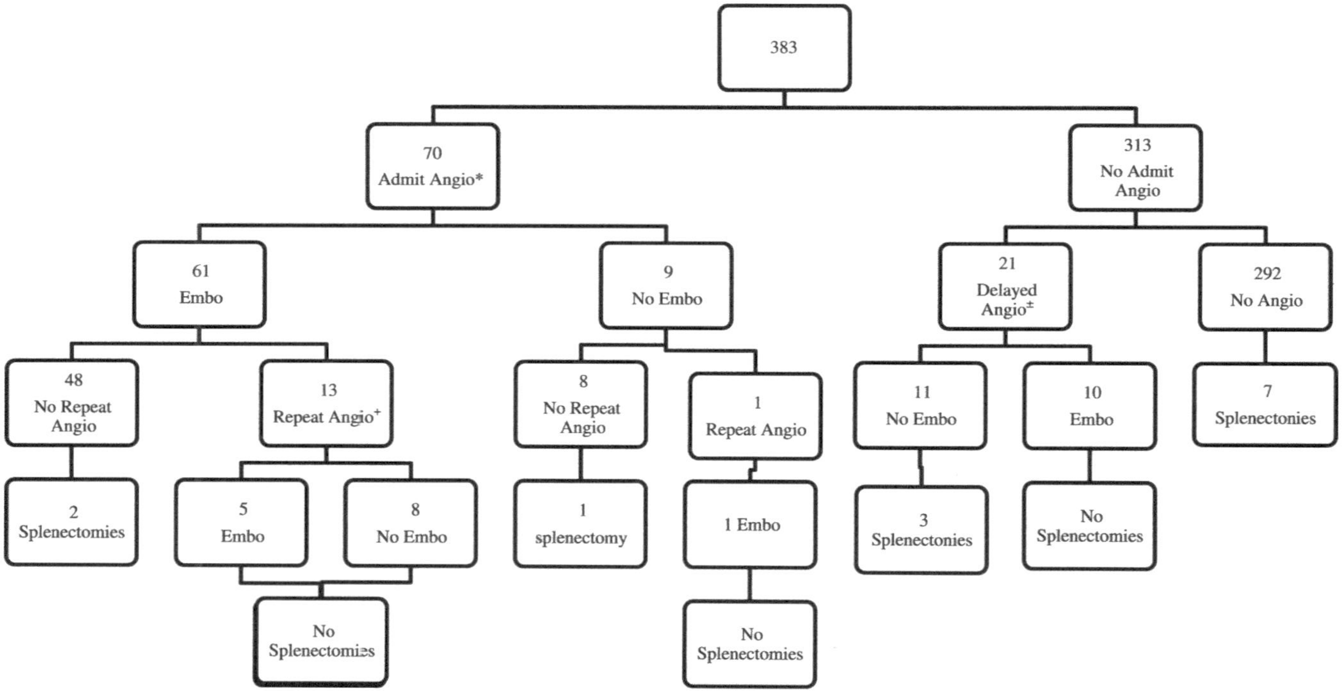

FIGURE 1.—Flow chart of patient outcomes. (Reprinted from Zarzaur BL, Kozar R, Myers JG, et al. The splenic injury outcomes trial: an American Association for the Surgery of Trauma multi-institutional study. *J Trauma Acute Care Surg.* 2015;79:335-342, with permission from Wolters Kluwer Health, Inc.)

embolization. This speaks for the need of additional multicenter trials to study this specific issue.

D. W. Mozingo, MD

Comorbidity-polypharmacy score predicts readmission in older trauma patients

Housley BC, Stawicki SPA, Evans DC, et al (The Ohio State Univ College of Medicine, Columbus)

J Surg Res 199:237-243, 2015

Background.—Hospital readmissions are considered to be a measure of quality of care, correlate with worse outcomes, and may soon lead to decreased reimbursement. The comorbidity-polypharmacy score (CPS) is the sum of the number of preinjury medications and comorbidities, and may estimate patient frailty more effectively than patient age. This study evaluates the association between CPS and readmission.

Methods.—Medical records for trauma patients ≥45 y evaluated between January 1 and December 31, 2008, at our American College of Surgeons-verified level 1 trauma center were reviewed to obtain information on demographics, injuries, preinjury comorbidities, and medications, and occurrences of readmission to our facility within 30 d of discharge. Chi-square and Kruskal–Wallis testing was used to evaluate differences between readmitted and nonreadmitted patients, with multiple logistic regression used to evaluate the contribution of independent risk factors for readmission.

Results.—A total of 879 patients were included; their ages ranged from 45–103 y (median 58), injury severity scores from 0–50 y (median 5), and CPS from 0–39 y (median 7). A total of 76 patients (8.6%) were readmitted to our facility within 30 d of discharge. The readmitted cohort had higher CPS (median, 9.5, range 0–32, $P = 0.031$) and injury severity score (median, 9, range 1–38, $P = 0.045$), but no difference in age (median, 59.5, range 47–99, $P = 0.646$). Logistic regression demonstrated independent association of higher CPS with increased risk of readmission, with each CPS point increasing readmission likelihood by 3.5% ($P = 0.03$).

Conclusions.—CPS appears to correlate well with readmissions within 30 d. Frailty defined by CPS was a significantly stronger predictor of readmission than was patient age. Early recognition of elevated CPS may improve discharge planning and help guide interventions to decrease readmission rates in older trauma patients (Fig 2).

▶ Unplanned hospital readmissions are considered an indicator of poor quality of care. They are associated with worse outcomes and may soon lead to decreased reimbursement from third-party payors. Despite the importance of this quality metric, known risk factors for readmission are not well defined. One important risk factor for readmission is patient age, and as the current

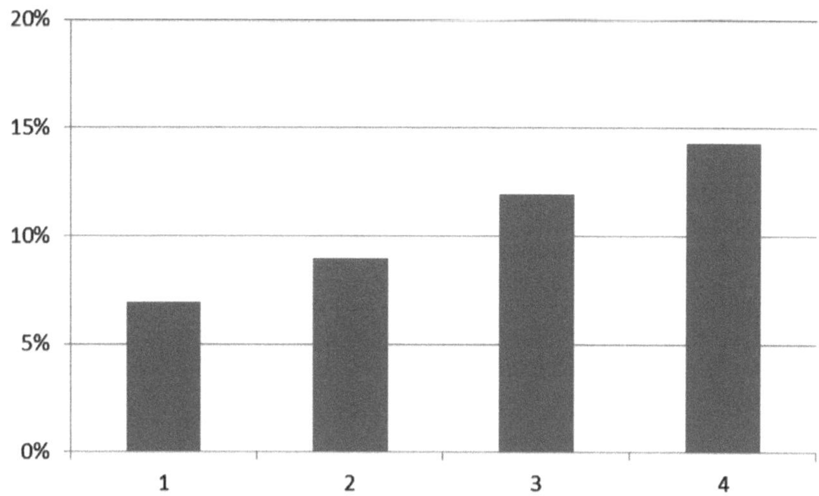

FIGURE 2.—Readmission rates per CPS group. CPS groups are defined as 1, "minor" (CPS, 0–7); 2, "moderate" (CPS, 8–15); 3, "severe" (CPS, 16–21); and 4, "morbid" (CPS ≥22). (Color version of figure is available online.) (Reprinted from Housley BC, Stawicki SPA, Evans DC, et al. Comorbidity-polypharmacy score predicts readmission in older trauma patients. *J Surg Res.* 2015;199:237-243, with permission from Elsevier Inc.)

population ages, a larger number of older individuals will be injured and require hospital care for traumatic injuries. Physiologic age or frailty may be more important to outcomes than chronologic age and portend an increased number of comorbidities. The comorbidity-polypharmacy score (CPS), developed by the authors of this study, is simply the number of drugs a patient takes added to the number of comorbidities present on admission. As the CPS in older individuals rises, an increased rate of complications after injury is observed. The authors use this simple tool to predict the risk of readmission after hospital discharge. It is much simpler than calculations of frailty and can be used to tailor discharge teaching and follow-up strategies in this vulnerable population. Fig 2 demonstrates nicely the correlation between increasing CPS and the rate of readmission.

D. W. Mozingo, MD

Role of computed tomography angiography in the management of Zone II penetrating neck trauma in patients with clinical hard signs

Schroll R, Fontenot T, Lipcsey M, et al (Tulane Univ School of Medicine, New Orleans; et al)

J Trauma Acute Care Surg 79:943-950, 2015

Background.—The Western Trauma Association (WTA) describes the management of Zone 2 penetrating neck trauma (PNT) and recommends neck exploration (NE) for patients with clinical hard signs (HS). We hypothesize that in stable patients with HS, the management of PNT augmented by computed tomography angiography (CTA) results in fewer negative NE results.

Methods.—This was a 4-year retrospective review of adult patients with Zone 2 PNT at a Level I trauma center. Stable patients with WTA-defined HS (airway compromise, massive subcutaneous emphysema/air bubbling through wound, expanding/pulsatile hematoma, active bleeding, shock, focal neurologic deficit, and hematemesis) who underwent CTA instead of emergent exploration were identified. Sensitivity, specificity, positive predictive value, and negative predictive value for CTA were calculated. A comparison was made between the rates of negative NE results in patients with HS who received a CTA versus the rate that would have occurred in the same patients if the WTA algorithm had been followed. Missed injury rates were also compared.

Results.—Of 183 PNT patients, 23 had HS and underwent CTA. Of the 23, 5 had a positive CTA findings and underwent NE, while 17 had a negative CTA findings and did not require NE. There was one false-negative in a patient who developed an expanding hematoma following negative neck CTA finding. Sensitivity, specificity, positive predictive value, and negative predictive value for CTA in the presence of HS were found to be 83%, 100%, 100%, and 94%, respectively. The addition of CTA to the WTA algorithm for this patient group significantly decreased the rate of negative NE (0 of 23 vs. 18 of 23, $p < 0.001$) without a significant increase in the rate of missed injury (1 of 23 vs. 0 of 23, $p = 0.323$). The use of CTA prevented 17 unnecessary NEs.

Conclusion.—CTA addition to the management of hemodynamically stable patients with HS in PNT significantly decreased the rate of negative NE result without increasing missed injury rate. Prospective study of CTA addition to the WTA algorithm is needed.

Level of Evidence.—Care management/therapeutic study, level IV.

▶ Physical examination has been the screening method of choice for penetrating neck trauma. This has led to the development of clinical treatment algorithms based on the presence of "hard signs" and "soft signs" of injury. Hard signs portend a higher likelihood of vascular or aerodigestive injuries requiring immediate operative intervention. Those patients presenting with soft signs proceed to further diagnostic evaluation and operative intervention only with positive diagnostic findings requiring surgical intervention. The authors of this selection have extended the indications for diagnostic workup to those patients with hard signs who are hemodynamically stable. They evaluated the role of computed tomography and geography in patients with Zone II injuries. Using this algorithm, 74% of the patients were spared an unnecessary neck exploration. Because this study was retrospective in nature, it is difficult to ascertain the underlying reasons that directed these patients to computed tomography and geography instead of neck exploration. A prospective study of computed tomography and geography in patients with Zone II neck injury, and hard signs would be useful to further validate these interesting results.

D. W. Mozingo, MD

The financial burden of emergency general surgery: National estimates 2010 to 2060

Ogola GO, Gale SC, Haider A, et al (Baylor Scott & White Health, Dallas, TX; East Texas Med Ctr, Tyler; Brigham and Women's Hosp, Boston, MA)

J Trauma Acute Care Surg 79:444-448, 2015

Background.—Adoption of the acute care surgery model has led to increasing volumes of emergency general surgery (EGS) patients at trauma centers. However, the financial burden of EGS services on trauma centers is unknown. This study estimates the current and future costs associated with EGS hospitalization nationwide.

Methods.—We applied the American Association for the Surgery of Trauma's DRG International Classification of Diseases—9th Rev. criteria for defining EGS to the 2010 National Inpatient Sample (NIS) data and identified adult EGS patients. Cost of hospitalization was obtained by converting reported charges to cost using the 2010 all-payer inpatient cost-to-charge ratio for all hospitals in the NIS database. Cost was modeled via a log-gamma model in a generalized linear mixed model to account for potential correlation in cost within states and hospitals in the NIS database. Patients' characteristics and hospital factors were included in the model as fixed effects, while state and hospital were included as random effects. The national incidence of EGS was calculated from NIS data, and the US Census Bureau population projections were used to estimate incidence for 2010 to 2060. Nationwide costs were obtained by multiplying projected incidences by estimated costs and reported in year 2010 US dollar value.

Results.—Nationwide, there were 2,640,725 adult EGS hospitalizations in 2010. The national average adjusted cost per EGS hospitalization was $10,744 (95% confidence interval [CI], $10,615–$10,874); applying these cost data to the national EGS hospitalizations gave a total estimated cost of $28.37 billion (95% CI, $28.03–$28.72 billion). Older age groups accounted for greater proportions of the cost ($8.03 billion for age ≥ 75 years, compared with $1.08 billion for age 18–24 years). As the US population continues to both grow and age, EGS costs are projected to increase by 45% to $41.20 billion (95% CI, $40.70–$41.7 billion) by 2060.

Conclusion.—EGS constitutes a significant portion of US health care costs and is expected to rise with the demographic changes in the population. Trauma centers should conduct careful financial analyses of their EGS services, based on their unique case mix and payer mix.

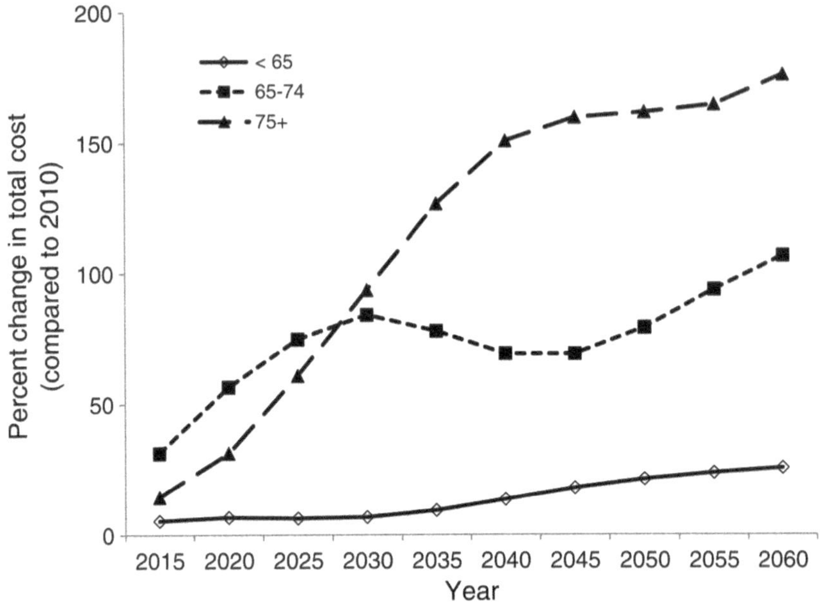

FIGURE 1.—Projected percent change in total costs (2010 as baseline) for EGS patients in the United States by age group, 2015 to 2060. (Reprinted from Ogola GO, Gale SC, Haider A, et al. The financial burden of emergency general surgery: National estimates 2010 to 2060. *J Trauma Acute Care Surg.* 2015;79:444-448, with permission from Wolters Kluwer Health, Inc.)

Level of Evidence.—Economic analysis, level III (Figs 1 and 2).

▶ Acute care surgery has developed as a specialty in the past 10 years to fill the increasing need of emergency surgical care in the United States. The 3 disciplines encompassed by acute care surgery are trauma, surgical critical care, and emergency general surgery. Although much is known about the incidence and costs of trauma and critical care, little is known about the public health impact of emergency general surgery. The authors of this selection acknowledge that the growing national population and its aging are expected to increase the burden of emergency general surgery over the decades. As more trauma centers use the acute care surgery model, the treatment of emergency general surgery patients on a regional level. This situation is likely to create a financial risk for trauma centers and other acute care hospitals because of the disproportionally low funding rates of this population. Fig 1 is included showing the projected costs over time for 3 age cohorts. Fig 2 is also included depicting the staggering direct cost of hospitalization for emergency general surgery compared with a number of other common clinical conditions. Emergency general surgery constitutes a significant financial burden on society and will continue to rise in the coming decades. Trauma centers that embrace this model

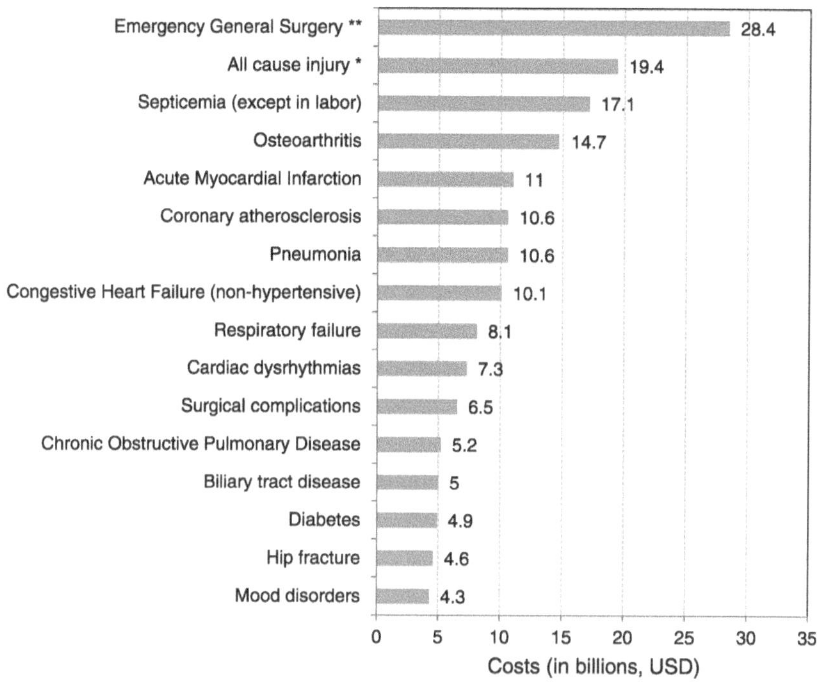

FIGURE 2.—Direct costs of hospitalization for EGS compared with other common conditions in the United States in 2010. *From Villaveces et al.[13] **Based on the current analysis. For other diseases with no asterisk, the reported costs are from Pfuntner et al.[14] *Editor's Note*: Please refer to original journal article for full references. (Reprinted from Ogola GO, Gale SC, Haider A, et al. The financial burden of emergency general surgery: National estimates 2010 to 2060. *J Trauma Acute Care Surg.* 2015;79:444-448, with permission from Wolters Kluwer Health, Inc.)

should undertake careful financial analysis of its emergency general surgery services bases on case and payer mix.

D. W. Mozingo, MD

Prophylactic Inferior Vena Cava Filter Placement Does Not Result in a Survival Benefit for Trauma Patients

Hemmila MR, Osborne NH, Henke PK, et al (Univ of Michigan, Ann Arbor; et al)

Ann Surg 262:577-585, 2015

Objective.—Trauma patients are at high risk for life-threatening venous thromboembolic (VTE) events. We examined the relationship between prophylactic inferior vena cava (IVC) filter use, mortality, and VTE.

Summary Background Data.—The prevalence of prophylactic placement of IVC filters has increased among trauma patients. However, there exists little data on the overall efficacy of prophylactic IVC filters with regard to outcomes.

Methods.—Trauma quality collaborative data from 2010 to 2014 were analyzed. Patients were excluded with no signs of life, Injury Severity Score <9, hospitalization <3 days, or who received IVC filter after occurrence of VTE event. Risk-adjusted rates of IVC filter placement were calculated and hospitals placed into quartiles of IVC filter use. Mortality rates by quartile were compared. We also determined the association of deep venous thrombosis (DVT) with the presence of an IVC filter, accounting for type and timing of initiation of pharmacological VTE prophylaxis.

Results.—A prophylactic IVC filter was placed in 803 (2%) of 39,456 patients. Hospitals exhibited significant variability (0.6% to 9.6%) in adjusted rates of IVC filter utilization. Rates of IVC placement within quartiles were 0.7%, 1.3%, 2.1%, and 4.6%, respectively. IVC filter use quartiles showed no variation in mortality. Adjusting for pharmacological VTE prophylaxis and patient factors, prophylactic IVC filter placement was associated with an increased incidence of DVT (OR = 1.83; 95% CI, 1.15–2.93, *P*-value = 0.01).

Conclusions.—High rates of prophylactic IVC filter placement have no effect on reducing trauma patient mortality and are associated with an increase in DVT events.

▶ Trauma patients often have a hypercoagulable state venous status due to immobility and endothelial damage outlining the 3 classic factors of Virchow's triad. Trauma patients are often at high risk for venous thromboembolism because of factors such as severity of injury, body region injured, immobilization, need for surgical interventions, and presence of inflammation and infection. In the high-risk patient who is not a suitable candidate for medical thromboembolic prophylaxis, inferior vena cava filters are found in many treatment algorithms. Prophylactic inferior vena cava filter placement has been increasing in trauma patients over the past decade, despite continued controversies regarding this approach. This study is important in that the authors showed that prophylactic inferior vena cava filter insertion varied widely within a statewide trauma quality collaborative. They also demonstrated that an inferior vena cava filter does not reduce the risk of mortality for trauma patients at the hospital level but is associated with an increased risk of subsequent deep venous thrombosis.

D. W. Mozingo, MD

Management of severe blunt hepatic injury in the era of computed tomography and transarterial embolization: A systematic review and critical appraisal of the literature

Melloul E, Denys A, Demartines N (Univ Hosp Lausanne, Switzerland)

J Trauma Acute Care Surg 79:468-474, 2015

Background.—During the last decade, the management of blunt hepatic injury has considerably changed. Three options are available as follows: nonoperative management (NOM), transarterial embolization (TAE), and surgery. We aimed to evaluate in a systematic review the current practice and outcomes in the management of Grade III to V blunt hepatic injury.

Method.—The MEDLINE database was searched using PubMed to identify English-language citations published after 2000 using the key words *blunt, hepatic injury, severe*, and *grade III to V* in different combinations. Liver injury was graded according to the American Association for the Surgery of Trauma classification on computed tomography (CT). Primary outcome analyzed was success rate in intention to treat. Critical appraisal of the literature was performed using the validated National Institute for Health and Care Excellence "Quality Assessment for Case Series" system.

Results.—Twelve articles were selected for critical appraisal (n = 4,946 patients). The median quality score of articles was 4 of 8 (range, 2–6). Overall, the median Injury Severity Score (ISS) at admission was 26 (range, 0.6–75). A median of 66% (range, 0–100%) of patients was managed with NOM, with a success rate of 94% (range, 86–100%). TAE was used in only 3% of cases (range, 0–72%) owing to contrast extravasation on CT with a success rate of 93% (range, 81–100%); however, 9% to 30% of patients required a laparotomy. Thirty-one percent (range, 17–100%) of patients were managed with surgery owing to hemodynamic instability in most cases, with 12% to 28% requiring secondary TAE to control recurrent hepatic bleeding. Mortality was 5% (range, 0–8%) after NOM and 51% (range, 30–68%) after surgery.

Conclusion.—NOM of Grade III to V blunt hepatic injury is the first treatment option to manage hemodynamically stable patients. TAE and surgery are considered in a highly selective group of patients with contrast extravasation on CT or shock at admission, respectively. Additional standardization of the reports is necessary to allow accurate comparisons of the various management strategies.

Level of Evidence.—Systematic review, level IV.

▶ The outcome of patients with severe blunt hepatic injury is closely related to the concomitant injuries. The primary management of hepatic injury is still debated, and this selection evaluates the 3 options available today: transarterial embolization, nonoperative management, or surgery. Because the majority of studies assessing these 3 management strategies include low-grade blunt hepatic injury and combine patients with blunt and penetrating liver injuries, it is difficult to extrapolate previous findings to patients with only high-grade blunt liver injury. The aim of this study was to assess in a systematic review the current practice and outcomes of the various treatments used in the treatment of Grade III to V blunt hepatic injuries. This study has several limitations that need to be addressed. The study was based on data collection from several heterogeneous retrospective series, precluding the use of prior meta-analyses. Unfortunately, randomized control trials in the setting of severe trauma can hardly be performed for ethical reasons. From this review, we can conclude that the nonoperative management of Grade III to V blunt hepatic injury should be considered as the first treatment strategy to manage hemodynamically stable patients. Transarterial embolization is indicated in patients with contrast extravasations on the angiographic CT at admission or in patients who failed nonoperative management. Surgery should be considered in only a highly selected group of patients with shock at the time of admission and/or suspicion of other abdominal organ injuries.

D. W. Mozingo, MD

Explaining the Paradoxical Age-Based Racial Disparities in Survival After Trauma: The Role of the Treating Facility

Hicks CW, Hashmi ZG, Hui X, et al (Johns Hopkins School of Medicine, Baltimore, MD; et al)

Ann Surg 262:179-183, 2015

Objective.—The objective of our study was to determine if differences in outcomes at treating facilities can help explain these age-based racial disparities in survival after trauma.

Background.—It has been previously demonstrated that racial disparities in survival after trauma are dependent on age. For patients younger than 65 years, blacks had an increased odds of mortality compared with whites, but among patients 65 years or older the opposite association was found.

Methods.—Data on white and black trauma patients were extracted from the Nationwide Inpatient Sample (2003–2009) using *International Classification of Diseases, Ninth Revision, Clinical Modification* diagnosis codes. Standardized observed-to-expected mortality ratios were calculated for individual treating facilities, adjusting for age, sex, insurance status, mechanism of injury, overall injury severity, head injury severity, and comorbid conditions. Observed-to-expected ratios were used to benchmark facilities as high-, average-, or low-performing facilities. Proportions and survival outcomes of younger (range, 16–64 years) and older (≥65 years) patients admitted within each performance stratum were compared.

Results.—A total of 934,476 patients from 1137 facilities (8.3% high-performing, 85% average-performing, and 6.7% low-performing) were analyzed. Younger black patients had a higher adjusted odds of mortality compared with younger white patients [odds ratio, 1.19; 95% confidence interval, 1.11–1.27], whereas older black patients had a lower odds of mortality compared with older white patients [odds ratio, 0.81; 95% confidence interval, 0.74–88]. A significantly greater proportion of younger black patients were treated at low-performing facilities compared with both younger white patients and older black patients (49.6% vs 42.2% and 38.7%, respectively; $P < 0.05$).

Conclusions.—Nearly half of all young black trauma patients are treated at low-performing facilities. However, facility-based differences do not

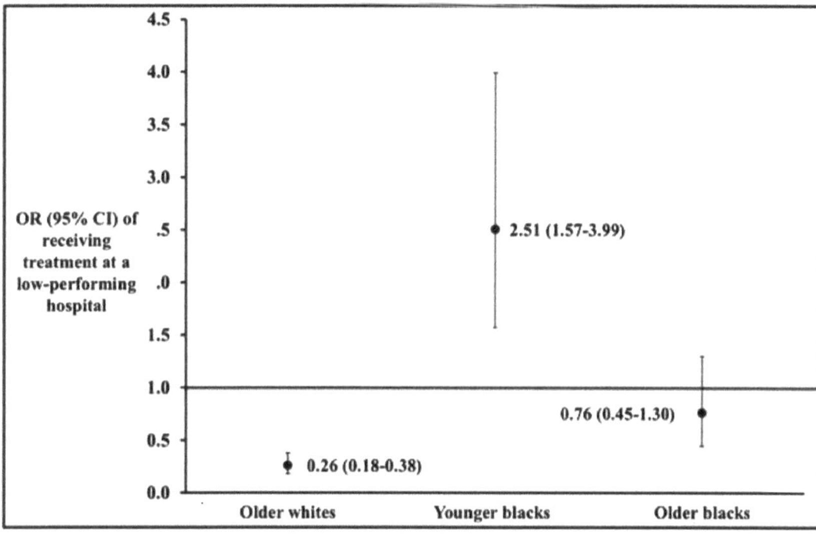

FIGURE 2.—Odds ratio (95% CI) of receiving treatment at a low-performing hospital versus at a high-performing hospital for older white, younger black, and older black patients compared with younger white patients (black line represents the odds ratio for the reference group, that is, younger white patients). Younger black patients had significantly higher odds of being treated at a low-performing facility compared with younger white patients. In contrast, older white patients had significantly lower odds of being treated at a low-performing facility compared with younger white patients. Older white patients also had lower odds of being treated at a low-performing facility than older black patients, who were no different from the younger white patient reference group. (Reprinted from Hicks CW, Hashmi ZG, Hui X, et al. Explaining the paradoxical age-based racial disparities in survival after trauma: the role of the treating facility. *Ann Surg.* 2015;262:179-183, with permission from Wolters Kluwer Health, Inc.)

seem to explain the paradoxical age-based racial disparities after trauma observed in the older population (Fig 2).

▶ The concept of racial disparities after trauma is not new, and the cause of this paradoxical difference in trauma outcomes remains unclear. There are some data to suggest hospital-based effects may play a role in race-based disparities after trauma within the younger population. Minority trauma patients have been shown to cluster at trauma centers with higher than expected mortality rates, which could explain the worse outcomes observed in this population. However, the relationship between trauma center performance and age-based racial disparities in mortality after traumatic injury is currently unknown, thus prompting this study. Their major findings are presented in Fig 2 presenting the odds ratio of being treated in a lower performing facility. Patient-level factors including comorbidities, mechanism of injury, frailty, and preinjury medical care might also play a role and are not captured in this study. Also, age-dependent racial disparities in trauma outcomes could reflect patient disease that is exacerbated by the traumatic event rather than directly related to the injury.

D. W. Mozingo, MD

Evaluation of diaphragm in penetrating left thoracoabdominal stab injuries: The role of multislice computed tomography

Yucel M, Bas G, Kulalı F, et al (Umraniye Training and Res Hosp, Istanbul, Turkey)

Injury 46:1734-1737, 2015

Introduction.—Penetrating left thoracoabdominal stab injuries are accompanied by diaphragmatic injury in 25–30% of cases, about 30% of which later develop into diaphragmatic hernia. This study aimed to determine the role of multislice computed tomography in the evaluation of left diaphragm in patients with penetrating left thoracoabdominal stab wounds.

Materials and Methods.—This study reviewed penetrating left thoracoabdominal stab injuries managed in our clinic between April 2009 and September 2014. The thoracoabdominal region was defined as the region between the sternum, fourth intercostal space, and arcus costa anteriorly and the vertebra, lower tip of scapula, and the curve of the last rib posteriorly. Unstable cases and cases with signs of peritonitis were operated with laparotomy; the remaining patients were closely monitored. Forty-eight hours later, a diagnostic laparoscopy was applied to evaluate the left hemidiaphragma in asymptomatic patients who did not need laparotomy. The preoperatively obtained multislice thoracoabdominal computed tomography images were retrospectively examined for the presence of left diaphragm injury. Then, operative and tomographic findings were compared.

Results.—This study included a total of 43 patients, 39 (91%) males and 4 (9%) females of mean age 30 years (range 15–61 years). Thirty patients had normal tomography results, whereas 13 had left diaphragmatic injuries. An injury to the left diaphragm was detected during the operation in 9 (1 in laparotomy and 8 in diagnostic laparoscopy) of 13 patients with positive tomography for left diaphragmatic injury and 2 (in diagnostic laparoscopy) of 30 patients with negative tomography. Multislice tomography had a sensitivity of 82% (95% CI: 48–98%), a specificity of 88% (71–96%), a positive predictive value of 69% (39–91%), and a negative predictive value of 93% (78–99%) for detection of diaphragmatic injury in penetrating left thoracoabdominal stab injury.

Conclusions.—Although diagnostic laparoscopy is the gold standard for diaphragmatic examination in patients with penetrating left thoracoabdominal stab wounds, multislice computed tomography is also valuable for detecting diaphragmatic injury (Fig 3).

▶ Penetrating injuries of the diaphragm are initially small, and majority of patients do not have visceral organ herniation into the thoracic cavity. It is often challenging to make the diagnosis by conventional CT. In this selection the authors describe their experience with multislice CT (MCT) to evaluate for diaphragm penetration. With MCT, a large region of interest can be rapidly scanned within a breath-holding interval. The shortened image acquisition time

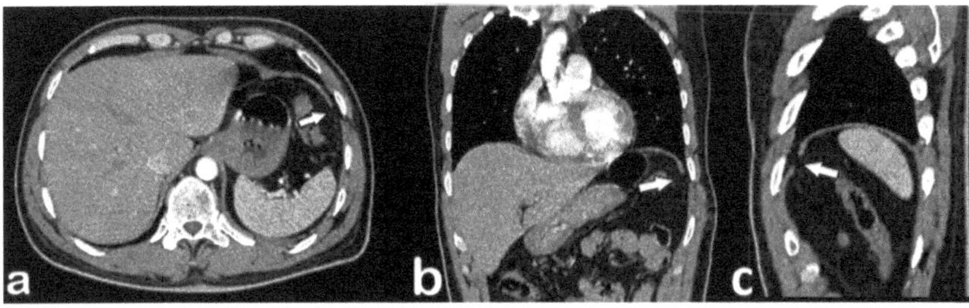

FIGURE 3.—Axial (a), coronal (b) and sagittal (c) plane views of the diaphragmatic injury in the same patient. (Reprinted from Yucel M, Bas G, Kulalı F, et al. Evaluation of diaphragm in penetrating left thoracoabdominal stab injuries: the role of multislice computed tomography. *Injury.* 2015;46:1734-1737, with permission from Elsevier Ltd.)

reduces the effects of patient movement and decreases the artifacts originating from breathing. Thinner sections with a better image quality can be obtained. Additionally, it is possible to perform coronal, sagittal, and oblique reconstructed images. Fig 3 is included demonstrating this finding. The use of MCT may allow some patients to avoid surgical therapy, and only patients with positive or equivocal findings would proceed to surgery, reducing the rate of nontherapeutic laparoscopy and the associated morbidity associated with this procedure.

D. W. Mozingo, MD

All the bang without the bucks: Defining essential point-of-care testing for traumatic coagulopathy

Goodman MD, Makley AT, Hanseman DJ, et al (Univ of Cincinnati, OH)
J Trauma Acute Care Surg 79:117-124, 2015

Background.—Rapid assessment and treatment of coagulopathy reduces postinjury morbidity and mortality. Although thrombelastography (TEG) may be more accurate and efficient than conventional coagulation tests, it requires significant financial and personnel investments. We hypothesized that point-of-care international normalized ratio (POC INR) may provide a rapid and accurate alternative to TEG.

Methods.—A retrospective review of sequential trauma patients who underwent both POC INR and rapid TEG (r-TEG) testing upon presentation to a Level I trauma center from July 2012 to December 2013 was performed. POC INR was compared with r-TEG values (*R* value, *K* time, α angle, maximum amplitude, percent clot lysis in 30 minutes) and transfusion requirements. Vital signs, admission laboratory values, and injury severity were analyzed. POC INR and venous blood gas testing was performed in the emergency department. All results and Pearson correlations noted were significant if $p < 0.05$.

Results.—We identified 628 trauma patients with concomitant r-TEG and POC INR testing. Median Injury Severity Score (ISS) was 13, 20%

arrived in shock (base value < −5), 21% were transfused, and 11% died. POC INR correlated with all r-TEG values, with stronger correlations for patients in shock. POC INR and r-TEG had similar correlations with blood products transfused at 4 hours and 24 hours, but only POC INR predicted substantial bleeding and massive transfusion. POC INR also correlated strongly with standard INR testing. POC INR test duration was less than 1 minute, compared with at least 30 minutes for r-TEG. Total cohort charges for POC INR were estimated at $21,980 versus $396,896 for r-TEG.

Conclusion.—POC INR testing is faster and cheaper than r-TEG. In addition, POC INR correlates not only with r-TEG values but also with acute blood product transfusions. POC INR provides a practical alternative for rapid coagulopathy assessment in the trauma patient at institutions that lack TEG capability.

Level of Evidence.—Diagnostic study, level III. Therapeutic/care management study, level IV (Table 5).

▶ Exsanguinating hemorrhage continues to be the leading cause of preventable death after traumatic injury. In addition to rapid surgical control of hemorrhage, identification and treatment of acute coagulopathy is necessary to prevent ongoing blood loss. The presence and severity of acute traumatic coagulopathy at presentation are associated with increased transfusion requirements and mortality in trauma patients. The rapid identification and treatment of coagulopathy by protocols and principles, such as damage-control resuscitation and newer transfusion strategies, may lessen the lethal effects of coagulopathy in traumatic hemorrhage. Timely recognition of traumatic coagulopathy may depend on the coagulation test performed upon arrival to the emergency department. Plasma-based conventional coagulation tests are traditionally used and include prothrombin time (PT) and its

TABLE 5.—Multiple Logistic Regression Analysis for Substantial Bleeding and Massive Transfusion

	Odds Ratio	95% Confidence Interval	*p*
Substantial bleeding			
r-TEG *R* value ≥ 55	1.70	0.721–4.006	0.23
r-TEG α angle ≤ 55	1.64	0.278–9.634	0.59
r-TEG MA ≤ 55	1.08	0.413–2.802	0.88
r-TEG LY30 > 3%	0.57	0.197–1.630	0.29
POC INR > 1.5	3.08	1.142–8.293	0.03*
Massive transfusion			
r-TEG *R* value ≥ 55	2.67	0.808–8.815	0.11
r-TEG α angle ≤ 55	3.42	0.538–21.694	0.19
r-TEG MA ≤ 55	1.71	0.491–5.927	0.40
r-TEG LY30 > 3%	1.84	0.541–6.225	0.33
POC INR > 1.5	5.12	1.192–21.975	0.03*

*Significance defined as $p < 0.05$.

Reprinted from Goodman MD, Makley AT, Hanseman DJ, et al. All the bang without the bucks: defining essential point-of-care testing for traumatic coagulopathy. *J Trauma Acute Care Surg*. 2015;79:117-124, with permission from Wolters Kluwer Health, Inc.

standardized international normalized ratio (INR), activated partial thromboplastin time, and fibrinogen level. Admission INR has further been identified as the most predictive individual trigger for any transfusion, including the need for massive transfusion. Recently, there has been increased interest in whole-blood viscoelastic hemostatic testing, such as thrombelastography (TEG), to address the need for rapid assessment of coagulopathy. Compared with standard coagulation testing, rapid TEG values have been shown to be faster and less expensive measures of coagulopathy. TEG strongly correlates with blood product transfusion in trauma patients; however, TEG and other viscoelastic tests are subject to a unique set of factors that can affect test reliability and reproducibility. In this selection, the authors evaluated a point-of-care test of INR as a predictor of severity of traumatic coagulopathy and compared their results to TEG and conventional tests of coagulopathy. Table 5 is included, which demonstrates the ability of the point-of-care test to discriminate the presence of substantial bleeding and the need for massive transfusion. Although retrospective in nature, this study suggests that point-of-care analysis is a rapid and accurate method of determining INR in the trauma population. Similar to the standard plasma-based INR test, point-of-care INR testing remains strongly associated with blood administration requirements in the actively bleeding trauma patient.

D. W. Mozingo, MD

Abdominal Injuries in the "Found Down": Is Imaging Indicated?

Ko A, Zaw AA, Barmparas G, et al (Cedars-Sinai Med Ctr, Los Angeles, CA)

J Am Coll Surg 221:17-24, 2015

Background.—We sought to investigate the incidence of abdominal injuries in "found down" trauma patients to better understand the value of emergency department (ED) imaging. Found down patients are at high risk for injuries to the head or neck and low risk to the abdomen or pelvis, so imaging with CT of the abdomen/pelvis (AP) or Focused Assessment with Sonography for Trauma (FAST) is of questionable value.

Study Design.—The trauma registry was queried over a 10-year period ending December 2013 for found down patients. Demographics, CT AP, FAST scans, and injuries were abstracted from the trauma registry and then through a confirmatory chart review. The primary outcome was significant abdominal or pelvis injury, defined as abdomen/pelvis Abbreviated Injury Scale (AIS) ≥3 or an abdominal injury that required operative intervention. The secondary outcome was mortality due to abdominal injury.

Results.—Of the 342 patients who met inclusion criteria, mean Glasgow Coma Scale (GCS) was 11.0, and 189 (60%) of those tested for alcohol were intoxicated. Abdominal imaging included: CT AP only, 88 (57%); FAST only, 37 (24%); and CT AP and FAST, 29 (19%). Neither CT AP nor FAST scan led to a change in treatment and no patient had abdomen/pelvis AIS ≥ 3. Overall mortality was 33 (10%). The 24 trauma deaths were attributed to serious head trauma (n = 16) or traumatic arrest in the ED (n = 8); the 9 medical deaths were due to cerebral vascular accident (n = 5) or sepsis (n = 4).

Conclusions.—Although patients found down have a high mortality, abdominal injuries identified by imaging are highly unlikely. Efforts should focus on rapidly identifying and treating other causes of mortality, especially trauma to the head and neck, or medical diagnoses such as cerebral vascular accident or sepsis.

▶ In patients who are "found down," or in those who fall from a standing position, the contextual information is often lacking, with no clear mechanism of injury. Found-down patients require significant resources to appropriately triage, diagnose, resuscitate, and treat definitively because of the relative high-acuity care needed to avoid delays and prevent misdiagnosis. To evaluate the found-down patient for abdominal or pelvic trauma or other intraabdominal cause of collapse, CT abdomen and pelvis is highly sensitive at detecting most injuries, evaluating solid organs, and identifying intraperitoneal air or fluid. Similarly, the focused assessment with sonography for trauma (FAST) ultrasound examination may be useful in such screening. The authors of this selection sought to investigate the incidence of abdominal injuries in found-down trauma patients to better understand the value of emergency department imaging. They determined that found-down patients are at much higher risk for injuries to the head or neck and low risk to the abdomen or pelvis. Imaging with CT of the abdomen/pelvis or FAST is of questionable value.

D. W. Mozingo, MD

Impact of preexisting opioid use on injury mechanism, type, and outcome

Pandya U, O'Mara MS, Wilson W, et al (Grant Med Ctr, Columbus, OH; Ohio Univ Heritage College of Osteopathic Medicine, Athens)

J Surg Res 198:7-12, 2015

Background.—The prevalence of prescription narcotic use in the United States is on the rise. Opioid use and its impact on the management of trauma patients has yet to be thoroughly studied. The aim of this study was to determine the prevalence of preinjury opioid use and its influence on specific outcomes among the trauma patient population.

Methods.—A retrospective review of all trauma patients presenting to a level 1 trauma center was performed from January 1, 2010–December 31, 2010. Patients who died within 24 h of presentation and those with incomplete medication data were excluded. Electronic medical record review of history and physical documentation and urine drug screen records were used to determine preinjury opioid status. Preexisting narcotic use, demographic data, injury mechanism and severity, injury type, and outcome variables were analyzed.

Results.—A total of 3953 patients met inclusion criteria. Among our sample, 644 (16.3%) were positive for preinjury opioid use. Patients in the preinjury opioid group were older (48 *versus* 41 y) and more likely to be female (37.9% *versus* 30.6%). The mechanism of injury was more often falls (32.8% *versus* 22.0%). Analysis of less severely injured patients (ISS <15) found a significantly increased length of stay (3.7 *versus* 2.9 d) in the narcotics group. Evaluation of injury type revealed that head injury, abdominal injury, and lower extremity and/or pelvic injuries had significantly increased length of stay.

Conclusions.—There is a considerable prevalence of preinjury opioid use in the trauma population. These patients have unique characteristics and causes of injury. Preinjury opioid use is predictive of increased length of stay, with important ramifications for patient care and health care costs.

▶ There has been an increasing prevalence of prescription opioid analgesics in the United States over the past decade. In addition, escalation of the use of illicit opioids has also contributed to the overall prevalence of narcotic use. With such an increase in the use of prescription narcotics, hospitals and trauma centers are faced with the challenge of managing acute pain in patients who have already developed some degree of tolerance. It would be reasonable to assume that the management of such patients would be more complex, resulting in potentially worse outcomes. A remarkable finding was that nearly 1 in 6 patients who presented as a trauma patient were recently taking opioid analgesics before injury. This compares with 1 in 20 taking opioid analgesics in the general population. Their findings suggest that preinjury opioid use has a significant impact on patient care. In the environment of increasing health care costs, a better understanding of the effect of opioid use on hospitalization and length of stay is needed.

D. W. Mozingo, MD

Contrast blush in pediatric blunt splenic trauma does not warrant the routine use of angiography and embolization

Bansal S, Karrer FM, Hansen K, et al (Cardinal Glennon Children's Med Ctr, St Louis, MO; Children's Hosp Colorado, Aurora)

Am J Surg 210:345-350, 2015

Background.—Splenic artery embolization (SAE) in the presence of contrast blush (CB) has been recommended to reduce the failure rate of nonoperative management. We hypothesized that the presence of CB on computed tomography has minimal impact on patient outcomes.

Methods.—A retrospective review was conducted of all children (<18 years) with blunt splenic trauma over a 10-year period at a level 1 pediatric trauma center. Data are presented as mean ± standard error of mean.

Results.—Seven hundred forty children sustained blunt abdominal trauma, of which 549 had an identified solid organ injury. Blunt splenic injury was diagnosed in 270 of the 740 patients. All patients were managed nonoperatively without SAE. CB was seen on computed tomography in 47 patients (17.4%). There were no significant differences in the need for blood transfusion (12.5% vs 11.1%) or length of stay (3.1 vs 3.3 days) or need for splenectomy when compared in children with or without CB.

Conclusion.—Pediatric trauma patients with blunt splenic injuries can be safely managed without SAE and physiologic response and hemodynamic stability should be the primary determinants of appropriate management.

▶ The management of pediatric blunt splenic trauma has undergone major change in the past 50 years. Nonoperative management is the current standard of care for hemodynamically stable children, with high success rates devoid of the morbidity and mortality associated with operative management. Also avoided are the long-term potential infectious complications from splenectomy. Guidelines for such conservative management of blunt splenic, hepatic, and renal trauma are well established. Presence of contrast blush on computed tomography has been cited as a risk factor for the failure of nonoperative management in adult trauma management, and splenic artery embolization is commonly performed in these cases. The authors cited that an increasing number of institutions continue to adopt a protocol using angiography and embolization in the presence of active extravasation of contrast on initial abdominal CT scan in children. They hypothesized that the presence of contrast blush on abdominal CT has little impact on patient outcomes in the pediatric trauma patient population. On the basis of this series, it seems clear that the presence of contrast blush does not mandate additional intervention, although it certainly indicates the need for observation in an intensive care unit. Pediatric trauma patients should be managed based on their hemodynamic status and their physiological response to resuscitation, rather than the radiologic appearance of the injury.

D. W. Mozingo, MD

Computed Tomographic Findings and Mortality in Patients With Pneumomediastinum From Blunt Trauma

Lee WS, Chong VE, Victorino GP (Univ of California, San Francisco—East Bay, Oakland)

JAMA Surg 150:757-762, 2015

Importance.—The care of most patients with pneumomediastinum (PNM) due to trauma can be managed conservatively; however, owing to aerodigestive tract injury and other associated injuries, there is a subset of patients with PNM who are at higher risk of mortality but can be difficult to identify.

Objective.—To characterize computed tomographic (CT) findings associated with mortality in patients with PNM due to blunt trauma.

Design, Setting, and Participants.—A retrospective review of medical records from January 1, 2002, to December 31, 2011, was conducted at a university-based urban trauma center. The patients evaluated were those injured by blunt trauma and found to have PNM on initial chest CT scanning. Data analysis was performed July 2, 2013, to June 18, 2014.

Main Outcomes and Measures.—In-hospital mortality.

Results.—During the study period, 3327 patients with blunt trauma underwent chest CT. Of these, 72 patients (2.2%) had PNM. Patients with PNM had higher Injury Severity Scores ($P < .001$) and chest Abbreviated Injury Scale scores ($P < .001$) compared with those without PNM. Pneumomediastinum was associated with higher mortality (9 [12.5%] vs 118 [3.6%] patients; $P < .001$) and longer mean (SD) hospital stays (11.3 [14.6] vs 5.1 [8.8] days; $P < .001$), intensive care unit stays (5.4 [10.2] vs 1.8 [5.7] days; $P < .001$), and ventilator days (1.7 [4.2] vs 0.6 [4.0] days; $P < .03$).We evaluated several chest CT findings that may have predictive value. Pneumomediastinum size was not associated with in-hospital mortality ($P = .22$). However, location of air in the posterior mediastinum was associated with increased mortality of 25% (7 of 28 patients; $P = .007$). Air in all mediastinal compartments was also associated with increased mortality of 40.0% (4 of 10 patients; $P = .01$). Presence of hemothorax along with PNM was associated with mortality of 22.2% (8 of 36 patients; $P = .01$).

Conclusions and Relevance.—Pneumomediastinum is uncommon in patients with injury from blunt trauma; however, CT findings of posterior PNM, air in all mediastinal compartments, and concurrent hemothorax are associated with increased mortality. These CT findings could be used as a triage tool to alert the trauma surgeon to a potentially lethal injury.

▶ In this selection, patients with pneumomediastinum were more severely injured compared with those without this finding. Patients with pneumomediastinum had a higher mean injury severity score of 23.8 compared with 11.7 in those without this finding. They also noted that the patients with pneumomediastinum tended to have lower Glasgow Coma Scale, lower systolic blood pressure, and higher heart rates.

They also noted that the size of the pneumomediastinum was not associated with increased mortality; however, patients were more likely to die if pneumomediastinum was identified posterior to the heart, was identified in all 3 mediastinal compartments, or was associated with hemothorax. They show that these findings on CT should alert the trauma surgeon that the patient has an increased risk of a lethal injury of up to 40%. When detected early on initial chest CT, the finding of a potentially lethal injury should warn the trauma surgeon to consider close monitoring in the intensive care unit, aggressive resuscitation, and the possible need of additional diagnostic studies to rule out injury to the aerodigestive tract.

D. W. Mozingo, MD

3 Burns

Morbidity and Survival Probability in Burn Patients in Modern Burn Care

Jeschke MG, the Inflammation and the Host Response to Injury Collaborative Research Program (Univ of Toronto, Ontario, Canada; Sunnybrook Health Sciences Centre, Toronto, Ontario, Canada; et al)
Crit Care Med 43:808-815, 2015

Objective.—Characterizing burn sizes that are associated with an increased risk of mortality and morbidity is critical because it would allow identifying patients who might derive the greatest benefit from individualized, experimental, or innovative therapies. Although scores have been established to predict mortality, few data addressing other outcomes exist. The objective of this study was to determine burn sizes that are associated with increased mortality and morbidity after burn.

Design and Patients.—Burn patients were prospectively enrolled as part of the multicenter prospective cohort study, Inflammation and the Host Response to Injury Glue Grant, with the following inclusion criteria: 0–99 years old, admission within 96 hours after injury, and more than 20% total body surface area burns requiring at least one surgical intervention.

Setting.—Six major burn centers in North America.

Measurements and Main Results.—Burn size cutoff values were determined for mortality, burn wound infection (at least two infections), sepsis (as defined by American Burn Association sepsis criteria), pneumonia, acute respiratory distress syndrome, and multiple organ failure (Denver 2 score > 3) for both children (<16 yr) and adults (16–65 yr). Five hundred seventy-three patients were enrolled, of which 226 patients were children. Twenty-three patients were older than 65 years and were excluded from the cutoff analysis. In children, the cutoff burn size for mortality, sepsis, infection, and multiple organ failure was approximately 60% total body surface area burned. In adults, the cutoff for these outcomes was lower, at approximately 40% total body surface area burned.

Conclusions.—In the modern burn care setting, adults with over 40% total body surface area burned and children with over 60% total body surface area burned are at high risk for morbidity and mortality, even in highly specialized centers (Fig 1).

▶ This is the first study to determine cutoff burn sizes linked to severe adverse outcomes, such as sepsis, infection, multiple organ failure, and mortality in burn patients in a multicenter setting. Predictors of survival were not analyzed in this study. The strength of this work is that it was carried out by 6 state-of-the-art

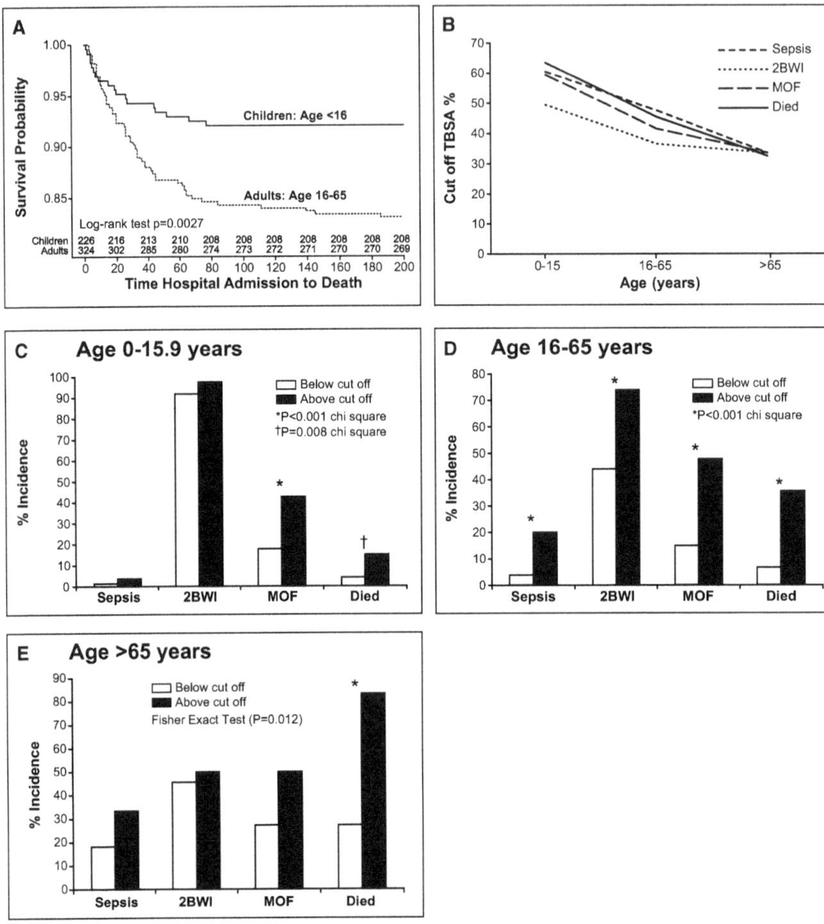

FIGURE 1.—A, Kaplan-Meier survival curve in pediatric and adult patients. Survival probability was greatest in pediatric patients and progressively worse in adult and elderly patients. *Significant difference between pediatric and adult patients ($p < 0.05$). B–E, Cutoff values for sepsis, burn wound infections (BWIs), multiple organ failure (MOF), and mortality, according to age. B, The cutoffs for sepsis, BWIs, MOF, and mortality are greatest in pediatric patients and then decrease to about 40% total body surface area (TBSA) burned in adults and 30% TBSA burned for elderly. C–E, Prevalence of patients with burns below or above the cutoff in the different age groups. *Significant difference between groups ($p < 0.05$). (Reprinted from Jeschke MG; the Inflammation and the Host Response to Injury Collaborative Research Program. Morbidity and survival probability in burn patients in modern burn care. *Crit Care Med.* 2015;43:808-815, with permission from the Society of Critical Care Medicine and Wolters Kluwer Health, Inc.)

burn centers following the same treatment protocols. Therefore, these findings may be applicable to other high-quality burn centers. Another major strength is the validity of the burn size assessment and that all of the collected data were validated. The authors found that pediatric patients had the best potential for survival, with survival being progressively worse in adult and elderly patients. The likelihood of developing severe adverse outcomes by age and cutoff value is included as Fig 1. A low number of elderly patients were enrolled in this trial, so they were excluded from the cutoff analysis. However, one can assume that the elderly have a much lower cutoff value for major complications and mortality than adults less than 65 years of age.

D. W. Mozingo, MD

Risk factors for the development of heterotopic ossification in seriously burned adults: A National Institute on Disability, Independent Living and Rehabilitation Research burn model system database analysis

Levi B, Jayakumar P, Giladi A, et al (Univ of Michigan, Ann Arbor; Massachusetts General Hosp, Boston; et al)

J Trauma Acute Care Surg 79:870-876, 2015

Background.—Heterotopic ossification (HO) is a debilitating complication of burn injury; however, incidence and risk factors are poorly understood. In this study, we use a multicenter database of adults with burn injuries to identify and analyze clinical factors that predict HO formation.

Methods.—Data from six high-volume burn centers, in the Burn Injury Model System Database, were analyzed. Univariate logistic regression models were used for model selection. Cluster-adjusted multivariate logistic regression was then used to evaluate the relationship between clinical and demographic data and the development of HO.

Results.—Of 2,979 patients in the database with information on HO that addressed risk factors for development of HO, 98 (3.5%) developed HO. Of these 98 patients, 97 had arm burns, and 96 had arm grafts. When controlling for age and sex in a multivariate model, patients with greater than 30% total body surface area burn had 11.5 times higher odds of developing HO ($p < 0.001$), and those with arm burns that required skin grafting had 96.4 times higher odds of developing HO ($p = 0.04$). For each additional time a patient went to the operating room, odds of HO increased by 30% (odds ratio, 1.32; $p < 0.001$), and each additional ventilator day increased odds by 3.5% (odds ratio, 1.035; $p < 0.001$). Joint contracture, inhalation injury, and bone exposure did not significantly increase odds of HO.

Conclusion.—Risk factors for HO development include greater than 30% total body surface area burn, arm burns, arm grafts, ventilator days, and number of trips to the operating room. Future studies can use these results to identify highest-risk patients to guide deployment of prophylactic and experimental treatments.

Level of Evidence.—Prognostic study, level III (Table 3).

▶ This is the first multicenter study of thermally injured patients to assess the clinical and epidemiologic predictors of heterotopic ossification. The majority of previous publications on burn-related heterotopic ossification have focused on single-center outcomes, making results difficult to interpret. Using the burn injury model system database, the authors were able to identify by multivariate

TABLE 3.—Multivariate Logistic Regression Model Results of Variables Related to Development of HO

Clinical Factor	OR	Effect on Development of HO 95% Confidence Interval	p
Arm burns requiring skin grafts	96.4*	1.19–7,806	0.04
TBS burn > 30%	11.5*	6.0–21.9	<0.001
No. trips to operating room (each trip)	1.32*	1.18–1.40	<0.001
No. days on ventilator (each day)	1.034*	1.03–1.04	<0.001
Contracture	6.26	0.79–49.5	0.082
Inhalation Injury	1.40	0.57–3.43	0.466
Bone exposure	1.52	0.36–6.44	0.569
Age	1.01	0.99–1.02	0.07
Sex (female)	0.64	0.38–1.12	0.11

*Significant, with $p < 0.05$.

Reprinted from Levi B, Jayakumar P, Giladi A, et al. Risk factors for the development of heterotopic ossification in seriously burned adults: a National Institute on Disability, Independent Living and Rehabilitation Research burn model system database analysis. *J Trauma Acute Care Surg.* 2015;79:870-876, with permission from Wolters Kluwer Health, Inc.

logistic regression those factors most closely associated with the development of heterotopic ossification. Predictors of heterotopic ossification included large burns greater than 30% of the total body surface area, arm burns requiring skin grafts, number of operating room procedures, and number of ventilator days. Some of these factors cannot be modified; however, early mobility and extubation would decrease ventilator days. Timely grafting of the arms would also be considered. Future studies can use this information to identify risk factors for heterotopic ossification formation and focus on prophylactic treatments in those patients with known risk factors.

D. W. Mozingo, MD

Revised Baux Score and updated Charlson comorbidity index are independently associated with mortality in burns intensive care patients

Heng JS, Clancy O, Atkins J, et al (Chelsea and Westminster Hosp, London, United Kingdom; et al)

Burns 41:1420-1427, 2015

Purpose.—The purpose of the current study was to utilise established scoring systems to analyse the association of (i) burn injury severity, (ii) comorbid status and (iii) associated systemic physiological disturbance with inpatient mortality in patients with severe burn injuries admitted to intensive care.

Methods.—Case notes of all patients with acute thermal injuries affecting ≥15% total body surface area (TBSA) admitted to the Burns Intensive Care Unit (BICU) at Chelsea and Westminster Hospital during a 10-year period were retrospectively reviewed. Revised Baux Score, Belgian Outcome in Burn Injury (BOBI) Score, Abbreviated Burn Severity Index

(ABSI), APACHE II Score, Sequential Organ Failure Assessment (SOFA) Score and Updated Charlson Comorbidity Index (CCI) were computed for each patient and analysed for association with inpatient mortality.

Results.—Ninety mechanically ventilated patients (median age 45.7 years, median % TBSA burned 36.5%) were included. 72 patients had full thickness burns and 35 patients had inhalational injuries. Forty-four patients died in hospital while 46 survived to discharge. In a multivariate logistic regression model, only the Revised Baux Score ($p < 0.001$) and updated CCI ($p = 0.014$) were independently associated with mortality. This gave a ROC curve with area under the curve of 0.920. On multivariate cox regression survival analysis, only the Revised Baux Score ($p < 0.001$) and the updated CCI ($p = 0.004$) were independently associated with shorter time to death.

Conclusion.—Our data suggest that the Revised Baux Score and the updated CCI are independently associated with inpatient mortality in patients admitted to intensive care with burn injuries affecting ≥15% TBSA. This emphasises the importance of comorbidities in the prognosis of patients with severe burn injuries.

▶ Burn severity scores remain the mainstay of prognostication in clinical studies and on burns units. The Revised Baux Score, which is the sum of the percent total body surface area burned plus 17, for the presence of inhalation injury is used commonly.

A standardized method to score chronic comorbidities is the Charlson Comorbidity Index, which was originally developed to predict the 1-year all-cause mortality in patients admitted to hospital medical services based on the presence of any of 17 comorbidities. The comorbidities included such conditions as congestive heart failure, chronic pulmonary disease, liver disease, diabetes, and metastatic cancer. An updated version of this index was subsequently validated for predicting inpatient mortality in large groups of patients but has not been evaluated in patients with burn injuries. The authors' data suggest that the Revised Baux Score and the Updated Charlson Comorbidity Index are independently associated with inpatient mortality in patients admitted to a burn intensive care with burn injuries involving greater than 15% of the total body surface area. This index emphasizes the importance of comorbidities in the prognosis of patients with severe burn injuries, unlike other burn scoring systems. As the elderly begin to make up a higher percentage of the population, the evaluation of comorbidities will become more important in addressing outcome analysis.

D. W. Mozingo, MD

Predictors of Discharge Disposition in Older Adults With Burns: A Study of the Burn Model Systems

Pham TN, Carrougher GJ, Martinez E, et al (Univ of Washington, Seattle; Univ of Colorado, Denver; et al)

J Burn Care Res 36:607-612, 2015

Older patients with burn injury have a greater likelihood for discharge to nursing facilities. Recent research indicates that older patients discharged to nursing facilities are two to three times as likely to die within a 3-year period relative to those discharged to home. In light of these poor long-term outcomes, we conducted this study to identify predictors for discharge to independent vs nonindependent living status in older patients hospitalized for burns. We retrospectively reviewed all older adults (age ≥ 55 years) who were prospectively enrolled in a longitudinal multicenter study of outcomes from 1993 to 2011. Patient, injury, and treatment outcomes data were analyzed. Recognizing that transfer to inpatient rehabilitation may have impacted final hospital discharge disposition: we assessed the likelihood of inpatient rehabilitation stay, based on identified predictors of inpatient rehabilitation. We subsequently performed a logistic regression analysis on the clustered, propensity-matched cohort to assess associations of burn and injury characteristics on the primary outcome of final discharge status. A total of 591 patients aged ≥55 years were treated and discharged alive from three participating U.S. burn centers during the study period. Mean burn size was 14.8% (SD 11.2%) and mean age was 66.7 years (SD 9.3 years). Ninety-three patients had an inpatient rehabilitation stay before discharge (15.7%). Significant factors predictive of inpatient rehabilitation included a burn >20% TBSA, mechanical ventilation, older age, range of motion deficits at acute care discharge, and study site. These factors were included in the propensity model. Four hundred seventy-one patients (80%) were discharged to independent living status. By matched propensity analysis, older age was significantly associated with a higher likelihood of discharge to nonindependent living ($P < .01$ in both the 65–74 age group and the oldest age group when compared with the 55–64 age group). Comorbidity ($P < .01$) and history of alcohol abuse ($P < 0.01$) were also predictive patient factors. Furthermore, clinical practice variations among the three study sites also constituted a significant factor in discharge disposition (both $P < .01$ when compared with the index study site). Older age remains an important risk factor for discharge to nonindependent living status, even after accounting for inpatient rehabilitation stay. This analysis, however, reveals significant variations in discharge disposition practices among the three participating study sites. We believe that these variations among burn centers need to be elucidated to better understand discharge disposition status in older patients with burns.

▶ Inpatient rehabilitation would seem to be a natural transition for older adults with severe burns. The Centers of Medicare and Medicaid Services requirements for rehabilitation center admission are stringent and include a need for multiple therapy services, an intensive rehabilitation therapy program that consists of at least 3 hours of therapy per day, and active patient participation. There should also be a reasonable expectation that the patient would benefit significantly from the program. Older adults who are frail or delirious may not qualify for such services. This study found that nearly 30% of older patients at University of Texas Southwestern (UTSW) had an inpatient rehabilitation stay that was 3 times that of University of Washington and Hopkins. Although numerous factors may account for this finding, it is most likely that the care protocols at UTSW contributed to the greater number of patients successfully qualifying for inpatient rehabilitation. UTSW has a long and extensive tradition of aggressive rehabilitation services for their burn patients. As such, other burn centers may benefit from reviewing and potentially modeling UTSW care protocols particularly relevant for older adult patients. Aggressive delirium prevention, patient mobilization during acute care, patient screening for rehabilitation transfer, and coordination among burn and rehabilitation services may improve the potential for these patients to be rehabilitation center candidates.

D. W. Mozingo, MD

Prevalence and Prediction of Prolonged Pruritus After Severe Burns
Gauffin E, Öster C, Gerdin B, et al (Uppsala Univ, Sweden)
J Burn Care Res 36:405-413, 2015

Years after injury, pruritus is a common and severe problem for many burn patients. However, its characteristics and consequences are often only partially described. The authors therefore performed a prospective detailed examination of burn- and individual-related factors and considered those in relation to pruritus severity. Sixty-seven consecutive burn patients were assessed during acute care, and at 3 and 12 months postburn regarding preburn psychiatric disorders, health-related quality of life, post traumatic stress disorder, and personality traits. Postburn pruritus was subsequently assessed 2 to 7 years postburn using the Questionnaire for Pruritus Assessment. Fifty-one individuals, 76% of the participants, reported burn pruritus any time after the burn. Thirty-three individuals, 49% of the participants, reported ongoing pruritus the last 2 months. Information on the characteristics of pruritus was obtained from 32 of these individuals. Most perceived pruritus as bothersome or annoying and as present every day, 16 (50%) were considered to have severe pruritus, and 11 (34%) scratched themselves to the point of bleeding. In logistic regressions, this was independently related to TBSA full-thickness burn and health-related quality of life at 3 months, and to TBSA full thickness burn and the personality trait impulsiveness, respectively. About half of the previous burn patients experienced ongoing pruritus on an average of 4.5 years after injury, and half of them had severe pruritus. Scratching oneself to the point of bleeding is linked both to a certain personality and to pruritus. It is suspected that many patients are left without access to the best available treatment.

▶ Severe pruritus is a common problem developing in postburn recovery. This study provides a detailed description and long-term perspective on the problem of pruritus after burn injury. The prospective design, interview assessments, and the use of validated and widely used instruments give strength to the conclusions from this study. The relatively small sample size prohibited some potential for subgroup analyses. Importantly, the individuals participating in this study had been treated in a national burn center an average of 4.5 years before this assessment. With few exceptions, these patients had left specialized burn care, making the observations in this study reasonably representative of the true situation for a larger numbers of patients who are not under specialty surveillance. These results suggest the need for better routines for the assessment of patients long term after their injury than is currently practiced. These long-term results have identified the need for high-quality treatment studies directed toward prolonged pruritus after burn injury.

D. W. Mozingo, MD

Does obesity affect outcomes of adult burn patients?

Ray JJ, Satahoo SS, Meizoso JP, et al (Univ of Miami Miller School of Medicine, FL)

J Surg Res 198:450-455, 2015

Background.—Obesity negatively affects outcomes after trauma and surgery; results after burns are more limited and controversial. The purpose of this study was to determine the effect of obesity on clinical and economic outcomes after thermal injury.

Methods.—The National Inpatient Sample was queried for adults from 2005–2009 with International Classification of Diseases-9 codes for burn injury. Demographics and clinical outcomes of obese and nonobese cohorts were compared. Univariate and multivariate analysis using logistic regression models were performed. Data are expressed as median (interquartile range) or mean ± standard deviation and compared at $P < 0.05$.

Results.—In 14,602 patients, 3.3% were obese (body mass index ≥30 kg/m^2). The rate of obesity increased significantly by year ($P < 0.001$). Univariate analysis revealed significant differences between obese and nonobese patients in incidence of wound infection (7.2% *versus* 5.0%), urinary tract infection (7.2% *versus* 4.6%), deep vein thrombosis in total body surface area (TBSA) ≥10% (3.1% *versus* 1.1%), pulmonary embolism in TBSA ≥10% (2.3% *versus* 0.6%), length of stay [6 d (8) *versus* 5 d (9)], and hospital costs ($10,122.12 [$18,074.72] *versus* $7892.07 [$17,191.96]) (all $P < 0.05$). Death occurred less frequently in the obese group (1.9% *versus* 4%, $P = 0.021$). Significant predictors of grouped adverse events (urinary tract infection, wound infection, deep vein

TABLE 3.—Significant Differences Observed Between Obese and Nonobese Patients

Outcome	Obese No	Obese Yes	P Value
Wound infection, %	5.00	7.20	0.04
UTI, %	4.60	7.20	0.009
DVT in TBSA ≥10%, %	1.10	3.10	0.039
PE in TBSA ≥10%, %	0.60	2.30	0.013
Discharged to home, %	66.60	57.70	<0.001
Disease severity, %	73.50	91.80	<0.001
LOS	5 d (9)	6 d (8)	<0.001
Hospital cost, $	7892.07 (17,191.96)	10,122.12 (18,074.72)	0.002
Died in hospital (all patients), %	4.00	1.90	0.021
Died in hospital (TBSA ≥20), %	22.7	10.3	0.025

Reprinted from Ray JJ, Satahoo SS, Meizoso JP, et al. Does obesity affect outcomes of adult burn patients? *J Surg Res.* 2015;198:450-455, with permission from Elsevier Inc.

thrombosis, and pulmonary embolism) on multivariate analysis include obesity, TBSA ≥20%, age, and black race (all $P \leq 0.05$).

Conclusions.—Obesity is an independent predictor of adverse events after burn injury; however, obesity is associated with decreased mortality. Our findings highlight the potential clinical and economic impact of the obesity epidemic on burn patients nationwide (Table 3).

▶ Obesity is a current global epidemic that is projected to worsen over time. More than one-third of the US population is affected, and this represents a major public health concern with significant clinical and economic implications in all patient populations. Previous reports in burn patients have shown some mixed results with respect to the effect of obesity on outcomes, but a trend toward more complications, higher costs, and longer length of hospital stay are noted most often. Mortality is generally not affected except in the morbidly obese population. This selection is significant in that the authors queried that national inpatient sample as their database. This is a much larger data set than has been used before and is able to provide a nationwide assessment. A summary of the patient characteristics is included as Table 3. The authors demonstrated that obesity is an independent predictor of adverse events effect of obesity approaching that of burns > 20% of the total body surface area. These findings highlight the potential clinical and economic impact of the obesity epidemic on burn patients nationwide. Obesity affects all aspects of burn management from resuscitation to patient care issues in the intensive care unit. With obesity afflicting more than one-third of our nation, special attention must be paid to this population in all facets of medical care. Specific therapeutic strategies and protocols should be considered to help decrease the excess risk posed by this condition in the burn patient.

D. W. Mozingo, MD

Alteration of Leukocyte Count Correlates With Increased Pulmonary Vascular Permeability and Decreased PaO_2:FiO_2 Ratio Early After Major Burns

Johansson J, Steinvall I, Herwald H, et al (Östersund Hosp, Sweden; Dept of Hand and Plastic Surgery and Intensive Care, Linköping, Sweden; Lund Univ, Sweden; et al)

J Burn Care Res 36:484-492, 2015

Leukocytes are activated systemically and their numbers increase soon after a burn followed by a rapid decline to low normal or subnormal levels, possibly by increased extravasation. Experimental data support that an important target for such extravasation is the lungs and that leukocytes when they adhere to endothelial cells cause an increase in vascular permeability. The authors investigated a possible relation between early increased pulmonary vascular permeability or a decreased PaO_2:FiO_2 ratio and the dynamic change in concentration of blood leukocytes after a burn. This is a prospective, exploratory, single-center study. The authors measured the dynamic changes of leukocytes in blood starting early after the burn, pulmonary vascular permeability index by thermodilution, and PaO_2:-FiO_2-ratios in 20 patients during the first 21 days after a major burn (>20% TBSA%). Median TBSA was 40% interquartile range (IQR, 25–52) and full thickness burn 28% (IQR, 2–39). There was a correlation between the early (<24 hours) alteration in white blood cell count and both early increased pulmonary vascular permeability ($r = .63$, $P = .004$) and the decreased oxygenation index defined as PaO_2:FiO_2 < 27 kPa ($P = .004$). The authors have documented a correlation between dynamic change of blood leukocytes and pulmonary failure early after burns (Fig 4).

▶ Lung function is affected soon after a major burn—not only by inhalation injury, but also by a condition that is similar to acute respiratory distress syndrome (ARDS). This is manifested by an increased pulmonary vascular permeability and decreased PaO_2:FiO_2 ratio. The exact mechanisms underlying these findings are not fully known; however, histamine, serotonin, oxygen radicals, and proinflammatory cytokines have been considered as possible mediators of this effect Polymorphonuclear cells sampled from burned patients have been shown to be systemically activated and the total leukocyte count increases within a few hours after burn injury. The total white blood cell count then falls to low normal or below normal levels within 24 to 48 hours. These changes in white blood cell (WBC) count after burns might reflect an early release of leukocytes from the bone marrow and subsequent trapping of leukocytes in the vessels of the lung and other vascular beds as well as the burn wound itself. In an earlier study, the authors of this selection examined ARDS and inhalation injury during the first week after a burn and found a correlation between changes in the WBC count and the development of respiratory failure.[1,2] The results of this study indicate that a change in the WBC count that is greater than 10 during the first 24 hours suggests a high probability of subsequent pulmonary failure.

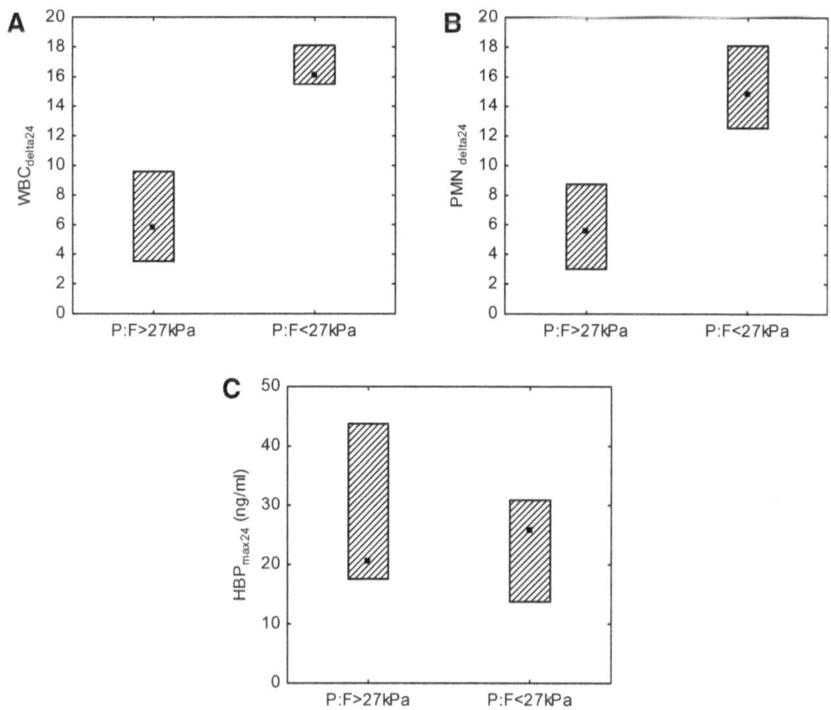

FIGURE 4.—A–C. The relation of $WBC_{\Delta 24}$ and of $PMN_{\Delta 24}$ with presence of PaO_2:FiO_2 < 27 kPa within 24 hours. The relation was significant (P = .004 and .003). There was no relation of HBP_{max24} with PaO_2:FiO_2 < 27 kPa (P = 1.0). *WBC*, white blood cell; *PMN*, polymorphonuclear leukocytes; *HBP*, heparin binding protein. Square and box indicate the median and interquartile range, respectively. (Reprinted from Johansson J, Steinvall I, Herwald H, et al. Alteration of leukocyte count correlates with increased pulmonary vascular permeability and decreased PaO_2:FiO_2 ratio early after major burns. *J Burn Care Res.* 2015;36:484-492, with permission from American Burn Association.)

Fig 4 demonstrating this finding is included here. Such a change could alert the physician to monitor more closely for changes in pulmonary function.

D. W. Mozingo, MD

References

1. Murray JF, Mattha MA, Luce JM, Flick MR. An expanded definition of the adult respiratory distress syndrome. *Am Rev Respir Dis.* 1988;138:720-723.
2. Bhatia RK, Pallister I, Dent C, Jones.

Aerobic Fitness Is Disproportionately Low in Adult Burn Survivors Years After Injury

Ganio MS, Pearson J, Schlader ZJ, et al (Univ of Texas Southwestern Med Ctr, Dallas; et al)

J Burn Care Res 36:513-519, 2015

A maximal aerobic capacity below the 20th percentile is associated with an increased risk of all-cause mortality. Adult Adult burn survivors have a lower aerobic capacity compared with nonburned adults when evaluated 38 ± 23 days postinjury. However, it is unknown whether burn survivors with well-healed skin grafts (ie, multiple years postinjury) also have low aerobic capacity. This project tested the hypothesis that aerobic fitness, as measured by maximal aerobic capacity (VO_{2max}), is reduced in well-healed adult burn survivors when compared with normative values from nonburned individuals. Twenty-five burn survivors (36 ± 12 years old; 13 females) with well-healed split-thickness grafts (median, 16 years post-injury; range, 1–51 years) covering at least 17% of their BSA (mean, 40 ± 16%; range, 17–75%) performed a graded cycle ergometry exercise to test volitional fatigue. Expired gases and minute ventilation were measured via a metabolic cart for the determination of VO_{2max}. Each subject's VO_{2max} was compared with sex- and age-matched normative values from population data published by the American College of Sports Medicine, the American Heart Association, and recent epidemiological data. Subjects had a VO_{2max} of 29.4 ± 10.1 ml O_2/kg body mass/min (median, 27.5; range, 15.9–53.3). The use of American College of Sports Medicine normative values showed that mean VO_{2max} of the subjects was in the lower 24th percentile (median, 10th percentile). A total of 88% of the subjects had a VO_{2max} below American Heart Association age-adjusted normative values. Similarly, 20 of the 25 subjects had a VO_{2max} in the lower 25% percentile of recent epidemiological data. Relative to nongrafted subjects, 80 to 88% of the evaluated skin-graft subjects had a very low aerobic capacity. On the basis of these findings, adult burn survivors are disproportionally unfit relative to the general U.S. population, and this puts them at an increased risk of all-cause mortality (Table 3).

▶ Relatively little is known about the cardiovascular fitness of adults who previously sustained severe burn injuries. Previous studies have been hampered by small sample size, wide variation in extent of burn, and inconsistent time of evaluation after recovery from burn injury. The purpose of this study was to examine the aerobic capacity, as indexed from VO_{2max}, of individuals with well-healed skin grafts involving 17% to 75% of their total body surface area. Using normal values of VO_{2max} from thousands of measurements published by the American College of Sports Medicine the authors of this selection demonstrated that 88% of the subjects evaluated were below age- and sex-matched normative values. Table 3 is included that depicts these findings with respect to burn size. With respect to population normative values, the VO_{2max} from subjects in the current investigation averaged in approximately the 25th percentile.

TABLE 3.—Classification of VO_{2max} Values Relative to Three Population Normative Data Sets

	AHA* n (% of Group)		ACSM† Mean ± SD (Median)	Aspenes‡ n in Each Quartile of VO_{2max}			
	Below Norm	Above Norm	Percentiles	0–25%	25–50%	50–75%	75–100%
% TBSA grafted classification							
20–35	12 (92%)	1 (8%)	22 ± 21 (10th)	10	2	0	1
40–55	7 (100%)	0	14 ± 5 (10th)	7	0	0	0
>60	3 (60%)	2 (40%)	44 ± 42 (20th)	3	0	0	2
Mean±SD for all subjects	22 (88%)	3 (12%)	24 ± 25 (10th)	20	2	0	3

Editor's Note: Please refer to original journal article for full references.
AHA, American Heart Association.
*From: Fletcher et al.[8]
†American College of Sports Medicine's (ACSM) Guidelines for Exercise Testing and Prescription.[11]
‡Aspenes et al.[12]
Reprinted from Ganio MS, Pearson J, Schlader ZJ, et al. Aerobic fitness is disproportionately low in adult burn survivors years after injury. *J Burn Care Res*. 2015;36:513-519, with permission from the American Burn Association.

The mechanism by which burn survivors have such low aerobic capacities remains unclear. Acute burn injury results in a catabolic state in which resting metabolic rate is increased for a period of time directly correlated with extent of body surface area burned. In severe cases, increased resting metabolic rate may persist for 1 year or more. This acute hypermetabolic state leads to substantial skeletal muscle loss. A lower skeletal muscle mass, compared with preinjury levels, leads to a reduction in the amount of aerobically active muscle mass. This will decrease maximal oxygen extraction across that muscle and may, in part, explain these findings. This assumes that the preinjury muscle mass is not recovered, a common clinical finding after major burn injury. Further studies that quantify muscle mass at the time of evaluation are warranted to further elucidate these important findings.

D. W. Mozingo, MD

Variation in Inpatient Rehabilitation Utilization After Hospitalization for Burn Injury in the United States

Greene NH, Pham TN, Esselman PC, et al (Duke Univ School of Medicine, Durham, NC; Univ of Washington, Seattle)
J Burn Care Res 36:613-618, 2015

Approximately 45,000 individuals are hospitalized annually for burn treatment. Rehabilitation after hospitalization can offer a significant improvement in functional outcomes. Very little is known nationally about rehabilitation for burns, and practices may vary substantially depending on the region based on observed Medicare posthospitalization spending amounts. This study was designed to measure variation in rehabilitation utilization by state of hospitalization for patients hospitalized with burn injury. This retrospective cohort study used nationally collected data over a 10-year period (2001 to 2010), from the Healthcare Cost and Utilization Project (HCUP) State Inpatient Databases (SIDs). Patients hospitalized for burn injury (n = 57,968) were identified by ICD-9-CM codes and were examined to see specifically if they were discharged immediately to inpatient rehabilitation after hospitalization (primary endpoint). Both unadjusted and adjusted likelihoods were calculated for each state taking into account the effects of age, insurance status, hospitalization at a burn center, and extent of burn injury by TBSA. The relative risk of discharge to inpatient rehabilitation varied by as much as 6-fold among different states. Higher TBSA, having health insurance, higher age, and burn center hospitalization all increased the likelihood of discharge to inpatient rehabilitation following acute care hospitalization. There was significant variation between states in inpatient rehabilitation utilization after adjusting for variables known to affect each outcome. Future efforts should be focused on identifying the cause of this state-to-state variation, its relationship to patient outcome, and standardizing treatment across the United States (Fig 1).

▶ Referral to impatient rehabilitation can provide an important intervention to improve recovery and independent living status after a burn injury. Burn patients who qualify for inpatient rehabilitation have more extensive burn, have had lengthy acute hospital stays, and are at a point in their recovery where they can participate in rehabilitation activities at least 3 hours per day.

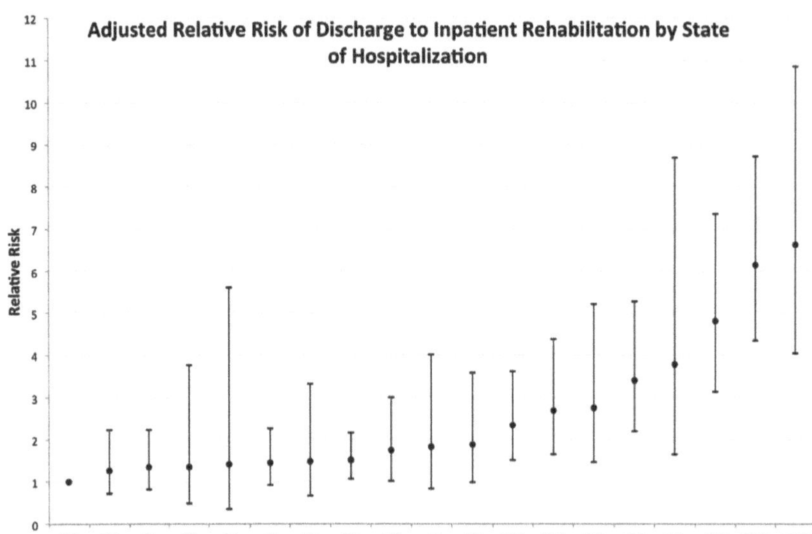

FIGURE 1.—Multivariate Poisson regression point estimates for relative risk by state of hospitalization with 95% confidence interval estimates, *$P < .05$. (Reprinted from Greene NH, Pham TN, Esselman PC, et al. Variation in inpatient rehabilitation utilization after hospitalization for burn injury in the United States. *J Burn Care Res.* 2015;36:613-618, with permission from the American Burn Association.)

Little is known about the inpatient rehabilitation rates for burn discharges in the United States. For this reason, the authors of this selection reviewed multiple national and state databases to assess rehabilitation center utilization. Year 1 is included, assessing the relative risk of discharge to an inpatient rehabilitation facility by state. The relative risk of discharge to inpatient rehabilitation varies widely on a national level. Future work could address whether increasing referral to inpatient rehabilitation will improve long-term outcomes such as survival and readmission rates. A more in-depth analysis at the state level may yield additional useful information.

D. W. Mozingo, MD

Are Visceral Proteins Valid Markers for Nutritional Status in the Burn Intensive Care Unit?

Shields BA, Pidcoke HF, Chung KK, et al (San Antonio Military Med Ctr, TX; U.S. Army Inst of Surgical Res, Fort Sam Houston, TX; et al)
J Burn Care Res 36:375-380, 2015

The aim of this study was to determine whether visceral protein levels increase under positive nitrogen balance during times of decrease in acute-phase reactant levels in patients with burn injury. This was a post hoc analysis of a prospective, interventional study approved by the local institutional review board. A total of 10 subjects between the ages of 18 and 72 with ≥20% total body surface area burn were enrolled over a 14-month period. Data were collected for five subjects (average age of 28 ± 8 years and total body surface area burn of 69 ± 15%) who met the inclusion criteria. Changes in visceral protein levels were examined along with nitrogen balance and acute-phase reactants when the subjects were on enteral nutrition, and the proteins were not examined during times of acute kidney injury. Descriptive statistics were performed, and linear regression was used to analyze the association of visceral proteins and nitrogen balance during times that acute-phase reactant levels were decreasing. The subjects received an average of 3044 ± 1613 kcal/day (39 ± 20 kcal/kg), meeting 72% of caloric goals and achieving positive nitrogen balance during 68% of the 40 weekly measurements, with 174 ± 85 g of protein intake per day (2.2 ± 1.1 g/kg). There was a weak relationship between nitrogen balance and changes in visceral protein levels during times that the acute-phase reactant levels were decreasing ($P > .05$). Visceral proteins were found to be poor markers of nutritional status. This study is unique because the subjects were able to achieve positive nitrogen balance despite severe burns (Fig 1).

► Nutrition plays an important role in improving outcomes in patients with thermal injury. Resting energy expenditure can increase 2-fold in patients with major burn injury, and protein loss may increase up to 3 times that of preinjury levels. Providing adequate nutrition is essential to decrease infection rates and to promote wound healing. Monitoring nutritional adequacy has always been a challenge in burn

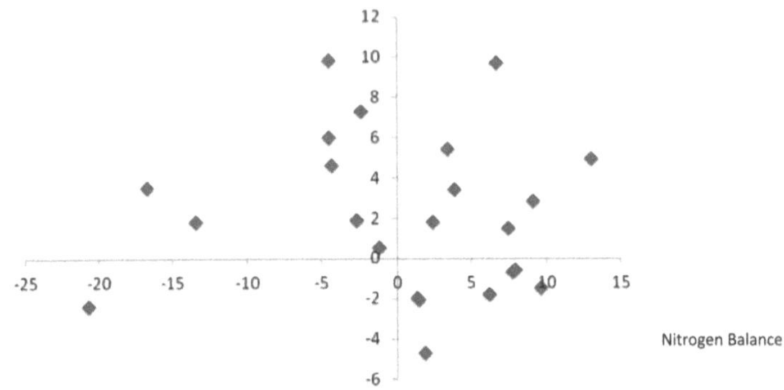

FIGURE 1.—Prealbumin and nitrogen balance values only including those when CRP are decreasing. (Reprinted from Shields BA, Pidcoke HF, Chung KK, et al. Are visceral proteins valid markers for nutritional status in the burn intensive care unit? *J Burn Care Res.* 2015;36:375-380, with permission from the American Burn Association.)

patients. The use of anthropometric measures is difficult due to edema formation and the slow rate that these changes manifest. Nutritional markers are commonly used in majority of burn centers; however, these measurements are unreliable because of the persistent inflammatory response after burn injury. Synthesis of hepatic proteins is reprioritized after burn injury. Acute-phase reactant levels, such as C-reactive protein, haptoglobin, and α-1-antitrypsin, are increased, and visceral protein levels, such as albumin, prealbumin, transferrin, and retinol binding protein, are decreased. Therefore, many have questioned the use of these nutritional markers in burn and trauma patients. The aim of this study was to determine the relationship between nutritional status and changes in visceral protein levels with regard to changes in acute-phase reactant levels. The experimental design in this study is unique because subjects were able to achieve positive nitrogen balance despite severe burns and because it allowed comparison of protein intake to changes in visceral protein and acute-phase reactant levels. The authors found visceral proteins to be poor markers of nutritional status, even in the presence of a positive nitrogen balance. Fig 1 demonstrates this lack of correlation. The clinical use of these markers in burn care has not been proven and may provide inaccurate information to clinicians regarding the patient's nutritional status. If visceral protein levels are not increasing, a decision to increase feeding could be made that could lead to overfeeding. The costs of obtaining routine test with limited value could also be considered. Clinical nutritional evaluation should probably focus on achieving positive nitrogen and caloric balance. Although the underlying mechanisms remain to be explored, this study demonstrated that high levels of protein intake are not associated with increases in visceral protein levels.

D. W. Mozingo, MD

Prevention of Hypophosphatemia After Burn Injury With a Protocol for Continuous, Preemptive Repletion

Kahn SA, Bell DE, Stassen NA, et al (Vanderbilt Univ Med Ctr, Nashville, TN; Univ of Rochester Med Ctr, New York; et al)

J Burn Care Res 36:e220-e225, 2015

Severe burn injury has been shown to result in hypophosphatemia. Hypophosphatemia can cause cardiac, hematologic, immunologic, and neuromuscular dysfunction. This study compares serum phosphate levels and outcomes in patients who were administered a continuous, preemptive phosphate repletion protocol vs those who only received phosphate supplementation after they developed hypophosphatemia. Records of patients with greater than 19% TBSA burn admitted to the intensive care unit from 2006 to 2010 were reviewed. Patients were divided into two groups: historical controls who received responsive repletion when serum phosphate levels were less than 2.5 mg/dl (2006–2008) and the experimental group that received 30 mmol intravenous every 6 hours starting at approximately 24 hours after injury as long as serum phosphate levels were less than 4 mg/dl (2008–2010). Patients with chronic kidney disease or acute kidney injury were excluded. Data collected included age, weight, burn size, age, all serum phosphate levels, and total amount of phosphate administered. Differences in groups were compared with Mann–Whitney *U* test and Fisher's exact test. A total of 30 patients were included in the study, 20 in the responsive repletion group and 10 in the continuous repletion group. No significant difference was detected in age, sex, burn size, or full thickness burn size between groups. The continuous group had a statistically lower percentage of hypophosphatemic lab values compared with the responsive group, 13 ± 14% vs 45 ± 21% ($P < .0001$). No difference was found in percent of observations reflecting hyperphosphatemia (median of 2% in each group, $P = .7$). Four patients in the continuous group suffered cardiac and/or infectious complications compared with 16 in the responsive group ($P = .04$). Continuous, pre-emptive repletion of phosphate prevents hypophosphatemia after severe burn injury when compared with responsive repletion in historical controls. The protocol resulted in less hypophosphatemia without increasing the risk of hyperphosphatemia. This study also suggests that continuous repletion may result in fewer complications, but this needs to be confirmed in larger, prospective studies.

▶ Hypophosphatemia following burn injury is a common occurrence. In thermally injured patients, decreases in serum phosphate levels occur via gastrointestinal tract losses, redistribution from extracellular to intracellular compartments, and from refeeding syndromes. The stress response, insulin, and topical mafenide acetate may also worsen hypophosphatemia after burn injury because they all contribute to intracellular ionic shifts. Maintaining normal serum phosphate is extremely important because hypophosphatemia may cause organ dysfunction and systemic complications. These include but are not limited to cardiac, hematologic, immunologic, and neuromuscular dysfunction. This selection was chosen to demonstrate that a practical, simple protocol for preemptive, continuous phosphate repletion to prevent hypophosphatemia without significantly increasing the incidence of hyperphosphatemia could be implemented. The authors noted a decrease in the infectious and cardiac complications in the infusion-treated group, but this needs further evaluation before assigning causation. This could be studied in larger, multi-institution, prospective studies to determine whether a true clinical benefit exists.

D. W. Mozingo, MD

Risk Factors in Hospitalized Patients With Burn Injuries for Developing Heterotopic Ossification—A Retrospective Analysis

Orchard GR, Paratz JD, Blot S, et al (The Univ of Queensland, Brisbane, Australia; Ghent Univ, Belgium; et al)

J Burn Care Res 36:465-470, 2015

The aims of this study were to identify the risk factors for developing heterotopic ossification in patients with burns injuries and, second, to review the outcomes associated with the treatment disodium etidronate. Patients with heterotopic ossification were identified using the burns unit computer database. The control group was the patients who were the next admission after admission of the patient who subsequently developed heterotopic ossification. Demographic and clinical data were collected. Univariate and multivariate techniques were used to identify risk factors for heterotopic ossification. We reviewed 337 patients admitted over a 5-year period and identified 19 patients with heterotopic ossification (5.6%). A further 19 burn injury patients were included as controls. Heterotopic ossification developed clinically and radiologically after a median time of 37 days (interquartile range [IQR], 30–40) and 49 days (IQR, 38–118), respectively. In univariate analysis, heterotopic ossification was associated with a greater %TBSA, inhalation injury, use of mechanical ventilation, number of surgical procedures, sepsis, and longer time to active movement. In a multivariate analysis that adjusted for severity of burn injury by means of the Belgian Outcome in Burn Injury score, time to active movement was recognized as an independent risk factor for heterotopic ossification (odds ratio 1.48, 95% confidence interval 1.09–2.01). Elevations in serum calcium concentrations were the only observed adverse effects for disodium etidonrate. This study has demonstrated that %TBSA, inhalation injury, and the need for ventilatory support and the use of multiple surgical procedures are predictive of the development of heterotopic ossification.

▶ Heterotopic ossification is the formation of lamella bone in connective tissue in which it normally should not exist. In their analysis, the authors of this selection identified statistically significant differences between many factors associated with the extent of injury in patients developing heterotopic ossification compared with those who did not develop this complication. After adjustment for severity of burn injury, logistic regression analysis identified delayed time to active movement as being independently associated with the risk of heterotopic ossification development. Heterotopic ossification carries significant morbidity during the recovery phase of burn care. It may also lengthen hospital stay and elevate health care costs. This study has confirmed that a prolonged period of inactivity is the main risk factor in the development of heterotopic ossification in burn patients. Multicenter trials to address the best prevention strategies are desperately needed because no one center will have the patient volume for adequate study material.

D. W. Mozingo, MD

Randomized controlled trial of three burns dressings for partial thickness burns in children

Gee Kee EL, Kimble RM, Cuttle L, et al (Univ of Queensland, Brisbane, Australia; et al)

Burns 41:946-955, 2015

Background.—This study compared the effects of three silver dressing combinations on small to medium size acute partial thickness burns in children, focusing on re-epithelialization time, pain and distress during dressing changes.

Method.—Children (0–15 years) with clean, ≤10% total body surface area (TBSA) partial thickness burns who met the inclusion criteria were included in the study. Children received either (1) Acticoat™; (2) Acticoat™ with Mepitel™; or (3) Mepilex Ag™ dressings. Measures of burn re-epithelialization, pain, and distress were recorded at dressing changes every 3–5 days until full re-epithelialization occurred.

Results.—One hundred and three children were recruited with 96 children included for analysis. No infections were detected for the course of the study. When adjusted for burn depth, Acticoat™ significantly increased the expected days to full re-epithelialization by 40% (IRR = 1.40; 95% CI: 1.11–1.73, $p < 0.01$) and Acticoat™ with Mepitel™ significantly increased the expected days to full re-epithelialization by 33% (IRR = 1.33; 95% CI: 1.08–1.63, $p < 0.01$) when compared to Mepilex Ag™. Expected FLACC scores in the Mepilex Ag™ group were 32% lower at dressing removal ($p = 0.01$) and 37% lower at new dressing application ($p = 0.04$); and scores in the Acticoat™ with Mepitel™ group were 23% lower at dressing removal ($p = 0.04$) and 40% lower at new dressing application ($p < 0.01$), in comparison to the Acticoat™ group. Expected Visual Analog Scale-Pain (VAS-P) scores were 25% lower in the Mepilex Ag™ group at dressing removal ($p = 0.04$) and 34% lower in the Acticoat™ with Mepitel™ group ($p = 0.02$) at new dressing application in comparison to the Acticoat™ group. There was no significant difference between the Mepilex Ag™ and the Acticoat™ with Mepitel™ groups at all timepoints and with any pain measure.

Conclusion.—Mepilex Ag™ is an effective silver dressing, in terms of accelerated wound re-epithelialization time (compared to Acticoat™ and Acticoat™ with Mepitel™) and decreased pain during dressing changes (compared to Acticoat™), for clean, <10% TBSA partial thickness burns in children.

▶ In children with partial thickness burns, it is critical to have their injuries fully re-epithelialize as quickly as possible and for them to have as little pain as possible during their dressing changes. Silver-impregnated creams have been the mainstay of therapy, but more recently silver-impregnated dressing have been used. The authors sought to determine which of 3 silver dressings would be best in children with more minor burn injuries. In this trial, 103 children were randomized to 1 of 3 dressing groups.

The results showed advantages in using a dressing with a silicone interface (Mepilex) compared with a dressing without (Acticoat). "Dressings that are silicone or have silicone interfaces, adhere to normal, intact skin and remain in situ on the surface of a wound but do not adhere to it, maintaining a moist wound environment while providing a less traumatic removal and subsequently less epidermal damage." Although the third group had a silicone interface, it was not as efficacious as the Mepilex dressing.

These types of trials are important in that they provide a foundation for studies in children with larger burn sizes and help to maximize the healing process in those with smaller burns.

J. M. Daly, MD, FACS, FRCSI (Hon), FRCSG (Hon)

Negative pressure wound therapy technologies for chronic wound care in the home setting: A systematic review

Rhee SM, Valle MF, Wilson LM, et al (Johns Hopkins Bayview Med Ctr, Baltimore, MD; Univ of Maryland, Baltimore; Johns Hopkins Univ Bloomberg School of Public Health, Baltimore, MD; et al)

Wound Repair Regen 23:506-517, 2015

The use of negative pressure wound therapy (NPWT) is increasing in both the inpatient and outpatient settings. We conducted a systematic review on the efficacy and safety of NPWT for the treatment of chronic wounds in the home setting. We searched MEDLINE, Embase, the Cochrane Central Register of Controlled Trials, and the Cumulative Index to Nursing and Allied Health Literature, up to June 2014. Two independent reviewers screened search results. Seven studies met our criteria for inclusion. Six of the studies compared NPWT devices to other wound care methods and one study compared two different NPWT technologies. Data were limited by variability in the types of comparator groups, methodological limitations, and poor reporting of outcomes. We were unable to draw conclusions about the efficacy or safety of NPWT for the treatment of chronic wounds in the home setting due to the insufficient evidence. Consensus is needed on the methods of conducting and reporting wound care research so that future studies are able inform decisions about the use of NPWT in the home environment for chronic wounds.

▶ This review of the literature focused on the use of negative pressure wound therapy (NPWT) in the home setting. Six studies were ultimately chosen for review. The bottom line is that "for each of the predefined five critical outcomes, across all wound etiologies, the strength of the evidence was insufficient to draw conclusions on the effectiveness and safety of NPWT compared with other wound care treatments." Why has this situation occurred since NPWT has been available in different forms since the 1980s? It has been assumed perhaps that because efficacy has been reported in the inpatient setting, that these results would occur in the home. However, the lack of well-done clinical studies in the home setting is not unusual due to the many variables involved, such as the type and duration of the wounds being treated, the comorbidities of the patients being treated, and the home settings and resources involved in such settings. It is disappointing, however, that such enormous health care expenditures continue to occur without better clinical evidence of efficacy. Clearly this is an area that begs for better science and support for prospective, randomized clinical trials.

J. M. Daly, MD, FACS, FRCSI (Hon), FRCSG (Hon)

Total Occlusive Ionic Silver-Containing Dressing vs Mupirocin Ointment Application vs Conventional Dressing in Elective Colorectal Surgery: Effect on Incisional Surgical Site Infection

Ruiz-Tovar J, Llavero C, Morales V, et al (Hosp Rey Juan Carlos, Madrid, Spain; Hosp Sureste, Madrid, Spain; Univ Hosp Ramon y Cajal, Madrid, Spain; et al)

J Am Coll Surg 221:424-429, 2015

Background.—Several pre- and intraoperative factors have been associated with incisional surgical site infection (SSI), but little is known about the influence of postoperative wound care and especially, the use of different dressings on incisional SSI. The aim of this study was to compare 3 methods of wound dressings (conventional dressing, silver-containing dressing, and mupirocin ointment dressing) for their ability to prevent SSI, as measured by SSI rates, in patients with colorectal cancer undergoing elective open surgery.

Study Design.—A prospective, randomized study was performed. Inclusion criteria were diagnosis of colorectal neoplasms and plans to undergo elective surgery with curative aims. Patients were randomized using a 1:1:1 allocation into 3 groups: patients receiving an ionic silver-containing dressing (ISD) (group 1), a mupirocin ointment application

(MOA) (group 2), and a conventional dressing (group 3 or standard dressing). The primary outcomes variable was occurrence of incisional SSI. Follow-up was 30 days postoperatively.

Results.—A total of 147 patients were included, 49 in each group. Incisional SSI occurred in 9 patients (18.4%) in the ISD group, 2 (4.1%) in the MOA group, and 10 (20.4%) in the standard dressing group ($p = 0.028$). Adjusting for multiple comparisons, there were no significant differences between ISD and standard dressing groups; a significant difference was observed between ISD and MOA (relative risk [RR] 4.5; 95% CI (1.1 to 19.8); $p = 0.046$) and between the standard group and the MOA group (RR 5; 95% CI (1.2 to 21.7); $p = 0.031$).

Conclusions.—Topical application of mupirocin ointment achieves better results for the prevention of SSI than ionic silver-containing dressing or standard dressing in patients undergoing elective open colorectal surgery.

▶ While surgical site infection (SSI) is uncommon in clean operative cases, it can occur in 5% to 15% of clean contaminated surgical procedures. As the authors note, "more than 25% of incisional SSIs after elective colorectal surgery are caused by gram-positive microorganisms, including *Streptococcus* spp and *Enterococcus* spp." Mupirocin is an antibiotic agent active against gram-positive bacteria. This prospective, randomized trial containing 147 patients compared postoperative standard wound dressings with silver-containing dressings and mupirocin dressings. All patients had staple skin closures, and the study wound observers were blinded to the treatment method.

Incisional SSI occurred in 9 patients (18.4%) in the ISD group, 2 (4.1%) in the MOA group, and 10 (20.4%) in the standard dressing group ($P < .028$). Results of this prospective trial suggest that postoperative wound dressings with mupirocin do decrease the occurrence of surgical site infections.

J. M. Daly, MD, FACS, FRCSI (Hon), FRCSG (Hon)

The Influence of Time Interval Between Preoperative Radiation and Surgical Resection on the Development of Wound Healing Complications in Extremity Soft Tissue Sarcoma

Griffin AM, Dickie CI, Catton CN, et al (Mount Sinai Hosp, Toronto, Ontario, Canada; Princess Margaret Cancer Centre, Toronto, Ontario, Canada; et al)
Ann Surg Oncol 22:2824-2830, 2015

Objective.—The aim of this study was to determine the relationship of the time interval between completion of preoperative radiation therapy (RT) and surgical resection on wound complications (WCs) in extremity soft tissue sarcoma (STS).

Methods.—Overall, 798 extremity STS patients were managed with preoperative RT and surgery from 1989 to 2013. WCs were defined as requiring secondary operations/ invasive procedures for wound care, use of vacuum-assisted closure, prolonged dressing changes, or infection within 120 days of surgery.

Results.—Mean tumor size was 8.8 cm. A total of 743 (93 %) tumors were primary presentations, 565 (71 %) patients had lower extremity tumors, and 238 patients (30 %) had a prior unplanned excision. Of 242 patients (30 %) who developed a WC, 206 (37 %) had lower extremity tumors and 36 (15 %) had upper extremity tumors. Mean time from RT completion to surgery was 41.3 (range 4–470) days; 42.0 (range 4–470) days for upper extremity cases, and 41.1 (range 4–109) days for lower extremity cases. Similarly, mean time interval for patients who developed a WC was 40.9 (range 4–100) days, and 41.5 (range 4–470) days for those who did not develop a WC ($p = 0.69$). Thirty-nine cases (5 %) had surgery within 3 weeks of RT; 15 (38 %) patients developed WCs versus 227 (30 %) patients who had their tumors excised after 3 weeks ($p = 0.28$). One hundred and twenty-nine (16 %) patients had surgery within 4 weeks, and 39 (30 %) patients developed WCs versus 203 (30 %) patients who had their tumors excised after 4 weeks ($p = 1.0$). A trend towards a higher rate of WCs was seen for those patients who had surgery after 6 weeks (28 % prior vs. 34 % after; $p = 0.08$). There was no difference in WCs with intensity-modulated RT (IMRT) versus non-IMRT cases ($p = 0.6$).

Conclusion.—The time interval between preoperative RT and surgical excision in extremity STS had minimal influence on the development of WCs. Four- or 5-week intervals showed equivalent complication rates between the two groups, suggesting an optimal interval to reduce potential WCs.

▶ The use of neoadjuvant therapy for patients with solid tumors has increased over time because these patients can undergo more focused radiation therapy, and it is possible that the primary tumor may decrease in size, resulting in less extensive operations. This retrospective report evaluated patients who received radiation treatment for soft tissue sarcomas and then underwent resection. The authors sought to understand whether the timing of operation after completion of radiation influenced the development of wound complications.

Overall, the wound complication rate after surgery was approximately 30% and was not affected by the time of operation after completion of radiation. In addition, the wound complication rate was not affected by the use of either primary closure or the use of local advancement flaps. The incidence of local recurrence also was not influenced by the timing of surgery after RT.

Clearly, more prospective study is required, along with different approaches to reduce the incidence of wound complications in those who receive preoperative radiation for treatment of soft tissue sarcomas; a 30% wound complication rate is unacceptable.

J. M. Daly, MD, FACS, FRCSI (Hon), FRCSG (Hon)

An open multicenter comparative randomized clinical study on chitosan

Mo X, Cen J, Gibson E, et al (Foshan United Med Technologies Ltd, Guangdong, China; Aspen Med Europe Ltd, Redditch, United Kingdom; et al)

Wound Repair Regen 23:518-524, 2015

Chitosan, a natural polysaccharide derivate from chitin, offers a promising alternative biomaterial for use in wound dressings. In this work, the safety and efficacy of a next-generation KA01 chitosan wound dressing in facilitating the healing of nonhealing chronic wounds was studied. This open multicenter comparative prospective randomized clinical study was conducted at three medical centers in China. A total of 90 patients (45 in test group and 45 in control group) with unhealed chronic wounds including pressure ulcers, vascular ulcers, diabetic foot ulcers, and wounds with minor infections, or at risk of infection, were treated with the next generation chitosan wound dressing as the test article or traditional vaseline gauze as a control. Baseline assessments were undertaken with the primary end point being wound area reduction. The secondary end points included pain reduction (using the NRS11 pain scale) at dressing change, wound exudate levels, wound depth and duration of the treatment. After 4 weeks treatment, the wound area reduction was significantly greater in the test group (65.97 ± 4.48%) than the control group (39.95 ± 4.48%). The average pain level in the test group was 1.12 ± 0.23 and 2.30 ± 0.23 in the control group. The wound depth was also lower in the test group 0.30 ± 0.48 cm than the control group 0.54 ± 0.86 cm. The level of exudate fell and the dressing could be removed integrally in both the test and control groups. The mean duration of the test group was 27.31 ± 5.37 days and control group 27.09 ± 6.44 days. No adverse events were reported in either group. In conclusion this open multicenter comparative prospective randomized clinical study has provided compelling evidence that the next generation chitosan wound dressing can enhance wound progression towards healing by facilitating wound reepithelialization and reducing the patients pain level. Furthermore the dressing was shown to be clinically safe and effective in the management of chronic wounds.

▶ Management of chronic wounds is an imprecise science because of the variety of wounds treated and the many comorbidities in patients. Previous standard therapies used standard Telfa gauze dressings with or without local antibacterial agents.

The authors note: "The advantage of advanced wound dressings, such as alginate and hydrocolloids are they exhibit high absorption and moisture retention capacity. Chitosan, a natural polysaccharide derivate from chitin, offers a promising alternative biomaterial for use in wound dressings due to its inherent ability to assist with wound pathophysiology." Chitosan is nontoxic, nonirritating, nonimmunogenic, biodegradable, and biocompatible. It has also been reported to provide a degree of hemostasis and bacteriostasis.

This prospective, open-label clinical trial used Chitosan as a dressing for a variety of wounds, demonstrating safety and efficacy. At week 4, there was a significant reduction in the mean sizes of treated versus control wounds; pain was significantly reduced as well. In future studies, it will be important to determine the time to complete healing as a major end point, to focus on similar wounds such as chronic venous ulcers or pressure ulcers and to use separate individuals to evaluate the wound healing from those that are applying the treatments.

J. M. Daly, MD, FACS, FRCSI (Hon), FRCSG (Hon)

Prediction of wound healing after minor amputations of the diabetic foot
Caruana L, Formosa C, Cassar K (Dept of Health, Malta; Univ of Malta)
J Diabetes Complications 29:834-837, 2015

Aim.—To identify any significant differences in physiological test results between healing and non healing amputation sites.

Methods.—A single center prospective non-experimental study design was conducted on fifty subjects living with type 2 diabetes and requiring a forefoot or toe amputation. Subjects underwent non-invasive physiological testing preoperatively. These included assessment of pedal pulses, preoperative arterial spectral waveforms at the ankle, absolute toe pressures, toe–brachial pressure index and ankle–brachial pressure index. After 6 weeks, patients were examined to assess whether the amputation site was completely healed, was healing, had developed complications, or did not heal.

Results.—There was no significant difference in ABPI between the healed/healing and the non-healing groups. Mean TBI ($p = 0.031$) and toe pressure readings ($p = 0.014$) were significantly higher in the healed/healing group compared to the non healing group. A significant difference was also found in ankle spectral waveforms between the two groups ($p = 0.028$).

Conclusions.—TBIs, toe pressures and spectral waveforms at the ankle are better predictors of likelihood of healing and non-healing after minor amputation than ABPIs. ABPI alone is a poor indicator of the likelihood of healing of minor amputations and should not be relied on to determine need for revascularization procedures before minor amputation.

▶ Prediction of healing after a surgical procedure such as amputation is critical in diabetic patients with lower limb ischemia. These patients have both distal vessel calcification and occlusion, as well as small vessel disease, both of which affect soft tissue healing. The ankle-brachial pressure index has been used as a predictor of healing after toe or forefoot amputation. This study evaluated additional physiologic tests to determine their accuracy in predicting outcomes in these patients.

This study shows that "TBPIs [toe–brachial pressure indexes] and toe pressures are better predictors of likelihood of healing after minor foot amputation than ABPIs [ankle–brachial pressure indexes]." Patients with diabetes may have relatively adequate ABPIs and yet have very poor perfusion to the toes.

Doppler waveforms are also predictive of wound healing. All patients with triphasic waveforms healed their amputation wounds within 6 weeks. Patients with monophasic continuous waveforms had a significantly higher risk of developing complications or failing to heal their amputation sites.

These are relatively simple and inexpensive tests to obtain and should be done before decisions regarding revascularization or minor or major amputations in diabetic patients.

J. M. Daly, MD, FACS, FRCSI (Hon), FRCSG (Hon)

Prospective Randomized Controlled Trial Comparing the Effects of Noncontact Low-Frequency Ultrasound with Standard Care in Healing Split-Thickness Donor Sites

Prather JL, Tummel EK, Patel AB, et al (Tampa General Hosp, FL; Univ of South Florida, Tampa)

J Am Coll Surg 221:309-318, 2015

Background.—Skin graft donor sites are notoriously painful, with potential complications of fluid loss, delayed healing, infection, and hypertrophic scarring, particularly in patients with burns or traumatic injury. In this population, rapid epithelialization is critical to reducing morbidity and cost.

Study Design.—This prospective, randomized controlled trial compared the effects of 40-kHz noncontact low-frequency ultrasound (NLFU) in addition to standard care (SC) with SC alone in subjects with split-thickness donor sites of 20 to 200 cm^2. Standard care consisted of cleansing and moist wound dressings. Outcomes measured were time to healing, defined as absence of drainage and full epithelialization; pain and itching scores; and recidivism rates.

Results.—Of 33 patients enrolled; 27 were randomized and received a minimum of 4 study treatments. Median age was 49 years, 69% were male, and 84% were burn patients. Comorbidities included hypertension (31%), coronary artery disease (22%), pulmonary disease (38%), anemia (31%), and diabetes (16%). Median donor site area was 136.0 cm^2. Noncontact low-frequency ultrasound and SC compared with SC demonstrated a mean time to heal of 12.1 days vs 21.3 days ($p = 0.04$). All NLFU+SC subjects had epithelialized by 4 weeks compared with only 71% in SC. Recidivism rates were 8% for NLFU+SC compared with 45% for SC. Pain scores were reduced and significant differences in itching were observed.

Conclusions.—Noncontact low-frequency ultrasound and SC compared with SC alone in the treatment of split-thickness donor sites demonstrated significant accelerated healing and reduced pain and itching. Noncontact low-frequency ultrasound subjects experienced a better quality of healing with less incidence of infection and recidivism.

▶ Patients with major body surface burns require maximum healing of donor sites to reutilize these areas to provide complete coverage of the patients' burned areas. This trial was a prospective randomized controlled, parallel-group, multicenter study that evaluated the healing outcomes of noncontact low-frequency ultrasound (NLFU) plus standard care (SC) compared with SC alone on split-thickness donor sites. The NLFU technology used in this trial, MIST Therapy (Celleration) was Food and Drug Administration–approved, indicated for promoting wound healing. "The system delivers low-frequency (40 kHz) ultrasound energy to the wound, via sterile saline as a conduit, and without direct contact with the patient. Noncontact low-frequency ultrasound energy penetrates into and below the wound bed tissue, stimulating changes within the microenvironment."

The primary end point of mean time to heal, defined per protocol as mean days to no drainage, was significantly shorter for NLFU plus standard care group at 12 days compared with 21 days for standard care alone ($P < .04$). Ninety-two percent of the NLFU plus standard care–treated donor sites had healed by day 14 compared with 64% with standard care alone. All NLFU plus standard care patients were healed by 4 weeks postoperatively compared with 71% of subjects in the standard care alone group.

In this trial, more than half of the SC subjects demonstrated increased odorous exudate and were treated for a suspected infection of the donor site. In contrast, only 1 NLFU subject experienced increased exudate and was treated for potential infection.

This interesting study showed the benefit of this new technology on would healing. Further clinical trials will be important to further define its usefulness.

J. M. Daly, MD, FACS, FRCSI (Hon), FRCSG (Hon)

Evidence-based chronic ulcer care and lower limb outcomes among Pacific Northwest veterans

Karavan M, Olerud J, Bouldin E, et al (VA Puget Sound Health Care System, Seattle, WA; Univ of Washington, Seattle; et al)

Wound Repair Regen 23:745-752, 2015

Evidence-based ulcer care guidelines detail optimal components of care for treatment of ulcers of different etiologies. We investigated the impact of providing specific evidence-based ulcer treatment components on healing outcomes for lower limb ulcers (LLU) among veterans in the Pacific Northwest. Components of evidence-based ulcer care for venous, arterial, diabetic foot ulcers/neuropathic ulcers were abstracted from medical records. The outcome was ulcer healing. Our analysis assessed the relationship between evidence-based ulcer care by etiology, components of care provided, and healing, while accounting for veteran characteristics. A minority of veterans in all three ulceretiology groups received the recommended components of evidence-based care in at least 80% of visits. The likelihood of healing improved when assessment for edema and infection were performed on at least 80% of visits (hazard ratio [HR] = 3.20, $p = 0.009$ and HR = 3.54, $p = 0.006$, respectively) in patients with venous ulcers. There was no significant association between frequency of care components provided and healing among patients with arterial ulcers. Among patients with diabetic/neuropathic ulcers, the chance of healing increased 2.5-fold when debridement was performed at 80% of visits ($p = 0.03$), and doubled when ischemia was assessed at the first visit ($p = 0.045$). Veterans in the Pacific Northwest did not uniformly receive evidence-based ulcer care. Not all evidence-based ulcer care components were significantly associated with healing. At a minimum, clinicians need to address components of ulcer care associated with improved ulcer healing.

▶ Evidence-based medicine has evolved to where the individual's diagnosis and associated comorbidities are fitted into simple or sometimes complex algorithms that define processes of care in an effort to improve outcomes. Although some may argue that evidence-based medicine can be "cookie-cutter" medicine, bringing standardized approaches to diagnostic testing, follow-up, and treatment have been shown to improve clinical care. Unfortunately, not all physicians understand, know, or follow "best practices" of evidence-based medicine. This retrospective study evaluated the utilization of evidence-based clinical care for veterans with chronic arterial insufficiency or chronic venous lower extremity ulcers.

Among veterans with a venous ulcer, 20% had edema assessment or moist wound healing elements in at least 80% of their visits. However, sharp debridement was not performed on at least 80% of visits for any veteran with venous ulcer, thus this variable was excluded from further venous ulcer components of care analysis. There was a significantly higher chance of healing among veterans receiving edema assessment on at least 80% of visits. Among veterans with arterial ulcers, 32% had infection assessment in at least 80% of visits, 56% had ischemia assessment on the first visit, and 39% had a vascular surgery evaluation within 30 days of ulcer presentation.

Clearly, when evidence-based best practices occur, clinical care is improved and patients ultimately do better. The goal must be to disperse information about these practices and, through clinical information systems, make it easier to for all physicians to practice evidence-based medicine.

J. M. Daly, MD, FACS, FRCSI (Hon), FRCSG (Hon)

Tobacco Use and Body Mass Index as Predictors of Outcomes in Patients Undergoing Breast Reduction Mammoplasty

Karamanos E, Wei B, Siddiqui A, et al (Wayne State Univ, Detroit, MI)

Ann Plast Surg 75:383-387, 2015

Background.—Breast reduction mammoplasty accounts for more than 60,000 procedures annually, but the literature is still sparse on outcomes, especially beyond the single institution perspective. The aim of this study was to seek a broader view by study breast reduction outcomes in the National Surgical Quality Improvement Program database.

Methods.—The National Surgical Quality Improvement Program data set was queried for the *Current Procedural Terminology* code 19318 from the years 2005 to 2010. The principal outcomes measured were wound complications, surgical site infections, and reoperations. Univariate and multivariate analysis was performed to identify significant relationships.

Results.—A total of 2779 patients were identified. The mean age was 42.7 (14.1) years and the mean body mass index (BMI) was 31.6 (7.0) kg/m^2. Tobacco use was associated with a higher rate of reoperation ($P = 0.02$). Body mass index was identified as an independent risk factor for wound complications (odds ratio, 1.85, $P = 0.005$). Patients with BMI greater than 40 kg/m^2 were significantly more likely to develop postoperative wound complications ($P = 0.02$).

Conclusions.—This study represents the largest sample on breast reduction in the literature. Age and surgeon specialty did not correlate with negative results. In contrast, tobacco use and BMI were associated with worse breast reduction outcomes.

▶ Complications of cosmetic surgery such as breast augmentation and reduction have been thought to be more prevalent in patients who smoke and who are obese compared with nonobese, nonsmokers. However, there are few large database studies to determine the exact relationship among these variables. National Surgical Quality Improvement Program data provides the opportunity to query the relationship among these factors in patients undergoing breast reduction surgery.

Patients with tobacco use were significantly more likely to require reoperation (3.8% for smokers vs 1.8% for nonsmokers, $P = .02$). After adjusting for differences between the 2 groups, smoking was not associated with increased odds of developing any surgical site infections or wound dehiscence. Patients with history of tobacco use were significantly more likely to require reoperation. Independent predictors of wound complications were proved to be wound classification at the end of the surgery, increasing body mass index (BMI), and increasing American Society of Anesthesiologists. An increase in BMI was linearly associated with an increase in probability of developing any wound complication.

Many organizations, such as the American College of Surgeons, recommends surgeons advise their patients to stop smoking before operations. This study provides greater emphasis for this counseling to occur preoperatively. Although obesity is more difficult to resolve, patients should understand the complications that may ensue after breast reduction operations.

J. M. Daly, MD, FACS, FRCSI (Hon), FRCSG (Hon)

Acceleration of diabetic wound healing using a novel protease–anti-protease combination therapy

Gao M, Nguyen TT, Suckow MA, et al (Univ of Notre Dame, IN)

Proc Natl Acad Sci U S A 112:15226-15231, 2015

Nonhealing chronic wounds are major complications of diabetes resulting in >70,000 annual lower-limb amputations in the United States alone. The reasons the diabetic wound is recalcitrant to healing are not fully understood, and there are limited therapeutic agents that could accelerate or facilitate its repair. We previously identified two active forms of matrix metalloproteinases (MMPs), MMP-8 and MMP-9, in the wounds of *db/db* mice. We argued that the former might play a role in the body's response to wound healing and that the latter is the pathological consequence of the disease with detrimental effects. Here we demonstrate that the use of compound ND-336, a novel highly selective inhibitor of gelatinases (MMP-2 andMMP-9) and MMP-14, accelerates diabetic wound healing by lowering inflammation and by enhancing angiogenesis and re-epithelialization of the wound, thereby reversing the pathological condition. The detrimental role of MMP-9 in the pathology of diabetic wounds was confirmed further by the study of diabetic MMP-9 knockout mice, which exhibited wounds more prone to healing. Furthermore, topical administration of active recombinant MMP-8 also accelerated diabetic wound healing as a consequence of complete re-epithelialization, diminished inflammation, and enhanced angiogenesis. The combined topical application of ND-336 (a small molecule) and the active recombinant MMP-8 (an enzyme) enhanced healing even more, in a strategy that holds considerable promise in healing of diabetic wounds.

▶ More than 300 million individuals have diabetes mellitus that significantly impairs wound healing through a variety of vascular physiologic and cellular biochemical mechanisms. Multiple studies have attempted to improve the healing of experimental wounds in diabetic animals through systemic and local administration of growth factors, use of local antibiotics and different cellular therapies. These investigators have previously shown alterations in matrix metalloproteinases in the wounds of genetically diabetic animals. They performed these experimental studies to evaluate a compound (ND-336) that selectively inhibits MMP-2, MMP-9, and MMP-14.

Because human wounds heal by reepithelialization, the authors evaluated the experimental wounds in diabetic mice with hematoxylin and eosin staining to visualize the epithelium. Treatment with ND-336 resulted in almost complete reepithelialization compared with partial reepithelialization in the ND-322 and vehicle-treated groups. This study confirmed that MMP-9 is involved in the pathology of diabetic wounds because in diabetic MMP-9–knockout mice both up-regulation of MMP-8 and absence of MMP-9 occurs.

Thus, these experimental studies demonstrate that matrix metalloproteinases are intimately involved with wound healing in diabetic animals. The next steps are to evaluate these processes in diabetic humans with inhibitors to these proteinases and evaluate their safety and effects.

J. M. Daly, MD, FACS, FRCSI (Hon), FRCSG (Hon)

Dual effects of atmospheric pressure plasma jet on skin wound healing of mice

Xu G-M, Shi X-M, Cai J-F, et al (Xi'an Jiaotong Univ, Shaanxi, People's Republic of China)

Wound Repair Regen 23:878-884, 2015

Cold plasma has become an attractive tool for promoting wound healing and treating skin diseases. This article presents an atmospheric pressure plasma jet (APPJ) generated in argon gas through dielectric barrier discharge, which was applied to superficial skin wounds in BALB/c mice. The mice ($n = 50$) were assigned randomly into five groups (named A, B, C, D, E) with 10 animals in each group. Natural wound healing was compared with stimulated wound healing treated daily with APPJ for different time spans (10, 20, 30, 40, and 50 seconds) on 14 consecutive days. APPJ emission spectra, morphological changes in animal wounds, and tissue histological parameters were analyzed. Statistical results revealed that wound size changed over the duration of the experimental period and there was a significant interaction between experimental day and group. Differences between group C and other groups at day 7 were statistically significant ($p < 0.05$). All groups had nearly achieved closure of the untreated control wounds at day 14. The wounds treated with APPJ for 10, 20, 30, and 40 seconds showed significantly enhanced daily improvement compared with the control and almost complete closure at day 12, 10, 7, and 13, respectively. The optimal results of epidermal cell regeneration, granulation tissue hyperplasia, and collagen deposition in histological aspect were observed at day 7. However, the wounds treated for 50 seconds were less well healed at day 14 than those of the control. It was concluded that appropriate doses of cold plasma could inactivate bacteria around the wound, activate fibroblast proliferation in wound tissue, and eventually promote wound healing. Whereas, over doses of plasma suppressed wound healing due to causing cell death by apoptosis or necrosis. Both positive and negative effects may be related to the existence of reactive oxygen and nitrogen species (ROS and RNS) in APPJ.

▶ Stimulation of wound healing in chronic nonhealing wounds remains the Holy Grail of scientists in the wound-healing arena. Many methods have been tried using biochemical, mechanical, cellular, and physiologic approaches. In this experimental mouse model of wound healing, atmospheric pressure plasma jet generated in argon gas was used for the treatment of cutaneous wounds in mice.

"Plasma is the fourth state of matter, the others being liquid, solid, and gas. As a term used in physics, it has an entirely different meaning to that of the term plasma used in biology to describe the noncellular fluid component of circulating blood. Plasma consists of many active components, including radicals (reactive species), ions, electrons, and photons. Cold plasma can be generated through electrical discharge with different work gases (air, argon, helium, etc.)." Results of this animal study showed that the wound healing effect with an atmospheric pressure plasma jet treatment time of 30 seconds was better than those with the treatment times of 10, 40, and 50 seconds. Similarly, the wound healing effect with a treatment time of 20 seconds was better than those with treatment times of 40 and 50 seconds.

This innovative approach for stimulation of wound healing will require much further study because the therapeutic window of treatment times appears quite narrow. In addition, there will need to be extensive safety studies carried out to be certain that adverse effects of atmospheric pressure plasma jet do not occur.

J. M. Daly, MD, FACS, FRCSI (Hon), FRCSG (Hon)

Wound healing and all-cause mortality in 958 wound patients treated in home care

Zarchi K, Martinussen T, Jemec GBE (Univ of Copenhagen, Roskilde, Denmark)

Wound Repair Regen 23:753-758, 2015

Skin wounds are associated with significant morbidity and mortality. Data are, however, not readily available for benchmarking, to allow prognostic evaluation, and to suggest when involvement of wound-healing experts is indicated. We, therefore, conducted an observational cohort study to investigate wound healing and all-cause mortality associated with different types of skin wounds. Consecutive skin wound patients who received wound care by home-care nurses from January 2010 to December 2011 in a district in Eastern Denmark were included in this study. Patients were followed until wound healing, death, or the end of follow-up on December 2012. In total, 958 consecutive patients received wound care by home-care nurses, corresponding to a 1-year prevalence of 1.2% of the total population in the district. During the study, wound healing was achieved in 511 (53.3%), whereas 90 (9.4%) died. During the first 3 weeks of therapy, healing was most likely to occur in surgical wounds (surgical vs. other wounds: adjusted hazard ratio [AHR] 2.21, 95% confidence interval 1.50–3.23), while from 3 weeks to 3 months of therapy, cancer wounds, and pressure ulcers were least likely to heal (cancer vs. other wounds: AHR 0.12, 0.03–0.50; pressure vs. other wounds: AHR 0.44, 0.27–0.74). Cancer wounds and pressure ulcers were further associated with a three times increased probability of mortality compared with other wounds (cancer vs. other wounds: AHR 3.19, 1.35–7.50; pressure vs. other wounds: AHR 2.91, 1.56–5.42). In summary, the wound type was found to be a significant predictor of healing and mortality with cancer wounds and pressure ulcers being associated with poor prognosis.

▶ Although patients with skin wounds are known to have increased morbidity and mortality as hospital inpatients, there is less information regarding their outcomes in the home setting. This article evaluates nearly 1000 patients in eastern Denmark for whom home care was initiated for the purpose of treating their skin wounds. Patients with diabetic foot ulcers and pressure sores are at increased risk of mortality because of their wounds and to their underlying condition. During the first 3 weeks of treatment, surgical wounds were most likely to heal compared to other types of wounds.

In contrast to the first 3 weeks, sex emerged as a significant predictor: wound healing was significantly more likely to occur in women than in men. Cancer wounds were significantly associated with reduced healing compared with other wounds, as were pressure ulcers compared with other wounds. This unique observational study provides a foundation to initiate more specific therapies and personnel for home patients with certain types of wounds to improve outcomes and reduce costs of care.

J. M. Daly, MD, FACS, FRCSI (Hon), FRCSG (Hon)

Peroxide-based oxygen generating topical wound dressing for enhancing healing of dermal wounds

Chandra PK, Ross CL, Smith LC, et al (Wake Forest Inst for Regenerative Medicine, Winston Salem, NC)

Wound Repair Regen 23:830-841, 2015

Oxygen generating biomaterials represent a new trend in regenerative medicine that aims to generate and supply oxygen at the site of requirement, to support tissue healing and regeneration. To enhance the healing of dermal wounds, we have developed a highly portable, in situ oxygen generating wound dressings that uses sodium percarbonate (SPO) and calcium peroxide (CPO) as chemical oxygen sources. The dressing continuously generated oxygen for more than 3 days, after which it was replaced. In the in vivo testing on porcine full-thickness porcine wound model, the SPO/CPO dressing showed enhanced wound healing during the 8 week study period. Quantitative measurements of wound healing related parameters, such as wound closure, reepithelialization, epidermal thickness and collagen content of dermis showed that supplying oxygen topically using the SPO/CPO dressing significantly accelerated the wound healing. An increase in neovascularization, as determined using Von Willebrand factor (vWF) and CD31 staining, was also observed in the presence of SPO/CPO dressing. This novel design for a wound dressing that contains oxygen generating biomaterials (SPO/CPO) for supplying topical oxygen, may find utility in treating various types of acute to chronic wounds.

▶ The presence of adequate oxygen and other nutrients in a wound are imperative to the cellular components of wound healing (macrophages, fibroblasts, etc). Using this concept, many attempts have been made in which additional oxygen has been focused on the local wound. Use of hyperbaric oxygen, inhalation of increased amounts of oxygen, and local wound perfusion with oxygen have been used in an attempt to improve healing and perhaps decrease the incidence of infection particularly with anaerobic bacteria.

As the authors noted, a "major drawback with most of the current devices is that they use gaseous oxygen as the source, which has several limitations, including having a constant supply of pure oxygen over the entire period of wound treatment (usually several days), physically attaching external oxygen supplying devices to the patients that restrict their daily activities and the overall cost of such treatments." Thus, they sought to provide a biochemical source of oxygen locally. The hydrogen peroxide (H_2O_2) produced decomposes in the presence of an alkaline environment to give oxygen, which diffuses through a gelatin layer to the wound tissue. This method of topical oxygen therapy demonstrated improvement in healing in their porcine model and showed that this process occurred even to depths of 6 mm in the dermis. Additional work is needed with this approach, but this innovative concept has merit and requires further testing because it may have good clinical applicability.

J. M. Daly, MD, FACS, FRCSI (Hon), FRCSG (Hon)

Inhibition of *Pseudomonas aeruginosa* biofilm formation on wound dressings

Brandenburg KS, Calderon DF, Kierski PR, et al (Univ of Wisconsin—Madison; et al)

Wound Repair Regen 23:842-854, 2015

Chronic nonhealing skin wounds often contain bacterial biofilms that prevent normal wound healing and closure and present challenges to the use of conventional wound dressings. We investigated inhibition of *Pseudomonas aeruginosa* biofilm formation, a common pathogen of chronic skin wounds, on a commercially available biological wound dressing. Building on prior reports, we examined whether the amino acid tryptophan would inhibit *P. aeruginosa* biofilm formation on the three-dimensional surface of the biological dressing. Bacterial biomass and biofilm polysaccharides were quantified using crystal violet staining or an enzyme linked lectin, respectively. Bacterial cells and biofilm matrix adherent to the wound dressing were visualized through scanning electron microscopy. D-/L-tryptophan inhibited *P. aeruginosa* biofilm formation on the wound dressing in a dose dependent manner and was not directly cytotoxic to immortalized human keratinocytes although there was some reduction in cellular metabolism or enzymatic activity. More importantly, D-/L-tryptophan did not impair wound healing in a splinted skin wound murine model. Furthermore, wound closure was improved when D-/L-tryptophan treated wound dressing with *P. aeruginosa* biofilms were compared with untreated dressings. These findings indicate that tryptophan may prove useful for integration into wound dressings to inhibit biofilm formation and promote wound healing.

▶ As noted by the authors, biofilms significantly delay normal healing by serving as a reservoir of bacterial cells that resist both antibiotic treatment and clearance by the immune system. Thus, it would be valuable to reduce or eliminate biofilm development in the healing wound. Debridement of wounds with necrotic tissues is the standard of care, but further biofilms often form afterward, resulting in a vicious cycle of infection and development of necrotic tissue requiring additional debridement.

To investigate the potential for inhibition of biofilm formation, the authors established a model for *Pseudomonas aeruginosa* biofilm formation on a commercially available biological wound dressing (Biobrane). The authors noted significant inhibition of biofilm formation with tryptophan in a dose-dependent manner, yet there was no inhibition of wound healing in an in vivo mouse model of injury.

It may be that tryptophan limits bacterial attachment or disrupts microcolony formation through altered bacterial motility as suggested by the authors.

This is a very interesting study because of its importance to wound healing and its suggestion that a relatively inexpensive amino acid, tryptophan, may be valuable when impregnated into biological dressings.

J. M. Daly, MD, FACS, FRCSI (Hon), FRCSG (Hon)

A comparison of an antibacterial sandwich dressing vs dressing containing silver

Krasowski G, Jawień A, Tukiendorf A, et al (Nutrikon, Krapkowice, Poland; Univ Hosp nr 1 Bydgoszcz, Poland; Oncology Ctr Inst Gliwice, Poland; et al)
Wound Repair Regen 23:525-530, 2015

The purpose of this study was to compare the efficacy of dressings containing octenidine vs. dressings containing silver in the wound healing in the course of a chronic venous disease. There were two groups of 40 patients who met the inclusion criteria and who did not meet the exclusion criteria. The patients were randomly assigned into the groups (envelope method). The first, "O group" was treated with octenidine-based dressings. The second, "S group" was treated with silver dressings. The study lasted for 56 days. All patients in the research were treated with medical compression stockings with cotton understockings. Microbiological eradication was observed on the 28th day of the study among 33% of patients in the treatment group vs. 6% in control group. On the 56th day of the treatment, these percentages equalled 72% and 35%. The rate of healing was faster in the 0 group than in the S group. In the wounds <10 cm^2 it was faster by 1.35 cm^2/week and in wounds >10 cm^2 it equalled 3.44 cm^2. The reduction of pain level was 37.5% higher in the O group, in contrast with the S group. One change of a dressing in the O group led to a 0.06 cm^2 greater wound size reduction and in the case of wounds >10 cm^2 to 0.29 cm^2 reduction compared with the S group. The presented results indicate that the efficacy of dressings containing octenidine is higher compared to silver dressings.

▶ Chronic venous ulcers are difficult wound management problems resulting in various degrees of disability for patients and often multiple hospital admissions for complications. Leg compression and some form of local antibacterial therapy are the mainstays of treatment. This prospective, randomized study compared a form of local antibacterial treatment with a standard therapy (silver impregnated solution). The first group of patients was treated with layers of octenidine-containing dressings. The skin surrounding the wound was covered with a thin layer of cholesterol ointment and the wound was rinsed with Octenilin (Schulke-Mayer, Norderstedt, Germany) solution. Subsequently, the wound was sprayed with Octenisept (Schulke-Mayer) antiseptic. Next, Octenilin gel was applied. The second group of patients was treated with silver dressings.

The investigators found that the experimental group healed significantly faster, had significantly reduced pain levels, and had significantly improved microbial reduction compared with the control (silver) group.

This is an important clinical trial because the stratification and randomization was adequate and the patients were followed closely with clinically relevant end points measured throughout the trial. It appears that actinide-based dressing is superior to standard silver-based dressing for chronic venous ulcers. Further studies should be done for burn injuries to determine whether such efficacy can be found in a broader array of injuries.

J. M. Daly, MD, FACS, FRCSI (Hon), FRCSG (Hon)

Hydrocellular foam dressing increases the leptin level in wound fluid

Yoshino S, Nakagami G, Ohira T, et al (Tokyo Univ of Agriculture, Japan; The Univ of Tokyo, Japan)

Wound Repair Regen 23:703-710, 2015

Hydrocellular foam dressing (HCF) absorbs excessive wound fluid, which contains various cytokines and growth factors, and ensures a moist environment to promote wound healing. However, the molecular mechanisms underlying the wound fluid component changes induced by HCF are poorly understood. In the present study, we examined the effect of HCF on wound healing and the associated regulatory mechanisms in relation to variations in cytokine levels in the wound fluid. We created full-thickness wounds on the dorsolateral skin of rats and collected the resulting wound fluid samples. HCF was immersed in a plate containing the wound fluids. HCF was then removed and the excess wound fluid remaining in the plate was examined by cytokine array and enzyme-linked immunosorbent assay. We also used a rat model and human dermal fibroblast cultures to examine the effect of wound fluid component changes during the wound healing process. Upon treatment with HCF, leptin levels were upregulated in the wound fluid. Fibroblast proliferation was enhanced and the effect was suppressed in the presence of leptin antagonist. In our in vivo model, HCF increased wound contraction compared with film dressings and this positive effect of HCF was suppressed by addition of leptin antagonist. Our results suggest that dermal fibroblast proliferation is upregulated by HCF due to increased leptin level at the wound surface, and these effects promote wound healing. We believe that the present study contributes to furthering the understanding of the mechanisms underlying the effects of HCF-induced wound healing.

▶ The wound-healing environment has been described in many ways: immunological, cellular, physiologic, and biochemical. Use of moist wound dressing has been proposed to improve the local wound environment to maximize the opportunity for complete wound healing. This experimental animal study evaluated hydrocellular foam dressing treatment of skin wounds in rats with particular emphasis on understanding local cytokine levels during the healing process. In previous studies, HCF was shown to contribute to wound healing by decreasing inflammation and increasing hyaluronan synthesis. Results of this study found that "fibroblast proliferation was upregulated in wound fluid pretreated with HCF while cell proliferation was blocked in the presence of leptin antagonist. This suggests that HCF-induced changes leptin levels at the wound may regulate fibroblast proliferation."

Experimental studies such as this are important to understand the basic science behind wound-healing processes. However, one must keep in mind that physiologic, cellular, and cytokine responses in rats may not be the same as those in humans Thus, further clinical basic science investigations are required to more fully understand our understanding of clinical wound healing.

J. M. Daly, MD, FACS, FRCSI (Hon), FRCSG (Hon)

Effect of Adhesive Strips and Dermal Sutures vs Dermal Sutures Only on Wound Closure: A Randomized Clinical Trial

Custis T, Armstrong AW, King TH, et al (Univ of California, Davis, School of Medicine, Sacramento; Univ of Colorado, Denver)

JAMA Dermatol 151:862-867, 2015

Importance.—Although applying adhesive strips to a wound closure has been shown to have outcomes equivalent to those with cuticular suturing, it is unknown whether adhesive strips provide additional benefit compared with dermal suturing alone.

Objective.—To determine whether the addition of adhesive strips to a wound closed with buried interrupted subcuticular sutures improves outcomes following wound closure.

Design, Setting, and Participants.—A prospective, randomized split-wound intervention was conducted between November 14, 2013, and May 16, 2014, in patients who underwent cutaneous surgical procedures at the University of California, Davis, outpatient dermatology clinic. Fifty-seven patients 18 years or older with postoperative defects of at least 3 cm, resulting from either Mohs micrographic surgical procedures or surgical excision, were screened for participation. Nine patients were excluded and 48 were enrolled.

Interventions.—Half of each wound was randomized to receive buried interrupted subcuticular sutures and overlying adhesive strips and the other half received buried interrupted subcuticular sutures only.

Main Outcomes and Measures.—At 3 months' follow-up, each patient and 2 blinded observers evaluated the wound using the Patient Observer Scar Assessment Scale.

Results.—The total mean (SD) Patient Observer Scar Assessment Scale score for observers for the side that received a combination of adhesive strips and buried interrupted subcuticular suturing (12.3 [4.8]) and the side that received sutures only (12.9 [6.3]) did not differ significantly at 3 months ($P = .32$). There was no significant difference in the total patient assessment scale score between the combination closure (14.0 [7.6]) and sutures only (14.7 [7.6]) sides at 3 months ($P = .39$). There was also no significant difference between the 2 closure methods in terms of mean (SD) scar width (both methods: 1.1 [0.8] mm, $P = .89$) at follow-up.

Conclusions and Relevance.—Combination closure with adhesive strips and buried interrupted subcuticular suturing was not significantly associated with improved overall scar assessment compared with buried interrupted subcuticular suturing alone when evaluated by blinded observers or the patients themselves. Our results do not support the use of adhesive strips as a means to improve cosmetic outcomes or reduce scar width.

Trial Registration.—clinicaltrials.gov Identifier: NCT01979497.

▶ It has been common surgical folklore that use of cutaneous stern-strips helps to minimize scar width and perhaps lead to improved wound healing. Although there have been studies to evaluate wound adhesives and cutaneous strips, there have not been good, randomized, prospective clinical trials to evaluate subcuticular closure compared with subcuticular closure plus cutaneous strips. This study randomized patients' wounds to have half the wound closed with subcuticular sutures and the other half closed using both modalities. Importantly, the evaluations done at 3 months were performed by blinded observers. The results showed no differences in outcomes for the different closure methods.

This is an important study and certainly changes my mind regarding the use of cutaneous strips. In addition to having no benefit, the use of cutaneous strips often leads to desquamation and a poorer wound outcome. Once again, science trumps folklore!

J. M. Daly, MD, FACS, FRCSI (Hon), FRCSG (Hon)

Comparative effectiveness of a bioengineered living cellular construct vs. a dehydrated human amniotic membrane allograft for the treatment of diabetic foot ulcers in a real world setting

Kirsner RS, Sabolinski ML, Parsons NB, et al (Univ of Miami Miller School of Medicine, FL; Sabolinski LLC, Franklin, MA; Organogenesis Inc., Canton, MA; et al)

Wound Repair Regen 23:737-744, 2015

We evaluated the comparative effectiveness of a bioengineered living cellular construct (BLCC) and a dehydrated human amnion/chorion membrane allograft (dHACM) for the treatment of diabetic foot ulcers (DFUs). Using a wound care–specific electronic medical record database, we assessed real-world outcomes in 218 patients with 226 DFUs receiving treatment in 2014 at 99 wound care centers. The analysis included DFUs ≥ 1 and $<25\ cm^2$ with duration $<=1$ year and area reduction $\leq 20\%$ in 14 days prior to treatment ($N=163$, BLCC; $N=63$, dHACM). The average baseline areas and durations were $6.0\ cm^2$ and 4.4 months for BLCC and $5.2\ cm^2$ and 4.6 months for dHACM, respectively. Patients treated with dHACM had more applications compared to those treated with BLCC (median 3.0 vs. 2.0) ($p=0.003$). A Cox model adjusted for key covariates including area and duration found the median time to closure for BLCC was 13.3 weeks compared to 26 weeks for dHACM, and the proportion of wounds healed were significantly higher for BLCC by 12 weeks (48% vs. 28%) and 24 weeks (72% vs. 47%) ($p=0.01$). Treatment with a bioengineered living cellular technology increased the probability of healing by 97% compared with a dehydrated amniotic membrane (hazard ratio $=1.97$ [95% confidence interval 1.17, 3.33], $p=0.01$).

► Management of diabetic foot ulcers is a major problem, resulting in patient morbidity, amputations, disability, and mortality. Surgical debridement and removing pressure from the affected area are the mainstays of therapy. However, there are newer products available that can be used for coverage that may accelerate healing. Of the few products studied in randomized controlled trials, one is a bioengineered living cellular construct (BLCC), which is composed of human neonatal keratinocytes and fibroblasts in an extracellular matrix of bovine and human collagen and other extracellular matrix proteins. BLCC was the first allogeneic cell-based product approved by the Food and Drug Administration and has approval for the treatment of nonhealing diabetic foot ulcers.

Another product is dehydrated human amniotic allograft (dHACM), which is a collagenous membrane derived from the submucosa of donated human placenta after a planned cesarean delivery. The product undergoes terminal sterilization and contains no living cells. This retrospective review found that the use of BLCC was associated with better wound closure of diabetic foot ulcers. Use of this type of analysis can describe "associations" but not necessarily "causations" so the results must be taken with this factor in mind. However, prospective trials are warranted to evaluate this issue further to perform a retrospective analysis comparing the effectiveness of BLCC versus dHACM for the treatment of DFUs.

J. M. Daly, MD, FACS, FRCSI (Hon), FRCSG (Hon)

Arachidonic acid-derived signaling lipids and functions in impaired healing

Dhall S, Wijesinghe DS, Karim ZA, et al (Univ of California, Riverside; Virginia Commonwealth Univ, Richmond; et al)

Wound Repair Regen 23:644-656, 2015

Very little is known about lipid function during wound healing, and much less during impaired healing. Such understanding will help identify what roles lipid signaling plays in the development of impaired/chronic wounds. We took a lipidomics approach to study the alterations in lipid profile in the LIGHT$^{-/-}$ mouse model of impaired healing which has characteristics that resemble those of impaired/chronic wounds in humans, including high levels of oxidative stress, excess inflammation, increased extracellular matrix degradation and blood vessels with fibrin cuffs. The latter suggests excess coagulation and potentially increased platelet aggregation. We show here that in these impaired wounds there is an imbalance in the arachidonic acid (AA) derived eicosonoids that mediate or modulate inflammatory reactions and platelet aggregation. In the LIGHT$^{-/-}$ impaired wounds there is a significant increase in enzymatically derived breakdown products of AA. We found that early after injury there was a significant increase in the eicosanoids 11-, 12-, and 15-hydroxyeicosa-tetranoic acid, and the proinflammatory leukotrienes (LTD4 and LTE) and prostaglandins (PGE_2 and $PGF_{2\alpha}$). Some of these eicosanoids also promote platelet aggregation. This led us to examine the levels of other eicosanoids known to be involved in the latter process. We found that thromboxane (TXA_2/B_2), and prostacyclins 6kPGF1α are elevated shortly after wounding and in some cases during healing. To determine whether they have an impact in platelet aggregation and hemostasis, we tested LIGHT$^{-/-}$ mouse wounds for these two parameters and found that, indeed, platelet aggregation and hemostasis are enhanced in these mice when compared with the control C57BL/6 mice. Understanding lipid signaling in impaired wounds can potentially lead to development of new therapeutics or in using existing nonsteroidal antiinflammatory agents to help correct the course of healing.

▶ Under ideal circumstances, wounds in humans go on to heal uneventfully. However, a variety of wound factors, such as the wound's magnitude, presence or absence of contamination type of wound, and host factors such as diabetes, previous radiation, malnutrition, and immunodeficiencies influence whether the healing process goes on to early completion or becomes a chronic problem.

As the authors noted, hallmarks of impaired and chronic wounds include increased oxidative stress, deregulated levels of growth factors, imbalance in cytokines and chemokines, sustained inflammation, leaky blood vessels, and uncontrolled function of proteases. Thus, they chose to study lipid signaling and biochemical products that predominate during an impaired healing process in a genetic mouse model. The results of these studies showed alterations in eicosanoids, thromboxanes, and prostacyclins that are associated with inflammation and platelet aggregation.

These studies offer an interesting view of the biochemical changes that occur in this animal model of impaired wound healing. It will be important to determine whether similar changes occur in the impaired healing of wounds in humans.

J. M. Daly, MD, FACS, FRCSI (Hon), FRCSG (Hon)

Elements affecting wound healing time: An evidence based analysis

Khalil H, Cullen M, Chambers H, et al (Monash Univ, Victoria, Australia; Latrobe Community Health Centre, Victoria, Australia)

Wound Repair Regen 23:550-556, 2015

The purpose of this study was to identify the predominant client factors and comorbidities that affected the time taken for wounds to heal. A prospective study design used the Mobile Wound Care (MWC) database to capture and collate detailed medical histories, comorbidities, healing times and consumable costs for clients with wounds in Gippsland, Victoria. There were 3,726 wounds documented from 2,350 clients, so an average of 1.6 wounds per client. Half (49.6%) of all clients were females, indicating that there were no gender differences in terms of wound prevalence. The clients were primarily older people, with an average age of 64.3 years (ranging between 0.7 and 102.9 years). The majority of the wounds (56%) were acute and described as surgical, crush and trauma. The MWC database categorized the elements that influenced wound healing into 3 groups—factors affecting healing (FAH), comorbidities, and medications known to affect wound healing. While there were a multitude of significant associations, multiple linear regression identified the following key elements: age over 65 years, obesity, nonadherence to treatment plan, peripheral vascular disease, specific wounds associated with pressure/friction/shear, confirmed infection, and cerebrovascular accident (stroke). Wound healing is a complex process that requires a thorough understanding of influencing elements to improve healing times.

▶ This population-based study evaluated wounds in a rural area in Australia with a population of 240 000. There were 3726 wounds documented from

2350 individuals. The majority of the wounds (56%) were acute wounds, described as surgical, crush, and trauma. Another 12.9% were associated with leg ulcers (venous, arterial, mixed, and neuropathic) and 9.4% were pressure ulcers to 10 conditions. Hypertension (52%) and diabetes (25%) were found to be the most prevalent comorbidities in those who were injured. Advanced age >65 years, obesity, nonadherence to treatment plan, peripheral vascular disease, pressure/friction/shear wound causation, confirmed wound infection, and cerebrovascular accident. The presence of hypertension significantly increased healing time of wounds.

Large population-based studies such as this one provide important insight as to expected healing durations and the local and systemic factors that can be responsible for delaying healing. Focusing on these variables can have important impacts on health care delivery, improving patient outcomes, and reducing expenditures.

J. M. Daly, MD, FACS, FRCSI (Hon), FRCSG (Hon)

Effects of rapid wound sealing on survival and blood loss in a swine model of lethal junctional arterial hemorrhage

St. John AE, Wang X, Lim EB, et al (Univ of Washington, Seattle)

J Trauma Acute Care Surg 79:256-262, 2015

Background.—Hemostatic gauzes, which must be packed into wounds and compressed for several minutes, may be of limited use for noncompressible wounds in junctional anatomic locations. Rapid mechanical wound sealing is an alternative approach that seals the wound at the skin, allowing internal clot formation. We evaluate wound sealing for junctional hemorrhage control using a hemostatic clamp (iTClamp).

Methods.—Severe junctional hemorrhage was induced in anesthetized immature female swine using a 5-mm femoral arteriotomy. After 30 seconds of free bleeding, animals were randomized to one of seven hemostatic interventions: no intervention (control), direct compression for 3 minutes (compression), plain gauze packing (packing), mechanical wound seal (seal), plain gauze packing + wound seal (packing + seal), plain gauze packing + compression (packing + compression), or hemostatic gauze packing (Combat Gauze) + compression (HS-packing + compression). All animals then received one 15-mL/kg bolus of Hextend, followed by lactated Ringer's solution for hypotension up to 100 mL/kg. Animals were monitored for 3 hours.

Results.—Survival was similar between control (3-hour survival, 0%) and compression (0%, Kaplan-Meier survival analysis and log-rank test [KM-LR], $p = 1.0$) but marginally improved with packing (12.5%, KM-LR, $p < 0.001$). Survival improved with seal (62.5%) versus control (KM-LR, $p < 0.001$) and with packing + seal (100%) versus packing alone (KM-LR, $p < 0.001$). Survival was similar between packing + compression (87.5%), HS-packing + compression (62.5%), and packing + seal (100%) (KM-LR, $p \geq 0.05$). Total hemorrhage volume was decreased for seal versus control ($p < 0.001$) and for packing + seal versus packing ($p < 0.001$). Hemorrhage was similar among packing + compression, HS-packing + compression, seal, and packing + seal (analysis of variance $p \geq 0.05$). Application times (mean [SD]) were significantly faster with packing+ seal (125.8 [56.2] seconds) than packing + compression (236.6 [7.2] seconds) and HS-packing + compression (223.0 [6.8] seconds) (analysis of variance, all $p < 0.001$).

Conclusion.—In this preclinical junctional hemorrhage model, rapid wound sealing improved survival and decreased hemorrhage in both packed and unpacked wounds and performed comparably with standard-of-care hemostatic bandages. Rapidly sealing junctional wounds may be a viable alternative to wound compression.

▶ In both civilian and military trauma, control of hemorrhage is of primary concern. When the injury occurs in the more distal limb, proximal occlusion can be lifesaving. However, as the authors point out, penetrating injuries to junctional points such as the neck, groin, and axilla can be difficult to control. In addition, the type of situation may preclude longer and continuous compression by health workers. Thus, the swine hemorrhage model was used to mimic the human penetrating trauma situation.

Hemorrhage control was best achieved by pressure with both plain and hemostatic gauze as well as by the wound seal device with or without plain gauze. Pressure and wound seal techniques independently improved survival.

Studies such as this lead to further investigations, such as when and how much fluid resuscitation should occur to maximize survival. We should also understand what are the consequences to the injured distal limb when tourniquets or wound-sealing devices are used. The model and hemostatic techniques clearly bear further study.

J. M. Daly, MD, FACS, FRCSI (Hon), FRCSG (Hon)

Mesenchymal stem cell—based therapy for nonhealing wounds: today and tomorrow

Li M, Zhao Y, Hao H, et al (Inst of Basic Med Science, Beijing, Peoples Republic of China; et al)

Wound Repair Regen 23:465-482, 2015

Although advancements have been made with traditional therapies, the treatment of chronic nonhealing wounds still remains a tough challenge. In the past two decades, mesenchymal stem cell (MSC)—based therapy has emerged as a promising therapeutic strategy for nonhealing wounds because of their characteristics including self-renewal and a multidirectional differentiation ability and their easy collection and weak immunogenicity. There is a growing body of basic scientific studies that shed light on the functional mechanism of MSCs in modulating nonhealing wounds. Furthermore, critical advances have been achieved using

MSC-based therapy in preclinical animal models as well as in clinics trials. In this present review, we summarize the mechanisms of MSCs and highlight the important preclinical and clinical trials of MSC therapy for non-healing wounds. In particular, the combination of MSCs transplantation and tissue-engineered skin is addressed as a new strategy to optimize the delivery efficiency and therapeutic potential. Additionally, the current drawbacks of MSC therapy and the potential to further optimize the use of MSCs are implied.

▶ Nonhealing chronic wounds result in major morbidity for patients, loss of productivity, and enormous health care expenditures. A large amount of basic and clinical research continues to investigate the processes of healing that is normal and processes that are interrupted and delayed. Standard approaches are often not successful once the nonhealing cascade begins because of systemic factors in the individual or local factors in the area of the wound. This review article nicely describes the use of mesenchymal stem cells (MSC) in the therapy of nonhealing wounds. Importantly, the review article describes the biochemical, growth factor, and physiologic consequences of MSC therapy. It also describes the potential harms (cancer development) that may occur. The future of MSC therapy for clinical treatment is not clear nor unanimous, but early studies are suggestive of benefit in patients with chronic nonhealing wounds. Can this therapy accelerate "normal" healing, perhaps not. However, there is an area that bears close watching.

J. M. Daly, MD, FACS, FRCSI (Hon), FRCSG (Hon)

Cost-effectiveness of becaplermin gel on wound healing of diabetic foot ulcers

Gilligan AM, Waycaster CR, Motley TA (Smith and Nephew, Inc., Fort Worth, TX; Univ of North Texas Health Sciences Ctr, Fort Worth)

Wound Repair Regen 23:353-360, 2015

We sought to determine the long-term cost effectiveness (payer's perspective) of becaplermin gel plus good wound care (BGWC) vs. good wound care (GWC) alone in terms of wound healing and risk of amputation in patients with diabetic foot ulcers (DFUs). Outcomes data were derived from a propensity score-matched cohort from the Curative Health Services database between 1998 and 2004, which was followed for 20 weeks. A four-state Markov model was used to predict costs and outcomes of wound healing and risk of amputation for BGWC vs. GWC alone over 1 year in patients with DFU. The primary outcome was closed-wound weeks. Transition probabilities for healing and amputation were derived from the aforementioned propensity score-matched cohorts. Ulcer recurrence was estimated from the medical literature. Utilization for becaplermin was calculated using the dosing algorithm in the product labeling. Of 24,898 eligible patients, 9.6% received BGWC. Based on the model, patients treated with BGWC had substantially more closed-wound weeks compared with GWC (16.1 vs. 12.5 weeks, respectively). More patients receiving BGWC had healed wounds at 1 year compared with those receiving GWC (48.1% vs. 38.3%). Risk of amputation was lower in the BGWC cohort (6.8% vs. 9.8%). Expected annual direct costs for DFU were $21,920 for BGWC and $24,640 for GWC. BGWC was economically dominant over GWC, providing better outcomes at a lower cost in patients with DFU. Compared with GWC alone, BGWC is more effective in healing wounds and lowering amputation risk, thereby decreasing long-term costs for DFU.

▶ There is little question that the presence of diabetes mellitus is a major comorbidity, leading to diabetic foot ulcers and major amputations, which lead to enormous economic health care expenditures, decreased quality of life, and loss of productivity. These investigators sought to determine the economic outcomes when becaplermin gel was used as an adjunct to good wound care versus good wound care alone for patients with diabetic foot ulcers. Becaplermin gel is platelet-derived growth factor that stimulates cellular growth and migration of granulation tissue, thereby promoting healing.

Controlling for mortality rates, ulcer recurrence, and amputation rates over 1 year, the projected healing rates were greater for the becaplermin gel plus good wound care (BGWC) group (48.4% vs 38.7%, respectively). In addition, the projected amputation rates were less for the BGWC group (6.8% vs 9.8%, respectively; $P < .0001$). Thus, it appears that use of this gel as an adjunct to good wound care helps patients and is economically superior to good wound care alone.

J. M. Daly, MD, FACS, FRCSI (Hon), FRCSG (Hon)

A topical aqueous oxygen emulsion stimulates granulation tissue formation in a porcine second-degree burn wound

Li J, Zhang Y-P, Zarei M, et al (Univ of Miami Miller School of Medicine, FL)
Burns 41:1049-1057, 2015

Background.—Oxygen is an essential substance for wound healing. Limited studies have shown that topical oxygen can influence healing. This study evaluated the effects of a Topical Oxygen Emulsion (TOE) on burn wound healing.

Methods.—A porcine second-degree burn wound model was used in the study. Burn wounds were randomly assigned to TOE, vehicle control, and no-treatment (air) groups. Effects of TOE on the granulation tissue formation and angiogenesis were studied using hematoxylin and eosin histological analysis. Protein production and gene expression of types I and III collagen and vascular endothelial growth factor (VEGF) were determined using immuno-fluorescent staining and Reverse Transcription and Polymerase Chain Reaction (RT-PCR), respectively.

Results.—The TOE treated wounds exhibited better angiogenesis and granulation tissue formation by histology examination. The immunofluorescence staining and RT-PCR analysis demonstrated that protein production and mRNA expression of VEGF and collagen III were significantly higher in TOE treatment group than vehicle alone and air control groups, while there was no significant difference in the level of collagen I.

Conclusions.—Our data demonstrate that TOE enhances burn wound healing via stimulating the expression of VEGF and type III collagen and strongly indicates the potential use of TOE in wounds.

▶ Rapid and complete healing of burn wounds is essential to reduce morbidity and mortality of patients. It is especially critical that second-degree burn wounds do not progress to third-degree wounds requiring excision and skin grafting. It is known that oxygen plays an important role in all aspects of wound healing through a variety of cellular mechanisms involving the host and local bacteria. In some instances, hyperbaric oxygen therapy has been used but is now indicated only for carbon monoxide poisoning and treatment of gas gangrene. The authors noted that "in a case-series study topical oxygen therapy (TOT) has shown no detrimental effects on wounds and showed beneficial indications in promoting wound healing. However, TOT has limited ability to penetrate the skin.

Topical Oxygen Emulsion (TOE) is a relative new technique which delivers emulsion-containing supersaturated oxygen to a wound and slowly releases additional oxygen. This technology is based on perfluorocarbon droplets being encapsulated within an aqueous continuous phase and has a high oxygen carrying capacity." In their pig burn model, the application of TOT significantly increased the expression of VEGF and type III collagen, suggesting this type of therapy should be further studied in this experimental model to actually determine its effects on the rate of healing, local bacterial colonization, and so on. If this treatment proves truly efficacious and without toxicity, then human trials may well be indicated.

J. M. Daly, MD, FACS, FRCSI (Hon), FRCSG (Hon)

Biodegradable soy wound dressings with controlled release of antibiotics: Results from a guinea pig burn model

Egozi D, Baranes-Zeevi M, Ullmann Y, et al (Kaplan Med Ctr, Rehovot, Israel; Tel-Aviv Univ, Israel; Technion – Israel Inst of Technology, Haifa; et al)

Burns 41:1459-1467, 2015

There is growing interest in the development of biodegradable materials from renewable biopolymers, such as soy protein, for biomedical applications. Soy protein is a major fraction of natural soybean and has the advantages of being economically competitive, biodegradable and biocompatible. It presents good water resistance as well as storage stability. In the current study, homogenous antibiotic-loaded soy protein films were cast from aqueous solutions. The antibiotic drug gentamicin was incorporated into the films in order to inhibit bacterial growth, and thus prevent or combat infection, upon its controlled release to the surrounding tissue. The current *in vivo* study of the dressing material in contaminated deep second-degree burn wounds in guinea pigs ($n = 20$) demonstrated its ability to accelerate epithelialization with 71% epithelial coverage compared to an unloaded format of the soy material (62%) and a significant improved epithelial coverage as compared to the conventional dressing material (55%). Our new platform of antibiotic-eluting wound dressings is advantageous over currently used popular dressing materials that provide controlled release of silver ions, due to its gentamicin release profile, which is safer. Another advantage of our novel concept is that it is based on a biodegradable natural polymer and therefore does not require bandage changes and offers a potentially valuable and economic approach for treating burn-related infections.

▶ Biodegradable burn wound dressings have a clear advantage in that they do not have to be removed as part of dressing changes, thus sparing the patient pain during or after this process. However, the polymer should be relatively inexpensive and have degradation properties that optimize the healing process. Impregnating the biodegradable dressing film with antibiotics can allow the slow release of the antibacterial reducing infection rates.

This interesting animal study evaluated a soy protein biodegradable dressing in an infected burn wound guinea pig model with and without gentamicin impregnated into the dressing. The results showed that the soy dressing itself had a major effect on the healing process with a slight improvement when gentamicin was added to the dressing. As the authors have noted, some individuals are allergic to soy protein, but they are in the minority. Additionally, depending on the magnitude of the burn injury, gentamicin levels could result in toxicity. Much further animal and clinical research is needed before these products are ready for clinical use, but this novel approach using relatively inexpensive soy protein may prove beneficial to patients.

J. M. Daly, MD, FACS, FRCSI (Hon), FRCSG (Hon)

Accelerated healing in NONcNZO10/LtJ type 2 diabetic mice by FGF-1

Blaber SI, Diaz J, Blaber M (Florida State Univ, Tallahassee)

Wound Repair Regen 23:538-549, 2015

The development of novel therapies to treat chronic diabetic ulcers depends upon appropriate animal models for early stage investigation. The NONcNZO10/LtJ mouse is a new polygenic strain developed to more realistically model human metabolic syndrome and obesity-induced type 2 diabetes; however, detailed wound healing properties have not been reported. Herein, we describe a quantitative wound healing study in the NONcNZO10/LtJ mouse using a splinted excisional wound.

The rate of wound healing is compared to various controls, and is also quantified in response to topical administration of normal and mutant fibroblast growth factor-1 (FGF-1). Quantitation of reepithelialization shows that the diabetic condition in the NONcNZO10/LtJ mouse is concomitant with a decreased rate of dermal healing. Furthermore, topical administration of a FGF-1/heparin formulation effectively accelerates reepithelialization. A similar acceleration can also be achieved by a stabilized mutant form of FGF-1 formulated in the absence of heparin. Such accelerated rates of healing are not associated with any abnormal histology in the healed wounds. The results identify the NONcNZO10/LtJ mouse as a useful model of impaired wound healing in type 2 diabetes, and further, identify engineered forms of FGF-1 as a potential "second-generation" therapeutic to promote diabetic dermal wound healing.

▶ The majority of diabetic patients in the Western world have type II diabetes associated with obesity. In these patients, wound healing is dramatically impaired resulting in untold medical costs both in the hospital and at home as well as impaired function and productivity. A number of diabetic animal models (genetic and biochemical) have been used to study the physiologic and biochemical processes involved in impaired wound healing. To develop new therapies to ameliorate healing deficits, the models themselves need to emulate the processes found in obesity-associated human diabetes.

In these studies, the investigators evaluated a novel polygenic mouse strain (NONcNZO10/LtJ) to determine the effects on a healing dermal wound. They noted acceleration of healing using local administration of fibroblast growth factor (FGF-1) with or without stabilization with heparin.

Further characterization of this mouse model will be important to fully determine all of the wound-healing processes to be sure they truly mimic healing events in the human, obese diabetic condition.

J. M. Daly, MD, FACS, FRCSI (Hon), FRCSG (Hon)

Effective use of Biobrane as a temporary wound dressing prior to definitive split-skin graft in the treatment of severe burn: A retrospective analysis

Tan H, Wasiak J, Paul E, et al (Monash Univ, Melbourne, Victoria, Australia)

Burns 41:969-976, 2015

Aims.—To report on the use of Biobrane, a synthetic skin substitute, as a temporary wound cover in patients with severe burn. In particular we wished to examine the role of Biobrane in maintaining a healthy wound bed following surgical excision and identify factors associated with regrafting.

Methods.—A retrospective case series review was performed on patients with severe burns (≥20% TBSA), admitted to the Victorian Adult Burns Service, in Melbourne, from January 2009 to June 2012. Logistic regression analysis was performed to identify factors associated with regrafting.

Results.—Out of 58 patients with median %TBSA burn of 30%, 22 patients (37.9%) required regrafting of at least one area previously treated with Biobrane and split-skin graft. On univariate analysis, need for regrafting was significantly associated with increasing %TBSA (OR 1.04, 95% CI: 1.01–1.08; $p = 0.02$); and after multivariate analysis to adjust for this effect, hospital LOS (OR 1.04, 95% CI: 1.02–1.07; $p = 0.001$); total operative time (OR 1.16, 95% CI; 1.06–1.28; $p = 0.002$) and total number of surgeries (OR 1.69, 95% CI: 1.27–2.26, $p < 0.001$) remained significantly associated with regrafting. Age, gender, time to surgical debridement and Biobrane application, and anatomical region were not found to be associated with regraft.

Conclusion.—At our institution, Biobrane has emerged as an alternative option to maintain a healthy wound bed after burn excision and prior to grafting. Our small number of extensive graft failures, small areas of regrafting and low infection rate following Biobrane application reflects our current experience with Biobrane. Precise indications and most appropriate methods for Biobrane use are yet to be established.

▶ In patients with major burn injury, coverage and complete healing of their wounds is critical to reducing their mortality. Donor sites may be unavailable for immediate split thickness skin grafts, and so artificial skin substitutes have been developed for use.

As the authors noted, "Biobrane is a bilaminate biosynthetic skin substitute composed of nylon mesh coated with collagen peptides bonded to a silicon membrane, designed to mimic the properties of the dermis and epidermis respectively. It therefore possesses many of the features of an ideal skin substitute such as wound adherence, protection from contamination, flexibility, good water vapor transmission, low cost, and ease of application and transparency for wound observation." This retrospective study evaluated 58 patients treated with Biobrane before split thickness skin grafting.

A total of 22 patients (38%) required a regraft of at least 2 area previously treated with Biobrane and autologous split thickness skin graft. Upon analysis, a higher rate of regraft was associated with larger burns, hospital length of stay, total operative time, and total number of operations.

This is an interesting study that unfortunately does not have a control group for comparison even with its retrospective analysis. It will be helpful for the authors to evaluate redraft rates in those not treated by Biobrane at their institution even if done in a different time period and to develop a prospective database that they can use to establish factors important in redrafting with and without Biobrane.

J. M. Daly, MD, FACS, FRCSI (Hon), FRCSG (Hon)

Effects of Botulinum Toxin A Injection on Healing and Tensile Strength of Ruptured Rabbit Achilles Tendons

Tuzuner S, Özkan Ö, Erin N, et al (Adana Numune Res and Training Hosp, Adana, Turkey)

Ann Plast Surg 74:496-500, 2015

Background.—Tendon lacerations are most commonly managed with surgical repair. Postoperative complications such as adhesions and ruptures often occur with immobilization. Early postoperative mobilization is therefore advised to minimize complications and time required to return to daily life. The aim of this study was to evaluate whether botulinum neurotoxin type-A (BoNT-A) can be used to enhance healing and prevent rupture in mobilized animals with Achilles tenotomy.

Methods.—Twenty-seven rabbits were divided into 3 groups, namely, I, II, and III, after surgical 1-sided Achilles tenotomy and end-to-end repair. The control group for biomechanical comparisons consisted of randomly selected contralateral (unoperated) healthy Achilles tendons. Group I received BoNT-A (4 U/kg) injection into the calf muscles. One week later, electromyographical confirmation was performed to establish the effects of injection. Surgery was then performed. Animals in the second group ($n = 9$, group II) were immobilized with a cast postoperatively. The third group ($n = 9$, group III) was mobilized immediately with no cast or BoNT-A. Tendons were harvested and gap formation or ruptures as well as strength of the repaired tendon were assessed 6 weeks after surgery.

Results.—Achilles tendons healed in all animals injected with BoNT-A, whereas all were ruptured in group III. All Achilles tendons of animals in groups I and II healed. However, group I repaired tendons were biomechanically equivalent to healthy tendons, whereas group II repaired tendons demonstrated significantly decreased tensile strength ($P = 0.009$).

Conclusions.—The present study suggests that local injection of BoNT-A can be used for treatment of tendon rupture and may replace the use of cast for immobilization. However, further studies are needed to determine whether BoNT-A injection can have a beneficial effect on the healing of tendon repairs in humans.

▶ Tissue repair, especially of tendons, is an inexact science in terms of the duration of immobilization and the type of physical therapy that results in maximum healing and function afterward. This animal study is interesting in that the 3 groups were chosen to mimic the clinical situation. Clearly, no repair resulted in no scar bridging and nonhealing of the tendon edges. Immediate repair resulted in healing, but tensile strength was worse when the limb was immobilized for a week postrepair. This result is in keeping with numerous other reports that some degree of tension is important to help align collagen fibrils and cross-linking, which maximizes strength. The use of botulinum toxin A to weaken the limb calf muscles in the short term offers a unique manner to diminish but not eliminate tension on the tendon repair and maximize tendon strength.

There is a great deal of more work to do before this approach becomes clinically applicable, but the concept merits further investigation.

J. M. Daly, MD, FACS, FRCSI (Hon), FRCSG (Hon)

Evaluation of Aquacel Ag for Autogenous Skin Donor Sites

Haith LR, Stair-Buchmann ME, Ackerman BH, et al (Crozer-Chester Med Ctr, Upland, PA)

J Burn Care Res 36:602-606, 2015

An ongoing objective of burn research is to evaluate wound dressings and develop new treatments to expedite wound healing. This was a single-center, prospective, randomized, controlled study to evaluate the effectiveness of Aquacel Ag as a dressing for autogenous skin donor sites compared with Xeroform. We hypothesized that donor sites treated with Aquacel Ag would heal faster. Patients were considered for enrollment if they required skin grafting with two donor sites >100 cm^2 at least 2 inches apart. Dressings were observed daily starting on post-op day #2 until discharge and then weekly in the outpatient burn clinic. Assessments evaluated pain, infection, and reapplication. Photographs were taken on post-op day #2, upon "90% re-epithelialization," and at post-op day #30–45. Scar assessments and blinded photographic reviews were completed to assess cosmetic healing. Twenty-nine patients completed the study. Re-epithelialization occurred faster with Xeroform (15.2 days vs 17.6 days). Daily pain scores were higher with Xeroform (6.72 vs 5.68) and Aquacel Ag needed to be replaced more often (1.72 times vs 0.10 times). Three patients developed donor site infections with Aquacel Ag. Scar scores between the donor sites were not statistically significant. The blinded photo review concluded that Xeroform had a better cosmetic outcome (24 vs 10%). Although patients complained of more pain with Xeroform, it demonstrated shorter healing times and better cosmetic outcomes. Aquacel Ag needed to be replaced more often and represented the only three donor site infections.

► A major condition of clinical practice is to continually evaluate our standard care practices to determine whether newer therapies can result in better outcomes for our patients. This study was a single-center, prospective, randomized, controlled study to evaluate the effectiveness of Aquacel Ag for the use as a dressing for autogenous skin donor sites compared with Xeroform, which was the standard treatment at the onset of this study. Although the newer therapy was thought to be an improvement, it turned out that Xeroform was superior as a donor site dressing except for donor site pain that the patients experienced. As noted, Xeroform required fewer dressing site changes, healed faster, and was cosmetically superior to the Aquacel Ag treatment. This study points out the importance of prospective trials that question our standard care protocols. Many such trials should be done to help us develop evidence-based medical care.

J. M. Daly, MD, FACS, FRCSI (Hon), FRCSG (Hon)

Delayed Primary Closure of Fasciotomy Incisions in the Lower Leg: Do We Need to Change Our Strategy?

Weaver MJ, Owen TM, Morgan JH, et al (Brigham and Women's Hosp, Boston, MA; Virginia Tech Carilion School of Medicine, Roanoke)

J Orthop Trauma 29:308-311, 2015

Objectives.—The primary purpose of this study is to determine whether a strategy of bringing patients back to the operating room for successive debridements allows for the eventual delayed primary closure (DPC) of fasciotomy wounds.

Design.—Retrospective cohort study. Data were collected from medical records and radiographs.

Setting.—Two urban level 1 trauma centers.

Patients.—One hundred four adult patients with acute compartment syndrome in the setting of a tibia fracture (open or closed).

Intervention.—All patients underwent decompressive fasciotomies with closure by either DPC or split-thickness skin grafting (STSG) during a subsequent surgical procedure.

Main Outcome Measure.—Number of fasciotomy wounds closed by DPC after the initial fasciotomy procedure.

Results.—Of the 104 patients brought to the operating room for their first debridement after their fasciotomies, 19 patients (18%) were treated with DPC, whereas 42 patients (40%) were closed with STSG because they were believed to be too swollen to allow for primary closure by the treating surgeon. Three of the remaining 43 patients were treated with DPC during their second debridement. No patients who underwent more than 2 washouts could be treated with DPC. No patients who sustained open fractures were able to be closed by DPC ($P = 0.02$). Patients who underwent STSG on their first postfasciotomy procedure had a significantly shorter hospital stay than patients who underwent additional procedures before closure (12.2 vs. 17.4 days; $P = 0.005$).

Conclusions.—Fasciotomy wounds that are not able to be primarily closed during their first postfasciotomy surgical procedure are rarely closed through DPC techniques. Early skin grafting of these wounds should be considered, especially in the clinical setting of an open injury, because it significantly decreases the length of hospital stay. Other techniques that avoid repeated debridements and attempted closures might also help reduce hospital stay.

▶ Patients who require fasciotomies for compartment syndrome after tibial fractures often have to be returned to the operating room for delayed primary closure because the leg is too swollen to attempt primary closure initially.

This process takes a lot of time, and the wound may become infected, resulting in tissue necrosis and further damage. These authors retrospectively reviewed their experiences at two institutions through chart review and learned that patients with attempted delayed primary closure spent significantly more time in the hospital and had great disability than those for whom a split thickness skin graft was placed early in the healing process.

One should realize that the choice of one treatment versus the other was done based on the injury and the recipient wound bed. It is certainly possible that split-thickness skin grafting was not possible because of infection or other factors and those repeated debridements and delayed primary closure was attempted. A next step would be to prospectively study this issue at the two institutions and perhaps perform a randomized trial to determine the best approach for treatment of these patients.

J. M. Daly, MD, FACS, FRCSI (Hon), FRCSG (Hon)

Effect of Fibroblast-Seeded Artificial Dermis on Wound Healing

Jang JC, Choi R-J, Han S-K, et al (Korea Univ College of Medicine, Seoul, Republic of Korea; Seoul Natl Univ, Republic of Korea)

Ann Plast Surg 74:501-507, 2015

In covering wounds, efforts should include use of the safest and least invasive methods with a goal of achieving optimal functional and cosmetic outcome. The recent development of advanced technology in wound healing has triggered the use of cells and/or biological dermis to improve wound healing conditions. The purpose of the study was to evaluate the effects of fibroblast-seeded artificial dermis on wound healing efficacy.

Ten nude mice were used in this study. Four full-thickness 6-mm punch wounds were created on the dorsal surface of each mouse (total, 40 wounds). The wounds were randomly assigned to one of the following 4 treatments: topical application of Dulbecco phosphate-buffered saline (control), human fibroblasts (FB), artificial dermis (AD), and human fibroblast-seeded artificial dermis (AD with FB). On the 14th day after treatment, wound healing rate and wound contraction, which are the 2 main factors determining wound healing efficacy, were evaluated using a stereoimage optical topometer system, histomorphological analysis, and immunohistochemistry.

The results of the stereoimage optical topometer system demonstrated that the FB group did not have significant influence on wound healing rate and wound contraction. The AD group showed reduced wound contraction, but wound healing was delayed. The AD with FB group showed decreased wound contraction without significantly delayed wound healing. Histomorphological analysis exhibited that more normal skin structure was regenerated in the AD with FB group. Immunohistochemistry demonstrated that the AD group and the AD with FB group produced less α-smooth muscle actin than the control group, but this was not shown in the FB group.

Fibroblast-seeded artificial dermis may minimize wound contraction without significantly delaying wound healing in the treatment of skin and soft tissue defects.

▶ Optimal wound healing should result in complete coverage that is cosmetically the best it can be. As the authors have noted, artificial dermis products have been developed to help accelerate wound healing while trying to maximize the cosmetic outcomes. This experimental animal study evaluated fibroblast impregnated dermis compared with dermis alone and standard saline control in nude mice. They measured wound healing rate and contracture and noted significantly improved results in both measures using the fibroblast seeded artificial dermis. Animal studies such as these are supportive of the fibroblast seeding of artificial dermis, but further prospective work is required in humans to be certain that the outcomes described translate from the nude mouse model, which has different dermal cellular composition than humans.

J. M. Daly, MD, FACS, FRCSI (Hon), FRCSG (Hon)

4 Critical Care

Maintaining an open trauma intensive care unit bed for rapid admission can be cost-effective

Fryman L, Talley C, Kearney P, et al (Univ of Kentucky HealthCare, Lexington)

J Trauma Acute Care Surg 79:98-104, 2015

Background.—In 2012, we implemented a ready open trauma intensive care unit (TICU) bed process. Our hypothesis was that this process would decrease emergency department (ED) length of stay (LOS) in a cost-effective manner without worsening clinical outcomes.

Methods.—We developed a charge nurse without a patient assignment to facilitate this open bed. We also provided team training for early ICU resuscitation. All Level 1 activations admitted directly to the TICU before and after the implementation were examined. Patients taken directly to the operating room from the ED, deaths within 24 hours of admission, and patients with nonsurvivable head injuries were excluded. Cost-effectiveness of the position was examined.

Results.—Age (mean [SD], 45.78 [18.71] years), sex (74.7% male), and Injury Severity Score (ISS) (mean [SD], 17.27 [9.26]) were not significantly different. Median ED LOS for the postimplementation group decreased from 230 minutes to 66 minutes ($p < 0.001$). Median ICU LOS (from 3.29 to 2.98 days, $p = 0.13$) and total median hospital LOS (from 10.71 to 7.98 days, $p = 0.06$) decreased but were not statistically significant. Controlling for age, ISS, sex, and mechanism of injury the postimplementation group had a 29% reduction in ICU LOS (2.12 days), a 28% reduction in hospital LOS (4.34), and a 54% reduction in ED LOS (154 minutes). The LOS decreased despite a small increase in ISS (from 15.89 to 18.37). Observed/expected mortality did not differ between the groups, preimplementation/postimplementation of 0.87 and 0.92. Nursing productivity increased one nurse after implementation at a cost of $624 per day. The ICU LOS decrease of 1.6 days at a rate of $1,144 average ICU daily cost of room and board totaled $1,830 per patient. The decreased ICU LOS dollars minus the increase nurse pay resulted in an overall savings of $1,206 per patient.

Conclusion.—Rapid access to the TICU made possible by the charge nurse without a direct assignment and team training has a potential cost savings without adversely affecting patient outcomes.

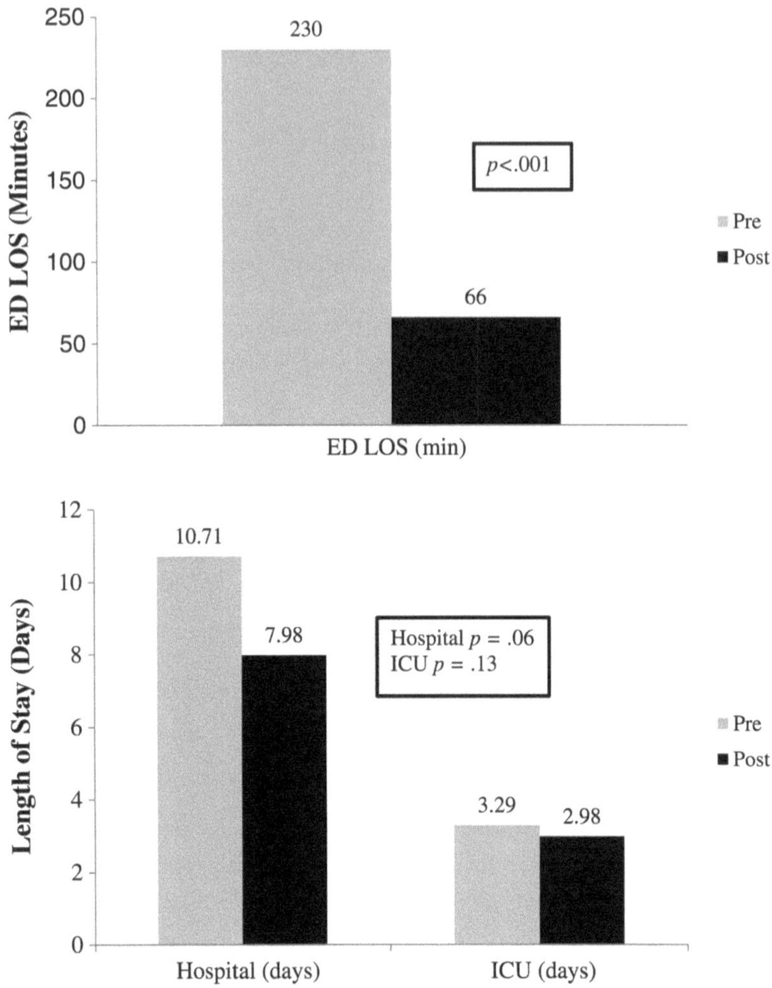

Note: Emergency Department (ED); Intensive Care Unit (ICU); hospital length of stay (LOS). ED LOS reported in minutes; ICU and hospital LOS reported in days.

FIGURE 2.—Median ED, hospital, and ICU LOS. (Reprinted from Fryman L, Talley C, Kearney P, et al. Maintaining an open trauma intensive care unit bed for rapid admission can be cost-effective. *J Trauma Acute Care Surg*. 2015;79:98-104, with permission from Wolters Kluwer Health, Inc.)

Level of Evidence.—Cost analysis, level III (Fig 2).

▶ An increase in emergency department length of stay can have a negative impact on overall patient outcomes and satisfaction. However, inpatient beds are decreasing as emergency department patient visits are increasing, causing a mismatch in patient volume and bed availability. Trauma centers around the country struggle with throughput issues, and one focus may be the rapid mobilization of the critically injured patient to the trauma intensive care unit. The authors of this selection describe their approach to maintaining intensive care unit availability. By using this approach, they dramatically reduce emergency department length of stay as well as hospital days and ICU days. These results are included as Fig 2. The study was somewhat limited by being retrospective in nature and did not address patients being admitted to units other than the trauma intensive care unit. Rapid access to the trauma intensive care unit was facilitated by the trauma intensive care unit charge nurse and trauma resuscitation team. This provided a potential cost savings without adversely affecting patient outcomes in this level 1 trauma center.

D. W. Mozingo, MD

Misclassification of acute respiratory distress syndrome after traumatic injury: The cost of less rigorous approaches

Hendrickson CM, Dobbins S, Redick BJ, et al (Univ of California, San Francisco)

J Trauma Acute Care Surg 79:417-424, 2015

Background.—Adherence to rigorous research protocols for identifying adult respiratory distress syndrome (ARDS) after trauma is variable. To examine how misclassification of ARDS may bias observational studies in trauma populations, we evaluated the agreement of two methods for adjudicating ARDS after trauma: the current gold standard, direct review of chest radiographs and review of dictated radiology reports, a commonly used alternative.

Methods.—This nested cohort study included 123 mechanically ventilated patients between 2005 and 2008, with at least one $Pa{O_2}/FI{O_2}$ less than 300 within the first 8 days of admission. Two blinded physician investigators adjudicated ARDS by two methods. The investigators directly reviewed all chest radiographs to evaluate for bilateral infiltrates. Several months later, blinded to their previous assessments, they adjudicated ARDS using a standardized rubric to classify radiology reports. A κ statistics was calculated. Regression analyses quantified the association between established risk factors as well as important clinical outcomes and ARDS determined by the aforementioned methods as well as hypoxemia as a surrogate marker.

Results.—The κ was 0.47 for the observed agreement between ARDS adjudicated by direct review of chest radiographs and ARDS adjudicated by review of radiology reports. Both the magnitude and direction of bias on the estimates of association between ARDS and established risk factors as well as clinical outcomes varied by method of adjudication.

Conclusion.—Classification of ARDS by review of dictated radiology reports had only moderate agreement with the current gold standard, ARDS adjudicated by direct review of chest radiographs. While the misclassification of ARDS had varied effects on the estimates of associations with established risk factors, it tended to weaken the association of ARDS with important clinical outcomes. A standardized approach to ARDS adjudication after trauma by direct review of chest radiographs will minimize misclassification bias in future observational studies.

Level of Evidence.—Diagnostic study, level II (Fig 2).

► Lack of adherence to a standard approach for identifying acute respiratory distress syndrome (ARDS) cases may contribute to substantial variability in even basic epidemiologic studies. A wide range of the incidence of ARDS has been reported, and it is difficult to predict and adjust for the bias created by highly variable approaches to outcome evaluation in observational studies. Thus, biased estimates of association can be driven by the misclassification of just a few patients. The authors of this selection hypothesized that relying on dictated radiology reports, rather than direct review of chest radiographs, would result in substantial misclassification of ARDS in a cohort of patients

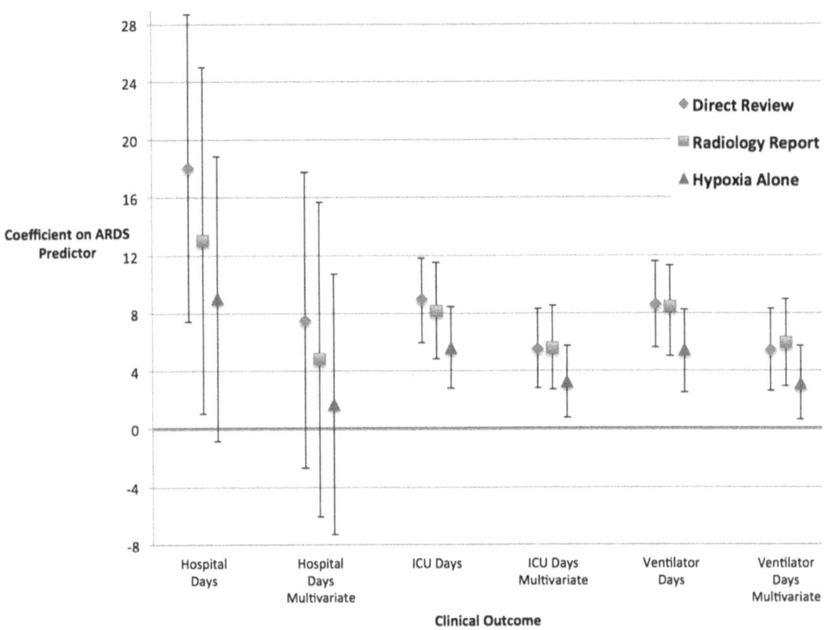

FIGURE 2.—Association of ARDS and clinical outcomes in linear regression models. Graphical presentation of findings from linear regression models showing the point estimates and 95% confidence interval of the β coefficients on the ARDS predictor variable for various clinical outcomes. All analyses excluded patients who died. Each style of marker represents a different method for adjudicating ARDS in hypoxemic trauma patients: direct review of chest radiographs, systematic evaluation of dictated reports of chest radiographs, and use of hypoxemia alone without consideration of chest radiograph findings. Multivariate models are adjusted for age and ISS. The findings for the outcome ventilator-free days were similar to ventilator days (Table 4, Clinical Outcomes Among Survivors in Univariate and Adjusted Linear Regression Models) but are not graphed here to streamline the visual presentation by limiting the range of values on the y-axis. *Editor's Note*: Please refer to original journal article for full references. (Reprinted from Hendrickson CM, Dobbins S, Redick BJ, et al. Misclassification of acute respiratory distress syndrome after traumatic injury: the cost of less rigorous approaches. *J Trauma Acute Care Surg.* 2015;79:417-424, with permission from Wolters Kluwer Health, Inc.)

with severe traumatic injuries who required mechanical ventilator support. They designed a protocol to evaluate the agreement between the 2 methods for ascertaining ARDS status: the current gold standard, direct review of chest radiographs by 2 clinician investigators, and a commonly used alternative, a systematic approach to review the radiology reports of the same chest radiographs. Fig 2 is included, which demonstrates their findings in a linear regression model. Although their findings are significant, the study has several limitations. The cohort evaluated is relatively small and was designed primarily to evaluate the agreement between the 2 methods of assigning the diagnosis of ARDS. Also, the small sample size likely contributes to the relatively large confidence intervals around the estimates of association.

D. W. Mozingo, MD

Acute kidney injury following severe trauma: Risk factors and long-term outcome

Eriksson M, Brattström O, Mårtensson J, et al (Karolinska Univ Hosp, Solna, Sweden; Karolinska Institutet, Stockholm, Sweden; et al)

J Trauma Acute Care Surg 79:407-412, 2015

Background.—The trauma patient sustains numerous potentially harmful insults that may contribute to a notable risk of acute kidney injury (AKI). The aim of this study was to investigate the incidence of and to identify risk factors for AKI in severely injured trauma patients admitted to the intensive care unit (ICU). The patients were followed up for 1 year with respect to survival and end-stage renal disease.

Methods.—Trauma patients admitted to the ICU for more than 24 hours at a Level I trauma center were included. The outcome measure was AKI diagnosed Days 2 to 7 of ICU treatment. Regression analysis was performed to identify factors associated with AKI development.

Results.—A quarter of the patients (103 of 413) developed AKI within the first week of ICU admission. AKI was associated with increased 30-day (17.5% vs. 5.8%) and 1-year (26.2% vs. 7.1%) mortality. Risk factors for AKI were male sex, age, nondiabetic comorbidity, diabetes mellitus, Injury Severity Score (ISS) greater than 40, massive transfusion, and volume loading with hydroxyethyl starch (HES) within the first 24 hours. Unexpectedly, sepsis before AKI onset, admission hypotension, and extensive contrast loading (>150 mL) were not associated with AKI development. None of the surviving AKI patients had developed end-stage renal disease 1 year after injury.

Conclusion.—AKI in ICU-admitted trauma patients is a common complication with substantial mortality. Diabetes, male sex, and severe injury were strong risk factors, but age, nondiabetic comorbidity, massive transfusion, and resuscitation with HES were also associated with postinjury AKI. Based on the results of the current study, volume resuscitation with HES cannot be recommended in trauma patients.

Level of Evidence.—Prognostic study, level III; therapeutic study, level IV (Fig 1).

▶ To what extent acute kidney injury (AKI) contributes to postinjury morbidity and mortality is not fully determined. Considering the frequent occurrence of this complication and the volume of severe trauma cases occurring annually, it is reasonable to assume that postinjury AKI may portend significant health problems. Thus, further insight into factors associated with strategies tailored to specific risk groups is needed. Until recently, the lack of a uniformly accepted definition of AKI has complicated research and comparison of studies. A new consensus definition merging the Risk, Injury, Failure, Loss, End stage (RIFLE) criteria and the Acute Kidney Injury Network (AKIN) definition, presented by the Kidney Disease Improving Global Outcomes (KDIGO) group, is now widely accepted. The aim of this study was to identify risk factors for postinjury AKI in intensive care unit–treated trauma patients. The authors of this selection used the new AKI definition in accordance with the consensus criteria. The patients who developed AKI were more likely to be male, were older, and had more comorbidity. They were more severely injured and exhibited signs

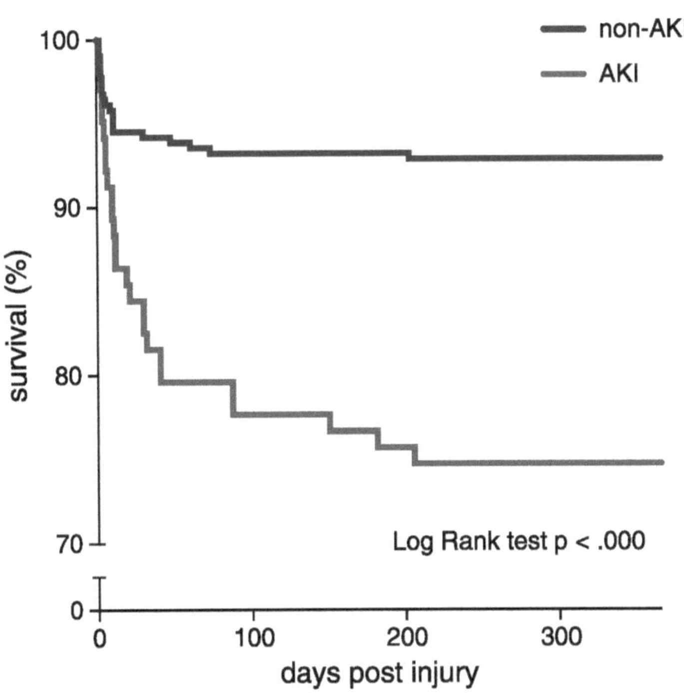

FIGURE 1.—One-year postinjury survival. Kaplan-Meier curves displaying 1-year postinjury survival for AKI (n = 103, *red line*) and non-AKI patients (n = 310, *blue line*). (For interpretation of the references to color in this figure legend, the reader is referred to web version of this article). (Reprinted from Eriksson M, Brattström O, Mårtensson J, et al. Acute kidney injury following severe trauma: risk factors and long-term outcome. *J Trauma Acute Care Surg.* 2015;79:407-412, with permission from Wolters Kluwer Health, Inc.)

of physiologic derangement on admission to a greater extent than those patients who did not develop AKI. Of note, patients with AKI had higher 30-day and 1-year postinjury mortality compared with the non-AKI cohort as noted in Fig 1. All deceased Swedish residents are recorded in the cause-of-death register. This register includes the cause and time of death and is updated yearly and linked to the patient charts, and therefore, no patients were lost to follow-up.

D. W. Mozingo, MD

Impact of advanced practice providers (nurse practitioners and physician assistants) on surgical residents' critical care experience

Kahn SA, Davis SA, Banes CT, et al (Vanderbilt Univ Med Ctr, Nashville, TN)
J Surg Res 199:7-12, 2015

Background.—Teaching hospitals often employ advanced practice providers (nurse practitioners and physician assistants or APPs) to counteract residents' work-hour restrictions. With increased utilization of APPs in labor-intense areas, such as intensive care units (ICUs), APPs may have an impact on resident education and experience. No studies have investigated the direct role an APP plays on the training experience of a surgical resident in the ICU.

Materials and Methods.—An institutional review board-approved survey was emailed to residents in Accreditation Council for Graduate Medical Education-accredited general surgery programs. Surveys asked about demographics, residency and/or ICU characteristics, and the effects of APPs on patient care, workflow, and educational experience. Regression analysis determined predictors of resident perception.

Results.—A total of 354 of 1178 residents responded to the survey (30%). Some residents felt that nurses calling APPs preferentially for patient-care issues interfered with education (17%) and residents' ability to follow patients (12%) and was associated with overall detrimental effects to ICU experience on regression (odds ratio, 3.7; confidence interval, 1.5−9.1). Most residents reported positive effects of APPs, such as reduced resident workload (79.8%), teaching protocols and/or guidelines (60.3%), enhanced patient care (60.3%), and enhanced communication (50.5%). When asked how APPs affected their overall ICU experience, 48.4% reported positive effects, 20.6% reported "no effect," and 31% reported detrimental effects.

Conclusions.—Only a minority of residents perceived that APPs detract from training, particularly those who felt excluded when nurses preferentially contact APPs with patientcare issues. APPs have the potential to enhance training and ICU experience, as reflected in many of the responses. Strategies to maintain direct nurse and resident communication

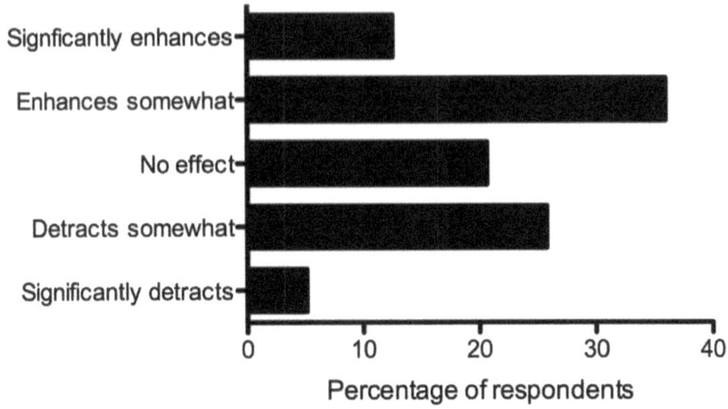

FIGURE 4.—Bar graph representing residents' perceptions of APPs effect on overall ICU experience: significantly enhance (12.5%), enhance somewhat (35.9%), no effect (20.6%), detract somewhat (25.8%), and significantly detract (5.2%). (Reprinted from Kahn SA, Davis SA, Banes CT, et al. Impact of advanced practice providers (nurse practitioners and physician assistants) on surgical residents' critical care experience. *J Surg Res.* 2015;199:7-12, with permission from Elsevier Inc.)

might preserve residents' perception of the educational value of APPs (Fig 4).

▶ Advanced practice providers have the potential to enhance training and foster a positive intensive care unit experience for physician trainees. Fig 4 from this selection is included, representing the residents' perceptions of advanced practice providers' effect on overall intensive care unit experience. Most of the respondents to this survey were in their second year of residency, and most intensive care unit rotations are scheduled for the residents in early years of training. It is likely that the advanced practice providers in mature programs have many years' experience in their roles providing intensive care for surgical patients. This could create a scenario in which the advanced practitioners have significantly more intensive care unit experience, potentially offering resident trainees valuable insight into the care and management of critically ill patients. In practices where the advanced practitioners are dedicated to specific intensive care units, they provide continuity of care that is difficult to obtain otherwise, compared with the continuous rotation of residents through the different intensive care settings.

D. W. Mozingo, MD

Mechanisms of early trauma-induced coagulopathy: The clot thickens or not?

Dobson GP, Letson HL, Sharma R, et al (James Cook Univ, Queensland, Australia; et al)

J Trauma Acute Care Surg 79:301-309, 2015

Traumatic-induced coagulopathy (TIC) is a hemostatic disorder that is associated with significant bleeding, transfusion requirements, morbidity

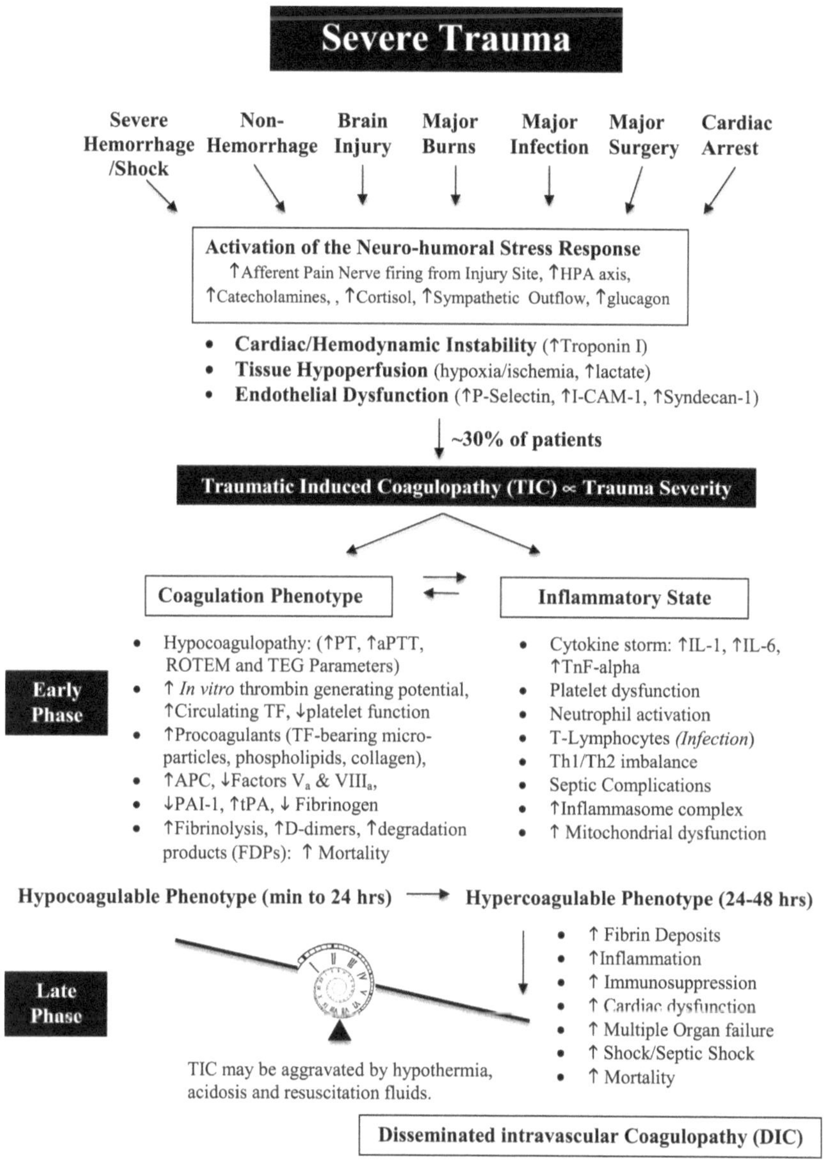

and mortality. A disorder similar or analogous to TIC was reported around 70 years ago in patients with shock, hemorrhage, burns, cardiac arrest or undergoing major surgery, and the condition was referred to as a "severe bleeding tendency," "defibrination syndrome," "consumptive disorder," and later by surgeons treating US Vietnam combat casualties as a "diffuse oozing coagulopathy." In 1982, Moore's group termed it the "bloody vicious cycle," others "the lethal triad," and in 2003 Brohi and colleagues introduced "acute traumatic coagulopathy" (ATC). Since that time, early TIC has been cloaked in many names and acronyms, including a "fibrinolytic form of disseminated intravascular coagulopathy (DIC)." A global consensus on naming is urgently required to avoid confusion. In our view, TIC is a dynamic entity that evolves over time and no single hypothesis adequately explains the different manifestations of the coagulopathy. However, early TIC is not DIC because an increased thrombin-generating potential in vitro does not imply a clinically relevant thrombotic state in vivo as early TIC is characterized by excessive bleeding, not thrombosis. DIC with its diffuse anatomopathologic fibrin deposition appears to be a latter phase progression of TIC associated with unchecked inflammation and multiple organ dysfunction (Fig 1).

▶ The authors of this review identify 2 forms of blood loss occurring from trauma or injury, namely, direct or anatomic bleeding from the site of injury and early coagulopathic bleeding. Early coagulopathic bleeding is a systemic oozing phenotype that is routinely diagnosed in trauma patients from prolonged plasma prothrombin time and activated partial thromboplastin time tests and reductions in clot strength and amplitude from rotational thromboelastometry and thromboelastography. Early trauma-induced coagulopathy does not seem to be a consumptive coagulopathy. Although the underlying mechanisms of trauma-induced coagulopathy are not well understood, the major drivers seem to be tissue hypoperfusion, endothelial injury, and inflammation. Fig 1 is included summarizing the mechanism of trauma induced coagulopathy. Finding the right balance in restoring homeostasis in vivo remains the ongoing challenge in the diagnosis and treatment of early coagulopathy following trauma. The authors of this selection summarize the existing knowledge of this complex problem identifying targets for future studies.

D. W. Mozingo, MD

FIGURE 1.—General scheme of TIC that occurs early after severe trauma. The upstream drivers of TIC seem to be the extent of tissue damage, hypoperfusion, and endothelial injury with different forms of trauma adding deep layers of complexity to its severity, progression, and clinical manifestation. Among the different types of trauma, severe burns exhibit the most dramatic hypermetabolic "stress response" of any injury. The early bleeding phenotype involves neurohormonal and cardiac/hemodynamic instabilities, leading to an imbalance among procoagulant factors, anticoagulant factors, platelets, the endothelium, inflammation, and fibrinolysis. Early TIC does not seem to be a consumptive coagulopathy but is characterized by multiple factors including prolonged clotting times, systemic anticoagulation, local factor V inhibition, a paradoxical increase in TF-initiated thrombin-generating potential, increased activated protein C, dysfibrinogenemia, impaired platelet function, red blood cells, and hyperfibrinolysis. TIC may be aggravated further by hypothermia, acidosis, and resuscitation fluids. There seems to be two phases of TIC, an early and late phase, which may evolve into DIC. Local and systemic inflammation plays an integral role in the progression of early coagulopathy. Potential biomarkers of endothelial injury include soluble P selectin (also a biomarker of platelet activation), intercellular adhesion molecule ICAM 1, and glycocalyx disruption indicator syndecan 1. Increased soluble ICAM-1 also reflects neutrophil activation and possible organ dysfunction. See text, Figure 2, and Table 1 for the major characteristics of TIC. It is important to note that specific infections (bacterial or viral) may cause distinct features in early coagulopathy. *Editor's Note*: Please refer to original journal article for full references. (Reprinted from Dobson GP, Letson HL, Sharma R, et al. Mechanisms of early trauma-induced coagulopathy: the clot thickens or not? *J Trauma Acute Care Surg*. 2015;79:301-309, with permission from Wolters Kluwer Health, Inc.)

Certified acute care surgery programs improve outcomes in patients undergoing emergency surgery: A nationwide analysis

Khalil M, Pandit V, Rhee P, et al (The Univ of Arizona, Tucson)

J Trauma Acute Care Surg 79:60-64, 2015

Background.—Differences in outcomes among trauma centers (TCs) and non-TCs (NTCs) in patients undergoing emergency general surgery (EGS) are well established. However; the impact of development of certified acute care surgery (ACS) programs on patient outcomes remains unknown. The aim of this study was to evaluate outcomes in patients undergoing EGS across TCs, NTCs, and TCs with ACS (ACS-TC).

Methods.—National estimates for EGS procedures were abstracted from the National Inpatient Sample database. Patients undergoing emergent procedures (appendectomy, cholecystectomy, hernia repair, as well as small and large bowel resections) were included. TCs were identified based on American College of Surgeons' verification. ACS-TC programs were recorded from the American Association for the Surgery of Trauma. Outcome measures were hospital length of stay, complications, and mortality. Regression analysis was performed after adjusting for age, sex, race, Charlson comorbidity index, and type of procedure.

Results.—A total of 131,410 patients undergoing EGS were analyzed. Patients managed in ACS-TCs had shorter hospital stay ($p = 0.045$) and lower complication rate ($p = 0.041$) compared with patients managed in both TCs and NTCs. There was no difference in mortality in patients managed across the groups; however, there was a trend toward lower mortality in patients managed in ACS-TCs in comparison with TCs ($p = 0.064$) and NTCs ($p = 0.089$). The overall hospital costs were lower for patients managed in ACS-TCs compared with TCs ($p = 0.036$).

Conclusion.—TCs with ACS have improved outcomes in EGS procedures compared with both TCs and non-TCs. ACS training with the associated infrastructure standards may contribute to these improved outcomes.

Level of Evidence.—Therapeutic/care management study, level IV (Table 2).

▶ The American College of Surgeons' Committee on Trauma and the American Association for the Surgery of Trauma redefined trauma surgery as "acute care surgery," encompassing the domains of trauma, critical care, and emergency general surgery. This model of acute surgical care is intended to address the shortage of physicians providing emergency surgical care and improve the continuity of care in acute surgical patients. To implement this model, the American Association for the Surgery of Trauma introduced an acute care surgery training fellowship in July 2008. Started initially, in a few centers, this program has now been implemented in 18 Level I trauma centers across the nation. The benefits of an acute care surgery model in improving system efficiency have been reported; however, the impact of verified acute care surgery training programs on patient-centered outcomes at a national level has not yet been reported.[1] The aim of this study was to assess the impact of verified acute care surgery programs

TABLE 2.—Outcomes

	NTC (n = 75,930)	TC (n = 47,753)	A-TC (n = 7,727)	*p*
Complications, % (n)	18.7 (14,199)	19.4 (9,264)	18.1 (1,398)	**0.04**
Urinary tract infection	6.8 (5,164)	7.2 (3,443)	6.5 (502)	**0.02**
Pneumonia	4.26 (3,241)	4.5 (2,153)	4.3 (322)	0.08
Surgical site infection	4.84 (3,681)	4.9 (2,331)	4.9 (379)	0.1
Sepsis	2.17 (1,648)	2 (955)	1.7 (131)	0.06
Reoperation	0.61 (465)	0.8 (382)	0.82 (64)	0.1
Hospital length of stay, mean (SD), d	7.9 (3.7)	8.5 (3.9)	7.2 (3.1)	**0.036**
Mortality, % (n)	2.4 (1,822)	2.2 (1,050)	2.1 (162)	0.12
Hospital cost, mean (SD), US dollars	69,561 (33,050)	67,554 (30,523)	59,928 (28,247)	**0.031**

Boldface indicates statistical significance.

Reprinted from Khalil M, Pandit V, Rhee P, et al. Certified acute care surgery programs improve outcomes in patients undergoing emergency surgery: a nationwide analysis. *J Trauma Acute Care Surg*. 2015;79:60-64, with permission from Wolters Kluwer Health, Inc.

on outcomes for patients undergoing emergency general surgery compared with trauma centers and nontrauma centers. Table 2 is included demonstrating these findings. The specialty of acute care surgery needs more studies like this to demonstrate at a local, regional, and national level that an acute care surgery hospital makes a clinical difference in terms of outcomes. Similar to the hospital designations for trauma, stroke, and cardiac disease, such designations often mandate a minimum amount of resources. This could be applied easily to acute care surgery as well.

D. W. Mozingo, MD

Reference

1. Britt RC, Weireter LJ, Britt LD. Initial implementation of an acute care surgery model: implications for timeliness of care. *J Am Coll Surg*. 2009;209:421-424.

Failure to clear elevated lactate predicts 24-hour mortality in trauma patients

Dezman ZDW, Comer AC, Smith GS, et al (Univ of Maryland, Baltimore)
J Trauma Acute Care Surg 79:580-585, 2015

Background.—Lactate clearance is a standard resuscitation goal in patients in nontraumatic shock but has not been investigated adequately as a tool to identify trauma patients at risk of dying. Our objective was to determine if trauma patients with impaired lactate clearance have a higher 24-hour mortality rate than patients whose lactate concentration normalizes.

Methods.—A retrospective chart review identified patients who were admitted directly from the scene of injury to an urban trauma center between 2010 and 2013 and who had at least one lactate concentration measurement within 24 hours. Transfers, patients without lactate measurement, and those who were dead on arrival were excluded. Of the

26,545 screened patients, 18,304 constituted the initial lactate measurement population, and 3,887 were the lactate clearance cohorts.

Results.—Initial lactate had an area under the receiver operating characteristic curve of 0.86 and 0.73 for mortality at 24 hours and in the hospital, respectively. An initial concentration of 3 mmol/L or greater had a sensitivity of 0.86 and a specificity of 0.73 for mortality at 24 hours. The mortality rate among patients with elevated lactate concentrations (n = 2,381; 5.6 [2.8] mmol/L) that did not decline to less than 2.0 mmol/L in response to resuscitative efforts (mean [SD] second measurement, 3.7 [1.9] mmol/L) was nearly seven times higher (4.1% vs. 0.6%, $p < 0.001$) than among those with an elevated concentration (n = 1,506, 5.3 [2.7] mmol/L) that normalized (1.4 [0.4] mmol/L). Logistic regression analysis showed that failure to clear lactate was associated with death more than any other feature (odds ratio, 7.4; 95% confidence interval, 1.5–35.5), except having an Injury Severity Score (ISS) greater than 25 (odds ratio, 8.2; 95% confidence interval, 2.7–25.2).

Conclusion.—Failure to clear lactate is a strong negative prognostic marker after injury. An initial lactate measurement combined with a second measurement for high-risk individuals might constitute a useful method of risk stratifying injured patients.

Level of Evidence.—Prognostic study, level III.

▶ The importance of the information provided in this selection is that after addressing other risk factors, the multivariate analysis demonstrated that failure to clear lactate was more predictive of death than age, hypotension, tachycardia, and mental obtundation. Only injuries severity scored greater than 25 had a greater predictive value. Trauma resuscitation techniques have changed dramatically in the past 20 years. The introduction of hypotensive resuscitation in patients with uncontrolled hemorrhage and damage control resuscitation limiting the volume of crystalloid administered and using blood and plasma early have been demonstrated to improve outcome. Serum lactate and base deficit have been shown to predict mortality in many studies, but the use of lactate clearance to identify patients at risk for early mortality is a novel approach. Limitations in this study include its retrospective nature and that the decision to order a second lactate was at the discretion of the clinician and not always performed, thus causing a selection bias in the identified cases.

D. W. Mozingo, MD

Optimal timing of tracheostomy after trauma without associated head injury

Keenan JE, Gulack BC, Nussbaum DP, et al (Duke Univ Med Ctr, Durham, NC; Duke Univ School of Medicine, Durham, NC)

J Surg Res 198:475-481, 2015

Background.—Controversy exists over optimal timing of tracheostomy in patients with respiratory failure after blunt trauma. The study aimed to determine whether the timing of tracheostomy affects mortality in this population.

Methods.—The 2008–2011 National Trauma Data Bank was queried to identify blunt trauma patients without concomitant head injury who required tracheostomy for respiratory failure between hospital days 4 and 21. Restricted cubic spline analysis was performed to evaluate the relationship between tracheostomy timing and the odds of inhospital mortality. The cohort was stratified based on this analysis. Unadjusted characteristics and outcomes were compared. Multivariable logistic regression was used to evaluate the effect of tracheostomy timing on mortality after adjustment for age, gender, race, payor status, level of trauma center, injury severity score, presentation Glasgow coma scale, and thoracic and abdominal abbreviated injury score.

Results.—There were 9662 patients included in the study. Restricted cubic spline analysis demonstrated a nonlinear relationship between timing of tracheostomy and mortality, with higher odds of mortality occurring with tracheostomy placement within 10 d of admission compared with later time points. The cohort was therefore stratified into early and delayed tracheostomy groups relative to this time point. The resulting groups contained 5402 (55.9%) and 4260 (44.1%) patients, respectively. After multivariable adjustment, the delayed tracheostomy group continued to have significantly reduced odds of mortality (Adjusted odds ratio, 0.82, 95% confidence interval, 0.71–0.95, C-statistic, 0.700).

Conclusions.—Among non–head injured blunt trauma patients with prolonged respiratory failure, tracheostomy placement within 10 d of admission may result in increased mortality compared with later time points (Fig 1).

▶ Given the lack of clear benefit with early tracheostomy versus delayed tracheostomy, it is not surprising that there is considerable variation in the timing of this procedure among critically ill trauma patients who develop prolonged respiratory failure, as depicted in Fig 1. Likely contributing to this variability are differing opinions among trauma surgeons and institutions regarding the optimal timing of the tracheostomy. The principal finding of this study therefore stands in contrast with the existing literature, which supports early tracheostomy to facilitate ventilator weaning, increase patient comfort, and improve pulmonary toilet. There are a number of potential explanations for this discrepancy. First, because this study focused specifically on blunt trauma patients with prolonged respiratory failure without concomitant head injury, it is possible that tracheostomy placement poses unique risks for this patient population compared with the ones that have been the focus of previous studies. The lack of detailed clinical information available in the national trauma data bank limits the ability to evaluate the factors that may have led to increased mortality with earlier tracheostomy. These findings should prompt additional prospective studies to investigate how the timing of tracheostomy influences mortality and

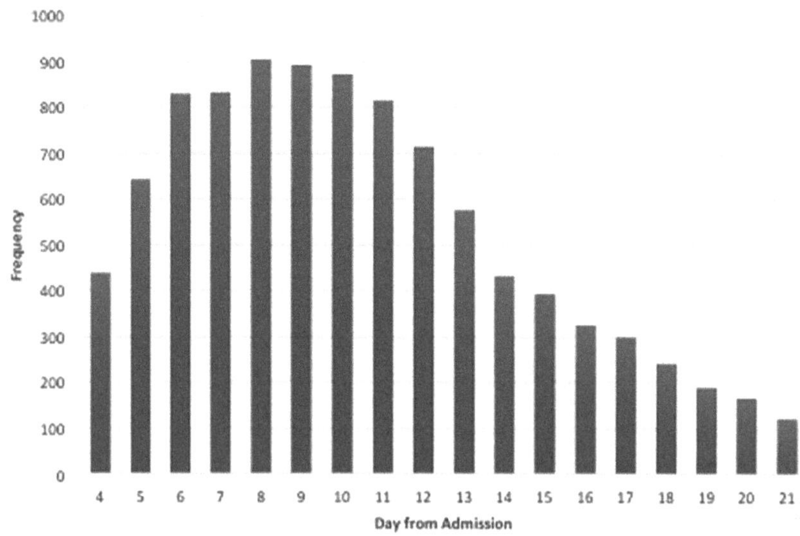

FIGURE 1.—Frequency of patients receiving tracheostomies with respect to day from admission. (Color version of the figure is available online.) (Reprinted from Keenan JE, Gulack BC, Nussbaum DP, et al. Optimal timing of tracheostomy after trauma without associated head injury. *J Surg Res.* 2015198:475-481, with permission from Elsevier Inc.)

other outcomes in this and other patients group to provide better guidance to clinicians on the optimal timing of tracheostomy.

D. W. Mozingo, MD

Factors associated with failure-to-rescue in patients undergoing trauma laparotomy

Joseph B, Zangbar B, Khalil M, et al (Univ of Arizona, Tucson)
Surgery 158:393-398, 2015

Introduction.—Quality improvement initiatives have focused primarily on preventing in-hospital complications. Patients developing complications are at a greater risk of mortality; however, factors associated with failure-to-rescue (death after major complication) in trauma patients remain undefined. The aim of this study was to identify risk factors associated with failure-to-rescue in patients undergoing trauma laparotomy.

Methods.—An -8-year, retrospective analysis of patients undergoing trauma laparotomy was performed. Patients who developed major in-hospital complications were included. Major complications were defined as respiratory, infectious, cardiac, renal, or development of compartment syndrome. Regression analysis was performed to identify independent factors associated with failure-to-rescue after we adjusted for demographics, mechanism of injury, abdominal abbreviated injury scale, initial vital signs, damage control laparotomy, and volume of crystalloids and blood products administered.

Results.—A total of 1,029 patients were reviewed, of which 21% ($n = 217$) patients who developed major complications were included. The mean age was 39 ± 18 years, 82% were male, 61% had blunt trauma, and median abdominal abbreviated injury scale was 25 [16–34, interquartile range]. Respiratory complications ($n = 77$) followed by infectious complications ($n = 75$) were the most common complications. The failure-to-rescue rate was 15.7% ($n = 34/217$). Age, blunt trauma, severe head injury, uninsured status, and blood products administered on the second day were independent predictor for failure-to-rescue.

Conclusion.—When major complications develop, age, uninsured status, severity of head injury, and prolonged resuscitation are associated independently with failure-to-rescue, whereas initial resuscitation, coagulopathy, and acidosis did not predict failure to rescue. Quality-of-care programs focus in patient level should be on improving the patient's insurance status, preventing secondary brain injury, and further development of resuscitation guidelines (Fig 2).

▶ Failure to rescue patients from complications of an underlying illness in the context of surgical treatment within the health care setting is a patient safety indicator (PSI4) of the Agency for Healthcare Research and Quality Indicator List. These events carry an increased potential for serious harm and appear often to be preceded by seemingly unrelated signals that clinicians may miss. Failure to rescue cases are typically regarded as preventable; however, clinicians may be presented with a varied or seemingly unrelated set of clinical deterioration signals, making for difficult diagnostic and treatment processes. Overreliance on studies in place of physical assessment, pursuing narrow diagnostic

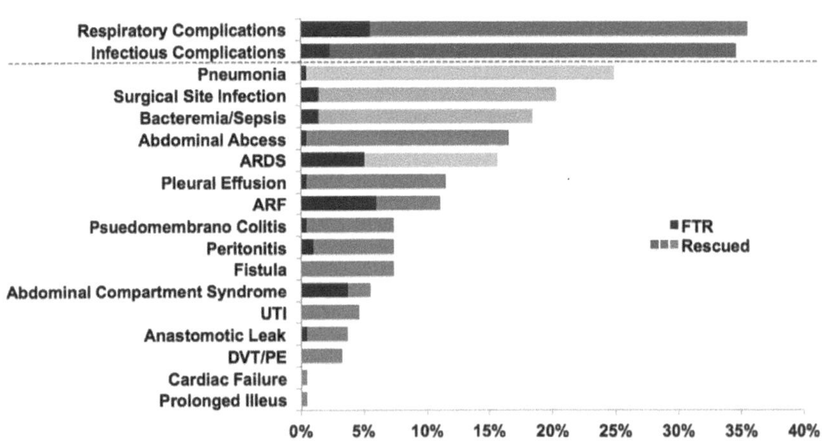

FIGURE 2.—Complications. (Reprinted from Joseph B, Zangbar B, Khalil M, et al. Factors associated with failure-to-rescue in patients undergoing trauma laparotomy. *Surgery.* 2015;158:393-398, with permission from Elsevier Inc.)

focus, lack of sense of urgency in critical situations, and general clinical inexperience are thought to be important targets to decrease failure to rescue situations. In this selection, the authors focused on complications occurring after trauma laparotomy. The complications that they tracked and the failure to rescue rates are included in Fig 2. They identified age, insurance status, severity of head injury, and prolonged resuscitation with an increased risk of failure to rescue. These factors should alert the clinician to prepare for an increased risk of complications in these populations. The study has several limitations, including the retrospective study design and the number of years over which the data were collected. It is also a single-center study, and most other analyses of failure to rescue have involved multiple hospital comparisons.

D. W. Mozingo, MD

Estimating the Effect of Palliative Care Interventions and Advance Care Planning on ICU Utilization: A Systematic Review

Khandelwal N, Kross EK, Engelberg RA, et al (Univ of Washington, Seattle)
Crit Care Med 43:1102-1111, 2015

Objective.—We conducted a systematic review to answer three questions: 1) Do advance care planning and palliative care interventions lead to a reduction in ICU admissions for adult patients with life-limiting illnesses? 2) Do these interventions reduce ICU length of stay? and 3) Is it possible to provide estimates of the magnitude of these effects?

Data Sources.—We searched MEDLINE, EMBASE, Cochrane Controlled Clinical Trials, and Cumulative Index to Nursing and Allied Health Literature databases from 1995 through March 2014.

Study Selection.—We included studies that reported controlled trials (randomized and nonrandomized) assessing the impact of advance care planning and both primary and specialty palliative care interventions on ICU admissions and ICU length of stay for critically ill adult patients.

Data Extraction.—Nine randomized controlled trials and 13 nonrandomized controlled trials were selected from 216 references.

Data Synthesis.—Nineteen of these studies were used to provide estimates of the magnitude of effect of palliative care interventions and advance care planning on ICU admission and length of stay. Three studies reporting on ICU admissions suggest that advance care planning interventions reduce the relative risk of ICU admission for patients at high risk of death by 37% (SD, 23%). For trials evaluating palliative care interventions in the ICU setting, we found a 26% (SD, 23%) relative risk reduction in length of stay with these interventions.

Conclusions.—Despite wide variation in study type and quality, patients who received advance care planning or palliative care interventions consistently showed a pattern toward decreased ICU admissions and reduced ICU length of stay. Although SDs are wide and study quality varied, the magnitude of the effect is possible to estimate and provides a basis for modeling impact on healthcare costs.

▶ In the United States, a significant proportion of health care resources are spent on the care of critically ill patients in the intensive care unit (ICU) setting. Furthermore, a significant and rising portion of these expenses are for patients who ultimately expire, and ICU stays in the previous 30 days of life have been increasing. The authors of this selection attempted to evaluate the effect of palliative care interventions and advanced care planning on ICU resource utilization by conducting a systematic review of the available literature. Despite an exhaustive review of highly variable studies, they were able to provide estimates of the magnitude of effect of advance care planning and palliative care interventions on ICU admission and ICU length of stay for patients with life-limiting illness. Their compound estimates may be more reliable for future studies of the potential effects of palliative care interventions on critically ill patients, regardless of the underlying condition. The primary rationale for advance care planning or palliative care interventions is to improve quality of care, ensure patients receive the care they would choose if fully informed, and improve patient and family outcomes. Understanding the potential for reduction in unwanted intensive care at the end of life will have important clinical and economic implications for how we approach end-of-life care in the inpatient setting.

D. W. Mozingo, MD

5 Transplantation

Introduction

The past year in solid organ transplantation has seen several recurrent themes with representative manuscripts in this chapter.

Kidney transplantation saw the establishment of the new Kidney Allocation System (KAS) on December 4, 2014. The OPTN/UNOS has updates on its websites looking at allocation numbers for each of the first six months of the new KAS with its more detailed one year evaluation due in early 2016. The major findings over the first six months were a large increase in the transplantation of highly sensitized recipients (CPRA 99 to 100%), up to 17% of all transplants at the beginning of the new KAS and then down to the 11% range at six months, a corresponding increase in Regional sharing of all kidney transplants to about one-third of all deceased donor renal transplantation, and a sharp increase in the proportion of African Americans transplanted with deceased donor grafts, higher than the percentage of Caucasians for the first time. The proportion of African Americans on the waiting list is just below that of Caucasians, so that would be the expected long term transplant ratios when the system stabilizes over time. (http://optn.transplant.hrsa.gov/learn/professional-education/kidney-allocation-system/)

In the kidney transplant literature review, I have included some long term outcome evaluation which suggests that donor specific antibody (DSA) does correlate with shortened graft survival and does appear to be causative in the shorter graft half-life (Wiebi et al). One paper demonstrates improved graft survival with early treatment of the discovery of DSA, though this treatment does not neutralize completely the negative effect of developing DSA (Orandi et al). Most authors point to the greater long term injury from Class II DSA. A bit of a PENDULUM SWING may be warranted, as perhaps our earlier allocation policies which rewarded more point for 'matching' were biologically more intelligent than our swing for greater access for all. The new KAS kept in a point per DR match, so at any given allocation, 0, 1, or 2 points are awarded to each candidate depending on DR matching. With the DSA evidence becoming very consistent concerning the hazards of developing Class II DSA, this decision by the OPTN Kidney Committee appears very appropriate despite some strong resistance by many in the community due to a desire to make the system more predictable. With the severe shortage of deceased donor organs, the transplant community needs to become stronger stewards of the precious gifts and perhaps begin siding with the HLA community who has been pushing against the decline in 0-mismatch allocation, mostly due to the increase in CPRA 100% candidates. The most highly matched candidates still have longer graft survival and optimizing the donated gifts is likely to become the next concentration of the Kidney Committee. Short and intermediate outcomes of the greatly increased highly sensitized transplants will help to shape this discussion in the coming years.

Living Kidney Donor risks review is highlighted in one article (Muzaale et al). It is vital to note that living kidney donation is relatively safe, but one to two donors on average die or have a severely morbid outcome from their donation operation. This must be told to each donor in a very clear manner. The push of some programs to utilize living donors with more co-morbidities must be followed very closely with very clear discussion with the donors and their families. Our historic good long term outcomes from living donation were in prior living donors with basically no co-morbidities. There is no logical reasoning to expect similar good outcomes with increased co-morbidities in some of today's living donors.

The discussion of DSA in kidney transplants has finally become more mainstream in liver transplantation. Our group published several cases of C4d peri-tubular staining with DSA and cholestatic liver disease which responded to removal of alloantibodies starting back in 2006.[1,2] We followed this with pathological descriptions of liver biopsies from various forms of procurement, reperfusion, cell mediated and antibody mediated injury.[3] Recently, large programs have raided their HLA freezers to demonstrate that the development of especially Class II DSA does lead to shortened liver allograft survival. A prospective study is reviewed in this chapter (Iacob et al). A referenced manuscript takes the next step and elutes DSA from liver biopsies from a patient with severe chronic antibody mediated rejection and graft loss (Neau-Cransac et al). Hypothermic and normothermic perfusion of liver grafts is also being discussed with a large European normothermic trial still under way.

Major news of interest in regards to liver allocation is referenced in two articles as the OPTN is looking at potential change in the geographic boundaries of liver allocation. The mathematical modeling being discussed by the OPTN was developed from a HRSA grant to Dr. Gentry. Dr. Gentry's group used some of the basics currently employed in defining school districts. Thus, re-districting is the current discussion topic in liver allocation. The arguments have been based on the definitions of 'need' – eg number of patients listed above a certain MELD score versus the number of people who die in a given area from that disease process – and supply – OPO efficiency versus overall eligible death rates. Without a doubt, if the new four or eight districts go into effect, surgeons will be traveling further and more often for organ procurements at an increased expense with no guarantee of reimbursement for the transplant program from private payers. The medical system as a whole may benefit from pre-transplant ICU shortened stays, but transplanting higher MELD patients has been proven to be more costly and is currently NOT reimbursed at a higher rate by any insurer. This is going to need to change for transplant programs to be able to survive financially as we tackle higher lab MELD score patients.

The difference between allocation and lab MELD scores and allocation is coming to light with the discussion of the new allocation thoughts. The current 'Share 35' was intended for acutely ill patient and gives them opportunity for Regional sharing (Massie et al). In some areas, exception MELD patients are entering this Regional sharing pool and this is not part of the original intent of the Share 35 policy. To correct this, exception points will stop at 34 and these exception point patients will not enter the Regional Share 35 pool (Heimbach et al). Also, an attempt to standardize the granting of exception points has improved with passage of 'Sodium MELD'. This will grant additional points for patients with hyponatremia in a standardized fashion starting in 2016 (http://optn.transplant.hrsa.gov/PublicComment/pubcommentPropSub_317.pdf). The OPTN Liver Committee is looking to nationalize the Review Boards so candidates are treated equally across the country.

The lung transplantation programs started the revolution in normothermic perfusion and are now publishing details on various algorithms for use of this technology, including when not to use it, such as the direct use of otherwise good appearing lung allografts from DCD donors (Sanchez et al, Cypel et al).

Frailty tests have been borrowed from geriatric medicine and applied to most solid organ recipient groups with striking predictability of outcomes (McAdams-DeMarco et al, Derck et al, Jha et al, Wilson et al, and Cron et al).

The initial reports of successful treatment of Hepatitis C in renal transplant recipients with the new non-interferon regimens are very promising to many transplant recipients (Kamar et al).

Kenneth A. Andreoni, MD, FACS

References

1. Watson R, Kozlowski T, Nickeleit V, et al. Isolated donor specific alloantibody-mediated rejection after ABO compatible liver transplantation. *Am J Transplant.* 2006;6:3022-3029.
2. Kozlowski T, Rubinas T, Nickeleit V, et al. Liver allograft antibody-mediated rejection with demonstration of sinusoidal C4d staining and circulating donor-specific antibodies. *Liver Transpl.* 2011;17:357-368.
3. Kozlowski T, Andreoni K, Schmitz J, Hayashi PH, Nickeleit V. Sinusoidal C4d deposits in liver allografts indicate an antibody-mediated response: diagnostic considerations in the evaluation of liver allografts. *Liver Transpl.* 2012;18:641-658.

Risk of End-Stage Renal Disease Following Live Kidney Donation

Muzaale AD, Massie AB, Wang M-C, et al (Johns Hopkins Univ School of Medicine, Baltimore, MD; Johns Hopkins Bloomberg School of Public Health, Baltimore, MD; et al)

JAMA 311:579-586, 2014

Importance.—Risk of end-stage renal disease (ESRD) in kidney donors has been compared with risk faced by the general population, but the general population represents an unscreened, high-risk comparator. A comparison to similarly screened healthy nondonors would more properly estimate the sequelae of kidney donation.

Objectives.—To compare the risk of ESRD in kidney donors with that of a healthy cohort of nondonors who are at equally low risk of renal disease and free of contraindications to live donation and to stratify these comparisons by patient demographics.

Design, Settings, and Participants.—A cohort of 96 217 kidney donors in the United States between April 1994 and November 2011 and a cohort of 20 024 participants of the Third National Health and Nutrition Examination Survey (NHANES III) were linked to Centers for Medicare & Medicaid Services data to ascertain development of ESRD, which was defined as the initiation of maintenance dialysis, placement on the waiting list, or receipt of a living or deceased donor kidney transplant, whichever was identified first. Maximum follow-up was 15.0 years; median follow-up was 7.6 years (interquartile range [IQR], 3.9-11.5 years) for kidney donors and 15.0 years (IQR, 13.7-15.0 years) for matched healthy nondonors.

Main Outcomes and Measures.—Cumulative incidence and lifetime risk of ESRD.

Results.—Among live donors, with median follow-up of 7.6 years (maximum, 15.0), ESRD developed in 99 individuals in a mean (SD) of 8.6 (3.6) years after donation. Among matched healthy nondonors, with median follow-up of 15.0 years (maximum, 15.0), ESRD developed in 36 nondonors in 10.7 (3.2) years, drawn from 17 ESRD events in the unmatched healthy nondonor pool of 9364. Estimated risk of ESRD at 15 years after donation was 30.8 per 10 000 (95% CI, 24.3-38.5) in kidney donors and 3.9 per 10 000 (95% CI, 0.8-8.9) in their matched healthy nondonor counterparts ($P < .001$). This difference was observed in both black and white individuals, with an estimated risk of 74.7 per 10 000 black donors (95% CI, 47.8-105.8) vs 23.9 per 10 000 black nondonors (95% CI, 1.6-62.4; $P < .001$) and an estimated risk of 22.7 per 10 000 white donors (95% CI, 15.6-30.1) vs 0.0 white nondonors ($P < .001$). Estimated lifetime risk of ESRD was 90 per 10 000 donors, 326 per 10 000 unscreened nondonors (general population), and 14 per 10 000 healthy nondonors.

Conclusions and Relevance.—Compared with matched healthy nondonors, kidney donors had an increased risk of ESRD over a median of 7.6 years; however, the magnitude of the absolute risk increase was small. These findings may help inform discussions with persons considering live kidney donation.

▶ This report on the long term outcome of living kidney donors provides important information for transplant professionals to relay to all potential living donors as they council them before donation. The authors followed living donors from 1994 to 2011 for up to 15 years with a mean of 8.6 years and compared them with matched healthy donors in the Third National Health and Nutrition Examination Survey study group. They also looked at the risk of ESRD in the unscreened general population. The donor population was 78% under age 50, 59% female and 74.6% white. Nine percent had a systolic blood pressure greater than 140 mm Hg with 24.2% smoking. Ninety-nine of 96 217 living donors developed ESRD over the 8.6 mean years of follow-up. Fifty of the 99 who developed end-stage renal disease (ESRD) were 18 to 39 years of age at the time of donation. In the healthy matched control group, there were 36 ESRD events with a mean of 10.7 years of follow-up. These results transformed into a cumulative incidence of ESRD in donors of 30.8 per 10 000, 3.9 per 10 000 in healthy nondonors.

Although there appears to be a numerical advantage for unrelated donors at 11 years, there was no statistical difference at 15 years after donation between biologically related versus unrelated donors. Racial/ethnic differences were evident with incidence of ESRD per 10 000 living donors being 75 for blacks, 33 for Hispanics, and 23 for whites; the relative proportions mirror the general population. Some of this risk for ESRD is obviously independent of kidney donation. For living donors, the risk of ERSD per 10 000 was 90, healthy individuals who did not donate had an incidence of 14 per 10 000, and the general population had a risk of 326 per 10 000. The conclusion is that there is a small increased risk of ESRD in those who donate a kidney. As in the general population, the risk is lowest for white women, then white men, black women, and finally black men.

There is clearly a risk to any person to donate a kidney for transplantation, but increasing knowledge on the quantity of the risks is vital to informed consent. With improved long-term follow-up, this information will hopefully be even more transparent in the future, and more applicable to an individual for their risks, not just a large group.

K. A. Andreoni, MD, FACS

A Cost-Benefit Analysis of Government Compensation of Kidney Donors

Held PJ, McCormick F, Ojo A, et al (Stanford Univ, CA; U.S. Economic and Financial Res, San Francisco, CA; Univ of Michigan Health Systems, Ann Arbor; et al)

Am J Transplant 16:877-885, 2016

From 5000 to 10 000 kidney patients die prematurely in the United States each year, and about 100 000 more suffer the debilitating effects of dialysis, because of a shortage of transplant kidneys. To reduce this shortage, many advocate having the government compensate kidney donors. This paper presents a comprehensive cost-benefit analysis of such a change. It considers not only the substantial savings to society because kidney recipients would no longer need expensive dialysis treatments—$1.45 million per kidney recipient—but also estimates the monetary value of the longer and healthier lives that kidney recipients enjoy—about $1.3 million per recipient. These numbers dwarf the proposed $45 000-per-kidney compensation that might be needed to end the kidney shortage and eliminate the kidney transplant waiting list. From the viewpoint of society, the net benefit from saving thousands of lives each year and reducing the suffering of 100 000 more receiving dialysis would be about $46 billion per year, with the benefits exceeding the costs by a factor of 3. In addition, it would save taxpayers about $12 billion each year.

▶ The inspiration from this article was a joint American Society of Transplant Surgeons and American Society of Transplantation workshop in June 2014, Increasing Organ Donation in the United States. The conclusion of the meeting was to remove disincentives to donation, explore opportunities to change or modify the National Organ Transplant Act as necessary, and work with other professionals to lay groundwork for the next steps in this effort. The authors present this comprehensive cost-benefit analysis of a proposed change in National Organ Transplant Act (2) to one that allows the government to compensate living kidney donors $45 000 for a donation and deceased donors $10 000.

The assumed benefits of having more living and deceased donors are ready access to the 100 000 patients on the Organ Procurement and Transplantation Networkkidney waiting list, with healthier recipients over time due to decreased wait time and less time on dialysis before transplant and better compatibility between donor and recipient that would increase the success rate. The authors used the value of $200 000 as the monetary value of a year of perfect health, with quality of life compared with "perfect health" 0.52 for dialysis and 0.75 for transplant. The cost of a kidney transplant including full organ acquisition charges was $145 000, with $32 000 estimated for a full year total medical cost after transplant, and $88 000 for a kidney graft failure event.

Findings were that taxpayers would save $12 billion each year if they supplemented donation and if this supplement increased the availability of available kidney allografts from 17 500 to 35 000 per year. The lifetime value of a kidney transplant to a recipient was $1.3 million. The savings from stopping dialysis was $1.45 million. Taxpayers save $403 000 for every dialysis patient who receives a kidney transplant. This analysis also resulted in a cost-effectiveness of dialysis and transplantation. The cost of a quality of life year via transplant was $49 000 compared with $186 000 from dialysis treatment.

The conclusion was simply that nearly any payment to increase organ donation would not only improve the lives of those who receive the transplants but would be a large cost savings to taxpayers because of the high cost of dialysis compared with transplantation.

K. A. Andreoni, MD, FACS

Variation in Cost and Quality in Kidney Transplantation

Nassir BA, Dean CE, Li S, et al (Hennepin County Med Ctr, Minneapolis, MN; Univ of Minnesota, Minneapolis; Minneapolis Med Res Foundation, MN; et al)

Transplantation 99:2150-2157, 2015

Background.—Bending the cost curve in medical expenses is a high national priority. The relationship between cost and kidney allograft failure has not been fully investigated in the United States.

Methods.—Using Medicare claims from the United States Renal Data System, we determined costs for all adults with Medicare coverage who underwent kidney transplant January 1, 2007, to June 30, 2009. We compared relative cost (observed/expected payment) for year 1 after transplantation for all transplant centers, adjusting for recipient, donor, and transplant characteristics, region, and local wage index. Using program-specific reports from the Scientific Registry of Transplant Recipients, we correlated relative cost with observed/expected allograft failure between centers, excluding small centers.

Results.—Among 19,603 transplants at 166 centers, mean observed cost per patient per center was $65,366 (interquartile range, $55,094-$71,624). Mean relative cost was 0.99 (±0.20); mean observed/expected allograft failure was 1.03 (±0.46). Overall, there was no correlation between relative cost and observed/expected allograft failure ($r = 0.096$, $P = 0.22$). Comparing centers with higher than expected costs and allograft failure rates (lower performing) and centers with lower than expected costs and failure rates (higher-performing) showed differences in donor and recipient characteristics. As these characteristics were accounted for in the adjusted cost and allograft failuremodels, they are unlikely to explain the differences between higher- and lower-performing centers.

Conclusions.—Further investigations are needed to determine specific cost-effective practices of higher- and lower-performing centers to reduce costs and incidence of allograft failure.

► Pay for performance and value-based reimbursement are key buzz words today in the new discussion of Medicare payment via Medicare Access and CHIP Reauthorization Act as the SGF has been repealed. The authors use the Scientific Registry of Transplant Recipients (SRTR) database with Medicare Claims Data to decide on the performance of centers using the SRTR Cox modeling for expected outcomes and the relative cost. The authors state that "Higher-performing centers (centers whose costs and incidence of allograft failure were both lower than expected) were more likely to have the following characteristics compared with lower-performing centers (centers whose costs and incidence of allograft failure were both higher than expected): fewer deceased donor transplants, more white recipients, fewer African American recipients, lower incidence of diabetes as the primary cause of ESRD, recipients with lower body mass index, less frequent retransplant, more frequent preemptive transplant, and lower incidence of congestive heart failure (CHF) (Table 3 in the original article). However, because these factors were accounted for in both the cost and the allograft failure models, they are likely not the drivers of the differences." Looking at the SRTR models, the AUC is only about 0.65, so one-third of the outcome is not explained by the model. Also, there are no interactive terms, and clinically we know several clinical factors, such as age and years of diabetes with degree of cardiac dysfunction are not isolated factors but are clearly interactive. I would argue strongly that the preceding findings of higher performing centers having more live donors, few African Americans, fewer patients with diabetes, lower body mass index, fewer retransplants, more preemptive transplants, and less congestive heart failure clearly explains why these centers had both better outcomes and cost less.

The SRTR, Organ Procurement and Transplantation Network, or any large database nationally has never been able to collect accurate interactive complex medical conditions. These factors described in this article are well known by all clinicians to describe outcomes and cost. Physicians need to heed the warnings of being involved with any statistical attempt to explain our outcomes that simply does not make clinical sense. Every statistical correlation must first stand the test of clinical common sense.

K. A. Andreoni, MD, FACS

Rates and Determinants of Progression to Graft Failure in Kidney Allograft Recipients With *De Novo* Donor-Specific Antibody

Wiebe C, Gibson IW, Blydt-Hansen TD, et al (Univ of Manitoba, Winnipeg, Canada; Univ of British Columbia, Vancouver, Canada; et al)

Am J Transplant 15:2921-2930, 2015

Understanding rates and determinants of clinical pathologic progression for recipients with *de novo* donor-specific antibody (*dn*DSA), especially subclinical *dn*DSA, may identify surrogate endpoints and inform clinical trial design. A consecutive cohort of 508 renal transplant recipients (n = 64 with *dn*DSA) was studied. Recipients (n = 388) without *dn*DSA or dysfunction had an eGFR decline of −0.65 mL/min/1.73 m^2/year. In recipients with *dn*DSA, the rate eGFR decline was significantly increased prior to *dn*DSA onset (−2.89 vs. −0.65 mL/min/1.73 m^2/year, $p < 0.0001$) and accelerated post-*dn*DSA (−3.63 vs. −2.89 mL/min/1.73 m^2/year, $p < 0.0001$), suggesting that *dn*DSA is both a marker and contributor to ongoing alloimmunity. Time to 50% post-*dn*DSA graft loss was longer in recipients with subclinical versus a clinical *dn*DSA phenotype (8.3 vs. 3.3 years, $p < 0.0001$). Analysis of 1091 allograft biopsies found that *dn*DSA and time independently predicted chronic glomerulopathy (cg), but not interstitial fibrosis and tubular atrophy (IFTA). Early T cell–mediated rejection, nonadherence, and time were multivariate predictors of IFTA. Independent risk factors for post-*dn*DSA graft survival available prior to, or at the time of, *dn*DSA detection were delayed graft function, nonadherence, *dn*DSA mean fluorescence intensity sum score, tubulitis, and cg. Ultimately, *dn*DSA is part of a continuum of mixed alloimmune-mediated injury, which requires solutions targeting T and B cells.

▶ The authors present long-term follow-up (median 75 months) of 508 adult and pediatric renal transplant recipients with good early graft function for the development of donor-specific antibody (dnDSA) as well as correlation among graft function and serologic, clinical, and histological characteristics. Most patients were on tacrolimus (82%; CsA 18%), mycophenolate mofetil, and prednisone. Only a third of patients had induction antibody therapy with basiliximab induction (23%) or thymoglobulin (9%). Subclinical dnDSA was <25% risk in SCr and <500 mg/d proteinuria within 2 months of dnDSA detection. Biopsies were done in 92% of clinical rejections. This patient cohort was low risk (95% first transplant, 85% PRA <25%) and showed dnDSA develop in 64 recipients at median of 49 months (6-143 months). Nonadherent patients were much more likely to develop dnDSA (72% vs 19% at 12 years). As demonstrated in other reports, class II DSA was more common (69% only class II, 17% both). Nine percent (6 of 64) dnDSA patients dropped their dnDSA MFI below positive cutoff with 1 recurring on later screen.

Clinically relevant take home points from this publication included the following:

1. Nine of 14 subclinical patients who developed antibody-mediated rejection on biopsy eventually developed graft failure at median of 24 months.
2. Despite equal baseline estimated glomerular filtration rate (eGFR) at 6 months posttransplant and at 6 months before dnDSA development, clinical dnDSA patients had lower eGFR by the time of dnDSA discovery. The clinical dnDSA patients had an initial eGFR decline at −6.18 ± 7.71 mL/min/1.73 m^2 that then stabilized at −5.61 mL/min/1.73 m^2, compared with subclinical dnDSA group at −3.15 mL/min/1.73 m^2. The best group of nondysfunction, no-dnDSA had a eGFR decline at −0.65 ± 3.94 mL/min/1.73 m^2 and the dysfunction, no-dnDSA group at −2.34 mL/min/1.73 m^2.
3. Proteinuria was more common after diagnosis of dnDSA (0.21 ± 0.48 vs 0.004 + 0.09 g/24H/y)
4. In multivariate analysis, dnDSA predicted chronic glomerulopathy (hazard ratio [HR] 4.42 for cg > 1, HR 10.36 for cg >2, HR 18.50 cg >3) with Banff cg score increasing by 1 grade every 3 years after dnDSA diagnosis.
5. After detection of clinical dnDSA, the remaining graft half-life was 3.3 years compared with 8.3 years in subclinical dnDSA patients. Graft loss patients tended to have higher MFI of dnDSA (15 018 vs 6998).

6. The patients with clinical dnDSA had the same HLA mismatch status with their donor as the other groups, 90% were documented to have nonadherence (compared with 24% of the subclinical dnDSA group) and had a higher incidence of cellular rejections.
7. Delayed graft function predicted shorter time to allograft loss in multivariate analysis for those who developed dnDSA.
8. The patients with clinical dnDSA had the same HLA mismatch status with their donor as the other groups; 90% were documented to have nonadherence (compared with 24% of the subclinical dnDSA group) and had a higher incidence of cellular rejections

The authors' major conclusions were that detection of dnDSA is a marker of ongoing alloimmunity, often preceded by the presence of T cell–mediated rejection. The dnDSA likely accelerates the immune process as it correlates strongly with cg, a major risk factor for graft loss. They argue that any dnDSA clinical study needs to address both forms of alloimmunity, cellular and humoral.

K. A. Andreoni, MD, FACS

Quantifying Renal Allograft Loss Following Early Antibody-Mediated Rejection

Orandi BJ, Chow EHK, Hsu A, et al (Johns Hopkins Univ School of Medicine, Baltimore, MD)

Am J Transplant 15:489-498, 2015

Unlike antibody-mediated rejection (AMR) with clinical features, it remains unclear whether subclinical AMR should be treated, as its effect on allograft loss is unknown. It is also uncertain if AMR's effect is homogeneous across donor (deceased/live) and (HLA/ABO) antibody types. We compared 219 patients with AMR (77 subclinical, 142 clinical) to controls matched on HLA/ABO-compatibility, donor type, prior transplant, panel reactive antibody (PRA), age and year. One and 5-year graft survival in subclinical AMR was 95.9% and 75.7%, compared to 96.8% and 88.4% in matched controls ($p = 0.0097$). Subclinical AMR was independently associated with a 2.15-fold increased risk of graft loss (95% CI: 1.19–3.91; $p = 0.012$) compared to matched controls, but not different from clinical AMR ($p = 0.13$). Fifty three point two percent of subclinical AMR patients were treated with plasmapheresis within 3 days of their AMR-defining biopsy. Treated subclinical AMR patients had no difference in graft loss compared to matched controls (HR 1.73; 95% CI: 0.73–4.05; $p = 0.21$), but untreated subclinical AMR patients did (HR 3.34; 95% CI: 1.37–8.11; $p = 0.008$). AMR's effect on graft loss was heterogeneous when stratified by compatible deceased donor (HR = 4.73; 95% CI: 1.57–14.26; $p = 0.006$), HLA-incompatible deceased donor (HR = 2.39; 95% CI: 1.10–5.19; $p = 0.028$), compatible live donor (no

AMR patients experienced graft loss), ABO-incompatible live donor (HR = 6.13; 95% CI: 0.55–67.70; $p = 0.14$) and HLA-incompatible live donor (HR = 6.29; 95% CI: 3.81–10.39; $p < 0.001$) transplant. Subclinical AMR substantially increases graft loss, and treatment seems warranted.

▶ As our ability to detect low levels of donor-specific antibodies (DSA) has improved and protocol renal biopsies have been increasing, especially in the background of known prior DSAs or after active desensitization of a recipient, the question of what to do with subclinical biopsy findings of mild antibody-mediated rejection (AMR) is more pertinent. The Johns Hopkins renal transplant group addressed this quandary by looking at long-term outcomes of their renal recipients over the past few years. They have an active desensitization program, as well as ABO incompatible program, and their program does routine protocol biopsies in additional to those for clinical cause. They looked at 2316 patients from 2000 to 2012 with the main outcome being AMR. Their treatment for AMR has a foundation in plasmapheresis with some use of rituximab and occasional eculizumab.

As in most desensitization programs, only patients with a living donor were allowed to have a positive cytotoxic crossmatch with their donor prior to desensitization. Nearly a third (30.7%) of their HLA incompatible living donor transplants had a positive cytotoxic crossmatch, with the majority (49.8%) flow crossmatch positive with negative cytotoxic crossmatch (PFNC), and 19.5% with Luminex beads positive, but flow crossmatch negative.

Of the diagnosed AMR biopsies, 35.2% were subclinical at a mean of 29 days posttransplant. Clinical AMR presented at a mean of 11 days posttransplant. Mean follow-up time was just under 4.5 years for the AMR patients.

Deceased donor and living donor HLA-compatible patients had a low AMR rates posttransplant of only 1.7% with 0.7%, respectively. Deceased donor HLA incompatible (PFNC) had a 44.7% rate of posttransplant AMR with 28.2% found on clinical presentation. Living donor HLA incompatible recipients had a 47.4% incidence of AMR with 29.3% on clinical presentation. Living donor ABO-incompatible recipients had 13.6% AMR with 11.1% on clinical presentation.

One major investigation of the study is the results and discussion of whether to treat subclinical AMR—that is, AMR on biopsy with no significant change in renal function. The authors show that their patients treated with plasmapheresis for subclinical AMR had no difference in outcomes compared with matched controls a statistically better 5-year death censored graft survival (74.9% vs 86.6%). They claim the untreated patients had decreased 5-year outcomes at 76.3% versus 90.6%. Comparing the outcomes directly, the treated patients had 1- and 5-year death censored graft survival of 94.6% and 74.9%, with the untreated patients 97.2% and 76.3%.

AMR overall had a 4.15-fold risk of graft loss. Subclinical AMR had a 2.15 risk of graft loss with clinical AMR 5.79-fold the risk compared with non-AMR transplants. One criticism of this article is that all graft loss is reported as "death censored graft loss" only. We know that there is an increase in patient death with aggressive AMR treatments, so presenting both the non—death censored and death censored results would be more clear to the reader to understand the true risk of AMR to the patient.

K. A. Andreoni, MD, FACS

Early Changes in Liver Distribution Following Implementation of Share 35

Massie AB, Chow EKH, Wickliffe CE, et al (Johns Hopkins Univ School of Medicine, Baltimore, MD; et al)

Am J Transplant 15:659-667, 2015

In June 2013, a change to the liver waitlist priority algorithm was implemented. Under Share 35, regional candidates with MELD ≥35 receive higher priority than local candidates with MELD <35. We compared liver distribution and mortality in the first 12 months of Share 35 to an equivalent time period before. Under Share 35, new listings with MELD ≥35 increased slightly from 752 (9.2% of listings) to 820 (9.7%, $p = 0.3$), but the proportion of deceased-donor liver transplants (DDLTs) allocated to recipients with MELD ≥35 increased from 23.1% to 30.1% ($p < 0.001$). The proportion of regional shares increased from 18.9% to 30.4% ($p < 0.001$). Sharing of exports was less clustered among a handful of centers (Gini coefficient decreased from 0.49 to 0.34), but there was no evidence of change in CIT ($p = 0.8$). Total adult DDLT volume increased from 4133 to 4369, and adjusted odds of discard decreased by 14% ($p = 0.03$). Waitlist mortality decreased by 30% among patients with baseline MELD >30 (SHR = 0.70, $p < 0.001$) with no change for patients with lower baseline MELD ($p = 0.9$). Posttransplant length-of-stay ($p = 0.2$) and posttransplant mortality ($p = 0.9$) remained unchanged. In the first 12 months, Share 35 was associated with more transplants, fewer discards, and lower waitlist mortality, but not at the expense of CIT or early posttransplant outcomes.

▶ Mandatory Regional Sharing for patients with a Model for End-Stage Liver Disease (MELD) score 35 or higher (Share 35) went into effect June 18, 2013. This article by Massie et al reviews the early results of this new national liver allocation policy change. The outcomes were analyzed only by allocation MELD, which is the higher of the MELD score from laboratory values or exception points. The early results showed no difference in posttransplant early outcome by allocation MELD, but the differences are not corrected for lab MELD independently of allocation MELD. In subsequent national discussions, as many as a third of patients in some high MELD waiting areas have allocation MELD from hepatocellular carcinoma (HCC) exception points, with subsequent much lower risk of early postoperative death.

Waitlist mortality of those with at MELD > 30 decreased by 30% with no change of those having lower MELDs. Some of the early data showing no change in length of stay or posttransplant mortality are somewhat hard to explain because subsequent data have emerged to show that the MELD ≥35 patients have higher posttransplant death rates than anyone else, including Status 1 patients.

Recent changes to the liver allocation system help to refine the early Share 35 system. On October 8, 2015, Organ Procurement and Transplantation Network (OPTN) policies 9.3.F and 9.3.f.vi went into effect. The first is known as "HCC [hepatocellular carcinoma] Delay" and attempts to prevent transplantation to patients with very high risk of HCC recurrence after transplant by mandating a 6-month waiting period from the time the patient first qualifies for HCC exception and is first listed with the OPTN to the time when the exception points of MELD 28 go into effect. This is in response to the observation that patients who were transplanted more quickly in lower MELD areas had higher rates of early HCC recurrence and death than in areas with higher MELD scare at transplant, thus making these HCC patients go through the test of time on the waiting list before transplantation. In some areas of the country, these HCC exception points were also enough to get these patients transplanted quickly and at a much higher rate of transplant than laboratory MELD patients. This advantage to access of organs was also considered to be inconsistent with the original intent of the HCC exception point policy. The second portion of this policy change addresses the fact that the original intent of Share 35 was to get liver transplant opportunities to acutely ill patients who were dying with high lab MELD score, not with high HCC exception MELD score. This second policy caps the HCC exception point MELD at 34.

The long-awaited Sodium MELD, or MELD corrected for hyponatremia, is expected to be implemented in January 2016. More information, including a table with additional MELD points depending on current laboratory MELD and degree of hyponatremia is available at the OPTN website: http://optn.transplant.hrsa.gov/news/meld-serum-sodium-policy-changes/.

K. A. Andreoni, MD, FACS

Delayed Hepatocellular Carcinoma Model for End-Stage Liver Disease Exception Score Improves Disparity in Access to Liver Transplant in the United States

Heimbach JK, Hirose R, Stock PG, et al (Mayo Clinic, Rochester, MN; Univ of California San Francisco; et al)

Hepatology 61:1643-1650, 2015

The current system granting liver transplant candidates with hepatocellular carcinoma (HCC) additional Model for End-Stage Liver Disease (MELD) points is controversial due to geographic disparity and uncertainty regarding optimal prioritization of candidates. The current national policy assigns a MELD exception score of 22 immediately upon listing of eligible patients with HCC. The aim of this study was to evaluate the potential effects of delays in granting these exception points on transplant rates for HCC and non-HCC patients. We used Scientific Registry of Transplant Recipients data and liver simulated allocation modeling software and modeled (1) a 3-month delay before granting a MELD exception score of 25, (2) a 6-month delay before granting a score of 28, and (3) a 9-month delay before granting a score of 29. Of all candidates waitlisted between January 1 and December 31, 2010 (n = 28,053), 2773 (9.9%) had an HCC MELD exception. For HCC candidates, transplant rates would be 108.7, 65.0, 44.2, and 33.6 per 100 person-years for the current policy and for 3-, 6-, and 9-month delays, respectively. Corresponding rates would be 30.1, 32.5, 33.9, and 34.8 for non-HCC candidates.

Conclusion.—A delay of 6-9 months would eliminate the geographic variability in the discrepancy between HCC and non-HCC transplant rates under current policy and may allow for more equal access to transplant for all candidates.

▶ The national liver transplant community has been divided on the exception points granted to patients with HCC within Milan Criteria. Rule in place until later in 2015 would grant newly listed patients with HCC within Milan Criteria 22 MELD points. Most of these patient had very low MELD lab scores, and some of these patients would have well-treated 2 to 3 cm solitary lesions with low chance of recurrence. Statistics show that these patients are often transplanted with far less burden of disease with regard to overall illness from their chronic liver dysfunction than patients with lab MELD scores only.

The Organ Procurement and Transplantation Network (OPTN) liver committee with their Scientific Registry of Transplant Recipients colleagues looked into the data from patients transplanted in 2010 with and without HCC MELD exception points. A major issue around the country is that some areas were transplanting these HCC exception patients quickly with their MELD 22 score or their first renewal to a score of 25, whereas in higher MELD transplant areas, the HCC patients would need to undergo several renewals to be competitive for organ allocation. The authors looked at several combinations of mandatory waiting and MELD HCC exception points. Comparing data from across the country, a 6- to 9-month waiting period between listing and granting exception points would make the transplant rates between HCC exception and lab MELD patients much closer, with dropout rates for both patient groups becoming similar. The findings of this article, a 6-month waiting period from listing with an eventual granting of 28 points via HCC exception, was accepted by the OPTN Liver Committee and then Board of Directors to make the disparity between transplant less for lab MELD candidates compared with HCC exception candidates across the country.

In related information, it is also well known that patients with HCC points who are transplanted very rapidly have a higher chance of early HCC recurrence. The long-term data from the University of California—San Francisco and other transplant centers who transplant at higher MELD scores showed that some of the early listed patients with HCC progressed rapidly and thus become noncandidates for transplant. Those who wait for at least several months with lack of progression after treatment have a more favorable biology of their cancer and lower recurrence after transplantation. This was another reason to support the 6-month wait in awarding HCC exception points. This new policy went into effect on October 8, 2015, as OPTN policy 9.3.F.

See http://optn.transplant.hrsa.gov/media/1200/optn_policies.pdf#nameddest=Policy_09.

K. A. Andreoni, MD, FACS

Gerrymandering for Justice: Redistricting U.S. Liver Allocation

Gentry S, Chow E, Massie A, et al (Johns Hopkins Univ School of Medicine, Baltimore, MD; et al)

Interfaces 45:462-480, 2015

U.S. organ allocation policy sequesters livers from deceased donors within arbitrary geographic boundaries, frustrating the intent of those who wish to offer the livers to transplant candidates based on medical urgency. We used a zero-one integer program to partition 58 donor service areas into between four and eight sharing districts that minimize the disparity in liver availability among districts. Because the integer program necessarily suppressed clinically significant differences among patients and organs, we tested the optimized district maps with a discrete-event simulation tool that represents liver allocation at a per-person, per-organ level of detail. In April 2014, the liver committee of the Organ Procurement and Transplantation Network (OPTN) decided in a unanimous vote of 22-0-0 to write a policy proposal based on our eight-district and four-district maps. The OPTN board of directors could implement the policy after the proposal and public-comment period. Redistricting liver allocation would save hundreds of lives over the next five years and would attenuate the serious geographic inequity in liver transplant offers.

▶ The discussion for changing the liver allocation system with respect to primary geographic units has been discussed in earnest for more than 15 years. Since the "liver wars" of the late 1990s, Health Resources and Services Administration has been lobbied and affected by politicians on both sides of the arguments. The major issues revolve around an agreed on method of measuring "need" or patient degree of illness, supply of allografts that includes local organ procurement agencies effectiveness in obtaining organs for transplantation, effects on short-term and long-term outcomes of transplanting increasing sicker recipients, and cost of doing so with more travel to obtain organs. Gentry et al obtained an HRSA grant to study this issue and developed new geographic sharing areas that they have termed districts. See "Modeling the Allocation System: Principles for Robust Design Before Restricting" by Mehrotra et al[1] for a response to the initial proposal by Gentry et al and the Organ Procurement and Transplantation Network (OPTN) Liver Committee.

The basis of need in their calculations is the number of wait-list candidates with a Model for End-Stage Liver Disease (MELD) score of 15 or greater. Arguments for and against this include that at a MELD of 15, there is a survival benefit for the average candidate versus listing practices around the country may not have every transplant center list's candidates at a MELD this low because they are highly unlikely to receive an offer until their MELD score is much higher. Centers in highly competitive areas may be forced by business practices to list all reasonable candidates as soon as possible. The counter-argument to Gentry el al is that these issues tend to make larger centers in large urban populations appear to have more need.

The liver committee of the OPTN/United Network for Organ Sharing has agreed to use the MELD score as a measure of patient disease urgency. MELD is a reasonable predictor of death on the wait list, but it does have geographic differences as discussed by several transplant centers form the Southeastern United States. Public health researchers from the Northeast have also discussed the great difference in the average patient's access to transplant services in urban versus rural areas. The apparent increased access to listed patients in the Southeast becomes the inverse when you take into account all patient deaths from liver disease in those states, not just listed patients. In this latter analysis, urban centers have better patient outcomes than rural areas despite transplant wait-list measurements. The OPTN liver committee argues it can only affect allocation to listed patients. The liver committee is rightfully making a strong push to make the granting of "exception points" more equal around the country. More than a third of high-allocation MELD patients have low laboratory MELD scores but have exception points, with the large majority of these for hepatocellular carcinoma.

The definition of "eligible donors" is believed by many to be too subjective to have meaningful discussions of organ procurement organizations (OPO) efficiency. Donor availability per patient population varies greatly around this country, with urban areas in general showing fewer donors per listed patient. However, the OPO in the Philadelphia/South Jersey/Delaware region is the blaring exception to this generality, because Gift of Life has been the most efficient OPO in the world at times over the past several years.

K. A. Andreoni, MD, FACS

Reference

1. Mehrotra. et al.

Modeling the Allocation System: Principles for Robust Design Before Restructuring

Mehrotra S, Kilambi V, Gilroy R, et al (Northwestern Univ, Evanston, IL; Univ of Kansas Med Ctr, Kansas City; et al)
Transplantation 99:278-281, 2015

The United Network for Organ Sharing is poised to resolve geographic disparity in liver transplantation and promote allocation based on medical urgency. At the time of writing, United Network for Organ Sharing is considering redistricting the organ procurement and transplantation network so that patient model for end-stage liver disease scores at transplant is more uniform across regions. We review the proposal with a systems-engineering focus and find that although the proposal is promising, it currently lacks evidence that it would perform effectively under realistic departures from its underlying data and assumptions. Moreover, we caution against prematurely focusing on redistricting as the only method to mitigate disparity. We describe system modeling principles which, if followed, will ensure that the redesigned allocation system is effective and efficient in achieving the intended goals.

▶ This article by Mehrotra et al, and the previous Gentry et al article on liver redistricting, discuss the potential changes to liver recipients in our country if the current Organ Procurement and Transplantation Network (OPTN 11) regions were changed. Gentry et al use a mathematical demand versus supply analysis to redistrict the country into 4 or 8 districts under some predefined rule by the OPTN liver committee. Mehrotra et al review their model and raise concerns with practical implementation and uncertainties in their modeling. A major focus of concern is how a modified allocation may change outcomes. Outcomes are challenging to discuss because the sickest patients, those with a very high Model of End Stage Liver Disease (MELD) score over 35, have a high personal benefit to attempted liver transplant because their chance of surviving otherwise is very low. The challenge comes in discussion of the great need for liver allografts compared with supply—the best use of organs in regard to the optimal outcome for the entire waiting list. There is no agreed on answer to the most pressing question in liver allocation: "What is an acceptable outcome in 1- and 5-year patient/graft survival in these most ill recipients, and when is the absolute outcome too low compared with what slightly less ill patients could achieve in terms of long-term outcomes?" In other words, when are patients too ill to receive a standard liver allograft offer because their outcomes, although personally far better for them than no transplant attempt, is not fair to the overall donor supply and national need? Today, our predictive modeling is lacking in all but the extremes of this discussion. Even then, the OPTN community has not been willing to create specific policy to address this issue, doing so only indirectly through outcome reviews of the entire program's patient population.

Cost is rather straightforward in this discussion. Transplanting more very ill patients is likely to decrease overall health care costs because earlier transplant will reduce the length of stay in expensive intensive care units; however, today, transplant program costs generally do not include entire patient life expense, but only the 24 hours before transplant. Therefore, for the vast majority of transplant events around the country, performing more transplants on more severely ill patients with many more donor procurement flights and for longer distances will increase the cost of the procedure to transplant centers and increase surgeon/procurement technician risks by flying more often in small aircraft. Also, an issue for discussion during the last liver forum meeting was that the Scientific Registry of Transplant Recipients (SRTR) simulations did not estimate more high-MELD patients to be transplanted if the new districts went into effect. This is counterintuitive because a significant percentage of high MELD patients become too ill to receive a transplant with current waiting times. If waiting times were decreased for the highest MELD candidates, more high-MELD patients would definitely receive offers/transplants. This important incorrect assumption in the SRTR simulations needs to be corrected, as does their method for estimating "lives saves." Their current estimations are over a short time horizon; over a longer period, the number of lives saved may be much smaller or reversed due to lower posttransplant survival in the high-MELD recipients as well as a significant percentage of deaths in mid-MELD candidates on the list before their transplant opportunities.

K. A. Andreoni, MD, FACS

De Novo Donor-Specific HLA Antibody Formation in Two Patients With Crigler-Najjar Syndrome Type I Following Human Hepatocyte Transplantation With Partial Hepatectomy Preconditioning

Jorns C, Nowak G, Nemeth A, et al (Karolinska Univ Hosp Huddinge, Stockholm, Sweden; et al)

Am J Transplant 16:1021-1030, 2016

Clinical hepatocyte transplantation is hampered by low engraftment rates and gradual loss of function resulting in incomplete correction of the underlying disease. Preconditioning with partial hepatectomy improves engraftment in animal studies. Our aim was to study safety and efficacy of partial hepatectomy preconditioning in clinical hepatocyte transplantation. Two patients with Crigler-Najjar syndrome type I underwent liver resection followed by hepatocyte transplantation. A transient increase of hepatocyte growth factor was seen, suggesting that this procedure provides a regenerative stimulus. Serum bilirubin was decreased by 50%, and presence of bilirubin glucuronides in bile confirmed graft function in both cases; however, graft function was lost due to discontinuation of immunosuppressive therapy in one patient. In the other patient, serum bilirubin gradually increased to pretransplant concentrations after ≈600 days. In both cases, loss of graft function was temporally associated with emergence of human leukocyte antigen donor-specific antibodies (DSAs). In conclusion, partial hepatectomy in combination with hepatocyte transplantation was safe and induced a robust release of hepatocyte growth factor, but its efficacy on hepatocyte engraftment needs to be evaluated with additional studies. To our knowledge, this study provides the first description of *de novo* DSAs after hepatocyte transplantation associated with graft loss.

► Hepatocyte transplantation or gene therapy for metabolic diseases has been a focus of many investigators for the past several decades. Jorns and his coinvestigators present 2 patients with Crigler-Najjar syndrome type I who received clinical hepatocyte allograft infusions after a left lateral segmentectomy to induce engraftment. The authors could demonstrate increased hepatocyte growth factor after the resection. The first patient received infusions from two deceased liver donors, and the second patient from 1 donor before the patient received a whole organ liver transplant due to increased bilirubin.

Both patients showed a transient decline in bilirubin signifying hepatocyte engraftment and function. The first patient stopped immunosuppression and had failure of his cellular transplant with new expression of donor specific antibodies (DSA). The second recipient had hepatocyte graft failure at about 600 days, also with new DSA detected.

Analysis of the liver tissue for donor hepatocytes showed very low percentage engraftment despite an infusion of hepatocytes with subsequent increase in portal pressures. The authors were hopeful further investigations with improved preconditioning and infusion techniques would lead to more success.

This study reminds us of the difficulty getting islets to engraft in liver tissue. Although the hepatocyte engraftment appeared to be fairly robust for some time, the immune system eventually ended both attempts at patient treatment. The presence of DSA is demonstrated for the first time in this hepatocyte cellular transplant model, but DSA has been shown in every human organ and cellular rejection series to date when properly investigated. Even the liver has been recently shown to be sensitize to decreased long-term survival in the presence of DSA, especially those to Class II antigens.

K. A. Andreoni, MD, FACS

Donor-Specific Anti-HLA Antibodies and Endothelial C4d Deposition—Association With Chronic Liver Allograft Failure

Iacob S, Cicinnati VR, Lindemann M, et al (Univ Hosp Münster, Germany; Univ Hosp Essen, Germany; et al)

Transplantation 99:1869-1875, 2015

Background.—The significance of humoral immune response for allograft survival after liver transplantation (LT) is still a matter of debate. The aim of this cross-sectional study was to assess immunological and clinical factors associated with advanced fibrosis (F3-F4) and chronic graft failure in LT recipients.

Methods.—Serum samples from 174 patients prospectively enrolled and followed up for 12 months were tested for anti-HLA antibodies and compared against donor HLA types. Immunohistochemical C4d staining was performed on formalin-fixed, paraffin-embedded liver tissue.

Results.—Mean time period from LT to enrollment was 66.9 ± 51.9 months. Independent predictive factors for graft failure included donor-positive cytomegalovirus serostatus ($P = 0.02$), donor-specific antibodies (DSA) against HLA class II ($P = 0.03$), donor age ($P = 0.01$), hepatitis C virus allograft reinfection ($P = 0.0008$), and biliary complications ($P = 0.003$). HLA class II DSA and HLA class I antibody positivity, hepatitis C virus reinfection, and mycophenolate mofetil-free regimens were significant risk factors for advanced fibrosis after LT. There was a significant association between C4d deposition on allograft endothelial cells and presence of class II DSA ($P < 0.0001$). Patients with C4d deposits had a 4.3 times higher risk of graft failure than those with negative staining and a significantly lower median time to graft failure (94.6 months [range, 3.6-158.9 months] vs 176.4 months [range, 9.4-217.8 months], $P < 0.0001$).

Conclusions.—Screening for HLA DSA might be useful for early identification of LT recipients at increased risk of graft failure who could benefit from closer surveillance and tailored immunosuppressive regimens.

▶ The past few years have seen a resurrection of antibody-mediated rejection (AMR)/injury in liver allografts as multiple groups have begun to apply state of the art C4d staining and donor-specific antibody (DSA) detection to liver transplant recipients. In this study from the University of Munster and University Hospital Essen, 174 patients were followed for at least a year with liver graft biopsies incorporating C4d staining, and serum determination for DSAs. Patients were an average of 67 ± 52 months from their transplant. Similar to findings in kidney allografts, the presence of Class II DSA was an independent predictor for graft failure. Both Class II and Class I DSA was a significant risk for advanced fibrosis. C4d staining was associated with Class II DSA. Patients that demonstrated C4d staining had nearly a 50% decrease in their graft longevity (94.6 vs 176.4 months). The authors found all patients positive for Class II DSA had high levels of antibody with MFI values ≥5000, and 64% with MFI values ≥10 000. All patients with Class II DSA had specificities against HLA-DQ, with 46% against HLA-DR.

Publications like this and others are making a dent in the historic belief that the liver is an immunologically privileged organ. Clearly, it is hardier against cellular and antibody-mediated rejections than the other solid organs transplanted, but its shields are not absolute. Multiple modern studies have demonstrated the association of DSA with C4d staining and liver graft loss, starting with a report from our group in 2006.[1] Other groups have associated both pre- and post-transplant DSA with graft injury, including de novo DSA at 1 year being correlated with both patient death and allograft loss.

The authors point to the potential benefit of long-term mycophenolate mofetil (MMF) in the liver recipient population, especially after detection of DSA. The lack of MMF in the chronic immunosuppressive regimen showed a 2.23 odds ratio of increased advanced fibrosis in the allograft. Although AMR is less frequent in liver allografts than kidney allografts, the presence of DSA in the multitude of publications over the past decade is now clearly associated with decreased graft longevity.

K. A. Andreoni, MD, FACS

Reference

1. Watson R, Kozlowski T, Nickeleit V, et al. Isolated donor specific alloantibody-mediated rejection after ABO compatible liver transplantation. *Am J Transplant.* 2006;6:3022-3029.

Evolution of serum and intra-graft donor-specific anti-HLA antibodies in a patient with two consecutive liver transplantations

Neau-Cransac M, Le Bail B, Guidicelli G, et al (Bordeaux Univ Hosp, France; et al)

Transpl Immunol 33:58-62, 2015

The current literature suggests that anti-HLA donor-specific antibodies (DSA) may have deleterious effects on liver grafts but there is no proof that they are directly involved in the graft lesions. We report the case of a donor HLA-sensitized patient who needed a second graft 6 months after the first transplantation owing to a progressive cholestatic disease that we could finally attribute to antibody-mediated rejection (AMR). We describe the longitudinal evolution of graft function, tissue histology, serum DSA and, for the first time, intra-graft DSA after elution from biopsies.

▶ Another report in the recent decade of rejuvenated interest in antibody mediated injury in liver allografts, this article describes not only donor-specific antibodies (DSA) in the serum of a patient during allograft loss but also eluted DSAs from both a liver allograft biopsy and, later, the allograft explant due to recurrent cirrhosis and the need for retransplantation. The authors were able to elute high levels of graft DSA (gDSA) from the allograft tissue itself while levels in the serum DSA (sDSA) were very low. The alloantibodies eluted from the graft were donor specific and did not contain third-party alloantibody that were high in serum at the time of the biopsy. The authors suggest that gDSA may be more sensitive than sDSA in determining antibody-mediated injury.

As shown in other reports in liver antibody-mediated rejection (AMR) and in other organs undergoing AMR, especially renal allografts, Class II DSA was more prominent in ongoing antibody mediated injury. The authors appropriately warn that this was only one patient, and similar studies need to be repeated in additional patients.

As liver recipients develop "chronic allograft dysfunction" of uncertain etiology, it will be interesting to see the percentage of biopsies that are positive for eluted DSA. Early determination of gDSA before severe fibrosis should lead to a change in immunosuppression to increase attempts to stop alloantibody formation, such as mycophenolic acid therapy. In severe acute liver graft dysfunction before cirrhosis, therapies used to salvage renal and heart allografts, such as plasmapheresis, rituximab, bortezomib, and eculizumab, may be warranted.

K. A. Andreoni, MD, FACS

International Society for Heart and Lung Transplantation Donation After Circulatory Death Registry Report

Cypel M, for the International Society for Heart and Lung Transplantation (International Society for Heart and Lung Transplantation Donation after Circulatory Death Registry, Dallas, TX)

J Heart Lung Transplant 34:1278-1282, 2015

Background.—The objective of this study was to review the international experience in lung transplantation using lung donation after circulatory death (DCD).

Methods.—In this retrospective study, data from the International Society for Heart and Lung Transplantation (ISHLT) DCD Registry were analyzed. The study cohort included DCD lung transplants performed between January 2003 and June 2013, and reported to the ISHLT DCD Registry as of April 2014. The participating institutions included 10 centers in North America, Europe and Australia. The control group was a cohort of lung recipients transplanted using brain-dead donors (DBDs) during the same study period. The primary end-point was survival after lung transplantation.

Results.—There were 306 transplants performed using DCD donors and 3,992 transplants using DBD donors during the study period. Of the DCD transplants, 94.8% were Maastricht Category III, whereas 4% were Category IV and 1.2% Category V (euthanasia). Heparin was given in 54% of the cases, donor extubation occurred in 90% of the cases, and normothermic ex vivo lung perfusion (EVLP) was used in 12%. The median time from withdrawal of life support therapy (WLST) to cardiac arrest was 15 minutes (5th to 95th percentiles of 5 to 55 minutes), and from WLST to cold flush was 33 minutes (5th to 95th percentiles of 19.5 to 79.5 minutes). Recipient age and medical diagnosis were similar in DCD and DBD groups ($p =$ not significant [NS]). Median hospital length of stay was 18 days in DCD lung transplants and 16 days in DBD transplants ($p = 0.016$). Thirty-day survival was 96% in the DCD group and 97% in the DBD group. One-year survival was 89% in the DCD group and 88% in the DBD group ($p =$ NS). Five-year survival was 61% in both groups ($p =$ NS). The mechanism of donor death within the DCD group seemed to influence recipient early survival. The survival rates through 30 days were significantly different by donor mechanism of death ($p = 0.0152$). There was no significant correlation between the interval of WLST to pulmonary flush with survival ($p = 0.11$).

Conclusion.—This large study of international, multi-center experience demonstrates excellent survival after lung transplantation using DCD donors. It should be further evaluated whether the mechanism of donor death influences survival after DCD transplant.

▶ Over the past couple of years, the lung transplant community has begun to embrace the use of lung allografts from donors after circulatory death (DCD). This registry report combines the largest centers in the world using these

DCD lungs. Three hundred and six DCD lung transplants were performed compared with 3992 donors after brain death (DBD) in this time period from 2003 through 2013. The overall outcomes from these DCD donor lung allografts are equivalent to standard DBD grafts. The authors were surprised to find any lack of correlation between outcome and multiple factors, such as heparinization before withdrawal, time from withdrawal to systolic blood pressure < 50, withdrawal to asystole, or withdrawal to start of pulmonary flush. Normothermic ex vivo lung perfusion (EVLP) was used in only 12% of the transplants performed.

The authors conclude that the use of DCD lung allografts is equivalent to DBD donors, and additional evaluation of the various time points during the DCD procurement process should be further investigated. Certainly the increased use of EVLP with its ability to evaluate lung function before implantation will allow more centers to be comfortable using these DCD lung allografts.

K. A. Andreoni, MD, FACS

Defining quality during ex vivo lung perfusion: The University of Maryland experience

Sanchez PG, Rajagopal K, Pham SM, et al (Univ of Maryland School of Medicine, Baltimore)

J Thorac Cardiovasc Surg 150:1376-1377, 2015

Background.—Lung transplant centers are encouraged to screen the unused donor pool with ex vivo lung perfusion (EVLP), assessing these organs for safety and suitability for transplantation. To improve conversion rates and maintain safety in light of the increased use of EVLP, the evaluation process is becoming more critical. Variables that should be considered when deciding whether to use lungs have been identified in clinical trials to be lung compliance and oxygenation, the level of lung parenchyma recruitment, and the surgeon's clinical assessment. The traditional most important indicator of lung donor quality has been gas exchange. The value of oxygen pressure (Po_2) in EVLP with an acellular perfusate may be unreliable because just a few molecules of oxygen can increase it significantly in plasmalike solutions. Lung compliance actually deteriorates earlier than Po_2 in acute lung injury. With these considerations in mind, a systematic approach was developed to refine the interpretation of the data provided by EVLP.

Procedure.—An algorithm was developed around the finding that lung compliance deteriorates earlier than other parameters in EVLP, making oxygenation secondary to compliance. A decision not to transplant is made based on close monitoring of the deterioration in lung compliance. If compliance falls but oxygenation is above a difference between Po_2 in the left atrium and that in the pulmonary artery (ΔPo_2) of at least 350 mm Hg, perfusion is continued for 1 hour, which generally reveals oxygenation decrease.

Transplantation is typically undertaken when lung compliance is stable or improving, but an additional consideration is a ΔPO_2 of at least 350 mm Hg and no significant new infiltrates or consolidation on the chest radiograph. Chest radiographs are obtained at hours 1 and 3. If lung compliance is stable or improving but ΔPO_2 is less than 350 mm Hg, the recruitment maneuver is repeated and gas values rechecked. If ΔPO_2 remains low, perfusion is done for an extra hour and the lung is reevaluated.

If two lungs are being assessed and only one has poor quality, compliance can be stable despite a low ΔPO_2. Selective vein gas values are obtained to evaluate oxygenation for each lung. If the better lung remains well oxygenated, a single-lung transplant is performed.

No lung is rejected solely on the basis of a surgeon's evaluation. A decision to reject a lung must be based on decreasing lung compliance and oxygenation that correlate with increasing opacities seen radiographically. These observations have been shown to correlate with decreased lung ventilator excursion, mainly of the lower lobes, and increased bogginess detected manually.

Results.—Of 17 donor lungs evaluated with EVLP, 11 were transplanted, for a conversion rate of 65%. The transplanted lungs all performed well, with patients exhibiting no signs of severe primary graft dysfunction after 72 hours.

Conclusions.—As new methods of measuring lung performance are developed, the current lung assessment protocol will require refinement. The evaluation of lungs with EVLP is an evolving process.

▶ This report from the University of Maryland lung transplant group discusses their findings on measured parameters of their deceased organs in the Normothermic Ex Vivo Lung Perfusion trial. The physiological variables they investigated were pulmonary arterial pressure, left atrial pressure, pulmonary vascular resistance, delta pO_2, peak airway pressure, mean airway pressure, and static lung compliance. They had 11 transplanted and 6 nontransplanted ex vivo lung perfusion (EVLP) lungs. Their decision algorithm starts with stable or improving lung compliance as a mandatory requirement. Then oxygenation over 350 mm Hg with stable or improving chest x-ray. Measurements were made at 1 and 3 hours on EVLP. All 11 transplanted lungs functioned well.

Clearly, the major question with this study is whether any of the unused EVLP lungs would have also performed well. As a basis of their prioritization of parameters on their algorithm, the group used reference to large animal studies where lung compliance was shown to be the first sign of acute lung injury, before that of decreased oxygenation.

EVLP has rapidly gained acceptance in the United States after groundbreaking reports from the Toronto lung transplant group. The ability to allow for organ injury repair, repeated therapeutic and diagnostic bronchoscopies, and serial evaluation of function and radiological findings are the key reasons for this rapid popularity. In addition to the potential cost of the per EVLP pump itself and the disposables for each lung with solutions is estimated to be approximately $40 000 per use. Some centers have purchased their own machines, whereas others are taking part in a study in which deceased donor lungs are retrieved and flown to a large regional facility in the Baltimore area, evaluated there, and then transported back to the original center that accepted the lungs for their patient for transplantation if deemed safe for transplant. Data are being actively accumulated by multiple centers using each of these methods.

In addition to normothermic lung perfusion for both evaluation and reconditioning of deceased donor organs, human transplants have also been performed after normothermic perfusion of livers, kidneys, and even hearts from donation after circulatory death donors. The ability to truly allow organs to repair injuries during the dying process and to thoroughly evaluate physiologic function in these organs are the obvious basis for excitement across all organ transplant specialists. The cost is the major barrier at this time because it is usually an additional unreimbursed expense to the transplant center at the current time. Hopefully with additional clinical evidence of normothermic perfusion for all organ types, this organ therapy may be reimbursed by insurers to allow for the use of more organs for transplant to the more than 100 000 candidates on the US organ waiting list alone.

K. A. Andreoni, MD, FACS

The Prevalence and Prognostic Significance of Frailty in Patients With Advanced Heart Failure Referred for Heart Transplantation

Jha SR, Hannu MK, Chang S, et al (St Vincent's Hosp, Sydney, New South Wales, Australia; Univ of Technology Sydney, Australia)

Transplantation 100:429-436, 2016

Background.—Frailty is a clinically recognized syndrome of decreased physiological reserve. The heightened state of vulnerability in these patients confers a greater risk of adverse outcomes after even minor stressors. Our aim was to assess the prevalence and prognostic significance of the frailty phenotype in patients referred for heart transplantation.

Methods. Consecutive patients referred or on the waiting list for heart transplantation from March 2013 underwent frailty assessment. Frailty was defined as a positive response to 3 or more of the following 5 components: weak grip strength, slowed walking speed, poor appetite, physical inactivity, and exhaustion. In addition, markers of disease severity were obtained, and all patients underwent cognitive (Montreal Cognitive Assessment) and depression (Depression in Medical Illness-10) screening.

Results.—One hundred twenty patients (83 men:37 women; age, 53 ± 12 years, range, 16-73 years; left ventricular ejection fraction, 27 ± 14%) underwent frailty assessment. Thirty-nine of 120 patients (33%) were assessed as frail. Frailty was associated with New York Heart Association class IV heart failure, lower body mass index, elevated intracardiac filling pressures, lower cardiac index, anemia, hypoalbuminemia, hyperbilirubinemia, cognitive impairment, and depression (all

$p < 0.05$). Frailty was independent of age, sex, heart failure duration, left ventricular ejection fraction, or renal function. Frailty was an independent predictor of increased all-cause mortality: 1 year actuarial survival was 79 ± 5% in the nonfrail group compared with only 54 ± 9% for the frail group ($P < 0.005$).

Conclusions.—Frailty is prevalent among patients with advanced symptomatic heart failure referred for heart transplantation and is associated with increased mortality.

▶ Frailty was assessed per 5 standard components on 120 consecutive patients referred for heart transplantation or waiting on the transplant list. Additionally, patients underwent cognitive and depression screening. One-third of the patients were frail, and these patients had associated New York Heart Association class IV heart failure and the others mentioned in the abstract. Most importantly, frailty was found to be an independent predictor of increased all-cause mortality to a substantial degree (54% ± 9% in frail vs 79% ± 5% 1-year survival in nonfrail group). The authors also found depression to be an independent predictor of mortality in their patients, although frail patients had a higher rate of depression than nonfrail patients.

It appears that the preoperative determination of frailty for most organ transplant candidates is important in predicting posttransplant patient survival. Goals of improving frailty before transplantation should be the next major push by the transplant community.

K. A. Andreoni, MD, FACS

Pretransplant frailty is associated with decreased survival after lung transplantation

Wilson ME, Vakil AP, Kandel P, et al (Mayo Clinic, Rochester, MN)

J Heart Lung Transplant 35:173-178, 2016

Background.—Frailty is a condition of increased vulnerability to adverse health outcomes. Although frailty is an important prognostic factor for many conditions, the effect of frailty on mortality in lung transplantation is unknown. Our objective was to assess the association of frailty with survival after lung transplantation.

Methods.—We performed a retrospective cohort analysis of all adult lung transplant recipients at our institution between 2002 and 2013. Frailty was assessed using the frailty deficit index, a validated instrument that assesses cumulative deficits for up to 32 impairments and measures the proportion of deficits present (with frailty defined as >0.25). We examined the association between frailty and survival, adjusting for age, sex, and bilateral (vs single) lung transplant using Cox proportional hazard regression models.

Results.—Among 144 lung transplant patients, 102 (71%) completed self-reported questionnaires necessary to assess the frailty deficit index within 1 year before lung transplantation. Frail patients ($n = 46$) had an increased risk of death, with an adjusted hazard ratio (HR) of 2.24 (95% confidence interval [CI], 1.22–4.19; $p = 0.0089$). Frailty was not associated with an increased duration of mechanical ventilation (median, 2 vs 2 days; $p = 0.26$), intensive care unit length of stay (median, 7.5 vs 6 days; $p = 0.36$) or hospital length of stay after transplantation (median, 14 vs 10.5 days; $p = 0.26$).

Conclusions.—Pre-transplant frailty was independently associated with decreased survival after lung transplantation. Pre-transplant frailty may represent an important area for intervention to improve candidate selection and lung transplant outcomes.

▶ The frailty deficit index was used in this publication looking retrospectively at lung transplant recipients from 2002 to 2013 at a single center. Of their 144 lung recipients, 102 patients had interpretable data from 1 year pretransplant. Forty-five percent were determined to be frail 1 year before lung transplant. These frail patients had an adjusted hazard ratio of increased risk of death of 2.24 despite having no difference in mechanical ventilation days, intensive care unit stay or hospital stay after transplantation. Again, the authors determine that frailty is an independent risk factor for patient death at 1 and 3 years post-transplant. The use of the 6-minute walk test was not able to reproduce the predictability of the frailty index.

The authors bring up the obvious point in the discussion of trying to improve frailty in patients pretransplant to determine whether this can improve post-transplant patient survival. Many lung transplant programs do currently use pre-operative conditioning as a critical component of their clinical program.

K. A. Andreoni, MD, FACS

Depression and Frailty in Patients with End-Stage Liver Disease Referred for Transplant Evaluation

Cron DC, Friedman JF, Winder GS, et al (Univ of Michigan Med School, Ann Arbor)

Am J Transplant 2015 [Epub ahead of print]

End-stage liver disease (ESLD) patients are believed to have a high prevalence of depression, although mental health in ESLD has not been studied comprehensively. Further, the relationship between depression and severity of liver disease is unclear. Using baseline data from a large prospective cohort study ($N = 500$) of frailty in ESLD patients, we studied the association of frailty with depression. Frailty was assessed with the 5-component Fried Frailty Index. Patients were assigned a composite score of 0 to 5, with scores ≥3 considered frail. Depression was assessed using the 15-question Geriatric Depression Scale, with a threshold of ≥6 indicating depression. 43.2% of patients were frail and 39.4% of patients were depressed (median score = 4, range 0-15). In multivariate analysis, frailty was significantly associated with depression (OR = 2.78, 95% CI: 1.87-4.15, $P < 0.001$), whereas model for end-stage liver disease score was not associated with depression. After covariate adjustment, depression prevalence was 3.6 times higher in the most-frail patients than the least-frail patients. In conclusion, depression is common in ESLD patients and is strongly associated with frailty but not with severity of liver disease. Transplant centers should address mental health issues and frailty; targeted interventions may lower the burden of mental illness in this population.

▶ In this study of frailty and its association to depression in end-stage liver disease (ESLD) patients, 43.2% of evaluated patients were frail, with these patients having higher Model for End-Stage Liver Disease (MELD) scores, lower sodium and albumin, and more encephalopathy. They also trended toward more ascites, diabetes, and chronic obstructive pulmonary disease. Furthermore, 39.4% of these patients were positive for depression. Frail patients had 1.5 times higher depression scores and 2-fold higher prevalence of depression (53.7% vs 28.5%), and more frail patients had substantially higher depression scores (7.5% vs 2.7%). Importantly, frailty and encephalopathy did not interact.

Other factors significantly associated with depression included younger age, never being listed for a transplant, hepatitis C, encephalopathy, and Medicare insurance type. Tobacco use trended toward significance. In addition, 1.5 times as many patients had a clinical diagnosis of depression if they were frail (35% vs 23%). MELD scores as a measure of disease severity did not correlate to depression scores.

The University of Michigan group points to their center's ongoing treatment of higher frailty general surgery patients, and now starting with ESLD patients, to see whether they can improve outcome and positively decrease depression. They also raise the question of whether depression treatment may decrease frailty development because the causal nature between the 2 are undefined.

K. A. Andreoni, MD, FACS

Quality of Life in Liver Transplant Candidates: Frailty Is a better Indicator Than Severity of Liver Disease

Derck JE, Thelen AE, Cron DC, et al (Univ of Michigan Med School, Ann Arbor)

Transplantation 99:340-344, 2015

Background.—In an effort to understand the diminished quality of life (QoL) exhibited by patients with end-stage liver disease (ESLD), we studied the association of frailty and severity of liver disease with quality of life in this patient population.

Methods.—In a prospective, single-center cohort study (N = 487), we assessed frailty and QoL in patients with ESLD referred for liver transplant. Frailty was measured on a scale from 0 to 5 by grip strength, gait speed, exhaustion, shrinkage, and physical activity, with scores of 3 or higher characterized as frail. Physical, mental, and combined overall quality of life scores ranging from 0 to 100 were assessed using Short Form 36. Pearson correlation and multiple linear regression were used to identify variables associated with QoL.

Results.—Quality of life was notably low in the study cohort (mean: physical, 42.9 ± 24.1; mental, 58.3 ± 23.2). In multivariate analysis adjusted for demographic and clinical characteristics, frailty was significantly negative associated with physical (slope, −22.55, 95% confidence interval, −26.39 to −18.71; $P < 0.001$) and mental QoL (slope, −17.59, 95% confidence interval, −21.47 to −13.71; $P < 0.001$). Model for ESLD (MELD) was not associated with QoL.

Conclusion.—In ESLD patient referred for liver transplant, diminished QoL appears to be significantly negatively associated with frailty and not with severity of liver disease as measured MELD. With further study, if frailty is shown to be a remediable condition, targeted programs may help decrease frailty and improve quality of life in ESLD patients.

▶ Frailty was measured as per "Frailty and mortality in kidney transplant recipients" on a 5-component instrument with each measurement 0 or 1. In addition to frailty, the SF-36 Quality of Life (QOL) questionnaire was used along with the Liver Disease Quality of Life (LDQoL) Questionnaire. The SF-36 and the LDQoL was found to be similar.

Frail patients had higher Model for End-Stage Liver Disease (MELD) scores, lower sodium and lower albumin, more ascites, encephalopathy, coronary artery disease, diabetes, and chronic obstructive pulmonary disease. Prior studies and this one show poor correlation between QoL and MELD. Physical QoL was more strongly associated with frailty than MELD. Frailty was not only a significant predictor of overall QoL but also of physical and mental QoL. MELD score was not a significant predictor of QoL in any of the models studied.

This study and others incorporating frailty measurements may be quantifying the clinician's subjective feeling of which patients have the ability to recover meaningful function after transplantation and reestablish what most of us consider to be a high quality of life.

K. A. Andreoni, MD, FACS

Frailty and Mortality in Kidney Transplant Recipients

McAdams-DeMarco MA, Law A, King E, et al (Johns Hopkins Univ School of Medicine, Baltimore, MD; et al)

Am J Transplant 15:149-154, 2015

We have previously described strong associations between frailty, a measure of physiologic reserve initially described and validated in geriatrics, and early hospital readmission as well as delayed graft function.

The goal of this study was to estimate its association with postkidney transplantation (post-KT) mortality. Frailty was prospectively measured in 537 KT recipients at the time of transplantation between November 2008 and August 2013. Cox proportional hazards models were adjusted for confounders using a novel approach to substantially improve model efficiency and generalizability in single-center studies. We precisely estimated the confounder coefficients using the large sample size of the Scientific Registry of Transplantation Recipients (n = 37 858) and introduced these into the single-center model, which then estimated the adjusted frailty coefficient. At 5 years, the survivals were 91.5%, 86.0% and 77.5% for nonfrail, intermediately frail and frail KT recipients, respectively. Frailty was independently associated with a 2.17-fold (95% CI: 1.01–4.65, $p = 0.047$) higher risk of death. In conclusion, regardless of age, frailty is a strong, independent risk factor for post-KT mortality, even after carefully adjusting for many confounders using a novel, efficient statistical approach.

▶ Frailty was measured in a single-center study of 537 kidney transplant recipients, and predicted patient survival at 5 years posttransplant independently, than the 30 other currently measured patient characteristics in the Scientific Registry of Transplant Recipients (SRTR) models. These SRTR models only account for about 67% of predicted outcome in the kidney transplants at 1 and 3 years (64%). Frailty is a measure of physiologic reserve, and this comes out of the geriatric literature in recent years. As our transplant patients both age and survive more years with chronic illnesses, the need to better predict in this higher risk population is obvious. Frailty was measured as previously defined in the literature as (1) shrinking—unintentional weight loss more than 10 lb in a year; weakness via grip strength; exhaustion, via self-report; low activity—kcals per week below an established cutoff; and slowed walking speed—walking time for 15 feet. Each of the 5 are scored 0 or 1 with nonfrail 0 or 1 total score, intermediate frailty 2, and frailty 3 or higher. In their patients who had a mean age of 53 ± 14 years, 33% were intermediately frail, and 19.9% were frail. Frailty had a marked independent prediction of mortality across all ages, even those under age 45. Frailty testing is becoming a useful objective method to determine posttransplant survival in many organ transplants as demonstrated in the other articles summarized in this chapter.

K. A. Andreoni, MD, FACS

Changes in Frailty After Kidney Transplantation

McAdams-DeMarco MA, Isaacs K, Darko L, et al (Bloomberg School of Public Health, Baltimore, MD; et al)

J Am Geriatr Soc 63:2152-2157, 2015

Objectives.—To understand the natural history of frailty after an aggressive surgical intervention, kidney transplantation (KT).

Design.—Prospective cohort study (December 2008–March 2014).
Setting.—Baltimore, Maryland.
Participants.—Kidney transplantation recipients (N = 349).
Measurements.—The Fried frailty score was measured at the time of KT and during routine clinical follow-up. Using a Cox proportional hazards model, factors associated with improvements in frailty score after KT were identified. Using a longitudinal analysis, predictors of frailty score changes after KT were identified using a multilevel mixed-effects Poisson model.
Results.—At KT, 19.8% of recipients were frail; 1 month after KT, 33.3% were frail; at 2 months, 27.7% were frail; and at 3 months, 17.2% were frail. On average, frailty scores had worsened by 1 month (mean change 0.4, $P < .001$), returned to baseline by 2 months (mean change 0.2, $P = .07$), and improved by 3 months (mean change −0.3, $P = .04$) after KT. The only recipient or transplant factor associated with improvement in frailty score after KT was pre-KT frailty (hazard ratio = 2.55, 95% confidence interval (CI) = 1.71–3.82, $P < .001$). Pre-KT frailty status (relative risk (RR) = 1.49, 95% CI = 1.29–1.72, $P < .001$), recipient diabetes mellitus (RR = 1.26, 95% CI = 1.08–1.46, $P = .003$), and delayed graft function (RR = 1.22, 95% CI = 1.04–1.43, $P = .02$) were independently associated with long-term changes in frailty score.
Conclusion.—After KT, in adult recipients of all ages, frailty initially worsens but then improves by 3 months. Although KT recipients who were frail at KT had higher frailty scores over the long term, they were most likely to show improvements in their physiological reserve after KT, supporting the transplantation in these individuals and suggesting that pretransplant frailty is not an irreversible state of low physiological reserve.

▶ Frailty score was compared from the time of kidney transplant to varying times after transplant. As expected after surgery, the patients were more frail at 1 month but equal to presurgical state by 2 months and improved over baseline by 3 months. Only patients who had frailty pretransplant improved posttransplant. The conclusion here is that pretransplant frailty may not be irreversible. These patients were only a mean of 53.3 ± 14.2 years old with only 19.2% diabetic. Average time on dialysis was only 2.1 years with 20% preemptive and 37.3% living donor recipients. Thus, this population was likely not as ill as the more worrisome portion of our waiting lists in whom we are considering frailty to be an important component of their survival postsurgery.

It needs to be noted that 11.7% of patients who were nonfrail at the time of surgery were frail at 3 months posttransplant, whereas 25.9% of frail patients at the time of transplant were still frail at 3 months; 33.4% of this frail group at the time of transplant were then nonfrail at 3 months, and 40.7% improved to intermediately frail. Diabetes was the greatest predictor of frailty after surgery in both the pretransplant frail and nonfrail population with prior transplant and age > 65 both next in importance. In a posttransplant model, delayed graft function was the most important predictor of frailty both in those with and without pretransplant frailty with diabetes second in importance.

Focusing on a multicenter subset of transplant candidates with comorbidities such as diabetes, a prior transplant, and being of increased age is likely to provide more evidence of factors that contribute to the progression across the stages of frailty before and after transplantation.

K. A. Andreoni, MD, FACS

Efficacy and Safety of Sofosbuvir-Based Antiviral Therapy to Treat Hepatitis C Virus Infection After Kidney Transplantation

Kamar N, Marion O, Rostaing L, et al (CHU Rangueil, Toulouse, France; et al)
Am J Transplant 2015 [Epub ahead of print]

There is no approved therapy for hepatitis C virus (HCV) infection after kidney transplantation, and no data regarding the use of new-generation direct antiviral agents (DAAs) have been published so far. The aims of this pilot study were to assess the efficacy and safety of an interferon-free sofosbuvir-based regimen to treat chronic HCV infection in kidney transplant recipients. Twenty-five kidney transplant recipients with chronic HCV infection were given, for 12 (n = 19) or 24 weeks (n = 6), sofosbuvir plus ribavirin (n = 3); sofosbuvir plus daclatasvir (n = 4); sofosbuvir plus simeprevir, with (n = 1) or without ribavirin (n = 6); sofosbuvir plus ledipasvir, with (n = 1) or without ribavirin (n = 9); and sofosbuvir plus pegylated-interferon plus ribavirin (n = 1). A rapid virological response, defined by undetectable viremia at week 4 after starting DAA therapy, was observed in 22 of the 25 patients (88%). At the end of therapy, HCV RNA was undetectable in all patients. At 4 and 12 weeks after completing DAA therapy, all had a sustained virological response. The tolerance to anti-HCV therapy was excellent and no adverse event was observed. A significant decrease in calcineurin inhibitor levels was observed after HCV clearance. New-generation oral DAAs are efficient and safe to treat HCV infection after kidney transplantation.

▶ Before the recent availability of the new class of anti–hepatitis C virus (HCV) medications, the traditional combination of interferon with ribavirin was rarely used to treat HCV after renal and other nonliver transplants because of the risk of rejection. The new generation direct antiviral agents (DAAs) such as sofosbuvir combined with daclatasvir, simeprevir, or ledipasvir, with or without ribavirin, have been shown to be highly effective in cirrhotic and noncirrhotic patients. The authors looked at various combinations of interferon-free sofosbuvir-based regimens to treat HCV RNA positive kidney transplant recipients.

With various combinations, 88% of kidney recipients became RNA negative by 4 weeks. By 12 weeks, all patients were HCV RNA negative, with therapy completed at 24 weeks. Eight patients of the 25 had complete follow-up data available and were sustained virological responders.

All kidney recipients had a GFR >30 mL/min. No change in renal function was observed during the therapy. Six patients had cryoglobulinemia and proteinuria at the start of treatment. Cryoglobulin levels decreased in all patients treated, but proteinuria remained stable at about 200 mg per day. No renal biopsies were required or performed, and hemoglobin levels were stable. Tacrolimus doses remained unchanged during therapy. However, with the stable tacrolimus dosing, levels did significantly decrease and remain lower after therapy was completed.

This study reveals that it is safe and efficacious to treat kidney transplant recipients with the new DAA drugs.

K. A. Andreoni, MD, FACS

6 Surgical Infections

Introduction

Many of the recent research on fighting surgical infections, particularly chronic wounds and foreign body infections, involves the understanding and treatment of bacterial biofilms. Multiple papers discussed in this chapter describe biofilms and examine different substances that can break down the extracellular polymeric substances (EPS) that are produced by the bacteria and create protection against subsequent antibiotics. Some of these substances have been described 1000 years ago (Harrison et al), and others are being designed today for hopeful clinical application in the near future (Batoni et al, Banerjee et al, Yadav et al). Engineers are attempting to create catheters that defoul themselves to decrease urinary tract infections (Levering et al), and perhaps this technology could apply to other devices in the future.

Meta-analyses fail to show a clear winner of chlorhexidine versus betadine in skin preparation, though the lean is going toward chlorhexidine in alcohol (Dumville et al). NSQIP database has brought back the 'old school' superiority of a mechanical and oral bowel prep prior to colorectal surgery (Kiran et al).

Sawyer et al demonstrate the success of 4 days of antibiotics after source control of intra-abdominal infections while Jarrell et al show the equivalence of 4 days of antibiotics to treat catheter associated UTIs in a trauma population.

Both Thakore et al and Bliss et al demonstrate the great expense of post surgical patients who have an infectious complication. They both show that there are no easily modifiable variable to prevent these infections and that financially punishing hospitals and physicians for infections in many of our populations after surgery needs to be carefully studied before implementation as this penalty is unlikely to change outcomes.

An interesting financial discussion of antibiotic treatment of uncomplicated appendicitis is discussed by Wu et al. Moghadamyeghaneh et al demonstrate the greater safety of elective treatment of diverticulitis compared to urgent or emergent treatment.

Kenneth A. Andreoni, MD, FACS

A 1,000-Year-Old Antimicrobial Remedy with Antistaphylococcal Activity

Harrison F, Roberts AEL, Gabrilska R, et al (Univ of Nottingham, United Kingdom; Texas Tech Univ Health Sciences Ctr, Lubbock)
MBio 6:e01129-15, 2015

Plant-derived compounds and other natural substances are a rich potential source of compounds that kill or attenuate pathogens that are resistant to current antibiotics. Medieval societies used a range of these natural substances to treat conditions clearly recognizable to the modern eye as microbial infections, and there has been much debate over the likely efficacy of these treatments. Our interdisciplinary team, comprising researchers from both sciences and humanities, identified and reconstructed a potential remedy for *Staphylococcus aureus* infection from a 10th century Anglo-Saxon leechbook. The remedy repeatedly killed established *S. aureus* biofilms in an *in vitro* model of soft tissue infection and killed methicillin-resistant *S. aureus* (MRSA) in a mouse chronic wound model. While the remedy contained several ingredients that are individually known to have some antibacterial activity, full efficacy required the combined action of several ingredients, highlighting the scholarship of premodern doctors and the potential of ancient texts as a source of new antimicrobial agents.

Importance.—While the antibiotic potential of some materials used in historical medicine has been demonstrated, empirical tests of entire remedies are scarce. This is an important omission, because the efficacy of "ancientbiotics" could rely on the combined activity of their various ingredients. This would lead us to underestimate their efficacy and, by extension, the scholarship of premodern doctors. It could also help us to understand why some natural compounds that show antibacterial promise in the laboratory fail to yield positive results in clinical trials. We have reconstructed a 1,000-year-old remedy which kills the bacteria it was designed to treat and have shown that this activity relies on the combined activity of several antimicrobial ingredients. Our results highlight (i) the scholarship and rational methodology of premodern medical professionals and (ii) the untapped potential of premodern remedies for yielding novel therapeutics at a time when new antibiotics are desperately needed.

▶ Old, old, old school.

Although modern medicine is rediscovering the importance of biofilms and how otherwise antibiotic susceptible organisms are protected within these complex structures, ancient practitioners had medications that used the ability of natural compounds to disrupt biofilms and allow for eradication of infection. The combination of various substances to prevent biofilm formation on implantable devices such as hernia mesh or orthopedic joints is being actively explored as multiresistant bacteria become the norm in modern health care facilities.

Perhaps one answer is to learn from the past and use more combinations of low-toxicity substances, which together break down the power of the biofilm.

K. A. Andreoni, MD, FACS

Antimicrobial peptides and their interaction with biofilms of medically relevant bacteria

Batoni G, Maisetta G, Esin S (Univ of Pisa, Italy)

Biochim Biophys Acta 1858:1044-1060, 2016

Biofilm-associated infections represent one of the major threats of modern medicine. Biofilm-forming bacteria are encased in a complex mixture of extracellular polymeric substances (EPS) and acquire properties that render them highly tolerant to conventional antibiotics and host immune response. Therefore, there is a pressing demand of new drugs active against microbial biofilms. In this regard, antimicrobial peptides (AMPs) represent an option taken increasingly in consideration. After dissecting the peculiar biofilm features that may greatly affect the development of new antibiofilm drugs, the present article provides a general overview of the rationale behind the use of AMPs against biofilms of medically relevant bacteria and on the possible mechanisms of AMP-antibiofilm activity. An analysis of the interactions of AMPs with biofilm components, especially those constituting the EPS, and the obstacles and/or opportunities that may arise from such interactions in the development of new AMP-based antibiofilm strategies is also presented and discussed. This article is part of a Special Issue entitled: Antimicrobial Peptides edited by Karl Lohner and Kai Hilpert.

▶ Biofilms are now acknowledged to be a major problem in successfully treating many types of infections, especially ones involving foreign bodies of some type. The bacteria protected within the biofilm are functionally resistant to antibiotics that would normally kill planktonic forms of the same bacteria. New approaches to fighting infection must include strategies to break down the extracellular polymeric substances so the bacteria can be successfully cleared with standard antibiotics. The use of antimicrobial peptides (AMPs) or host defense peptides may be a new approach to preventing and treating biofilm infections. The article reviews the microenvironment of biofilms and how these AMPs may work to help prevent or break down biofilms.

K. A. Andreoni, MD, FACS

Spectrum of bacteria associated with diabetic foot ulcer and biofilm formation: A prospective study

Banu A, Noorul Hassan MM, Rajkumar J, et al (Bangalore Med College and Res Inst, India)

Australas Med J 8:280-285, 2015

Background.—India has the world's largest number of diabetics. Non-traumatic lower limb amputation is the most common devastating complication of diabetes, primarily due to diabetic foot ulcers (DFU) and diabetic foot infections (DFI). In India, the incidence of foot ulcers ranges from 8–17 per cent. DFIs are predominantly polymicrobial and multidrug-resistant (MDR) with the ability to form biofilm, which is an important virulence factor and results in treatment failure.

Aims.—The main objectives of the study are to identify the spectrum of multidrug-resistant bacteria associated with these infections, their antibiotic sensitivity pattern, and to detect the biofilm formation.

Methods.—This was a prospective study at a tertiary care hospital. One hundred patients over the age of 18, having chronic diabetic foot ulcer, and attending the surgery outpatient department were included. Samples of pus were collected from deep wounds and processed using standard techniques for culture and sensitivity. Biofilm detection was done. Results were compiled and statistically analysed.

Results.—One hundred samples were processed and 82 yielded positive cultures. *Staphylococcus aureus* was the predominant organism, followed by *Pseudomonas aeruginosa*. Biofilm formation was seen in 38 (46.34 per cent) of the organisms. Biofilms were formed predominantly by *Staphylococcus aureus* (20 per cent).

Conclusion.—The organisms causing chronic diabetic foot ulcers were commonly multidrug-resistant; this was also observed among biofilm formers. Therefore, screening for biofilm formation, along with the usual antibiogram, needs to be performed as a routine procedure in chronic diabetic ulcers to formulate effective treatment strategies for these patients.

▶ This prospective study of diabetic foot ulcers of more than 3 months' duration yielded biofilm-producing bacteria in 46% of positive cultures. The cultures were all of a single bacterium, and nearly all were multidrug resistant. Routine culturing of these diabetic foot ulcers may help direct therapy, especially with biofilm production. The presence of biofilms requires aggressive debridement to decrease colony count and allow for wound healing.

K. A. Andreoni, MD, FACS

The Small Molecule DAM Inhibitor, Pyrimidinedione, Disrupts *Streptococcus pneumoniae* Biofilm Growth *In Vitro*

Yadav MK, Go YY, Chae S-W, et al (Korea Univ College of Medicine, Seoul, South Korea; et al)

PLoS One 10:e0139238, 2015

Streptococcus pneumoniae persist in the human nasopharynx within organized biofilms. However, expansion to other tissues may cause severe infections such as pneumonia, otitis media, bacteremia, and meningitis, especially in children and the elderly. Bacteria within biofilms possess increased tolerance to antibiotics and are able to resist host defense systems. Bacteria within biofilms exhibit different physiology, metabolism, and gene expression profiles than planktonic cells. These differences underscore the need to identify alternative therapeutic targets and novel antimicrobial compounds that are effective against pneumococcal biofilms. In bacteria, DNA adenine methyltransferase (Dam) alters pathogenic gene expression and catalyzes the methylation of adenine in the DNA duplex and of macromolecules during the activated methyl cycle (AMC). In pneumococci, AMC is involved in the biosynthesis of quorum sensing molecules that regulate competence and biofilm formation. In this study, we examine the effect of a small molecule Dam inhibitor, pyrimidinedione, on *Streptococcus pneumoniae* biofilm formation and evaluate the changes in global gene expression within biofilms via microarray analysis. The effects of pyrimidinedione on *in vitro* biofilms were studied using a static microtiter plate assay, and the architecture of the biofilms was viewed using confocal and scanning electron microscopy. The cytotoxicity of pyrimidinedione was tested on a human middle ear epithelium cell line by CCK-8. *In situ* oligonucleotide microarray was used to compare the global gene expression of *Streptococcus pneumoniae* D39 within biofilms grown in the presence and absence of pyrimidinedione. Real-time RT-PCR was used to study gene expression. Pyrimidinedione inhibits pneumococcal biofilm growth *in vitro* in a concentration-dependent manner, but it does not inhibit planktonic cell growth. Confocal microscopy analysis revealed the absence of organized biofilms, where cell-clumps were scattered and attached to the bottom of the plate when cells were grown in the presence of pyrimidinedione. Scanning electron microscopy analysis demonstrated the absence of an extracellular polysaccharide matrix in pyrimidinedione-grown biofilms compared to control-biofilms. Pyrimidinedione also significantly inhibited MRSA, MSSA, and *Staphylococcus epidermidis* biofilm growth *in vitro*. Furthermore, pyrimidinedione does not exhibit eukaryotic cell toxicity. In a microarray analysis, 56 genes were significantly up-regulated and 204 genes were significantly down-regulated. Genes involved in galactose metabolism were exclusively up-regulated in pyrimidinedione-grown biofilms. Genes related to DNA replication, cell division and the cell cycle, pathogenesis, phosphate-specific transport, signal transduction, fatty acid biosynthesis, protein folding, homeostasis, competence, and biofilm formation were down regulated in pyrimidinedione-grown biofilms. This study demonstrated that the small molecule Dam inhibitor, pyrimidinedione, inhibits pneumococcal biofilm growth *in vitro* at concentrations that do not inhibit planktonic cell growth and down regulates important metabolic-, virulence-, competence-, and biofilm-related genes. The identification of a small molecule (pyrimidinedione) with *S. pneumoniae* biofilm-inhibiting capabilities has potential for the development of new compounds that prevent biofilm formation.

▶ This study looks at a specific inhibitor of a gene whose expression is necessary to regulate biofilm formation within bacteria during the activated methyl cycle (AMC). DNA adenine methyltransferase (Dam) activates this AMC cycle. The authors used a small molecule DAM inhibitor, pyrimidinedione, to study its effects on biofilm production by several bacteria important in nasopharyngeal infections. The pyrimidinedione was able to completely inhibit extracellular polysaccharide matrix production by several bacteria under in vitro conditions. This agent did not result in any direct bacterial killing or growth inhibition, nor did it break down established biofilms. The authors demonstrated no direct cell toxicity of this compound to eukaryotic cell cultures.

This type of compound, which is aimed at genes unique to the prokaryotic cell formation of biofilms, has obvious benefits in terms of likely safety to mammals. Such agents are useful only in preventing the formation of biofilms and thus would appear to be ideal for incorporating within implantable devices or applying to chronic wounds after debriding procedures.

K. A. Andreoni, MD, FACS

The antimicrobial agent, Next-Science, inhibits the development of *Staphylococcus aureus* and *Pseudomonas aeruginosa* biofilms on tympanostomy tubes

Banerjee D, Tran PL, Colmer-Hamood JA, et al (Texas Tech Univ Health Sciences Ctr, Lubbock; et al)

Int J Pediatr Otorhinolaryngol 79:1909-1914, 2015

Objective.—The purpose of this study was to determine if the recently developed novel antimicrobial/antibiofilm agent Next-Science (NS) inhibits biofilm development by *Staphylococcus aureus* or *Pseudomonas aeruginosa* on tympanostomy tubes (TT) and to define the concentration of NS at which this inhibition occurs.

Methods.—Preliminary titration experiments determined the effective concentrations of NS that completely inhibit the planktonic growth of *S. aureus* and *P. aeruginosa*. Since NS has the potential to inhibit both planktonic growth and biofilm development, we examined the antibiofilm effect using the established concentrations that inhibited planktonic growth. Biofilms developed on TT using the microtiter plate assay were assessed quantitatively by determining the number of microorganisms per tube (CFU/tube) and qualitatively by visualization with confocal laser scanning microscopy (CLSM).

Results.—Planktonic growth of *S. aureus* and *P. aeruginosa* was inhibited by 20.3 μg/mL and 325 μg/mL of NS, respectively. While *S. aureus* and *P. aeruginosa* formed well-developed biofilms on TT at 24 h without treatment, addition of the indicated concentrations of NS at the time of inoculation of the TT inhibited the formation of biofilms by both organisms. CLSM confirmed the absence of biofilms on either the inner or outer surface of the treated TTs. At 8 h post-inoculation, *P. aeruginosa* formed a partial biofilm on the TT when untreated. In comparison, the NS-treated biofilms failed to develop further and the CFU/TT were significantly reduced.

Conclusion.—The novel antimicrobial agent NS inhibited the development of *S. aureus* and *P. aeruginosa* biofilms on TTs. The same concentrations of NS inhibited both planktonic growth and biofilm development.

▶ This proprietary compound, Next-Science (NS), is a combination antimicrobial/antibiofilm agent that destroys both the extracellular polymeric substance (EPS) matrix of the biofilm and kills bacteria within the biofilm. The authors had previously used organoselenium to inhibit biofilm production by multiple bacteria on the surface of TTs. Although this was purely an in vitro study, the NS agent was able to penetrate and destabilize an existing biofilm and kill the released bacteria. This agent destabilizes the EPS by chelating calcium, and thus its use in various animal models will need to be explored to both ensure its safety in the living mammal as well as show that NS retains its ability to destroy local biofilm production without having a greater affinity for normal cells and tissues. Even in its current form, it appears as though the use of substances such as NS that can destroy both biofilms and the bacteria within is promising for control of at least topical applications, such as the inner ear, and likely chronic wounds. Long-term safety on more internal uses should also be explored.

K. A. Andreoni, MD, FACS

Urinary catheter capable of repeated on-demand removal of infectious biofilms via active deformation

Levering V, Cao C, Shivapooja P, et al (Duke Univ, Durham, NC)
Biomaterials 77:77-86, 2016

Biofilm removal from biomaterials is of fundamental importance, and is especially relevant when considering the problematic and deleterious impact of biofilm infections on the inner surfaces of urinary catheters. Catheter-associated urinary tract infections are the most common cause of hospital-acquired infections and there are over 30 million Foley urinary catheters used annually in the USA. In this paper, we present the design and optimization of urinary catheter prototypes capable of on-demand removal of biofilms from the inner luminal surface of catheters. The urinary catheters utilize 4 intra-wall inflation lumens that are pressure-actuated to generate region-selective strains in the elastomeric urine lumen, and thereby remove overlying biofilms. A combination of finite-element modeling and prototype fabrication was used to optimize the catheter design to generate greater than 30% strain in the majority of the luminal surface when subjected to pressure. The catheter prototypes are able to remove greater than 80% of a mixed community biofilm of *Proteus mirabilis* and *Escherichia coli* on-demand, and furthermore are able to remove the biofilm repeatedly. Additionally, experiments with the prototypes demonstrate that biofilm debonding can be achieved upon application of both tensile and compressive strains in the inner surface of the catheter. The fouling-release catheter offers the potential for a nonbiologic, non-antibiotic method to remove biofilms and thereby for impacting the thus far intractable problem of catheter-associated infections.

▶ Why direct all your efforts into developing a better Foley catheter? Just ask Willie Sutton: "Because that's where most of the hospital acquired infections are." These engineers developed a catheter with 4 separate inflation lumens that generate deformation in the lumen resulting in sluffing of the biofilm. The catheters were able to remove 80% of the biofilms using both tensile and compressive strains in the inner surface of the catheter.

This novel engineering attempt to remove biofilms and decrease urinary catheter associated urinary tract infections deserves a close look in clinical trial, and this concept is worthy of consideration in applications to other catheter lumens and implantable devices.

In other areas of surgery, engineering attempts to decrease the adherence of bacteria and biofilms is gaining more interest. This is being attempted through both intelligent material design as well as various coatings. The National Academy of Sciences sponsored a roundtable through its Biomedical Engineering Materials and Applications group on October 19, 2015, titled "Implications of Biofilms in Medical Device Applications." International representation was present to discuss this challenging medical problem with new insights into the biology of the biofilm and material design to help prevent fouling.

K. A. Andreoni, MD, FACS

Preoperative skin antiseptics for preventing surgical wound infections after clean surgery

Dumville JC, McFarlane E, Edwards P, et al (Univ of Manchester, United Kingdom; Natl Inst for Health and Clinical Excellence, Manchester, United Kingdom; Univ of York, United Kingdom; et al)

Cochrane Database Syst Rev 4:CD003949, 2015

Background.—Surgical site infection rates in the month following clean surgery vary from 0.6% (knee prosthesis) to 5% (limb amputation). Due to the large number of clean surgical procedures conducted annually the costs of these surgical site infections (SSIs) can be considerable in financial and social terms. Preoperative skin antisepsis using antiseptics is performed to reduce the risk of SSIs by removing soil and transient organisms from the skin where a surgical incision will be made. Antiseptics are thought to be toxic to bacteria and therefore aid their mechanical removal. The effectiveness of preoperative skin preparation is thought to be dependent on both the antiseptic used and the method of application, however, it is unclear whether preoperative skin antisepsis actually reduces postoperative wound infection, and, if so, which antiseptic is most effective.

Objectives.—To determine whether preoperative skin antisepsis immediately prior to surgical incision for clean surgery prevents SSI and to determine the comparative effectiveness of alternative antiseptics.

Search Methods.—For this third update we searched just the Cochrane Wounds Group Specialised Register (searched 27 January 2015); The Cochrane Central Register of Controlled Trials (CENTRAL) (*The Cochrane Library* 2014, Issue 12).

Selection Criteria.—Randomised controlled trials evaluating the use of preoperative skin antiseptics applied immediately prior to incision in clean surgery. There was no restriction on the inclusion of reports based on language of publication, date or publication status.

Data Collection and Analysis.—Data extraction and assessment of risk of bias were undertaken independently by two review authors.

Main Results.—There were no new studies added to the review in the third update.

Thirteen studies were included in this review (2,623 participants). These evaluated several different types of skin antiseptics - leading to 11 different comparisons being made. Although the antiseptics evaluated differed between studies, all trials involved some form of iodine. Iodine in alcohol was compared to alcohol alone in one trial; one trial compared povidone iodine paint (solution type not reported) with soap and alcohol. Six studies compared different types of iodine-containing products with each other and five compared iodine-containing products with chlorhexidine-containing products.

There was evidence from one study suggesting that preoperative skin preparation with 0.5% chlorhexidine in methylated spirits led to a reduced risk of SSI compared with an alcohol based povidone iodine solution: RR 0.47 (95% CI 0.27 to 0.82). However, it is important to note that the trial does not report important details regarding the interventions (such as the concentration of povidone iodine paint used) and trial conduct, such that risk of bias was unclear.

There were no other statistically significant differences in SSI rates in the other comparisons of skin antisepsis. Overall the risk of bias in included studies was unclear.

A mixed treatment comparison meta-analysis was conducted and this suggested that alcohol-containing products had the highest probability of being effective - however, again the quality of this evidence was low.

Authors' Conclusions.—A comprehensive review of current evidence found some evidence that preoperative skin preparation with 0.5% chlorhexidine in methylated spirits was associated with lower rates of SSIs following clean surgery than alcohol-based povidone iodine paint. However this single study was poorly reported. Practitioners may therefore elect to consider other characteristics such as costs and potential side effects when choosing between alternatives.

The design of future trials should be driven by the questions of high priority to decision makers. It may be that investment in at least one large trial (in terms of participants) is warranted in order to add definitive and hopefully conclusive data to the current evidence base. Ideally any future trial would evaluate the iodine-containing and chlorhexidine-containing solutions relevant to current practice as well as the type of solution used (alcohol vs. aqueous).

▶ This Cochrane review was a meta-analysis of 13 published studies looking at surgical site infection after clean surgery. Most studies used 1 type of iodine, many with chlorhexidine, in both alcohol- and aqueous-based solutions. The authors concluded that there still is no definite evidence that one type of skin preparation is superior to another in clean wounds. They point to the Darouiche 2010 study of patients with clean contaminated cases that showed deep incisional infections were fewer with chlorhexidine in alcohol than aqueous povidone iodine. Other meta-analyses that incorporate this study suggest the same. However, the role of alcohol here cannot be isolated.

The authors suggest that a large well-performed randomized trial with povidone and chlorhexidine in aqueous- and alcohol-containing preparations needs to be performed to answer this important clinical question.

K. A. Andreoni, MD, FACS

Combined Preoperative Mechanical Bowel Preparation With Oral Antibiotics Significantly Reduces Surgical Site Infection, Anastomotic Leak, and Ileus After Colorectal Surgery

Kiran RP, Murray ACA, Chiuzan C, et al (Columbia Univ Med Ctr, New York; Columbia Univ, New York)

Ann Surg 262:416-425, 2015

Objectives.—To clarify whether bowel preparation use or its individual components [mechanical bowel preparation (MBP)/oral antibiotics] impact specific outcomes after colorectal surgery.

Methods.—National Surgical Quality Improvement Program–targeted colectomy data initiated in 2012 capture information on the use/type of bowel preparation and colorectal-specific complications. For patients undergoing elective colorectal resection, the impact of preoperative MBP and antibiotics (MBP+/ABX+), MBP alone (MBP+/ABX−), and no bowel preparation (no-prep) on outcomes, particularly anastomotic leak, surgical site infection (SSI), and ileus, were evaluated using unadjusted/adjusted logistic regression analysis.

Results.—Of 8442 patients, 2296 (27.2%) had no-prep, 3822 (45.3%) MBP+/ABX−, and 2324 (27.5%) MBP+/ABX+. Baseline characteristics were similar; however, there were marginally more patients with prior sepsis, ascites, steroid use, bleeding disorders, and disseminated cancer in no-prep. MBP with or without antibiotics was associated with reduced ileus [MBP+/ABX+: odds ratio (OR) = 0.57, 95% confidence interval

(CI): 0.48–0.68; MBP+/ABX–: OR = 0.78, 95% CI: 0.68–0.91] and SSI [MBP+/ABX+: OR = 0.39, 95% CI: 0.32–0.48; MBP+/ABX–: OR = 0.80, 95% CI: 0.69–0.93] versus no-prep. MBP+/ABX+ was also associated with lower anastomotic leak rate than no-prep [OR = 0.45 (95% CI: 0.32–0.64)]. On multivariable analysis, MBP with antibiotics, but not without, was independently associated with reduced anastomotic leak (OR = 0.57, 95% CI: 0.35–0.94), SSI (OR = 0.40, 95% CI: 0.31–0.53), and postoperative ileus (OR = 0.71, 95% CI: 0.56–0.90).

Conclusions.—These data clarify the near 50-year debate whether bowel preparation improves outcomes after colorectal resection. MBP with oral antibiotics reduces by nearly half, SSI, anastomotic leak, and ileus, the most common and troublesome complications after colorectal surgery.

► Old school wins again! It took the American College of Surgeons National Surgical Quality Improvement Program to reverse the hands of time and show that mechanical bowel prep (MBP) with oral antibiotics (ABX) IS superior to no prep or single-component prep in regard to fewer surgical site infections (SSIs), lower anastomotic leak rates, and lower incidence of postoperative ileus. Over the years, there have been many studies for and against MBP and/or ABX. Several years ago, the pendulum swung to no MBP or ABX, and with this study, it should swing in the other direction.

The 3 groups (no prep, MPB+/ABX–, and MBP+/ABX+) did differ in race (more whites in MPB+/ABX+), body mass index (more >30 in both MPB+ groups), previous sepsis, and cancer. Controlling for these differences in multivariate logistic analyses did show significant improvement it the MBP+/ABX+ group regarding SSI, anastomotic leak, and ileus. The authors note they were not able to follow for later *Clostridium difficile* infection, although subsequent study has not shown any effect from oral antibiotics and MBP. ABX+ alone did not show significance in multivariate analysis. The study did confirm that laparoscopic procedures also had lower SSI rates, anastomotic leaks, and ileus than open procedures.

What was not controlled for was the surgeon. Do surgeons who prefer bowel preps have improved outcomes?

K. A. Andreoni, MD, FACS

Wound Edge Protectors in Open Abdominal Surgery to Reduce Surgical Site Infections: A Systematic Review and Meta-Analysis

Mihaljevic AL, Müller TC, Kehl V, et al (Technische Universität München, Munich, Germany)

PLoS One 10:e0121187, 2015

Importance.—Surgical site infections remain one of the most frequent complications following abdominal surgery and cause substantial costs, morbidity and mortality.

Objective.—To assess the effectiveness of wound edge protectors in open abdominal surgery in reducing surgical site infections.

Evidence Review.—A systematic literature search was conducted according to a prespecified review protocol in a variety of data-bases combined with hand-searches for randomized controlled trials on wound edge protectors in patients undergoing laparotomy. A qualitative and quantitative analysis of included trials was conducted.

Findings.—We identified 16 randomized controlled trials including 3695 patients investigating wound edge protectors published between 1972 and 2014. Critical appraisal uncovered a number of methodological flaws, predominantly in the older trials. Wound edge protectors significantly reduced the rate of surgical site infections (risk ratio 0.65; 95% CI, 0.51–0.83; $p = 0.0007$; $I^2 = 52\%$). The results were robust in a number of sensitivity analyses. A similar effect size was found in the subgroup of patients undergoing colorectal surgery (risk ratio 0.65; 95% CI, 0.44–0.97; $p = 0.04$; $I^2 = 56\%$). Of the two common types of wound protectors double ring devices were found to exhibit a greater protective effect (risk ratio 0.29; 95% CI, 0.15–0.55) than single-ring devices (risk ratio 0.71; 95% CI, 0.54–0.92), but this might largely be due to the lower quality of available data for double-ring devices. Exploratory subgroup analyses for the degree of contamination showed a larger protective effect in contaminated cases (0.44; 95% CI, 0.28–0.67; $p = 0.0002$, $I^2 = 23\%$) than in clean-contaminated surgeries (0.72, 95% CI, 0.57–0.91; $p = 0.005$; $I^2 = 46\%$) and a strong effect on the reduction of superficial surgical site infections (risk ratio 0.45; 95% CI, 0.24–0.82; $p = 0.001$; $I^2 = 72\%$).

Conclusions and Relevance.—Wound edge protectors significantly reduce the rate of surgical site infections in open abdominal surgery. Further trials are needed to explore their effectiveness in different risk constellations.

▶ This is a systemic literature review of randomized trials looking at the ability of wound edge protectors to decrease surgical site infections (SSIs) in open abdominal procedures. Utilizing 16 randomized control studies with 3695 patients between 1972 and 2014, a significant reduction in SSIs was seen (relative risk [RR] 0.65; 95% confidence interval [CI], 0.51-0.83). This protection also held performing a subset analysis with colorectal cases only. The double ring devices were found to be superior to the single ring devices. The rings helped to a greater extent in decreasing the amount of wound contamination in contaminated cases (RR 0.44) than clean-contaminated cases (RR 0.72), and this resulted in a significant decrease in SSIs (hazard ratio 0.45; 95% CI, 0.24-0.82).

The authors also discuss reasons for why some apparently well-conducted recent trials have shown no benefit. They review that another author group mentioned the lack of universally changing gloves after removing the ring devices and before fascial closure in the studies that showed no advantage. Most of us can recall using these devices over the years depending on the preference of the attending surgeon. Now it appears that there is reasonable evidence we should consider the double ring wound protectors, especially in contaminated cases.

K. A. Andreoni, MD, FACS

Trial of Short-Course Antimicrobial Therapy for Intraabdominal Infection

Sawyer RG, Claridge JA, Nathens AB, et al (Univ of Virginia Health System, Charlottesville; Case Western Reserve Univ, Cleveland, OH; Univ of Toronto, Ontario, Canada; et al)

N Engl J Med 372:1996-2005, 2015

Background.—The successful treatment of intraabdominal infection requires a combination of anatomical source control and antibiotics. The appropriate duration of antimicrobial therapy remains unclear.

Methods.—We randomly assigned 518 patients with complicated intraabdominal infection and adequate source control to receive antibiotics until 2 days after the resolution of fever, leukocytosis, and ileus, with a maximum of 10 days of therapy (control group), or to receive a fixed course of antibiotics (experimental group) for 4 ± 1 calendar days. The primary outcome was a composite of surgical-site infection, recurrent intraabdominal infection, or death within 30 days after the index source-control procedure, according to treatment group. Secondary outcomes included the duration of therapy and rates of subsequent infections.

Results.—Surgical-site infection, recurrent intraabdominal infection, or death occurred in 56 of 257 patients in the experimental group (21.8%), as compared with 58 of 260 patients in the control group (22.3%) (absolute difference, −0.5 percentage point; 95% confidence interval [CI], −7.0 to 8.0; $P = 0.92$). The median duration of antibiotic therapy was 4.0 days (interquartile range, 4.0 to 5.0) in the experimental group, as compared with 8.0 days (interquartile range, 5.0 to 10.0) in the control group (absolute difference, −4.0 days; 95% CI, −4.7 to −3.3; $P < 0.001$). No significant between group differences were found in the individual rates of the components of the primary outcome or in other secondary outcomes.

Conclusions.—In patients with intraabdominal infections who had undergone an adequate source-control procedure, the outcomes after fixed-duration antibiotic therapy (approximately 4 days) were similar to those after a longer course of antibiotics (approximately 8 days) that extended until after the resolution of physiological abnormalities. (Funded by the National Institutes of Health; STOP-IT ClinicalTrials.gov number, NCT00657566.)

▶ This study focuses on the duration of appropriate antibiotics after source control in surgical patients. The authors warn that there is a reported 20% rate of clinically significant infectious complications after standard antibiotic course treatment, but they hypothesize that this is due to inadequate source control. Their study looks at antibiotic duration after obtaining confirmed source control with an intervention in patients with complicated intraabdominal infections. The durations are defined in the abstract.

Patients had a mean APACHE (Acute Physiology and Chronic Health Evaluation) II score 10 ± 0.3 with most common source from colon or rectum and one-third treated with percutaneous drainage. Forty-seven of 211 patients in the short course treatment group received antibiotics for more than 4 days because of laboratory or clinical abnormalities. Median duration of antibiotics was 4.0 days in the short course treatment group and 8.0 days in the control group. The groups did not differ in rates of *Clostridium difficile*, extraabdominal infection or secondary infections with resistant organisms. The control group did display a longer time to surgical site infection and recurrent intraabdominal infection. The mortality rate was only 1% with both groups, better than predicted per APACHE score. It appears as though successful aggressive source control was more important than antibiotic duration in these patients, and that the use of fewer days of antibiotics was safe. My hospital surgical intensive care unit is using this study to decrease days of antibiotic use in hope of decreasing overall rates of resistant organisms.

K. A. Andreoni, MD, FACS

Short-duration treatment for catheter-associated urinary tract infections in critically ill trauma patients

Jarrell AS, Wood GC, Ponnapula S, et al (The Johns Hopkins Hosp, Baltimore, MD; Univ of Tennessee Health Science Ctr, Memphis; VA Tennessee Valley Healthcare System, Murfreesboro)

J Trauma Acute Care Surg 79:649-653, 2015

Background.—The optimal treatment duration for catheter-associated urinary tract infection (CA-UTI) in critically ill patients is unclear. The Infectious Diseases Society of America recommends up to 14 days of therapy; however, short-duration therapy (SDT) for 3 days to 5 days is often used in trauma intensive care unit (ICU) patients at our center. The efficacy of SDT for CA-UTI has not been studied in this population. The objective was to evaluate the efficacy of SDT for CA-UTI in trauma ICU patients.

Methods.—This retrospective study of patients with CA-UTI in a trauma ICU included patients with a urine culture growing bacteria of 100,000 CFU/mL or greater and definitive antibiotic treatment. Urine cultures were collected as part of standard workups for suspected sepsis. Duration of therapy was at the discretion of the trauma team. Exclusion criteria included concomitant infection, renal replacement therapy, or pregnancy. Clinical success and microbiologic success were evaluated.

Results.—One hundred ninety-two patients were evaluated, and 77 patients with SDT were included. Mean (SD) age was 49 (22) years, median Injury Severity Score (ISS) was 27 (interquartile range, 18–34), and median ICU stay was 17 days (interquartile range, 1–33 days). Mean (SD) duration of CA-UTI therapy was 4 (1) days (range, 3–5 days) with most patients (42%) receiving 5 days. The most common organisms were *Escherichia coli*, *Enterococcus* species, and *Pseudomonas* species. The clinical success rate was 82% (63 of 77), and the microbiologic success rate was 75% (36 of 48). Overall mortality was 4%, but no deaths were CA-UTI related.

Conclusion.—SDT provided an acceptable clinical success rate in critically ill trauma patients, which was similar to studies of CA-UTI in other populations. These results suggest that SDT could be considered an option for treating CA-UTIs in trauma ICU patients.

Level of Evidence.—Therapeutic study, level V.

▶ Shorter duration of antibiotic therapy after source control has become the new theme with the rapid emergence of multiresistant bacteria in our intensive care units (ICUs). The Foley catheter was replaced in these patients at the start of antibiotic therapy. Antibiotics were adjusted when necessary or possible on the basis of culture results. These patients were critically ill and in a trauma ICU with a mean age of 49 ± 22 and 49% men. Time from admission to diagnosis was a median of 5 days and treatment duration was 4 ± 1 days. Only 8% were started on inappropriate antibiotics after final culture results were available.

The authors point out that their success rate of about 82% clinical and 75% microbiologic is consistent with traditional longer courses of therapy. Another study of short- versus long-course oral antibiotics in a VA study showed an advantage of less *Clostridium difficile* infection and fewer late recurrent infections in short-course recipients with no difference in short-term success. The authors do point out that it may not be possible to extrapolate the results in this trauma population to older and more chronically ill populations.

K. A. Andreoni, MD, FACS

Surgical site infection in orthopedic trauma: A case–control study evaluating risk factors and cost

Thakore RV, Greenberg SE, Shi H, et al (Vanderbilt Univ, Nashville, TN)

J Clin Orthop Trauma 6:220-226, 2015

Background.—With the shift of our healthcare system toward a value-based system of reimbursement, complications such as surgical site infections (SSI) may not be reimbursed. The purpose of our study was to investigate the costs and risk factors of SSI for orthopedic trauma patients.

Methods.—Through retrospective analysis, 1819 patients with isolated fractures were identified. Of those, 78 patients who developed SSIs were compared to 78 uninfected control patients. Patients were matched by fracture location, type of fracture, duration of surgery, and as close as possible to age, year of surgery, and type of procedure. Costs for treatment during primary hospitalization and initial readmission were determined and potential risk factors were collected from patient charts. A Wilcoxon test was used to compare the overall costs of treatment for case and control patients. Costs were further broken down into professional fees and technical charges for analysis. Risk factors for SSIs were analyzed through a chi-squared analysis.

Results.—Median cost for treatment for patients with SSIs was $108,782 compared to $57,418 for uninfected patients ($p < 0.001$). Professional fees and technical charges were found to be significantly higher for infected patients. No significant risk factors for SSIs were determined.

Conclusions.—Our findings indicate the potential for financial losses in our new healthcare system due to uncompensated care. SSIs nearly double the cost of treatment for orthopedic trauma patients. There is no single driver of these costs. Reducing postoperative stay may be one method for reducing the cost of treating SSIs, whereas quality management programs may decrease risk of infection.

▶ This matched case-control study is very timely in regard to information on both patient risks that increase orthopedic traumas surgical site infections (SSIs) in a level 1 trauma center population, as well as costs of these SSIs. The authors allude to the increasing financial risks hospitals and physicians will be taking as reimbursement moves nationally from fee-for-service to value-based reimbursement. Medicare's authoritarian decree that certain complications are "never events" gives them license to refuse payment, or even decrease standard payment, if these negative events occur. As all clinicians know, in surgery, wound complications and SSIs occur at a given frequency mostly dependent on wound class, type of operation, presence of devitalized tissue in cases of trauma or severe vascular disease, and other important patient characteristics. There is likely *never* to be a day when SSIs are rare events. The average increased cost for a wound infection in their trauma population was $51 000, nearly double the cost of care for a noninfected patient. More than 80% of the costs were "technical costs" such as hospital room, tests, and the like, and not physician fees. Most importantly in this study, they could not find significant risk factors to delineate the patients who would develop infections from those who did not. Even diabetes only approached significance at 0.07, likely because of the overall low number of diabetics in their trauma population. Being a past smoker and having a cardiac dysrhythmia also trended toward a difference. The authors point to a recent similar study of increased cost with infection after elective orthopedic surgery that demonstrated a 300% increase in costs with 2 more weeks in the hospital for the infected patients.

As this country moves to a value-based payment system, the physicians and hospitals must be at the table when payment methodologies are constructed. Complications are a given in some subset of patients for every operative or otherwise invasive procedure. Bringing careful consideration for how insurers allow for the expected frequency of complications via reimbursement is the only way hospitals and providers will continue to offer services where a significant risk of complications with increased costs exists. The increasing age and comorbidities in our US population will also lead to increased complication rates through the years if a large public health campaign does not reverse the growing diabetes and obesity rates in even our youngest citizens. If these additional costs for complications are not appropriately factored into future payments, access to many of these necessary services will be difficult for many future patients.

K. A. Andreoni, MD, FACS

Readmission After Resections of the Colon and Rectum: Predictors of a Costly and Common Outcome

Bliss LA, Maguire LH, Chau Z, et al (Beth Israel Deaconess Med Ctr, Boston, MA; Massachusetts General Hosp, Boston; UMass Memorial Med Ctr, Worcester, MA; et al)

Dis Colon Rectum 58:1164-1173, 2015

Background.—Readmission rates are a measure of surgical quality and an object of clinical and regulatory scrutiny. Despite increasing efforts to improve quality and contain cost, 6% to 25% of patients are readmitted after colorectal surgery.

Objective.—The aim of this study is to define the predictors and costs of readmission following colorectal surgery.

Design.—This is a retrospective cohort study of patients undergoing elective and nonelective colectomy and/ or proctectomy in the Healthcare Cost and Utilization Project Florida State Inpatient Database 2007 to 2011. Readmission is defined as inpatient admission within 30 days of discharge. Univariate analyses were performed of sex, age, Elixhauser score, race, insurance type, procedure, indication, readmission diagnosis, cost, and length of stay. Multivariate analysis was performed by logistic regression. Sensitivity analysis of nonemergent admissions was conducted.

Settings.—This study was conducted in Florida acutecare hospitals.

Patients.—Patients undergoing colectomy and proctectomy from 2007 to 2011 were included.

Intervention(S).—There were no interventions.

Main Outcome Measure(S).—The primary outcomes measured were readmission and the cost of readmission.

Results.—A total of 93,913 patients underwent colectomy; 14.7% were readmitted within 30 days. From 2007 to 2011, readmission rates remained stable (14.6%–14.2%, trend $p = 0.1585$). After multivariate adjustment, patient factors associated with readmission included nonwhite race, age <65, and a diagnosis code other than neoplasm or diverticular disease ($p < 0.0001$). Patients with Medicare or Medicaid were more likely to be readmitted than those with private insurance ($p < 0.0001$). Patients with longer index admissions, those with stomas, and those undergoing all procedures other than sigmoid or transverse colectomy were more likely to be readmitted ($p < 0.0001$). High-volume hospitals had higher rates of readmission ($p < 0.0001$). The most common reason for readmission was infection (32.9%). Median cost of readmission care was $7030 (intraquartile range, $4220–$13,247). Fistulas caused the most costly readmissions ($15,174; intraquartile range, $6725–$26,660).

Limitations.—Administrative data and retrospective design were limitations of this study.

Conclusions.—Readmissions rates after colorectal surgery remain common and costly. Nonprivate insurance, IBD, and high hospital volume are significantly associated with readmission.

▶ Analyzing a retrospective database, 14.7% of patients who underwent colectomy were readmitted within 30 days. As expected, the most common reason for readmission was infection (32%). Inflammatory bowel disease with fistula formation was the most expensive reason for readmission, nearly twice the cost of infection. Patients under age 65 had an adjusted hazard ratio (HR) for readmission of 1.2, with nonwhite patients at HR 1.103, Medicare patients at 1.357, and Medicaid patients 1.516. Total colectomy (HR 1.842), abdominoperineal resection (HR 1.516), and a stoma formation (HR 1.333) were the most likely procedures to result in readmission. Indication for colectomy from ischemia (HR 1.467) was the most likely cause for readmission with neoplasm and diverticular disease the lowest. Surprisingly, and in contradiction to 2 previous large studies, high-volume hospitals had a higher rate of readmission (HR 1.133), even despite multivariate adjustment. Despite the great push for decreased length of stay over the past several years, there was no improvement in readmission rates from 2007 to 2011. The authors conclude that many factors correlated with readmission are not easily modifiable, such as age, race, comorbidities, and indication for procedure. The pressure to decrease readmissions in colorectal surgery has not resulted in any significant improvement in readmission rates. The authors state that perhaps longer initial length of stays may decrease readmission rates coupled with more intense outpatient care of the higher risk patients. Again, politics alone cannot legislate less expensive or improved health care. Additional outpatient services are likely a fundamental tool in decreasing hospital readmissions of all types, particularly after surgery. These services are currently not adequately available because they are under- or unfunded, and they are more challenging in rural population areas.

K. A. Andreoni, MD, FACS

Cost effectiveness of nonoperative management versus laparoscopic appendectomy for acute uncomplicated appendicitis

Wu JX, Dawes AJ, Sacks GD, et al (UCLA David Geffen School of Medicine, Los Angeles, CA; et al)

Surgery 158:712-721, 2015

Background.—Appendectomy remains the gold standard in the treatment of acute, uncomplicated appendicitis in the United States. Nonetheless, there is growing evidence that nonoperative management is safe and efficacious.

Methods.—We constructed a decision tree to compare nonoperative management of appendicitis with laparoscopic appendectomy in otherwise healthy adults. Model variables were abstracted from a literature review, data from the Healthcare Cost and Utilization Project data, the Medicare Physician Fee schedule, and the American College of Surgeons Surgical Risk Calculator. Uncertainty surrounding parameters of the model was assessed via 1-way and probabilistic sensitivity analyses.

Results.—Operative management cost $12,213 per patient. Nonoperative management without interval appendectomy (IA) was the dominant strategy, costing $1,865 less and producing 0.03 more quality-adjusted life-years (QALYs). Nonoperative management with IA cost $4,271 more than operative management, but yielded only 0.01 additional QALY. One-way sensitivity analysis suggested operative management would become the preferred strategy if the recurrence rate was >40.5% or the total cost of appendectomy was decreased to <$5,468. Probabilistic sensitivity analysis confirmed nonoperative management without IA was the preferred strategy in 95.6% of cases.

Conclusion.—Nonoperative management without IA is the least costly, most effective treatment for acute, uncomplicated appendicitis and warrants further evaluation in a disease thought to be definitively surgical.

► Nonoperative management (3 days of inpatient antibiotics followed by 7 days of oral outpatient antibiotics) may save significant amounts every year as the average appendectomy in the United States costs near $9000. Some studies suggest that up to 20% of patients treated nonoperatively at first may require subsequent surgery. Would delayed surgery lead to an overall offset of the initial cost savings due to more complicated surgery and longer length of stay in delayed surgical care patients? The authors estimated that nonoperative hospitalization was $1865 less than a surgical admission. Nonoperative management with later interval appendicitis (IA) was obviously the least cost-effective strategy at $4271 more than conventional initial surgery. Using literature data and Medicare costs, the authors estimated that failure of medical care would need to be around 40% in all situations (initial medical hospitalization, recurrence with 30 days of discharge or recurrence, or recurrence of appendicitis without IA). The estimates the authors used from the literature were 12.5% for initial antibiotic failure, 10.5% for failure within 30 days of discharge, and 6% for failure of second antibiotic course. Emergency expenses and estimates of more complicated delayed surgery are included in the analysis. The authors do discuss clearly that their estimates of antibiotic failure are for uncomplicated appendicitis, which excludes appendicoliths. In complicated cases, recurrence has been reported at 39%. The quality of life estimates are minimal, and the patient effect of preventable perforation and ostomy may be undervalued in this study.

We must be attentive to the fact that surgeons should continue to be the primary caregivers in acute appendicitis. Early operative intervention in cases of antibiotic failure are necessary both for optimal patient outcomes and fiscal outcomes. Future studies should investigate the value of daily surgical evaluation of the uncomplicated acute appendicitis patient undergoing attempts at non-surgical management.

K. A. Andreoni, MD, FACS

A comparison of outcomes of emergent, urgent, and elective surgical treatment of diverticulitis

Moghadamyeghaneh Z, Carmichael JC, Smith BR, et al (Univ of California, Irvine, CA)

Am J Surg 210:838-845, 2015

Background.—There is a controversy regarding the best urgent surgical treatment of colonic diverticulitis. We sought to compare outcomes of patients who underwent surgery for diverticulitis by the type of admission.

Methods.—The National Surgical Quality Improvement Program databases were used to examine the clinical data of patients who underwent colorectal resection for diverticulitis during 2012 to 2013. Multivariate regression analysis was performed to identify outcomes of patients.

Results.—We sampled a total of 13,510 patients admitted for diverticulitis who underwent colorectal resection, of which 7.8% had emergent and 19.7% had urgent operation. Patients with perforation (adjusted odds ratio [AOR] 188.56, $P < .01$) and preoperative sepsis (AOR 28.17, $P < .01$) had significantly higher rates of emergent surgery. Patients who underwent emergent operation had higher mortality (AOR 4.08, $P = .04$) and morbidity (AOR 2.14, $P < .01$). Emergent operations had a significantly higher risk of anastomosis leakage compared with elective operation (AOR 3.92, $P = .02$).

Conclusions.—Emergent treatment of diverticulitis is associated with a high morbidity and mortality. In the setting of emergent treatment of diverticulitis, colonic anastomosis without a stoma has a high risk of anastomosis leakage.

▶ With one-third of the US population having diverticulosis and 20% of those developing diverticulitis, this large National Surgical Quality Improvement Program 2012-2013 database study is highly informative for both patient outcomes and cost of surgery for emergent, urgent, and elective treatment of diverticulitis. Of the 19% of all diverticulitis patients, 18% of those required emergent surgery; 7.8% of those who had a colon resection were emergent with 19.7% urgent and the remaining 72.5% elective surgery. For emergent procedures, resection and colostomy without anastomosis was performed in 83.6% of patients and in 58% of those with urgent surgery. Most importantly, mortality rates were 6.9%, 3.5%, and 0.2% for emergent, urgent, and elective cases. Similarly, postoperative complications were a similar trend, as was prolonged length of stay and hemorrhagic complications. Emergent surgery also had a higher anastomotic leak rate in the relatively fewer patients who had that procedure. Patients who had laparoscopic surgery did better, but risk factors that prevented laparoscopic surgery (only 8.1% of emergent cases) also correlated with overall complications and mortality, as expected. Sixty-one percent of emergent surgical patients had postoperative morbidity, consistent with prior reports.

The authors did find that patients admitted with high white blood cell counts and American Society of Anesthesiologists classification score > 2 had a high rate of emergency surgery, and further studies are warranted to determine whether these patients should go to surgery more quickly to improve postoperative complications. Because of the high rate of anastomotic leak in nonelective patients, an ileostomy proximal to primary anastomosis may be most prudent in urgent cases. Perhaps this could be a strategy in a larger percentage of emergent cases, although a randomized study is necessary to answer this question.

With the recent move toward more medical treatment of even recurrent diverticulitis, a lifetime risk-benefit with cost analysis study needs to be done. If a significant number of these medically managed patients later present as nonelective surgical patients, a subset of these medically managed patients may warrant safer and less costly elective resection.

K. A. Andreoni, MD, FACS

Long-term Mortality After Rapid Screening and Decolonization of Staphylococcus Aureus Carriers: Observational Follow-up Study of a Randomized, Placebo-controlled Trial

Bode LGM, van Rijen MML, Wertheim HFL, et al (Erasmus Univ Med Ctr, Rotterdam, the Netherlands; Amphia Hosp, Breda, the Netherlands; et al)

Ann Surg 263:511-515, 2016

Objective.—To identify patients who benefit most from Staphylococcus aureus screening and decolonization treatment upon admission.

Background.—*S. aureus* carriers are at increased risk of developing surgical-site infections with *S. aureus*. Previously, we demonstrated in a randomized, placebo-controlled trial (RCT) that these infections can largely be prevented by detection of carriage and decolonization treatment upon admission. In this study, we analyzed 1- and 3-year mortality rates in both treatment arms of the RCT to identify patient groups that should be targeted when implementing the screen-and-treat strategy.

Methods.—Three years after enrolment in the RCT, mortality dates of all surgical patients were checked. One- and 3-year mortality rates were calculated for all patients and for various subgroups.

Results.—After 3 years, 44 of 431 (10.2%) and 43 of 362 (11.9%) patients had died in the mupirocin/chlorhexidine and placebo groups, respectively. No significant differences in mortality rates were observed between the treatment groups or the subgroups according to type of surgery. In the subgroup of patients with clean procedures (382 cardiothoracic, 167 orthopedic, 61 vascular, and 56 other), mupirocin/chlorhexidine reduced 1-year mortality: 11 of 365 (3.0%) died in the mupirocin/chlorhexidine versus 21 of 301 (7.0%) in the placebo group [hazard ratio = 0.38 (95% CI: 0.18–0.81)].

Conclusions.—Detection and decolonization of *S. aureus* carriage not only prevents *S. aureus* surgical-site infections but also reduces 1-year mortality in surgical patients undergoing clean procedures. Such patients with a high risk of developing *S. aureus* infections should therefore be the primary target when implementing the screen-and-treat strategy in clinical practice.

▶ The authors discuss that decolonizing patients who are carriers of *Staphylococcus aureus* with mupirocin nasal ointment and washing with chlorhexidine soap resulted in half as many patients (3.4%) with surgical site infections (SSIs) compared with (7.7%) of those in the placebo group (randomized double-blind placebo-controlled multicenter trial with 1251 *S aureus* carriers discovered). The authors followed these patients to see whether protection from SSI resulted in a mortality benefit at 1 and 3 years. The cumulative mortality rates were the same, but those who underwent a clean operation at their initial hospitalization had far fewer SSIs and subsequent mortality if they were decolonized on admission versus those in the placebo group (3% vs 7% at 1 year, 7.4% vs 10% at 3 years). The survival curves stayed separated to the 10-year follow-up.

Other studies have shown chlorhexidine soap can prevent colonization with resistant organisms while in the hospital. With all of our hospitals having larger populations of patients carrying *S aureus* and other more resistant organisms, preoperative screening may become more common in hopes of improving 1- and 3-year mortality.

K. A. Andreoni, MD, FACS

Clinical recommendations and practical guide for negative pressure wound therapy with instillation

Gupta S, Gabriel A, Lantis J, et al (Loma Linda Univ School of Medicine, CA; PeaceHealth Med Group Plastic Surgery, Vancouver, WA; Mount Sinai St. Luke's Roosevelt Hosp, New York)
Int Wound J 13:159-174, 2016

Effective wound management involves a comprehensive assessment of the patient and the wound to determine an optimal wound treatment plan. It is critical to identify and address factors that may impair wound healing, prior to selecting the most appropriate therapy for each patient. Negative pressure wound therapy (NPWT) is a well-established advanced therapy that has been successful in adjunctive management of acute and chronic wounds. In recent years, the introduction of topical wound solution delivery in combination with NPWT has provided further benefits to wound healing. A commercially available system now offers automated, volumetric control of instilled topical wound solutions with a dwell time in combination with NPWT (NPWTi-d; V.A.C. VeraFlo™ Therapy, KCI, an Acelity company, San Antonio, TX). This NPWTi-d system differs from other instillation systems in that a timed, predetermined volume of topical wound solution is intermittently delivered (versus continuously fed) and allowed to dwell in the wound bed (without NPWT), for a user-selected period of time before NPWT is resumed. This added accuracy and process simplification of solution delivery in tandem with NPWT have prompted use of NPWTi-d as first-line therapy in a wider subset of complex wounds. However, considerably more research is required to validate efficacy of NPWTi-d in various wound types. The purpose of this review is to provide a relevant overview of wound healing, describe current literature supporting the adjunctive use of NPWTi-d, propose a clinical approach for appropriate application of NPWTi-d and conclude with case studies demonstrating successful use of NPWTi-d. Based on this review, we conclude that either a large case series examining effects of NPWTi-d on different wound types or possibly a large prospective registry evaluating NPWTi-d with real-world topical wound solutions versus immediate debridement and closure would be valuable to the medical community in evaluating the efficacy of this promising therapy.

▶ The authors discuss the advantages of wound irrigation in difficult-to-heal wounds, such as wound hydration and helping to remove deep cellular debris, wound exudate, and metabolic wastes. Negative pressure wound therapy (NPWT) increases blood flow and granulation tissue formation but has not been shown to improve bioburden. The authors review the logic behind combining NPWT with solution instillation with a set dwell time (NPWTi-d) to help improve wounds with high bioburden. Prior studies have shown that instillation of fluid with later removal via NPWT removes wound exudate and decreases planktonic bacteria burden while increasing granulation tissue formation. Results have also been show to improve outcome with decreased time to final surgical procedure, fewer operative procedures, shorter hospital stays, and faster wound healing. The fluid instillation also results in increased patient comfort with dressing changes. Some studies calculated a cost savings of $8143 per patient attributable to fewer operative debridements with the NPWTi-d system.

Former studies also show that periodic instillation cover the wound much more equally than continuous irrigation, especially in allowing the solution to reach undermined regions of the wound. Two types of solution have been suggested by an expert panel: Prontosan (ie, polyhexamethylene biguanide with betaine and water) and Microcyn/Dermacyn. Others have used Dakin's solution with saline with good effect.

Defining which wounds truly benefit from the initially more expensive NPWTi-d technology will be an important discussion to allow appropriate use of this technology for difficult wound treatment.

K. A. Andreoni, MD, FACS

Deaths from necrotizing fasciitis in the United States, 2003–2013

Arif N, Yousfi S, Vinnard C (Drexel Univ College of Medicine, Philadelphia, PA)

Epidemiol Infect 144:1338-1344, 2016

Necrotizing fasciitis (NF) is a life-threatening infection requiring urgent surgical and medical therapy. Our objective was to estimate the mortality burden of NF in the United States, and to identify time trends in the incidence rate of NF-related mortality. We obtained data from the National Center for Health Statistics, which receives information from death certificates from all states, including demographic information and cause of death. The U.S. Multiple Cause of Death Files were searched from 2003 to 2013 for a listing of NF (ICD-10 code M72.6) as either the underlying or contributing cause of death. We identified a total of 9871 NF-related deaths in the United States between 2003 and 2013, corresponding to a crude mortality rate of 4·8 deaths/1 000 000 person-years, without a significant time trend. Compared to white individuals, the incidence rate of NF-associated death was greater in black, Hispanic, and American Indian individuals, and lower in Asian individuals. Streptococcal infection was most commonly identified in cases where a pathogen was reported. Diabetes mellitus and obesity were more commonly observed in NF-related deaths compared to deaths due to other causes. Racial differences in the incidence of NF-related deaths merits further investigation.

▶ As expected, streptococcal infection was the most common infection identified. There was no trend in frequency of death from necrotizing fasciitis (NF) over the duration of the study period from 2003 to 2013. The highest risk factors for NF associated death were obesity (hazard ratio [HR] 2.83) and diabetes (HR 2.37) with renal failure a close third (HR 2.31). Age was a strong risk factor for death from NF.

This study suffers from the standard weaknesses of a death certificate retrospective study. The accuracy of the comorbid conditions was not checked against Medicare-available information or the like for accuracy. A more detailed electronic health record of NF may be warranted to have a clearer idea of degree of diabetic control, amount of obesity, and stage of renal dysfunction. I would have thought that the association with diabetes would have been stronger, but again, a more detailed review of electronic health records may help with this clinical observation made in the past.

K. A. Andreoni, MD, FACS

Daptomycin for the treatment of osteomyelitis and orthopaedic device infections: real-world clinical experience from a European registry

Malizos K, Sarma J, Seaton RA, et al (Univ of Thessalia, Larissa, Greece; North Tyneside General Hosp, North Shields, United Kingdom; Queen Elizabeth Univ Hosp, Glasgow, United Kingdom; et al)

Eur J Clin Microbiol Infect Dis 35:111-118, 2016

Osteomyelitis is a serious infection predominantly caused by Gram-positive bacteria, including methicillinresistant *Staphylococcus aureus* (MRSA). Orthopaedic device-related infections are complex and require a careful combination of surgical intervention and antimicrobial therapy. Daptomycin, a cyclic lipopeptide, effectively penetrates soft tissue and bone and demonstrates rapid concentration-dependent bactericidal activity against Gram-positive pathogens. This retrospective, non-interventional study evaluated clinical outcomes in patients with osteomyelitis or orthopaedic device infections treated with daptomycin from the European Cubicin® Outcomes Registry and Experience (EU-CORE^{SM}) study. Patients were treated between January 2006 and April 2012, with follow-up to 2014. Clinical outcomes were assessed as success (cured or improved), failure or nonevaluable. Of 6,075 patients enrolled, 638 (median age, 63.5 years) had primary infections of osteomyelitis or orthopaedic device infections, 224 had non-prosthetic osteomyelitis, 208 had osteomyelitis related to a permanent or temporary prosthetic device, and 206 had orthopaedic device infections. The most commonly isolated pathogen was *S. aureus* (214 [49.1%]; 24.8% were MRSA). Overall, 455 (71.3%) patients had received previous antibiotic therapy. Patients underwent surgical interventions, including tissue (225 [35.3%]) and bone (196 [30.7%]) debridement, as part of their treatment. Clinical success rates were 82.7% and 81.7% in *S. aureus* and coagulase-negative staphylococcal infections. Adverse events (AEs) and serious AEs assessed as possibly related to daptomycin were observed in 6.7% and 1.9% of patients, respectively. Daptomycin was discontinued by 5.5% of patients due to AEs and 10 (1.6%) deaths were reported. In conclusion, daptomycin was effective and safe in patients with osteomyelitis or orthopaedic device infections.

▶ The authors provide background that osteomyelitis is most commonly caused by *Staphylococcus aureus*, with coagulase-negative staphylococci the most common in prosthetic joint and device-related infection. Because of biofilm production on bone or prosthetics, cure often involves surgical debridement/removal of infected material and appropriate antibiotics. In appropriately treated cases, good responses are seen in 80% to 90% of patients; however, relapse rates can be high. In particular, the authors note the synergistic effect of daptomycin and rifampin to inhibit biofilm production and possibly reduce formation of resistance to antibiotics.

High rates of clinical success were seen with both first-line (80.1%) and second-line (83.1%) daptomycin treatment. In combination with rifampin, successful treatment trended upward to 86.8% versus 80.3% with single therapy. Median duration of therapy was 14 days for inpatients, 27 days for outpatients, and only 6 days for intensive care unit patients. Adverse events (AEs; 6.7%) and serious AEs (1.9%) were low. Three rhabdomyolysis cases occurred, possibly related to daptomycin. Two-year follow-up showed little late recurrence. The authors conclude that the combination of daptomycin and oral rifampin is highly effective with low rates of AEs in this patient population. There was no mention of infusion catheter use or complications of intravenous access.

With the added expense of intravenous formulation, a comparison with intravenous transitioned to oral linezolid is the obvious next topic of study in this patient population.

K. A. Andreoni, MD, FACS

Validated prediction model for severe groin wound infection after lower extremity revascularization procedures

Bennett KM, Levinson H, Scarborough JE, et al (Duke Univ Med Ctr, Durham, NC)

J Vasc Surg 63:414-419, 2016

Background.—Groin wound infection is a costly and morbid event after lower extremity revascularization. To date, a comprehensive and validated method for identifying patients who are at greatest risk for this complication has yet to be developed.

Methods.—Our retrospective analysis included all patients at a single institution who underwent lower extremity revascularization using a groin incision from 2009 through 2012. Patients were randomly assigned to one of two groups: a test group, which was used to develop a predictive model for our primary outcome; and a validation group, which was used to test that model. The primary outcome for our analysis was severe groin wound infection, which we defined as postoperative groin infection that required operative intervention. Multimodel inference methods were used to evaluate all possible combinations, interactions, and transformations of potential predictor variables from the test group of patients. The resulting model that exhibited the lowest Akaike information criterion was then selected for testing with the validation group of patients.

Results.—A total of 284 patients who underwent lower extremity revascularization procedures were included in our study (140 in the test group, 144 in the validation group). In the test group, 17 patients (12.1%) developed severe groin wound infection requiring operative intervention. The best-fit predictive model developed from this group identified the following independent risk factors for severe groin wound infection: prior ipsilateral groin incision, female gender, body mass index, end-stage renal disease, malnutrition, and urgent or emergency procedure status. The correct classification rate of this model in the test group was 88.6%. The incidence of severe groin wound infection in the validation group was 13.9%, and application of our predictive model to this group yielded a correct classification rate of 86.1%.

Conclusions.—We have developed and validated a statistical model that accurately predicts those patients who are likely to sustain severe groin wound infection after lower extremity revascularization.

▶ The authors used their single-center data to find a predictive model for severe groin infection after lower extremity revascularization procedures. The independent risk factors were not unexpected: prior ipsilateral groin incision, female gender, body mass index, end stage renal disease, malnutrition, and urgent or emergent surgery. Prophylactic muscle flap coverage is identified as a potential useful procedure at the time of bypass if one could predict which patients would benefit upfront.

Their patients had a 13% rate of severe groin infection requiring reoperation. They had a correlation of 88% with their test patients and 86% with their validation patients of predicting severe groin wounds requiring reoperation. They plan on using this model to perform prophylactic muscle flap coverage on their highest risk patients.

Because multiple studies are showing that we cannot prevent most surgical wound infections with our current strategies, tools to help surgeons predict with high accuracy which wounds are most at risk may allow additional prophylactic maneuvers, such as a muscle flap in groin wounds, or may convince surgeons to apply negative pressure wound therapy or pack other types of wounds to allow either delayed primary or secondary closure.

K. A. Andreoni, MD, FACS

7 Endocrine

Defining contralateral adrenal suppression in primary aldosteronism: implications for diagnosis and outcome

Kline GA, Chin A, So B, et al (Univ of Calgary, Alberta, Canada)

Clin Endocrinol (Oxf) 83:20-27, 2015

Objective.—Unilateral primary aldosteronism (PA) should have a contralaterally normal and therefore suppressed adrenal zona glomerulosa. However, there is no validated definition of adrenal suppression. We created two biochemical hypotheses of adrenal suppression based upon measurements taken during adrenal vein sampling (AVS) to determine whether either proved useful for interpretation of AVS or prediction of hypertension outcome in operated cases.

Design.—Retrospective database analysis.

Patients.—Ninety-nine cases of PA from a tertiary hypertension unit.

Measurements.—Hypothesis 1 was the proportional suppression of the uninvolved/lowest $adrenal_{aldo/cortisol}$ to $IVC_{aldo/cortisol}$ ratio pre- and post cosyntropin. Hypothesis 2 was the absolute decrease in the uninvolved $adrenal_{aldo/cortisol}$ ratio after cortrosyn injection. ROC analysis performed using lateralization and hypertension resolution as the outcomes of interest.

Results.—Hypothesis 1 proved highly predictive of lateralization with a ROC AUC of 0·958, $P < 0 \cdot 0001$, giving $adrenal_{aldo/cortisol}$: $IVC_{aldo/cortisol}$ <1·4 as the optimized criterion (sensitivity 90%, specificity 94%). For blood pressure outcomes in the surgical subgroup ($n = 52$), hypertension resolution was most commonly seen among subjects with adrenal suppression by both definitions although there was significant overlap with subjects requiring ongoing medication.

Conclusions.—Post cosyntropin suppression of the uninvolved adrenal-to-IVC ratio is a highly useful definition of adrenal suppression that accurately predicts unilateral PA. This may be particularly useful in a case where AVS fails to catheterize one of the adrenal veins but suppression is seen on the other side. Adrenal suppression may also predict blood pressure outcome, however, a much larger PA database is likely necessary to determine the relative contribution of this predictor.

▶ Adrenal vein sampling (AVS) has slowly become a standard part of the diagnostic algorithm for almost all patients who face a diagnosis of primary hyperaldosteronism. A lateralization index >4 has been the most widely accepted cutoff for a localizing study. However, it is not uncommon to have a borderline lateralization index (LI) and the authors address this scenario in this article. The study is a multicenter study, which is important because patients had some difference in technique used for the AVS. It appears that all centers used a cosyntropin stimulation, but half of the centers used just a bolus and half a bolus followed by an infusion. Contralateral suppression was documented with a lateralization index > 2.6 and a ratio of plasma aldosterone to cortisol in the nondominant side compared with the ratio in the vena cava < 1. Of the 29 patients operated on with a LI < 4, those in the group with contralateral suppression had excellent outcomes, comparable to those with a LI > 4, whereas those in the group without suppression had normalization of hypokalemia—that is, evidence that there was a beneficial effect, but only approximately half had normalization of the aldosterone to renin ratio postoperatively. The argument for AVS in patients with primary aldosteronism is compelling. This study significantly enhances the argument for surgery in patients who have borderline AVS and contralateral suppression. How to advise patients who have borderline AVS and do not meet criteria for contralateral suppression remains a difficult problem because it is clear from the resolution of the hypokalemia that these patients also benefited in some way from the surgery. Finally, it is somewhat surprising that the authors conclude by advocating including findings on CT scan in the final decision on whether to operate. The results of the AVS really should be paramount in this decision.

T. J. Fahey III, MD

A Meta-Analysis of Somatic KCNJ5 K$^+$ Channel Mutations In 1636 Patients With an Aldosterone-Producing Adenoma

Lenzini L, Rossitto G, Maiolino G, et al (Univ of Padua, Italy; et al)
J Clin Endocrinol Metab 100:E1089-E1095, 2015

Context.—Due to selection biases and inadequate statistical power, individual studies may fail to identify the clinical features of patients with an aldosterone-producing adenoma (APA) harboring KCNJ5 mutations. When this failure occurs, meta-analysis can provide significant outcome data.

Objective.—The objective was to determine the clinical features of these APA patients.

Design.—We systematically searched the PubMed, Scopus, Web of Science, and Cochrane databases library in January 2015 applying the Population, Intervention, Comparison, and Outcome (PICO) strategy. The standardized differences in mean and corresponding 95% confidence interval of continuous variables were computed by random-effects modeling.

Setting.—We performed a meta-analysis of all available studies on somatic KCNJ5 mutations in APA.

Patients.—We could identify 13 studies that recruited 1636 patients (age 49 ± 4 years; 55% females).

Main Outcomes and Measures.—Differences between APA with and without KCNJ5 mutations in gender, plasma renin activity, plasma aldosterone, tumor size, serum potassium, and blood pressure were investigated.

Results.—The overall prevalence of KCNJ5 mutations was 43% (range = 12–80%). Their rate was lower ($P < .003$) in the studies done in Europe, the United States, and Australia (35%) than in Japan and China (63%); it correlated ($r = 0.60$, $P = .029$) with the mean daily urinary sodium excretion. Compared with the wild-type, the mutated APA patients were younger (45 ± 3 vs 52 ± 5 yrs), had higher plasma aldosterone (42 ± 8 vs 33 ± 8 ng/dl), larger tumors (16.1 ± 6.4 versus 14.9 ± 7.4 mm), and were more often females (67% vs 44%) (all $P < .05$).

Conclusions.—Meta-analysis showed that more pronounced hyperaldosteronism, young age, female gender, and larger tumors are the phenotypic features of APA patients with KCNJ5 mutations. No significant differences in blood pressure and serum K^+ was found, which suggests that these clinical features do not help in identifying mutated APA patients.

▶ Primary hyperaldosteronism is the most common endocrine cause for hypertension. These authors performed a meta-analysis of published studies analyzing the presence of KCNJ5 in the adrenal nodules from patients who underwent surgery for primary hyperaldosteronism. KCNJ5 mutations are now the most commonly recognized mutation in patients with primary hyperaldosteronism. The most notable finding is that the identification of the KCNJ5 mutation occurs twice as often in studies from Asia than in the United States, Europe, or Australia (approximately two-thirds of Asian patients and one-third of patients in United States, Europe, and Australian studies). Unfortunately, although the study confirms the importance of KCJN5 mutations in the pathogenesis of unilateral hyperaldosteronism, it leaves many questions unanswered. Are these differences genetically or environmentally determined? Because the clinical presentation of the disease is similar between patients with a mutation and without, is this important to know? And finally, if a drug targeting the mutation (similar to Sensipar for primary hyperparathyroidism) is developed, what will the role of medical management be, especially for patients who are currently managed nonsurgically? Unfortunately, the incidence of mutations in these patients (with bilateral hyperplasia) is not well characterized. Further studies are needed to try to identify a cause or predisposition to developing a KCJN5 mutation.

T. J. Fahey III, MD

Screening Tests for Cushing's Syndrome: Urinary Free Cortisol Role Measured by LC-MS/MS

Ceccato F, Barbot M, Zilio M, et al (Univ-Hosp of Padova, Italy)

J Clin Endocrinol Metab 100:3856-3861, 2015

Introduction and Aim.—As initial screening for Cushing's syndrome (CS), The Endocrine Society guidelines recommend one of the following: the 1-mg dexamethasone suppression test (DST) or late-night salivary cortisol (LNSC) or urinary free cortisol (UFC) measurement. We examined the diagnostic performance of the above-mentioned tests in a series of patients.

Materials and Methods.—We retrospectively analyzed 137 patients with clinical conditions suggestive of hypercortisolism: 38 with confirmed CS diagnosis and 99 without (termed non-CS). UFC was measured by liquid chromatography tandem-mass spectrometry, whereas LNSC by the radioimmunometric method and serum cortisol were measured by a chemiluminescence immunoassay.

Results.—Comparing CS vs non-CS, a cutoff of 138 nmol/L after 1-mg DST revealed the best specificity (SP; 97%), whereas the 50-nmol/L cutoff confirmed the best sensitivity (SE; 100%); the SE and SP for LNSC greater than 14.46 nmol/L were, respectively, 84% and 89%, whereas the SE and SP for UFC greater than 170 nmol per 24 hours, they were 97% and 91%. Overall, UFC revealed both a combined higher positive and a lower negative likelihood ratio among first-line tests (respectively 10.7 and 0.03). Computing a receiver-operating curve-contrast analysis to compare the power of each single test with that of the others, alone or combined (DST + LNSC, DST + UFC, and LNSC + UFC) or with that of all the tests together (DST + LNSC + UFC), the UFC assay was at least as good as all the other possible combinations.

Conclusions.—Measuring UFC by liquid chromatography tandem-mass spectrometry achieves the best accuracy in diagnosing CS among patients presenting with suspected hypercortisolism.

▶ Work-up of patients with adrenal incidentalomas or patients referred with possible Cushing syndrome must include an assessment of cortisol levels. Currently, there are 3 basic options, excluding serum cortisol, which should never be used as a screening test for Cushing syndrome. These options are the 1 mg dexamethasone suppression test, a single late-night salivary cortisol assay, or 24-hour urine collection for urinary free cortisol. Traditionally the 24-hour urinary free cortisol level was reported to have the highest specificity for Cushing syndrome, although some recent reports that used an antibody detection method for cortisol have been less accurate. Here the authors report that the 24-hour urine collection, when measured by liquid chromatography with mass spectrometry, is the best overall test (Table 1 in the original article). However, it is important to realize that the sensitivity and specificity of these tests is highly dependent on where you set the cutoff as diagnostic for Cushing. This is highlighted by the data included on the 1-mg dexamethasone suppression test that indicates a higher threshold allows for higher specificity although lower sensitivity. It is worth noting that in our population of patients in the United States (this study was conducted in northern Italy), the specificity for the 1-mg dexamethasone suppression test is usually even lower because of the higher percentage of obese and overweight patients. Another lesson to be learned from this study is to be sure that the laboratory you are sending your sample to is one that uses the chromatography-mass spectrometry technique. Finally, the authors suggest in the conclusion that urinary free cortisol can be used as the screening test and confirmed with the 1-mg dexamethasone suppression test. Many endocrinologists whom I have worked with would feel more comfortable with the reverse order, although I routinely order the urinary free cortisol as the first and usually only test.

T. J. Fahey III, MD

Features Associated With Metastases Among Well-Differentiated Neuroendocrine (Carcinoid) Tumors of the Appendix: The Significance of Small Vessel Invasion in Addition to Size

Kleiman DA, Finnerty B, Beninato T, et al (Weill Cornell Med College, New York)

Dis Colon Rectum 58:1137-1143, 2015

Background.—The risk of metastatic disease among carcinoid tumors of the appendix increases with tumor size. However, it is unclear if any features other than size are also associated with an increased risk of metastatic disease.

Objective.—The aim of this study was to review the characteristics of appendiceal carcinoid tumors and determine if other histologic features besides size should guide surgical decision making.

Design.—This study involved a retrospective case series.

Settings.—This study was conducted at a single tertiary acute care hospital.

Patients.—Patients diagnosed with an appendiceal carcinoid tumor between 2000 and 2014 were identified. Goblet cell carcinoids, adenocarcinomas with neuroendocrine features, and tumors from other primary locations were excluded.

Interventions.—Simple appendectomy or segmental/total colectomy with lymphadenectomy was performed.

Main Outcome Measures.—The primary outcomes measured were metastases, recurrence, and overall survival.

Results.—Seventy-nine patients were included. The overall incidence of metastatic disease was 10%. Patients with metastatic disease were more likely to be male (75% vs 28%, $p = 0.008$), have small-vessel invasion (43% vs 5%, $p = 0.001$), and have larger tumors (median 2.0 cm vs 0.5 cm, $p < 0.001$). Among tumors <2 cm, the incidence of metastases among tumors with small-vessel invasion was 60% compared with 0% among those without smallvessel invasion ($p < 0.001$). Among tumors ≥2 cm, the incidence of metastases was 50% irrespective of smallvessel invasion. If small-vessel invasion was used as a second indication for performing a right hemicolectomy along with size ≥2 cm, both the sensitivity and negative predictive value would have been 100% compared with 63% and 96% if size was used alone. Patients with metastatic disease had a higher incidence of recurrence (13% vs 0%, $p = 0.003$), but overall survival was 100% in both groups.

Limitations.—Small sample size, retrospective design, and limited long-term follow-up were the limitations of this study.

Conclusions.—Carcinoid tumors of the appendix <2 cm with small-vessel invasion have similar metastatic potential as tumors ≥2 cm. Therefore, a recommendation for a right hemicolectomy should be considered for tumors <2 cm with small-vessel invasion. Additional prospective multicenter studies are warranted.

▶ The dilemma about when to go back and do more radical surgery when an appendiceal carcinoid is found on appendectomy persists. This is particularly true for appendiceal carcinoids between 1 and 2 cm. Although the metastatic potential of these tumors is generally recognized to be low, and the mortality for appendiceal carcinoid tumors between 1 and 2 cm rare, the decision as to whether additional surgery is necessary for these lesions is difficult for both doctors and patients largely because inadequate data are available. This report adds support to the histologic finding of small vessel invasion as an important prognosticator of the presence of metastases in tumors in the gray-zone of 1 to 2 cm in diameter. Although this is clearly not the only factor that should be taken into consideration, the absence of small vessel invasion histologically was associated with 0% chance of lymph node metastases. The study is large for a single-center study on appendiceal carcinoids, but it remains a small series, and thus validation of the results should be sought in much larger clinical series.

T. J. Fahey III, MD

Clinical value of ^{68}Ga-DOTATATE-PET/CT compared to stand-alone contrast enhanced CT for the detection of extra-hepatic metastases in patients with neuroendocrine tumours (NET)

Albanus DR, Apitzsch J, Erdem Z, et al (Univ Hosp RWTH Aachen, Pauwelsstraße, Aachen, Germany; et al)

Eur J Radiol 84:1866-1872, 2015

Purpose.—To compare and outline the beneficial skills of combined ^{68}Ga-DOTATATE positron emission tomography (PET) with concurrent contrast enhanced X-ray computed tomography (ceCT) against stand-alone ceCT in 54 patients with neuroendocrine tumours (NET).

Methods.—Patients with histologically confirmed NET and available follow-up of at least 6 months (median 12.6 months; range 6.1–23.2) were included. PET/CT and ceCT images were initially analyzed separately by two blinded nuclear medicine physicians and two radiologists, respectively. In a second step all four physicians reviewed all detected lesions together reaching a consensus-grading for PET/ceCT. The results were then compared to the reference standard consisting of clinical follow-up data.

Results.—With regard to true positive lesions, PET/ceCT vs. stand alone ceCT detected 139 vs. 48 bone-lesions, 106 vs. 71 lymph node metastases and 26 vs. 26 pulmonary lesions. On a per-patient basis, PET/ceCT achieved a higher sensitivity (100% vs. 47%) and specificity (89% vs. 49%) for bone lesions than ceCT. For lymph nodes the effect was similar (sensitivity 92% vs. 64% and specificity 83% vs. 59%). For the detection of pulmonary lesions the sensitivity was identical (100%) while specificity of PET/ceCT was superior to ceCT-alone (95% vs. 82%).

Conclusion.—In summary, the use of ^{68}Ga-DOTATATE PET/ceCT leads to an increase in sensitivity and specificity in the detection of extra-hepatic NET metastases compared to stand-alone ceCT. Therefore, ^{68}Ga-DOTATATE PET/ceCT should be the imaging modality of choice in patients with NET.

► Imaging neuroendocrine tumors, especially metastases, has been a vexing problem. Here the authors demonstrate that ^{68}gallium DOTATATE is superior to standard contrast enhanced CT for identifying metastatic disease in patients with neuroendocrine tumors (NETs), and particularly for metastases to bone or lymph nodes. DOTATATE is a pharmacologically modified octreotide analog that binds to the somatostatin receptor. The use of ^{68}gallium DOTATATE will become increasingly important because it is likely that patients with metastatic NETs will be candidates for treatment with peptide receptor radionuclide therapy (PRRT) such as lutetium dotatoc. The authors do acknowledge that there are some limitations with their study design here. First, only patients who were not adequately imaged by CT alone were likely referred for DOTATATE imaging. Second, there really was no way to eliminate false-positive scans in the DOTATATE studies because not all of these lesions were confirmed by biopsy. The biggest problem facing patients and their physicians is that the gallium DOTATATE scans are not widely available. However, it is likely that as PRRT becomes Food and Drug Administration approved, more centers will provide Gallium DOTATATE scans for patients with NETs.

T. J. Fahey III, MD

Hyperparathyroidism Associated with Long-Term Proton Pump Inhibitors Independent of Concurrent Bisphosphonate Therapy in Elderly Adults

Hinson AM, Wilkerson BM, Rothman-Fitts I, et al (Univ of Arkansas for Med Sciences, Little Rock)

J Am Geriatr Soc 63:2070-2073, 2015

Objectives.—To measure the effect of proton pump inhibitors (PPIs), with and without concurrent bisphosphonates, on parathyroid hormone (PTH), vitamin D, and calcium.

Design.—Retrospective chart review of individuals 60 years and older. Subjects with reduced renal function (creatinine >1.3 mg/dL) and low vitamin D (<30 ng/mL) were excluded.

Setting.—Academic geriatric outpatient center in southern midwest.

Participants.—Individuals aged 60 and older with concurrent calcium, PTH, vitamin D, and creatinine laboratory measurements ($N = 80$) meeting labeled criteria.

Measurements.—Serum calcium, PTH, vitamin D, and creatinine.

Results.—Chronic PPI exposure was associated with statistically significantly higher PTH (65.5 vs 30.3 pg/mL, $P < .001$; normal range 10–55 pg/mL) and lower calcium (9.1 vs 9.4 mg/dL, $P = .02$; normal range 8.5–10.5 mg/dL) than no PPI exposure. Chronic PPI exposure with concurrent BP therapy was associated with statistically significantly higher PTH (65.2 vs 43.4 pg/mL, $P = .05$) and lower calcium (9.2 vs 9.6 mg/dL, $P = .04$) than BP therapy only.

Conclusion.—Based on the present study, chronic PPI exposure in elderly adults is associated with mild hyperparathyroidism regardless of concurrent oral BP administration (Fig 2).

► This is an interesting study that links chronic proton pump inhibitors (PPI) use with higher parathyroid hormone (PTH) levels in older adults. The study is retrospective and relatively small (20 patients in each of 4 arms), but as shown in Fig 2, the PTH levels in the patients taking PPIs for more than 6 months had substantially higher PTH levels regardless of whether they were also taking bisphosphonates. The authors propose a number of possible explanations to explain this observed effect, including chronic calcium malabsorption induced by PPIs, leading to a secondary type of hyperparathyroidism. This is supported by the fact that calcium levels were statistically lower on average,

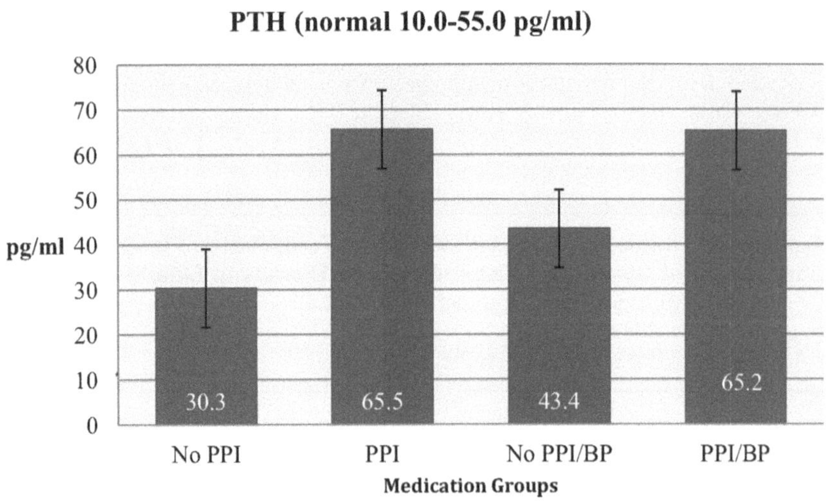

FIGURE 2.—Parathyroid hormone (PTH) levels (normal range 10–55 pg/mL) were significantly higher ($P < .001$) in the proton pump inhibitor (PPI) group (65.5 ± 31.7 pg/mL) than in the group not taking a PPI (30.3 ± 18.0 pg/mL). In the presence of bisphosphonates (BP), PTH levels were significantly higher ($P = 0.05$) in the PPI group (65.2 ± 36.3 pg/mL) than in the group taking a BP alone (43.4 ± 31.1 pg/mL). The error bars denote 1 standard deviation from the mean. (Reprinted from Hinson AM, Wilkerson BM, Rothman-Fitts I, et al. Hyperparathyroidism associated with long-term proton pump inhibitors independent of concurrent bisphosphonate therapy in elderly adults. *J Am Geriatr Soc.* 2015;63:2070-2073, with permission from The American Geriatrics Society.)

even if only by 0.3 to 0.4 mg/dL. There is also some evidence in animal models that PPIs can directly induce higher PTH gene expression. The finding that the elevation in PTH is also found in patients on concurrent bisphosphonates provides an interesting possible link to fracture risk in patients on chronic PPIs. It raises the possibility that both medicines contribute synergistically to disordered bone formation. Certainly additional data need to be accrued to evaluate this possibility. The data presented give additional pause to recommending PPIs on a chronic basis and stimulate further research into the relationship into PPIs and eucalcemic elevations in parathyroid hormone.

T. J. Fahey III, MD

Normocalcaemic, vitamin D-sufficient hyperparathyroidism – high prevalence and low morbidity in the general population: A long-term follow-up study, the WHO MONICA project, Gothenburg, Sweden

Kontogeorgos G, Trimpou P, Laine CM, et al (Univ of Gothenburg, Sweden)

Clin Endocrinol (Oxf) 83:277-284, 2015

Objective.—There is limited knowledge about the natural history of normocalcaemic, vitamin D-sufficient hyperparathyroidism (nHPT). The aim was to study the prevalence of nHPT and its relation to morbidity.

Design.—Cross-sectional and retrospective study at the Sahlgrenska University Hospital, Gothenburg, Sweden.

Subjects.—A random population of 608 men and women, age 25–64 years, was studied in 1995 as part of the WHO MONICA study and reinvestigated in 2008 ($n = 410$, of whom 277 were vitamin D sufficient).

Measurements.—A serum intact parathyroid hormone (S-PTH) ≥60 ng/l was considered as HPT, S-calcium 2·15–2·49 mmol/l as normocalcaemia and S-25(OH)D ≥ 50 nmol/l as vitamin D sufficiency. Data on fractures, stroke and myocardial infarction were retrieved until 2013, that is a 17-year follow-up.

Results.—The prevalence of nHPT was 2·0% in 1995 (age 25–64) and 11·0% in 2008 (age 38–79). S-PTH was positively correlated with age and BMI. After adjustment for these variables, a high S-PTH level (≥60 ng/l) at follow-up was associated with previously low S-25(OH)D, high osteocalcin, S-PTH and both past and presently treated hypertension. No relation was seen with creatinine, cystatin C, malabsorption markers, thyroid function, glucose, insulin, lipids, calcaneal quantitative ultrasound, fractures, myocardial infarction, stroke or death at follow-up.

Conclusions.—This small random population study showed that nHPT was common, 11% at follow-up. Only one individual developed mild hypercalcaemia in 13 years. Previous S-PTH was predictive of nHPT and hypertension was prevalent, but no increase in hard end-points was seen over a 17-year period.

▶ Management of patients with eucalcemia and elevation in their serum parathyroid hormone levels is complex. Usually patients referred for consideration of surgery with eucalcemia and elevated parathyroid hormone (PTH) levels have some possible complication that can be attributed to possible early hyperparathyroidism. These cases must be treated on an individual basis because there is no exact formula that can predict benefit. This article suggests that patients with eucalcemic hyperparathyroidism (designated nHPT in this article) have little if any morbidity that can be attributed to their elevated parathyroid hormone levels. The major problem with this study is the very small number of patients that fit into the nHPT group. Only 25 patients make up the 2% group that had normal serum calcium and elevated PTH levels, and only 12 of these could truly be characterized as nHPT because 13 of the 25 had low 25-OH vitamin D levels. Ultimately 5 of these 12 patients either died or were lost to follow-up. Additionally, the authors analyzed only fracture incidence and major cardiovascular events as outcomes. Interestingly 1 of the 13 patients with low vitamin D and nHPT died from suicide. So any conclusions drawn here have to be considered with a high degree of circumspection. Thus, although I am not advocating for routine neck exploration for patients with isolated nHPT, this article does not eliminate concerns about these patients, and further study is needed.

T. J. Fahey III, MD

No Need to Abandon Focused Unilateral Exploration for Primary Hyperparathyroidism with Intraoperative Monitoring of Intact Parathyroid Hormone

Day KM, Elsayed M, Monchik JM (Rhode Island Hosp, Providence, RI)
J Am Coll Surg 221:518-523, 2015

Background.—We investigated the rate of persistent and recurrent hyperparathyroidism after focused unilateral exploration (UE) with intraoperative monitoring of intact parathyroid hormone (IOPTH).

Study Design.—A prospective cohort of 915 patients with primary hyperparathyroidism (PHP) underwent parathyroid surgery by a single surgeon from January 2003 to September 2013. A total of 556 patients with at least a single positive preoperative localization by ultrasound (US) and/or sestamibi scan (STS) underwent UE with IOPTH. The criterion for completion of surgery was an IOPTH fall of 50% from the highest intraoperative level and into the normal range 5 to 10 minutes after resection of the localized gland.

Results.—Fifteen patients had either persistent or recurrent PHP, yielding a 2.7% (95% CI 1.6% to 4.4%) overall recurrence rate based on the refined Wilson method with continuity correction. Four patients had persistent PHP. Three of these patients were cured with reoperation, and the fourth patient was followed nonoperatively. Eleven patients had recurrent PHP, with 5 corrected by surgery and 6 patients followed nonoperatively. The mean postoperative serum calcium (Ca) level was 9.4 mg/dL over a mean follow-up interval of 44.0 months. Preoperative localization rates by each localization study were: US 74.3% (n = 413), STS 86.9%

(n = 483), and US and STS 71.4% (n = 397). There was no difference in the preoperative study that localized the hyperfunctional parathyroid gland in recurrent vs nonrecurrent patients by the Fisher's exact test (US, $p = 1.00$; STS, $p = 0.65$; US and STS, $p = 1.00$).

Conclusions.—The low rate of recurrent PHP after focused unilateral exploration with IOPTH suggests that this procedure should not be abandoned.

▶ This is a simple retrospective report analyzing a single surgeon's experience with focused parathyroid explorations over a 10-year period. Recent literature, most notably from Jim Norman's group in Tampa, has strongly advocated for routine bilateral exploration to achieve the lowest recurrence rates. Others have maintained that a focused exploration using intraoperative parathyroid hormone monitoring remains a valid approach. This article by Dr Monchik documents excellent outcomes over the 10-year period with a persistence/ recurrence rate combined of < 3%. It is worth noting that not all patients over the 10 years underwent a focused exploration; only approximately 60% of patients were deemed appropriate for unilateral focused exploration by preoperative imaging and intraoperative PTH results. The outcomes reported here are similar to the report from the Miami group some years ago and confound the findings reported by the Cleveland Clinic group that indicate that up to 25% of patients slated to undergo unilateral exploration may have additional enlarged glands identified at the time of surgery. Although the pendulum has definitely swung back toward bilateral exploration for primary hyperparathyroidism, for the well-localized patient with a single identified gland, a unilateral exploration with intraoperative PTH remains a valid option. I find that this is particularly important for patients who are having surgery under a local anesthetic because routine bilateral exploration is considerably more uncomfortable for patients if they are awake.

T. J. Fahey III, MD

Parathyroidectomy Halts the Deterioration of Renal Function in Primary Hyperparathyroidism

Tassone F, Guarnieri A, Castellano E, et al (Santa Croce and Carle Hosp, Cuneo, Italy; et al)

J Clin Endocrinol Metab 100:3069-3073, 2015

Objective.—Decreased renal function has been consistently included among factors prompting recommendation for surgery in primary hyperparathyroidism (PHPT). However, most retrospective studies addressing this issue did not show an improvement in renal function after parathyroidectomy (PTX). The aim of this study was to investigate changes in renal function after PTX in PHPT patients subdivided according to renal function at diagnosis.

Design.—This was a retrospective cross-sectional study.

Patients and Methods.—We studied 109 consecutive PHPT patients before and after PTX. Biochemical evaluation included fasting total and ionized serum calcium, phosphate, creatinine, immunoreactive intact PTH, and 25-hydroxyvitamin D3 levels. Glomerular filtration rate (GFR) was assessed with the Chronic Kidney Disease Epidemiology Collaboration (CKD-EPI) equation.

Results.—Mean (± SD) CKD-EPI estimated GFR (eGFR) at diagnosis was 82.4 ± 19.3 mL/min/1.73 m^2 (median, 84.8 mL/min/1.73 m^2; interquartile range, 68.5–94.2 mL/min/1.73 m^2). Patients with eGFR equal to or higher than 60 mL/min/1.73 m^2 (group 1, $n = 95$) were significantly younger than patients with eGFR lower than 60 mL/min/1.73 m^2 (group 2, $n = 14$; $P < .0003$). After PTX, eGFR did not change in patients of group 2 ($P = .509$), whereas it was significantly reduced in patients of group 1 ($P < .0002$). The difference in eGFR between baseline and post-PTX values was correlated negatively with baseline serum creatinine ($R = -0.27$; $P = .0052$) and positively with baseline CKD-EPI eGFR ($R = 0.32$; $P = .00062$). At multiple regression analysis, only systolic blood pressure and baseline CKD-EPI eGFR were independent predictors of GFR variation.

Conclusion.—Surgical cure of PHPT halts renal function deterioration in patients with coexisting renal disease. Our study thus supports the indication for surgery in patients with eGFR less than 60 mL/min/1.73 m^2, as recommended by current guidelines. Moreover, our data show that presurgical renal function is a relevant predictor of renal function after PTX.

▶ One of the criteria used to refer patients with biochemical hyperparathyroidism for surgery is altered renal function, but data supporting improvement or interruption of continued decline are lacking. This study does provide some support, but the numbers are surprisingly small, and the data somewhat sparse. In addition to the small number of patients (only 14) in the group of patients with a glomerular filtration rate (GFR) <60 (the standard criteria for renal impairment), the timing of the post-parathyroidectomy GFR calculation was fairly short: only a little over 2 years. Thus, although the data presented can certainly lend support for a role for parathyroidectomy in preventing further deterioration of renal function in patients whose renal function is already compromised, a larger study with longer follow-up remains desirable. Finally, it is not at all clear why patients with normal renal function should have a decline in GFR following parathyroidectomy. The decline reported here is not dramatic, but it was statistically significant and thus cannot be ignored. Further study will be necessary to address this question.

T. J. Fahey III, MD

Parathyroidectomy and survival among Japanese hemodialysis patients with secondary hyperparathyroidism

Komaba H, Taniguchi M, Wada A, et al (Tokai Univ School of Medicine, Isehara, Japan; Committee of Renal Data Registry of the Japanese Society for Dialysis Therapy, Tokyo, Japan)

Kidney Int 88:350-359, 2015

Parathyroidectomy (PTx) drastically improves biochemical parameters and clinical symptoms related to severe secondary hyperparathyroidism (SHPT) but the effect of PTx on survival has not been adequately investigated. Here we analyzed data on 114,064 maintenance hemodialysis patients from a nationwide registry of the Japanese Society for Dialysis Therapy to evaluate the associations of severity of SHPT and history of PTx with 1-year all-cause and cardiovascular mortality. We then compared the mortality rate between 4428 patients who had undergone PTx and 4428 propensity score—matched patients who had not despite severe SHPT. During a 1-year follow-up, 7926 patients of the entire study population died, of whom 3607 died from cardiovascular disease. Among patients without a history of PTx, severe SHPT was associated with an increased risk for all-cause and cardiovascular mortality. However, such an increased risk of mortality was not observed among patients with a history of PTx. In the propensity score—matched analysis, patients who had undergone PTx had a 34% and 41% lower risk for all-cause and cardiovascular mortality, respectively, compared to the matched controls. The survival benefit associated with PTx was robust in several sensitivity analyses and consistent across subgroups, except for those who had persistent postoperative SHPT. Thus, successful PTx may reduce the risk for all-cause and cardiovascular mortality in hemodialysis patients with severe, uncontrolled SHPT (Fig 4).

▶ Referral for parathyroidectomy for patients with secondary hyperparathyroidism declined substantially after the introduction of cinacalcet. Currently, most dialysis patients are maintained on cinacalcet unless their PTH levels become dramatically elevated or they are not tolerating the cinacalcet. This article presents a comprehensive analysis of a large database that strongly advocates for parathyroidectomy in the management of patients with renal secondary hyperparathyroidism as shown best in Fig 4. The study does have some flaws, and these are delineated nicely in an accompanying commentary on the article.[1] Perhaps the most important limitation is that the design of the study looks at mortality starting a variable length of time after parathyroidectomy but always more than several months after surgery, and thus postoperative surgical mortality is excluded from the equation. Perioperative mortality has been estimated to be around 3% after parathyroidectomy for this patient population, so this is not a trivial exclusion. Additionally, although the authors match the patients with controls, some bias may be introduced in this study design because patients who do not undergo surgery may have

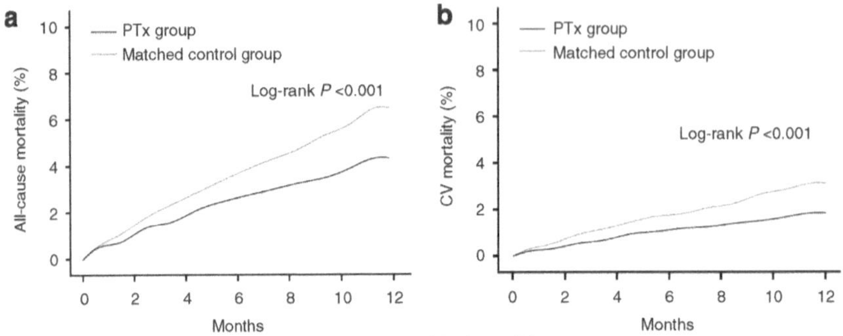

Number at risk							
PTx	4428	4395	4356	4317	4293	4270	4231
Control	4428	4378	4322	4274	4234	4189	4136

Number at risk							
PTx	4428	4395	4356	4317	4293	4270	4231
Control	4428	4378	4322	4274	4234	4189	4136

FIGURE 4.—Kaplan–Meier analysis of all-cause and cardiovascular mortality in the propensity score–matched cohort comparing patients who had undergone PTx with those who had not undergone PTx. (**a**) All-cause mortality. (**b**) Cardiovascular mortality. CV, cardiovascular; PTx, parathyroidectomy. (Reprinted from Komaba H, Taniguchi M, Wada A, et al. Parathyroidectomy and survival among Japanese hemodialysis patients with secondary hyperparathyroidism. *Kidney Int.* 2015;88:350-359, with permission from International Society of Nephrology.)

been sicker and thus more prone to mortality than those eligible to undergo surgery. Despite these potential biases, the data support a return to a more aggressive surgical approach to dialysis-dependent patients with significantly elevated PTH levels—at least until better medical therapy becomes available.

T. J. Fahey III, MD

Reference

1. Scialla JJ, Wolf M. When there will never be a randomized controlled trial. *Kidney Int.* 2015;88:220-222.

How Well Does Renal Transplantation Cure Hyperparathyroidism?

Lou I, Foley D, Odorico SK, et al (Univ of Wisconsin, Madison)
Ann Surg 262:653-659, 2015

Background.—Most patients with end-stage renal disease will develop hyperparathyroidism (HPT). Transplantation reportedly resolves HPT in most cases. Currently, guidelines recommend a watchful waiting approach to HPT for the first 12 months after the transplantation to allow maximal allograft function. The purpose of our study is to examine the incidence and impact of HPT, defined as an elevated parathyroid hormone (PTH) level, after renal transplantation in a contemporary cohort.

Methods.—Primary kidney transplantation was performed on 1609 patients from January 1, 2004, to June 6, 2012. Patients were stratified by timing of achieving normal serum PTH levels, and a multivariate logistic regression was constructed to determine predictive variables.

Kaplan–Meier analysis was then performed on overall graft survival based on PTH normalization.

Results.—Four hundred eighty-eight (30.3%) patients achieved normal PTH within 1 year posttransplant. Four hundred twenty-seven (26.6%) attained normal PTH between 1 and 2 years, with the remaining 694 (43.1%) categorized as having HPT. Patients achieving normal PTH within 12 months of transplantation had a significantly longer median graft survival (7.33 years) compared with those patients who normalized between 12 and 24 months (4.92 years, $P < 0.001$), and those with HPT (5.13 years, $P < 0.001$). Comparing normalization of PTH by 2 years to HPT patients, obesity ($P < 0.001$), months on dialysis ($P < 0.001$), and delayed graft failure ($P = 0.006$) were predictive of nonnormalization. Overall, allograft survival analysis revealed a survival advantage for patients who normalize PTH within 24 months of transplantation ($P = 0.038$).

Conclusions.—Renal transplant resolves HPT in 56.9% of patients at 2 years. Resolution within the first year portends longer graft survival. Therefore, earlier intervention for HPT should be considered.

▶ A previous article reviewed here found that parathyroidectomy in dialysis patients with secondary hyperparathyroidism was associated with decreased mortality.[1] This report supports a role for parathyroidectomy in the posttransplant patient if their parathyroid (PTH) hormone levels do not normalize within 1 year to improve graft survival. The report comes from one of the largest transplant centers, and so the numbers for a single center are quite good for such an analysis. However, the big question that remains after reading the article is what, if any, is the mechanism behind this association. Unfortunately, the authors did not provide data on serum calcium levels during this time and did not have preoperative PTH levels available. Furthermore, it is not known from the data presented whether the patients with elevated PTH had worse graft function thereby causing the elevated PTH levels (as pointed out by Dr. Quan Duh in the discussion of the article). The authors also note in the discussion that only 13% of their patients were managed with cinacalcet while on dialysis—a number that seems very low. This raises the question as to whether the patient population here started with significantly higher pretransplant PTH levels and could explain the fairly low percent (56%) of patients who did resolve their elevated PTH within the first 2 years after transplant. The article is an excellent example of how initial observations frequently raise more questions than they answer.

T. J. Fahey III, MD

Reference

1. Komaba H, Taniguchi M, Wada A, Iseki K, Tsubakihara Y, Fukagawa M. Parathyroidectomy and survival among Japanese hemodialysis patients with secondary hyperparathyroidism. *Kidney Intl.* 2015;88:350-359.

Intramuscular and subcutaneous forearm parathyroid autograft hyperplasia in renal dialysis patients: A retrospective cohort study

Hsu Y-C, Hung C-J (Natl Cheng Kung Univ, Tainan, Taiwan; et al)

Surgery 158:1331-1338, 2015

Background.—Intramuscular and subcutaneous forearm parathyroid autograft are proved to have compatible short-term outcome. However, long-term clinical courses have not been studied.

Methods.—A single-surgeon retrospective cohort study of parathyroid autograft hyperplasia from August 1998 to January 2013 was performed. According to the location of their parathyroid autograft, patients were divided into an Intramuscular group and a Subcutaneous group. Clinical parameters were analyzed to assess the risk factors and clinical course of autograft hyperplasia.

Results.—There were 888 consecutive patients who underwent total parathyroidectomy with forearm autotransplantation for renal hyperparathyroidism during the period. The median age at the time of total parathyroidectomy with forearm autotransplantation was 54.2 years (range, 12–86) and the median follow-up time was 4.0 years (range 0.1–16). Autograftectomy was performed on 29 of 888 patients. The incidence of autograftectomy was 15 of 65 in the Intramuscular group and 14 of 823 in the Subcutaneous group; the incidence of repeated autograftectomy was 4 of 65 in the Intramuscular group and 1 of 823 in the Subcutaneous group. The cumulative frequency of autograftectomy was greater in the Intramuscular group than that in the Subcutaneous group (11.6 vs 3.1% at 6 years, $P < .001$). The location of the autograft was the only significant factor affecting the autograftectomy frequency ($P = .002$). The Intramuscular group reoperation patients experienced a longer period between their first operation and the autograftectomy (6.6 vs 3.3 years, $P = .003$), longer operating times (79 vs 37 minutes, $P = .002$), and a greater level of pre-autograftectomy systemic intact parathyroid hormone (1,044 vs 559 ng/L, $P = .014$) than the Subcutaneous group.

Conclusion.—Intramuscular parathyroid autotransplantation results in a high incidence of autograftectomy, repeated autograftectomy, and a high cumulative frequency of autograftectomy.

► This report has a major design flaw, and yet it presents some very interesting data from a large experience with parathyroid autotransplantation in surgery for renal secondary hyperparathyroidism. The authors compare a small series of intramuscular forearm parathyroid autografts to a very large number of subcutaneous forearm parathyroid autografts and find a high incidence of reoperation in the intramuscular group. The problem is that all of the intramuscular grafts were done in the first 5 years of the 15-year study. The authors acknowledge that this is a potential major confounder but note that although this bias cannot be eliminated, the data still strongly favor the subcutaneous site for autografting. Anyone who has had to go back to excise a parathyroid autograft from the brachioradialis muscle knows that this is sometimes a laborious and inexact procedure as the parathyroid cells have frequently insinuated themselves into the surrounding muscle fibers. A subcutaneous pocket is both easier to approach if an autograft must be excised and a more complete job can be accomplished. Finally, the data in the article support the subcutaneous position as equally effective when examining the postautograft parathyroid levels. Thus, although the article has a major design flaw, the data support migration to a subcutaneous site for parathyroid autografts.

T. J. Fahey III, MD

The Natural History of Benign Thyroid Nodules

Durante C, Costante G, Lucisano G, et al (Università di Roma Sapienza, Italy; Università di Catanzaro Magna Graecia, Italy; Ctr for Outcomes Res and Clinical Epidemiology, Pescara, Italy; et al)

JAMA 313:926-935, 2015

Importance.—Detection of asymptomatic thyroid nodules has increased. Consensus is lacking regarding the optimal follow-up of cytologically proven benign lesions and sonographically nonsuspicious nodules. Current guidelines recommend serial ultrasound examinations and reassessment of cytology if significant growth is observed.

Objective.—To determine the frequency, magnitude, and factors associated with changes in thyroid nodule size.

Design, Setting, and Participants.—Prospective, multicenter, observational study involving 992 consecutive patients with 1 to 4 asymptomatic, sonographically or cytologically benign thyroid nodules. Patients were recruited from 8 hospital-based thyroid-disease referral centers in Italy between 2006 and 2008. Data collected during the first 5 years of follow-up, through January 2013, were analyzed.

Main Outcomes and Measures.—Baseline nodule growth (primary end point) was assessed with yearly thyroid ultrasound examinations. Size changes were considered significant for growth if an increase of 20% or more was recorded in at least 2 nodule diameters, with a minimum increase of 2 mm. Baseline factors associated with growth were identified. Secondary end points were the sonographic detection of new nodules and the diagnosis of thyroid cancer during follow-up.

Results.—Nodule growth occurred in 153 patients (15.4% [95% CI, 14.3%-16.5%]). One hundred seventy-four of the 1567 original nodules (11.1% [95% CI, 10.3%-11.9%]) increased in size, with a mean 5-year largest diameter increase of 4.9 mm (95% CI, 4.2-5.5 mm), from 13.2 mm (95% CI, 12.1-14.2 mm) to 18.1 mm (95% CI, 16.7-19.4 mm). Nodule growth was associated with presence of multiple nodules (OR, 2.2 [95% CI 1.4-3.4] for 2 nodules; OR, 3.2 [95% CI, 1.8-5.6 for 3 nodules; and OR, 8.9 [95% CI, 4.4-18.0] for 4 nodules), main nodule volumes larger than 0.2 mL (OR, 2.9 [95% CI, 1.7-4.9] for volumes >0.2 to <1 mL and OR, 3.0 [95% CI, 1.8-5.1] for volumes ≥1 mL), and male sex (OR, 1.7 [95% CI, 1.1-2.6]), whereas an age of 60 years or older was associated with a lower risk of growth than age younger than 45 years (OR, 0.5 [95% CI 0.3-0.9]). In 184 individuals (18.5% [95% CI, 16.4%-20.9%]), nodules shrank spontaneously. Thyroid cancer was diagnosed in 5 original nodules (0.3% [95% CI, 0.0%-0.6%]). Only 2 had grown. An incidental cancer was found at thyroidectomy in a nonvisualized nodule. New nodules developed in 93 patients (9.3% [95% CI, 7.5%-11.1%]), with detection of one cancer.

Conclusions and Relevance.—Among patients with asymptomatic, sonographically or cytologically benign thyroid nodules, the majority of nodules exhibited no significant size increase during 5 years of follow-up and thyroid cancer was rare. These findings support consideration of revision of current guideline recommendations for follow-up of asymptomatic thyroid nodules.

▶ This study provides sound evidence for recommendations that advocate for decreasing the surveillance of benign thyroid nodules. The recent American Thyroid Association guidelines for managing benign thyroid nodules bases the recommendation at least in part on the appearance of the nodule on ultrasound. Unfortunately, the authors here did not characterize the nodules by ultrasound features into low, intermediate, or high suspicion. Nevertheless, for those of us who have traditionally recommended yearly follow-up ultrasound for benign nodules, this study adds to the growing body of evidence that benign nodules can safely be monitored less frequently. Future studies incorporating the ultrasound characteristics will likely further clarify who can simply be referred back to their primary care physicians and told to return only if there is a change detected on physical examination.

T. J. Fahey III, MD

Efficacy and Safety of Radiofrequency Ablation Versus Observation for Nonfunctioning Benign Thyroid Nodules: A Randomized Controlled International Collaborative Trial

Deandrea M, Sung JY, Limone P, et al ("Umberto I" Hosp, Turin, Italy; Daerim St. Mary's Hosp, Seoul, Korea; et al)

Thyroid 25:890-896, 2015

Background.—Percutaneous radiofrequency thermal ablation (RFA) has been reported as an effective tool for the management of benign thyroid nodules (BTN). However, large, randomized controlled trials (RCTs) are lacking.

Objective.—The aims of this study were to assess the volume reduction of BTN after a single RFA performed using the moving-shot technique and to compare the volume reduction obtained in patients treated in two centers with different experience of the moving-shot technique.

Method.—This study was an international prospective RCT. It was carried out at the Mauriziano Hospital (Turin, Italy) and the Asan Medical

Center (Seoul, Korea). Eighty patients harboring solid, compressive, nonfunctioning BTN (volume 10–20 mL) were enrolled. Twenty patients in each country were treated by RFA using a 18-Gauge internally cooled electrode (group A); 20 nontreated patients in each country were followed as controls (group B).

Results.—At six months, BTN volume significantly decreased in group A (15.1 ± 3.1 mL vs. 4.2 ± 2.7 mL; $p < 0.0001$), whereas it remained unchanged in group B (14.4 ± 3.3 mL vs. 15.2 ± 3.5 mL). The baseline volume was larger in the Italian series (16.4 ± 2.5 mL vs. 13.9 ± 3.3 mL, $p = 0.009$). However, at six months, there was no significant difference between the Korean group and the Italian group (3.7 ± 2.9 mL vs. 5.5 ± 2.2 mL). Both cosmetic and compressive symptoms significantly improved (3.6 ± 0.5 vs. 1.7 ± 0.4 and 3.6 ± 1.9 vs. 0.4 ± 0.7, respectively; $p < 0.001$). No side effects occurred.

Conclusions.—RFA was effective in reducing the volume of BTN. The outcome was similar in centers with different experience in the moving-shot technique.

▶ Benign thyroid nodules can usually be simply observed. However, some nodules cause local compressive symptoms, and some are cosmetically unacceptable to the patient. The use of radiofrequency ablation (RFA) to treat thyroid nodules has been slowly gaining acceptance in many countries, notably in Europe and Korea. This modest-sized study from Italy and South Korea demonstrates that thyroid nodule RFA is effective and results in a large reduction in the size of the thyroid nodule. Furthermore, although there have been reports of complications, including nerve injury and vocal cord paralysis, it appears to be a generally very safe technique. Long-term follow-up is not provided in this article, but as can be seen from Table 3 in the original article, the 6-month outcomes are impressive. We can expect that RFA will become a part of the armentarium of the endocrine surgeon in treating locally symptomatic or cosmetically unacceptable benign thyroid nodules. One of the chief roadblocks to doing thyroid nodule RFA in the United States appears to be insurance reimbursement because there is currently no code to assign to this procedure, and it may not be recognized and therefore reimbursed. However, this obstacle can and should be overcome in the future.

T. J. Fahey III, MD

Performance of the Afirma Gene Expression Classifier in Hürthle Cell Thyroid Nodules Differs from Other Indeterminate Thyroid Nodules

Brauner E, Holmes BJ, Krane JF, et al (Massachusetts General Hosp, Boston; Brigham and Women's Hosp, Boston, MA; et al)

Thyroid 25:789-796, 2015

Background.—The recently introduced Afirma gene expression classifier (AGEC) provides binary results (benign or suspicious) to guide management of cytologically indeterminate thyroid nodules. The AGEC is intended to reduce unnecessary surgeries for benign nodules, and management algorithms favor surgery for suspicious results. Limited data are available on the performance of this test for Hürthle cell nodules (HCNs). This study hypothesized that a predominance of Hürthle cells leads to an increased rate of suspicious AGEC results with a potential for overtreatment, despite a relatively low risk of malignancy.

Methods.—The pathology databases from three tertiary care facilities were queried from 2010 to 2014 for fine-needle aspirates (FNAs) diagnosed as suspicious for Hürthle cell neoplasm (SHCN) or atypia of undetermined significance/follicular lesion of undetermined significance concerning for Hürthle cell neoplasm (AFHCN). Cytology diagnoses were rendered internally prior to AGEC testing. The patient demographics, FNA diagnosis, AGEC result, surgical procedure, and pathologic outcomes were recorded.

Results.—The cohort consisted of 134 patients with HCNs. Prior to AGEC availability, 62 patients underwent surgery: 81% (50/62) of patients had surgery, and 34% (17/50) of the resected index nodules were malignant. After introduction of the AGEC, 72 patients underwent AGEC testing: 65% (47/72) of patients had surgery, and 13% (6/46) of the resected nodules were malignant. Thirty-two percent (23/72) of patients had a benign AGEC result and did not undergo surgery, and 4% (3/72) had surgery despite a benign AGEC result with benign final pathology, whereas 63% (45/72) of patients had suspicious AGEC results, with 96% of these patients (43/45) undergoing surgery, and 14% (6/43) of these index nodules were malignant.

Conclusions.—While 32% of tested patients declined surgery based on a benign AGEC, 86% of patients with suspicious AGEC findings had unnecessary surgery, reflecting a substantially lower rate of malignancy from what was previously reported for all indeterminate nodules. Given the approximate pretest malignancy risk of 25–35% for an FNA diagnosis of SHCN or AFHCN, a suspicious AGEC diagnosis does not increase the probability of malignancy in an HCN, and patients should be counseled accordingly.

▶ Molecular testing continues to refine who should have surgery for thyroid nodules and will continue to evolve for years to come. This article highlights the problem of gene expression analysis in Hurthle cell nodules. If an Afirma assay calls a Hurthle cell nodule benign, the nodule is still highly likely to be benign. The problem is what to do about nodules deemed suspicious on the Afirma assay. As noted in Table 3 in the original article (included), a Bethesda III or IV nodule deemed suspicious on Afirma has only a 7.5% chance of being malignant. This was a problem that we predicted would develop based on our analysis of Hurthle cell nodules by gene expression analysis published more than 10 years ago.[1] For reasons that remain to be explained; even benign Hurthle cell nodules frequently have a gene expression profile similar to that of papillary thyroid cancer. When faced with this dilemma in the clinic, I base my recommendation on the clinical factors associated with the nodule, not just the Afirma result. These include the size of the nodule (there is a well-described relationship between the size of Hurthle cell lesions and the incidence of malignancy) and the presence or absence of chronic thyroiditis. Small Hurthle cell nodules, even when suspicious on Afirma, are rarely, if ever, malignant.

T. J. Fahey III, MD

Reference

1. Finley DJ, Zhu B, Fahey TJ 3rd. Molecular analysis of Hurthle cell neoplasms by gene profiling. *Surgery*. 2004;136:1160-1168.

The Value of Repeat Thyroid Fine-Needle Aspiration Biopsy in Patients with a Previously Benign Result: How Often Does It Alter Management?

Singh Ospina N, Sebo TJ, Morris JC, et al (Mayo Clinic, Rochester, MN)

Thyroid 25:1121-1126, 2015

Background.—Thyroid nodules are prevalent and mostly benign, being present in up to 67% of the population when assessed by ultrasound. Due to the variable diagnostic performance of ultrasound-guided fine-needle aspiration biopsy (USFNA) of the thyroid and the possibility of a false-negative result, current clinical guidelines recommend ultrasonographic follow-up of benign thyroid nodules. The objective of this study was to evaluate the clinical relevance of a repeat fine-needle aspiration (rFNA) in patients with an initial benign fine-needle aspiration biopsy (iFNA).

Methods.—A retrospective review was conducted of medical records of patients seen at the Mayo Clinic between January of 2003 and December of 2013 who had undergone rFNA of a nodule with benign iFNA. The outcome measured was the result of the rFNA and histopathological correlation, when available.

Results.—Three hundred and thirty-four nodules with benign iFNA underwent rFNA during the 10-year study period. The rFNA was most commonly reported as benign (85.3%), followed by suspicious (7.2%), nondiagnostic (5.7%), and malignant (1.8%). The rFNA changed clinical management in 9.5% of the cases. The prevalence of thyroid malignancy ranged from 4.1% to 1.2% based on the gold standard used (histology vs. long-term follow-up, 4.0–2.3 years).

Conclusion.—In the majority of patients with a benign iFNA, results of the rFNA were unchanged. However, in a small group of patients, the rFNA may differ from the initial results, and alter management. Even so, the prevalence of malignancy remains very low, ranging from 1.2% to 4.1% depending on the gold standard.

▶ When a thyroid nodule is deemed benign on initial cytology, does it require repeat fine-needle aspiration (FNA) biopsy? The American Thyroid Association guidelines indicate that this decision should be based on the characteristics of the nodule on ultrasound (US): highly suspicious nodules should have repeat FNA in 12 months, whereas nodules with low or intermediate suspicion on US can just undergo US in 12 to 24 months and only require repeat FNA if there is at least 20% increase in 2 of the nodule dimensions.[1] However, the data supporting these guidelines are relatively weak, particularly the data regarding low and intermediate suspicion nodules. This report takes a retrospective look at nodules that underwent repeat FNA over a 10-year period and finds that nearly 10% of patients who underwent repeat FNA had a change in management as a result, which is essentially summarized in Fig 2 in the original article. The study provides some important data for helping to guide management of initially benign thyroid nodules. However, it is possible that the study is overestimating the frequency with which nodules change because the reason for the repeat biopsy was entirely up to the treating physician. Additionally, the follow-up period is relatively short. However, it is clear that stable benign nodules do not require yearly biopsy to ensure that they remain benign. The study highlights the fact that clinical follow-up remains necessary for thyroid nodules, but the vast majority of the time, initially benign nodules will remain benign—at least for the short term.

T. J. Fahey III, MD

Reference

1. Haugen BR, Alexander EK, Bible KC, et al. 2015 American Thyroid Association management guidelines for adult patients with thyroid nodules and differentiated thyroid cancer: the American Thyroid Association Guidelines Task Force on thyroid Nodules and differentiated thyroid cancer. *Thyroid*. 2016;26:1-133.

Impact of the Multi-Gene ThyroSeq Next-Generation Sequencing Assay on Cancer Diagnosis in Thyroid Nodules with Atypia of Undetermined Significance/Follicular Lesion of Undetermined Significance Cytology

Nikiforov YE, Carty SE, Chiosea SI, et al (Univ of Pittsburgh Cancer Inst, PA; et al)

Thyroid 25:1217-1223, 2015

Background.—Fine-needle aspiration (FNA) cytology is a common approach to evaluate thyroid nodules. It offers definitive diagnosis of a benign or malignant nodule in the majority of cases. However, 10–25% of nodules yield one of three indeterminate cytologic diagnoses, leading to suboptimal management of these patients. Atypia of undetermined significance/follicular lesion of undermined significance (AUS/FLUS) is a common indeterminate diagnosis, with the cancer risk ranging from 6% to 48%. This study assessed whether a multi-gene next-generation sequencing (NGS) assay can offer significant improvement in diagnosis in AUS/ FLUS nodules.

Methods.—From May 2014 to March 2015, 465 consecutive FNA samples with the cytologic diagnosis of AUS/ FLUS underwent prospective molecular testing using the ThyroSeq v2.1 panel. The panel included 14 genes analyzed for point mutations and 42 types of gene fusions occurring in thyroid cancer. In addition, eight genes were assessed for expression in order to evaluate the cell composition of FNA samples. Ninety-eight (21%) of these nodules had definitive surgical ($n = 96$) or nonsurgical ($n = 2$) follow-up and were used to determine the assay performance.

Results.—Among 465 AUS/FLUS nodules, three were found to be composed of parathyroid cells and 462 of thyroid follicular cells. Of the latter, 31 (6.7%) were positive for mutations. The most frequently mutated genes were *NRAS* and *HRAS*, and overall point mutations in seven different genes and five types of gene fusions were identified in these nodules. Among 98 nodules with known outcome, histologic analysis revealed 22 (22.5%) cancers. ThyroSeq v2.1 was able to classify 20/22 cancers correctly, showing a sensitivity of 90.9% [confidence interval (CI) 78.8–100], specificity of 92.1% [CI 86.0–98.2], positive predictive value of 76.9% [CI 60.7–93.1], and negative predictive value of 97.2% [CI 78.8–100], with an overall accuracy of 91.8% [CI 86.4–97.3].

Conclusions.—The results of the study demonstrate that the ThyroSeq v2.1 multi-gene NGS panel of molecular markers provides both high sensitivity and high specificity for cancer detection in thyroid nodules with AUS/FLUS cytology, which should allow improved management for these patients.

▶ The dilemma about how to manage patients with Bethesda III nodules (atypia of undetermined significance/follicular lesion of undermined significance) is rapidly becoming clearer with the recent advances in molecular diagnostics. The Thyroseq v2.1 test will likely become the standard of care for patients with indeterminate thyroid nodules. The most important finding in this article is probably that in these Bethesda III nodules the risk of missing a malignancy in a Thyroseq mutation negative nodule is less than 3% (Fig 1 in the original article). These data make it difficult to justify operating on patients with mutation negative nodules to rule out malignancy, and operation can be avoided unless there are other indications to do the surgery (local symptoms for instance). The bigger question down the road will be whether mutation analysis should be applied to the diagnosis of all thyroid nodules. It is also interesting to note that the risk of malignancy in *NRAS*-mutated Bethesda III nodules is now closer to historical series (60%), which does raise the dilemma about whether a hemithyroidectomy is preferred over a total thyroidectomy in these patients. Finally, although the Thyroseq test does appear to offer outstanding results, the data really need to be validated outside of Pennsylvania.

T. J. Fahey III, MD

RAS mutations in AUS/FLUS Cytology: Does it Have an Additional Role in BRAF^{V600E} Mutation-Negative Nodules?

Yoon JH, Kwon HJ, Lee HS, et al (Res Inst of Radiological Science, Seoul, South Korea; Yonsei Univ, College of Medicine, Seoul, South Korea; Yonsei Univ, College of Medicine, Seoul, South Korea)
Medicine (Baltimore) 94:e1084, 2015

The object of this study is to evaluate the additional role of *RAS* mutation in detecting thyroid malignancy among BRAF^{V600E} mutation-negative nodules diagnosed as atypia of undetermined significance/follicular lesion of undetermined significance (AUS/FLUS) on cytology.

From December 2009 to December 2011, 202 BRAF^{V600E} mutation-negative thyroid nodules diagnosed as AUS/FLUS cytology in 201 patients were included in this study. *RAS* mutation analysis was performed using residual material from ultrasonography-guided fine needle aspiration (USFNA) cytology testing for *K-RAS*, *N-RAS*, and *H-RAS* codons 12/13 and 61 point mutations. The authors evaluated the association between *RAS* mutation status and cytopathologic characteristics.

Of the 202 BRAF^{V600E} mutation-negative thyroid nodules with AUS/FLUS cytology, 4 were considered insufficient for mutation analysis. Of the 198 thyroid nodules, 148 (74.7%) were confirmed as benign and 50 (25.3%) as malignant. Thirty-one (15.7%) of the 198 thyroid nodules were positive for any *RAS* mutation, 4 positive for *K-RAS* 12/13, 26 for *N-RAS* 61, and 1 positive for *H-RAS* 61. Seven (22.6%) of the *RAS* mutation positive nodules were malignant, 1 with *K-RAS* 12/13, 6 with *N-RAS* 61. Twenty-four (77.4%) of the 31 nodules positive for *K-RAS* 12/13 (N = 3), *N-RAS* 61 (N = 20), or *H-RAS* 61 (N = 1) mutations were proven benign. None of the 198 thyroid nodules were positive for *K-RAS* 61, *N-RAS* 12/ 13, or *H-RAS* 12/13 mutations.

N-RAS 61 mutation is the most common mutation detected among BRAF^{V600E} mutation-negative nodules with AUS/FLUS cytology. *RAS* mutation has limited value in predicting malignancy among BRAF^{V600E} mutation-negative thyroid nodules with AUS/FLUS cytology and further, investigation is anticipated to evaluate the true role of *RAS* mutation in thyroid malignancy.

▶ Mutation analysis in thyroid nodules has become more widely possible because of the development of RNA sequencing technology. The Pittsburgh group has been at the forefront of applying this technology to the molecular diagnosis of thyroid nodules, with great success. One of the factors contributing to their overall accuracy rates has been the high frequency with which Ras-mutated tumors have proven to be malignant in their reports. This report from Korea challenges the utility of detecting Ras mutations in indeterminate thyroid nodules—and in particular in the group that is most troublesome for the patient and treating physician. The risk of malignancy in Ras-mutated thyroid nodules in this report is essentially the inverse of that reported by the Pittsburgh group (see report by Yip et al, reviewed earlier in this chapter).[1] Why the discrepancy? There could be a number of factors: can the effect of Ras mutations be different in different ethnic backgrounds? Are pathologists in Pittsburgh more liberal in their designation of thyroid cancer in these atypical follicular lesions? Or could it be that the nodules described in the article are smaller and thus more likely to be benign on that basis? These are questions that will have to be answered in future studies to determine how best to advise our patients with Bethesda III nodules and a Ras mutation.

T. J. Fahey III, MD

Reference

1. Yip, et al.

Role of BRAF V600E mutation as an indicator of the extent of thyroidectomy and lymph node dissection in conventional papillary thyroid carcinoma

Kim SK, Woo J-W, Lee JH, et al (Sungkyunkwan Univ School of Medicine, Seoul, South Korea; Sungkyunkwan Univ School of Medicine, Changwon, South Korea)

Surgery 158:1500-1511, 2015

Background.—The extent of surgery for papillary thyroid carcinoma (PTC) is associated strongly with disease persistence, recurrence, and mortality. It is difficult, however, to determine the optimal extent for surgery. The BRAF mutation is well known for its diagnostic and prognostic value in PTC. Among the variants of PTC, the clinical importance of the BRAF mutation has been associated particularly with conventional PTC. The goal of this study was to clarify the role of the BRAF mutation as a determinant for the operative extent in conventional PTC.

Methods.—Histopathology and BRAF mutation status of 3,019 patients with conventional PTC were analyzed. With regard to the extent of surgery in PTC, focus was given to the factors of tumor bilaterality, central lymph node metastasis (CLNM), and lateral lymph node metastasis. In addition, the prognostic impact of BRAF mutation on loco-regional recurrence was investigated.

Results.—The BRAF mutation was found to be an independent indicator of tumor bilaterality (odds ratio [OR] 1.484, $P = .010$); however, it was not an independent indicator of CLNM (OR 1.167, $P = .254$) or lateral lymph node metastasis (OR 0.647, $P = .384$). Moreover, it was not an independent indicator of CLNM in either the therapeutic or prophylactic central neck dissection. Finally, BRAF mutation positivity did not increase the risk of loco-regional recurrence (adjusted hazard ratio = 0.829, $P = .523$).

Conclusion.—The BRAF mutation is a possible indicator for determining the extent of thyroidectomy required but not for the extent of lymph node dissection and prognosis in patients with conventional PTC (Table 1).

▶ This single-center study runs counter to the data published in the Xing et al study[1] previously discussed. The authors looked at more than 3000 patients and found that the presence of a *BRAF* mutation was not associated with either central neck or lateral neck metastasis. What is different? Although the authors do not discuss this, perhaps the biggest difference is the size of the tumors. It would appear from Table 1 that less than one-third of the patients had tumors greater than 1 cm. Although micro-papillary thyroid carcinoma (PTC) have been found to metastasize to lymph nodes up to 40% of the time, larger tumors have a higher rate of lymph node mets. To really tease out this potential relationship more directly, it would have been nice to see a separate analysis of microPTC versus typical classical PTC. However, the main figure from the article analyzes recurrence-free survival and demonstrates that there were no differences in recurrence between *BRAF*-positive and -negative tumors regardless of the type and extent of surgery—lobectomy versus total thyroidectomy or with or without central or lateral neck dissection. This article reinforces my conviction that treatment decisions (except,

TABLE 1.—Associations Between BRAF Mutation and Clinicopathologic Characteristics of Patients with Conventional PTC

	BRAF Mutation, No. (%)			
	Negative	*Positive*	*OR (95% CI)*	*P Value*
Total number	522 (17.3)	2,497 (82.7)		
Age >45 y	290 (55.6)	1,397 (55.9)	1.016 (0.840–1.228)	.870
Male	78 (14.9)	542 (21.7)	1.578 (1.218–2.044)	.001
Size >1 cm	148 (28.4)	858 (34.4)	1.323 (1.075–1.628)	.008
Multifocality	97 (18.6)	600 (24.0)	1.386 (1.091–1.760)	.007
ETE	211 (40.4)	1,284 (51.4)	1.560 (1.288–1.890)	<.001
CLT	192 (36.8)	613 (24.5)	0.559 (0.458–0.683)	<.001
Operative approach				
Endoscopic/robotic	102 (19.5)	404 (16.2)		
Open	420 (80.5)	2,093 (83.8)	1.258 (0.989–1.601)	.062
Operative extent				
Lobectomy	210 (40.2)	818 (32.8)		
Total thyroidectomy	312 (59.8)	1,679 (67.2)	1.382 (1.138–1.677)	.001
CND	468 (89.7)	2,320 (92.9)	1.512 (1.098–2.084)	.011
LND	63 (12.1)	271 (10.9)	0.887 (0.662–1.188)	.421
LRR	15 (2.9)	65 (2.6)	0.903 (0.497–1.666)	.726
RAI	1,219 (79.8)	1,278 (85.7)	1.521 (1.256–1.842)	<.001
Mean RAI dose, mCi	38.1 (±59.4)	49.2 (±63.6)	NA	<.001

CI, Confidence interval; *CLT*, chronic lymphocytic thyroiditis; *CND*, central neck dissection; *ETE*, extrathyroidal extension; *LND*, lateral neck dissection; *LRR*, locoregional recurrence; *NA*, not available; *OR*, odds ratio; *PTC*, papillary thyroid carcinoma; *RAI*, radioactive iodine.

as the authors of this article note, regarding hemi vs total thyroidectomy) cannot yet be made based on mutation analysis and that clinicopathologic features must remain the gold standard until prospective studies can address this issue.

T. J. Fahey III, MD

Reference

1. Xing M, Alzahrani AS, Carson KA, et al. Association between BRAF V600E mutation and recurrence of papillary thyroid cancer. *J Clin Oncol.* 2015;33: 42-50.

Association Between *BRAF* V600E Mutation and Recurrence of Papillary Thyroid Cancer

Xing M, Alzahrani AS, Carson KA, et al (Johns Hopkins Univ School of Medicine, Baltimore, MD; Johns Hopkins Univ Bloomberg School of Public Health, Baltimore, MD; et al)

J Clin Oncol 33:42-50, 2015

Purpose.—To investigate the prognostic value of *BRAF* V600E mutation for the recurrence of papillary thyroid cancer (PTC).

Patients and Methods.—This was a retrospective multicenter study of the relationship between *BRAF* V600E mutation and recurrence of PTC in 2,099 patients (1,615 women and 484 men), with a median age of 45 years (interquartile range [IQR], 34 to 58 years) and a median follow-up time of 36 months (IQR, 14 to 75 months).

Results.—The overall *BRAF* V600E mutation prevalence was 48.5% (1,017 of 2,099). PTC recurrence occurred in 20.9% (213 of 1,017) of *BRAF* V600E mutation–positive and 11.6% (125 of 1,082) of *BRAF* V600E mutation–negative patients. Recurrence rates were 47.71 (95% CI, 41.72 to 54.57) versus 26.03 (95% CI, 21.85 to 31.02) per 1,000 person-years in *BRAF* mutation–positive versus –negative patients ($P < .001$), with a hazard ratio (HR) of 1.82 (95% CI, 1.46 to 2.28), which remained significant in a multivariable model adjusting for patient sex and age at diagnosis, medical center, and various conventional pathologic factors. Significant association between *BRAF* mutation and PTC recurrence was also found in patients with conventionally low-risk disease stage I or II and micro-PTC and within various subtypes of PTC. For example, in *BRAF* mutation–positive versus –negative follicular-variant PTC, recurrence occurred in 21.3% (19 of 89) and 7.0% (24 of 342) of patients, respectively, with recurrence rates of 53.84 (95% CI, 34.34 to 84.40) versus 19.47 (95% CI, 13.05 to 29.04) per 1,000 person-years ($P < .001$) and an HR of 3.20 (95% CI, 1.46 to 7.02) after adjustment for clinicopathologic factors. *BRAF* mutation was associated with poorer recurrence-free probability in Kaplan-Meier survival analyses in various clinicopathologic categories.

Conclusion.—This large multicenter study demonstrates an independent prognostic value of *BRAF* V600E mutation for PTC recurrence in various clinicopathologic categories.

▶ The importance of the *BRAF* V600E mutation as an independent prognostic indicator in patients with papillary thyroid cancer (PTC) continues to be debated. Here Dr Xing has put together a large international consortium to try to answer this question, and the authors conclude that the *BRAF* mutation is associated with increased risk of recurrence in PTC. The *BRAF* mutation has been largely associated with classical and tall cell variant PTCs. Many have argued previously that the increase in recurrence seen in association with *BRAF*-mutated tumors simply reflects the difference in recurrence between classical and follicular-variant PTC (FVPTC), and although this may represent an effect of the BRAF mutation, it is not a valuable observation clinically because the vast majority of classical PTCs are *BRAF* mutated. This report attempts to overcome that as the authors specifically analyzed FVPTC with and without the *BRAF* mutation and found that *BRAF*-mutated FVPTC had a significantly higher recurrence rate than BRAF-normal FVPTC. Furthermore, *BRAF*-mutated classical PTCs had a higher recurrence than BRAF WT PTCs. Fig 2 in the original article shows the Kaplan-Meier curves for recurrence-free survival of the effect of the *BRAF* mutation. Interestingly, as seen in Fig 2B in the original article, the effect of extrathyroidal extension on recurrence-free survival mirrors that for the presence of BRAF mutation, suggesting that pathologic features continue to have an important prognostic impact. Although the authors make a convincing argument for an independent prognostic role for the *BRAF* mutation, it remains to be determined whether treatment strategies should change simply on the basis of a *BRAF* mutation.

T. J. Fahey III, MD

Tumor Genotype Determines Phenotype and Disease-related Outcomes in Thyroid Cancer: A Study of 1510 Patients

Yip L, Nikiforova MN, Yoo JY, et al (Univ of Pittsburgh, PA)

Ann Surg 262:519-525, 2015

Objectives.—To correlate thyroid cancer genotype with histology and outcomes.

Background.—The prognostic significance of molecular signature in thyroid cancer (TC) is undefined but can potentially change surgical management.

Methods.—We reviewed a consecutive series of 1510 patients who had initial thyroidectomy for TC with routine testing for *BRAF*, *RAS*, *RET/PTC*, and *PAX8/PPARG* alterations. Histologic metastatic or recurrent TC was tracked for 6 or more months after oncologic thyroidectomy.

Results.—Papillary thyroid cancer (PTC) was diagnosed in 97% of patients and poorly differentiated/anaplastic TC in 1.1%. Genetic alterations were detected in 1039 (70%); the most common mutations were *BRAFV600E* (644/1039, 62%), and *RAS* isoforms (323/1039, 31%). *BRAFV600E*-positive PTC was often conventional or tall cell variant (58%), with frequent extrathyroidal extension (51%) and lymph node metastasis (46%). Conversely, *RAS*-positive PTC was commonly follicular variant (87%), with infrequent extrathyroidal extension (4.6%) and lymph node metastasis (5.6%). *BRAFV600E* and *RET/PTC*-positive PTCs were histologically similar. Analogously, *RAS* and *PAX8/PPARG*-positive PTCs were histologically similar. Compared with *RAS* or *PAX8/PPARG*-positive TCs, *BRAFV600E* or *RET/PTC*-positive TCs were more often associated with stage III/IV disease (40% vs 15%, $P < 0.001$) and recurrence (10% vs 0.7%, $P < 0.001$; mean follow-up 33 ± 21 mo). Distant metastasis was highest in patients with *RET/PTC*-positive TC (10.8%, $P = 0.02$).

Conclusions.—In this large study of prospective mutation testing in unselected patients with TC, molecular signature was associated with distinctive phenotypes including cancers, with higher risks of both distant metastasis and early recurrence. Preoperative genotype provides valuable prognostic data to appropriately inform surgery.

▶ This article from the Pittsburgh group is a definitive study on mutation analysis in patients with thyroid cancer at this point, but it will soon be eclipsed by another using expanded mutation analysis (Thyroseq 2). It establishes in a large series the association of B-Raf mutations with classical PTC and ras mutations with FV-PTC. The authors make the argument that delineation of mutation profile preoperatively may lead to better initial treatment of patients with thyroid cancer and ultimately to cost savings, but this has yet to be proven in a prospective study. It is interesting to note that the mutations tested—the most common ones in differentiated thyroid cancers—were only detected in 69% of the 1500 cancers tested. We must wait for the more detailed analysis that I expect to see once the more advanced mutation panel is available to know whether preoperative mutation testing really can or should change management. Nevertheless, this is a great starting point for future prospective studies looking at the role of mutation analysis in determining treatment and follow-up in thyroid nodules and differentiated thyroid cancers.

T. J. Fahey III, MD

Lateral Neck Lymph Node Characteristics Prognostic of Outcome in Patients with Clinically Evident N1b Papillary Thyroid Cancer

Wang LY, Palmer FL, Nixon IJ, et al (Memorial Sloan Kettering Cancer Ctr, New York)

Ann Surg Oncol 22:3530-3536, 2015

Purpose.—To identify lateral lymph node (LN) characteristics predictive of outcome in papillary thyroid cancer patients with clinically evident nodal disease.

Methods.—A total of 438 patients with lateral neck metastases from papillary thyroid cancer were identified from an institutional database of 3,664 differentiated thyroid cancers. The number of positive LNs, size of the largest LN, number of positive LNs to total number of LNs removed (LN burden), and presence of extranodal spread (ENS) were recorded. Cutoffs for continuous variables were determined by receiver operating characteristic curves. LN variables predictive of recurrence free survival and disease-specific survival (DSS) were identified by the Kaplan–Meier method and the Cox proportional hazard model.

Results.—The median age was 41 years (range 5–86 years). The median follow-up was 65 months (range 1–332 months). Fifty-nine patients developed disease recurrence; these were local in five, regional in 40, and distant in 30 patients. Fifteen patients died of disease. Receiver operating characteristic cutoffs were >10 positive LNs and a LN burden >17 %. No lateral LN characteristics were predictive of DSS. In patients <45 years old, univariate predictors of recurrence were >10 positive nodes ($p = 0.049$) and LN burden >17 % ($p < 0.001$). In patients ≥45 years old, >10 positive nodes, LN burden >17 %, and presence of ENS were predictive of recurrence ($p = 0.019$, $p = 0.019$, and $p = 0.029$, respectively).

Conclusions.—LN burden >17 % (1 positive LN in 6 LNs removed) in the lateral neck is predictive for recurrence in patients of all ages, whereas ENS is also prognostic for recurrence in older patients.

▶ This article analyzes the impact of lymph node metastases in papillary thyroid cancer (PTC) in a single-institution cohort of patients with lateral neck metastases. The findings here focus on recurrence-free survival and provide more evidence that recurrence is impacted by lymph node metastases in PTC. Although extranodal spread in lymph node metastases has long been associated with a higher chance of recurrence, the finding that this is not as important as the number of lymph node metastases in younger patients is noteworthy. In contrast to the data presented through analysis of the large national databases examining survival in patients with lymph node metastases from Sosa's group,[1] here the impact appears to be associated with a larger burden of disease. It is difficult to reconcile why these findings appear to be contradictory; however, the data in this article intuitively make sense—a larger burden of disease is associated with a higher risk of recurrence. The authors also report in the body of the article that the development of distant metastases was influenced by metastatic lymph node burden. So taking these 2 papers together, despite the fact that the impact on survival for young patients remains overall very small, the likelihood of requiring additional treatment for PTC if you are a younger patient with lymph node metastases, at least in the lateral neck, is not trivial.

T. J. Fahey III, MD

Reference

1. Adam MA, Pura J, Goffredo P, et al. Presence and number of lymph node metastases are associated with compromised survival for patients younger than age 45 years with papillary thyroid cancer. *J Clin Oncol*. 2015;33:2370-2375.

Presence and Number of Lymph Node Metastases Are Associated With Compromised Survival for Patients Younger Than Age 45 Years With Papillary Thyroid Cancer

Adam MA, Pura J, Goffredo P, et al (Duke Clinical Res Inst, Durham, NC)
J Clin Oncol 33:2370-2375, 2015

Purpose.—Cervical lymph node metastases are recognized as a prognostic indicator only in patients age 45 years or older with papillary thyroid cancer (PTC); patients younger than age 45 years are perceived to have low-risk disease. The current American Joint Committee on Cancer staging for PTC in patients younger than age 45 years does not include cervical lymph node metastases. Our objective was to test the hypothesis that the presence and number of cervical lymph node metastases have an adverse impact on overall survival (OS) in patients younger than age 45 years with PTC.

Patients and Methods.—Adult patients younger than age 45 years undergoing surgery for stage I PTC (no distant metastases) were identified from the National Cancer Data Base (NCDB; 1998-2006) and from SEER 1988-2006 data. Multivariable models were used to examine the association of OS with the presence of lymph node metastases and number of metastatic nodes.

Results.—In all, 47,902 patients in NCDB (11,740 with and 36,162 without nodal metastases) and 21,855 in the SEER database (5,188 with and 16,667 without nodal metastases) were included. After adjustment, OS was compromised for patients with nodal metastases compared with patients who did not have them (NCDB: hazard ratio (HR), 1.32; 95% CI, 1.04 to 1.67; $P = .021$; SEER: HR, 1.29; 95% CI, 1.08 to 1.56; $P = .006$). After adjustment, increasing number of metastatic lymph nodes was associated with decreasing OS up to six metastatic nodes (HR, 1.12; 95% CI, 1.01 to 1.25; $P = .03$), after which more positive nodes conferred no additional mortality risk (HR, 0.99; 95% CI, 0.99 to 1.05; $P = .75$).

Conclusion.—Our results suggest that cervical lymph node metastases are associated with compromised survival in young patients, warranting consideration of revised American Joint Committee on Cancer staging. A change point of six or fewer metastatic lymph nodes seems to carry prognostic significance, thus advocating for rigorous preoperative screening for nodal metastases.

▶ Before analysis of large administrative databases was possible, the presence of lymph node metastases were actually reported to be associated with increased survival in patients with differentiated thyroid cancer. Recent reports have indicated that this is not the case for patients older than 45 years. This report now extends those findings to patients younger than age 45. There are a couple of important points to consider though. First, as shown in Fig 1 in the original article, the overall deaths from thyroid cancer in this large cohort of patients was very small. The 10-year survival rates were 98.2% for patients who did not have nodal metastases and 97.8% for patients who did have nodal metastases. So the impact of lymph node metastases on survival is very small and only because this is a very large data set can it be teased out. As with all analysis of large administrative data sets, there are also problems. One issue that cannot be addressed is who was getting lymph nodes removed and how this affects the outcome. For instance, does this analysis apply to patients who have prophylactic central neck dissection and microscopic lymph node metastases present in their central neck compartment? Or is the analysis really more applicable to patients with clinically or radiologically apparent lateral neck metastases? Nevertheless, the fact that metastatic disease in papillary thyroid cancer—even to "just lymph nodes"—does have some (even if very small) impact on survival makes sense. But it is important to remind our patients (who may discover this article on the Internet) that the overall survival for younger patients with papillary thyroid cancer remains excellent.

T. J. Fahey III, MD

Cancer Incidence and Mortality in Patients Treated Either With RAI or Thyroidectomy for Hyperthyroidism

Ryödi E, Metso S, Jaatinen P, et al (Tampere Univ Hosp, Finland; Univ of Tampere, Finland; et al)

J Clin Endocrinol Metab 100:3710-3717, 2015

Context.—Some previous studies have suggested increased cancer risk in hyperthyroid patients treated with radioactive iodine (RAI). It is unclear whether the excess cancer risk is attributable to hyperthyroidism, its treatment, or the shared risk factors of the two diseases.

Objective.—The objective was to assess cancer morbidity and mortality in hyperthyroid patients treated with either RAI or surgery.

Patients.—We identified 4334 patients treated surgically for hyperthyroidism in Finland during 1986–2007 from the Hospital Discharge Registry and 1814 patients treated with RAI for hyperthyroidism at Tampere University Hospital. For each patient, three age- and gender-matched controls were chosen. Information on cancer diagnoses was obtained from the Cancer Registry. The follow-up began 3 months after the treatment and ended at cancer diagnosis, death, emigration, or the common closing date (December 31, 2009).

Results.—The overall cancer incidence was not increased among the hyperthyroid patients compared to their controls (rate ratio [RR], 1.05; 95%confidence interval [CI], 0.96–1.15). However, the risk of cancers of the respiratory tract (RR, 1.46; 95% CI, 1.05–2.02) and the stomach (RR, 1.64; 95% CI, 1.01–2.68) was increased among the patients. The overall cancer mortality did not differ between the patients and the controls (RR, 1.08; 95% CI, 0.94–1.25). The type of treatment did not affect the overall risk of cancer (hazard ratio for RAI vs thyroidectomy, 1.03; 95% CI, 0.86–1.23) or cancer mortality (hazard ratio, 1.04; 95% CI, 0.91–1.21).

Conclusions.—In this cohort of Finnish patients with hyperthyroidism treated with thyroidectomy or RAI, the overall risk of cancer was not increased, although an increased risk of gastric and respiratory tract cancers was seen in hyperthyroid patients. Based on this large-scale, long-term follow-up study, the increased cancer risk in hyperthyroid patients is attributable to hyperthyroidism and shared risk factors, not the treatment modality.

▶ If you manage enough patients with thyroid cancer, you will occasionally see someone who presents with a thyroid cancer some time after radioactive iodine (RAI) treatment for Graves disease. Is there a connection? If it is early after treatment (within 1 year), it is highly likely that a nodule existed before treatment and was not adequately assessed before RAI. For patients who are seen many years (10+) after RAI for the treatment of Graves, there is always a question of whether the cancer arose secondary to treatment with RAI or independent of the treatment. Or what if someone is treated with RAI for hyperthyroidism and develops a second malignancy years later? Postoperative RAI in the management of thyroid cancer has been linked to an increased risk of secondary malignancies, particularly of the salivary glands and leukemia. This study attempts to answer these questions. The authors conclude that any increased cancer risk is attributable to the underlying diagnosis of hyperthyroidism and not whether they were treated by surgery or RAI. However, the data to support this are hard to find in the article. None of the five tables in the article include data comparing surgery to RAI. There is one line that states that the type of treatment was note associated with the risk for thyroid cancer. Furthermore, the total proportion of deaths in patients treated with RAI (28% over the course of the study) was more than twice the proportion of deaths in the surgically treated group, although this is likely explained by the fact that the patients treated with RAI were on average 13 years older than those treated surgically.

Overall, this article will probably be used to support those who believe that there is no long-term risk when RAI is used to treat patients with hyperthyroidism but will do little to convince those of us who find it hard to reconcile an increased risk of RAI ablation for thyroid cancer and no additional risk for those treated with RAI for hyperthyroidism.

T. J. Fahey III, MD

Increased Risk of Leukemia After Radioactive Iodine Therapy in Patients with Thyroid Cancer: A Nationwide, Population-Based Study in Korea

Seo GH, Cho YY, Chung JH, et al (Health Insurance Review and Assessment Service, Seoul, Korea; Sungkyunkwan Univ School of Medicine, Seoul, Korea)

Thyroid 25:927-934, 2015

Background.—The use of radioactive iodine therapy (RAIT) is increasing in thyroid cancer management. The association between RAIT at high doses and leukemia is well known, but studies of this association in a large population are lacking. This study aims to investigate the association between RAIT and leukemia in the context of current practice.

Methods.—Retrospective analysis of a 542,845 person-year (PY) follow-up of thyroid cancer patients was conducted using the Korean National Health Insurance claims database between January 2008 and December 2013. Patients were categorized according to RAIT dose (no RAI; low dose, ≤30 mCi; moderate dose, 31–100 mCi; high dose, 101–150 mCi; and very high dose, >150 mCi).

Results.—Among 211,360 thyroid cancer patients, 72 (0.03%) patients developed leukemia during follow-up (median 877 days). The cumulative incidence of leukemia per 10^5 person-year (PY) was 9.8 in the no RAI [95% confidence interval (CI) 6.4–14.4]; 6.1 [CI 1.7–15.7] in the low-dose; 8.6 [CI 3.2–18.7] in the moderate-dose; 29.5 [CI 18.3–45.1] in the high-dose; and 20.9 [CI 11.7–34.4] in the very high-dose groups. The hazard ratios were elevated significantly in the high- and very high-dose groups (HR 3.1 and 2.1, respectively, $p < 0.001$) when compared with the no RAI group.

Conclusions.—RAIT exceeding 100 mCi was strongly associated with the development of leukemia in a nationwide, population-based study, while lower RAIT doses were not. Considering the favorable survival of patients with thyroid cancer and the potential harm of RAIT, physicians need to consider the pros and cons of RAIT when using this treatment option.

▶ There have been a number of reports of increased risk of secondary malignancy associated with radioactive iodine (RAI) treatment for patients with differentiated (papillary and follicular) thyroid cancer. These include leukemia and salivary gland cancers. This has been the heart of the move to reduce the use of RAI routinely after surgery for differentiated thyroid cancers, and there is an increased recognition that RAI has potential deleterious effects. This report has as a significant strength the ability to gather data from an essentially closed system. Thus, it is unlikely that there were many cases of either thyroid cancer or leukemia that were missed during this time frame. The advantage of studying hematopoietic cancers is that there is a shorter lag time to development: leukemias are thought to arise within 5 years of exposure, whereas the risk is thought to be around 10 years for solid tumors. Unfortunately, the authors found that the risk of leukemia is more closely associated with higher doses. I say unfortunately because the patients who really are likely to benefit most from RAI are those who need the higher doses. One could argue that in many cases, lower doses, for "ablation," may not really be necessary. There is some promise that mutation profiling may help us to better design RAI treatment in the future so that similar effects can be achieved with lower doses of RAI.

T. J. Fahey III, MD

8 Nutrition

Immunonutrition Support for Patients Undergoing Surgery for Gastrointestinal Malignancy: Preoperative, Postoperative, or Perioperative? A Bayesian Network Meta-Analysis of Randomized Controlled Trials

Song G-M, Tian X, Zhang L, et al (Tianjin Hosp, China; Tianjin Univ of Traditional Chinese Medicine, China)

Medicine (Baltimore) 94:e1225, 2015

Enteral immunonutrition (EIN) has been established to be as a significantly important modality to prevent the postoperative infectious and noninfectious complications, enhance the immunity of host, and eventually improve the prognosis of gastrointestinal (GI) cancer patients undergoing surgery. However, different support routes, which are the optimum option, remain unclear. To evaluate the effects of different EIN support regimes for patients who underwent selective surgery for resectable GI malignancy, a Bayesian network meta-analysis (NMA) of randomized controlled trials (RCTs) was conducted.

A search of PubMed, EMBASE, and the Cochrane Central Register of Controlled Trials (CENTRAL) was electronically searched until the end of December 2014. Moreover, we manually checked reference lists of eligible trials and review and retrieval unpublished literature. RCTs which investigated the comparative effects of EIN versus standard enteral nutrition (EN) or different EIN regimes were included if the clinical outcomes information can be extracted from it.

A total of 27 RCTs were incorporated into this study. Pair-wise meta-analyses suggested that preoperative (relative risk [RR], 0.58; 95% confidence interval [CI], 0.43–0.78), postoperative (RR, 0.63; 95% CI, 0.52–0.76), and perioperative EIN methods (RR, 0.46; 95% CI, 0.34–0.62) reduced incidence of postoperative infectious complications compared with standard EN. Moreover, perioperative EIN (RR, 0.65; 95% CI, 0.44–0.95) reduced the incidence of postoperative noninfectious complications, and the postoperative (mean difference [MD], −2.38; 95% CI, −3.4 to −1.31) and perioperative EIN (MD, −2.64; 95% CI, −3.28 to −1.99) also shortened the length of postoperative hospitalization compared with standard EN. NMA found that EIN support effectively improved the clinical outcomes of patients who underwent selective surgery for GI cancer compared with standard EN.

Our results suggest EIN support is promising alternative for operation management in comparison with standard EN, and perioperative EIN regime is the optimum option for managing clinical status of patients who underwent selective surgery for GI cancer.

▶ Although meta-analysis of previous studies has shown benefit of preoperative enteral immunonutrition (EIN) in patients undergoing surgery for gastrointestinal malignancies, there continues to be interest in defining which nutrients may be involved in creating these positive results. In this meta-analysis, the authors identified 7 eligible trials that directly evaluated the comparative effects of preoperative EIN diet versus standard enteral nutrition (EN), and all were incorporated into this traditional pairwise meta-analysis. Fifteen eligible studies that included 1524 participants directly compared the effects of postoperative EIN related with standard EN in terms of postoperative infectious complications. Six trials, including 758 patients, evaluated perioperative EIN and standard EN groups and reported the incidence of postoperative infectious complications. The pairwise meta-analysis revealed that perioperative immunonutrition method was better than the standard EN in decreasing incidence of postoperative noninfectious complications. A similar trend was obtained by Bayesian analysis. In terms of length of hospitalization, the meta-analysis indicated a significant difference and the postoperative EIN was better than standard EN.

Statistical analytic studies such as this are important in that they rigorously evaluate previous published trials to evaluate outcomes that are important to patient care.

J. M. Daly, MD, FACS, FRCSI (Hon), FRCSG (Hon)

Volume-Based Feeding in the Critically Ill Patient

McClave SA, Saad MA, Esterle M, et al (Univ of Louisville School of Medicine, KY; et al)

JPEN J Parenter Enteral Nutr 39:707-712, 2015

Introduction.—Critically ill patients placed on enteral nutrition (EN) are usually underfed. A volume-based feeding (VBF) protocol designed to adjust the infusion rate to make up for interruptions in delivery should provide a greater volume of EN than the more common fixed hourly rate-based feeding (RBF) method.

Methods.—This single-center, randomized (3:1; VBF/RBF) prospective study evaluated critically ill patients on mechanical ventilation expected to receive EN for ≥3 days. Once goal rate was achieved, the randomized feeding strategy was implemented. In the VBF group, physicians used a total goal volume of feeds to determine an hourly rate. For the RBF group, physicians determined a constant hourly rate of infusion to meet goal feeds.

Results.—Sixty-three patients were enrolled in the study with a mean age of 52.6 years (60% male). Six patients were excluded after randomization because of early extubation. The VBF group (n = 37) received 92.9%

of goal caloric requirements with a mean caloric deficit of −776.0 kcal compared with the RBF group (n = 20), which received 80.9% of goal calories (P = .01) and a caloric deficit of −1933.8 kcal (P = .01). Uninterrupted EN was delivered for 51.7% of all EN days in VFB patients compared with 54.5% in RBF patients. On days when feeding was interrupted, VFB patients overall received a mean 77.6% of goal calories (while RBF patients received 61.5% of goal calories, P = .001). No vomiting, regurgitation, or feeding intolerance occurred due to VBF.

Conclusions.—A VBF strategy is safe and improves delivery to better meet caloric requirements than the standard more commonly used rate-based strategy.

▶ It is often difficult to provide adequate enteral nutrition for critically ill patients in the intensive care unit, particularly in those receiving mechanical ventilation, because of the many interruptions of feeding that occur for a variety of reasons, such as medication administration, instability, and radiologic studies. As the authors have noted, the most common method of feeding simply returns the rate of feeding back to its original rate. This prospective randomized trial compared rate-based with volume-based feeding.

Overall, study patients in the volume-based feeding group received a significantly greater volume of enteral nutrition, providing 93% of their caloric goal requirements for the study period, compared with control patients in the rate-based feeding group who received 81% of goal calories (P = .01). Importantly, the volume-based feeding group had no major complications related to the feeding regime. Next steps would be to determine that this method of feeding improves biochemical (serum albumin levels) and clinical (infections, morbidity/mortality, etc) outcomes.

J. M. Daly, MD, FACS, FRCSI (Hon), FRCSG (Hon)

Adequate enteral protein intake is inversely associated with 60-d mortality in critically ill children: a multicenter, prospective, cohort study

Mehta NM, Bechard LJ, Zurakowski D, et al (Boston Children's Hosp, MA; et al)

Am J Clin Nutr 102:199-206, 2015

Background.—The impact of protein intake on outcomes in pediatric critical illness is unclear.

Objective.—We examined the association between protein intake and 60-d mortality in mechanically ventilated children.

Design.—In a prospective, multicenter, cohort study that included 59 pediatric intensive care units (PICUs) from 15 countries, we enrolled consecutive children (age: 1 mo to 18 y) who were mechanically ventilated for ≥48 h. We recorded the daily and cumulative mean adequacies of energy and protein delivery as a percentage of the prescribed daily goal during the PICU stay ≤10 d. We examined the association of the adequacy of protein delivery with 60-d mortality and determined variables that predicted protein intake adequacy.

Results.—We enrolled 1245 subjects (44% female) with a median age of 1.7 y (IQR: 0.4, 7.0 y). A total of 985 subjects received enteral nutrition, 354 (36%) of whom received enteral nutrition via the postpyloric route. Mean ± SD prescribed energy and protein goals were 69 ± 28 kcal/kg per day and 1.9 ± 0.7 g/kg per day, respectively. The mean delivery of enteral energy and protein was 36 ± 35% and 37 ± 38%, respectively, of the prescribed goal. The adequacy of enteral protein intake was significantly associated with 60-d mortality ($P < 0.001$) after adjustment for disease severity, site, PICU days, and energy intake. In relation to mean enteral protein intake <20%, intake ≥60% of the prescribed goal was associated with an OR of 0.14 (95% CI: 0.04, 0.52; $P = 0.003$) for 60-d mortality. Early initiation, postpyloric route, shorter interruptions, larger PICU size, and a dedicated dietitian in the PICU were associated with higher enteral protein delivery.

Conclusions.—Delivery of >60% of the prescribed protein intake is associated with lower odds of mortality in mechanically ventilated children. Optimal prescription and modifiable practices at the bedside might enhance enteral protein delivery in the PICU with a potential for improved outcomes. This trial was registered at clinicaltrials.gov as NCT02354521.

▶ It is of major importance that critically ill children receive adequate protein and calorie nutritional support during their episode of illness because less than adequate support is associated with higher morbidity and mortality. However, it is often difficult to provide adequate enteral nutritional support to these children when they are critically ill. This prospective multi-institutional study enrolled consecutive children (aged 1 month to 18 years) admitted to the pediatric critical care unit (PICU) with anticipated stay >48 hours and who required mechanical ventilatory support were eligible for enrollment. Data from 1245 subjects (44% female; 42% surgical) were analyzed from 59 PICUs across 15 countries.

The multivariable analysis for predictors of enteral protein adequacy showed that enteral protein adequacy was significantly and directly associated with the early initiation of EN, use of the postpyloric route, decreased duration of EN interruption, PICU size (>20 beds), and a dedicated dietitian per 10 patients in the PICU. Studies such as this one are important because of the large number of patients, PICUs, countries, and its prospective nature. Clearly more needs to be done to intervene early in critically ill children and to have adequate dietetic resources to assure adequate nutrient intake in accordance with each child's needs.

J. M. Daly, MD, FACS, FRCSI (Hon), FRCSG (Hon)

Impact of Parenteral Fat Composition on Cholestasis in Preterm Infants

Teng J, Arnell H, Bohlin K, et al (Karolinska Institutet, Stockholm, Sweden)

J Pediatr Gastroenterol Nutr 60:702-707, 2015

Objectives.—Parenteral nutrition–associated liver disease (PNALD) is frequently detected in neonatal intensive care units. Parenteral lipid emulsion (PLE) content has been implicated in its pathogenesis. We aimed to study the effect on incidence and outcome of PNALD by replacing soy-based PLE with olive oil–based PLE in a population-based group of preterm infants.

Methods.—All infants in Stockholm County with gestational age (GA) <30 weeks were included (n = 615). Infants who died before 28 days of age or were referred to or from other regions were excluded (n = 97). PNALD was defined as conjugated serum bilirubin ≥30 μmol/L and exceeding 20% of the total fraction on at least 2 occasions. Two different 2-year time periods were compared: before (SOY period) and after (OLIVE period) switching PLE. For each PNALD case, 2 GA-matched controls were randomly identified.

Results.—PNALD incidence was 14.8% (37/250) in the SOY period and 12.7% (34/268) in the OLIVE period ($P = 0.52$). The OLIVE infants with PNALD had more risk factors, such as lower GA and longer periods of parenteral nutrition, for developing PNALD than the SOY infants. Nevertheless, treatment during the SOY period was an independent risk factor for PNALD in logistic regression analysis.

Conclusions.—Population-based incidence of PNALD is 1 of 7 in preterm infants with GA <30 weeks. Changing from soy oil to olive oil–based PLE did not decrease the incidence of PNALD significantly. Olive oil–based PLE carries an equal or slightly decreased risk to develop PNALD compared with soy oil–based PLE.

► As the authors have noted, prolonged total parenteral nutrition is the most important risk factor for parenteral nutrition–associated lived disease (PNALD), and other risk factors include low birth weight, low gestational age, necrotizing enterocolitis (NEC), intestinal malformations, and intestinal surgery. These authors performed a population-based cohort study with retrospective review of hospital charts to evaluate the effect on cholestasis following the change from soy oil–based to olive oil–based parenteral lipid emulsion.

The incidence of cholestasis was 14.8% in the SOY population compared with 12.7% in the OLIVE population. The rate of NEC was higher among cholestatic OLIVE infants, 74%, compared with 43% among the SOY infants with PNALD. The potential beneficial effect of changing from soy oil–based to olive oil–based lipid emulsion is at best moderate. Reducing the incidence of cholestasis in infants requiring total parenteral nutrition is critical to reduce their morbidity and mortality. It may be that dietary nutrients such as omega-3 fatty acids have some effect, but so do the comorbidities of NEC, among other factors.

J. M. Daly, MD, FACS, FRCSI (Hon), FRCSG (Hon)

Standardized Slow Enteral Feeding Protocol and the Incidence of Necrotizing Enterocolitis in Extremely Low Birth Weight Infants

Viswanathan S, McNelis K, Super D, et al (Case Western Reserve Univ, Cleveland, OH)

JPEN J Parenter Enteral Nutr 39:644-654, 2015

Background.—Compared with early enteral feeds, the delayed introduction and slow advancement of enteral feedings to reduce the incidence of necrotizing enterocolitis (NEC) are not well studied in extremely low birth weight (ELBW) infants.

Objective.—To study the effects of a standardized slow enteral feeding (SSEF) protocol in ELBW infants.

Methods.—ELBW infants who followed an SSEF protocol (September 2009 to December 2012) were compared with a similar group of historical controls (January 2003 to July 2009). Short-term outcomes between the 2 groups were compared by propensity score (PS) analysis.

Results.—One hundred twenty-five infants in the SSEF group were compared with 294 historical controls. Compared with the controls, feeding initiation day, full enteral feeding day, parenteral nutrition (PN) days, and total central line days were longer in the SSEF group. There was no significant difference in overall NEC (5.6% vs 11.2%, respectively; $P = .10$) or surgical NEC (1.6% vs 4.8%, respectively; $P = .17$) between the SSEF group and controls. However, in infants with birth weight <750 g, NEC (2.1% vs 16.2%, respectively; $P < .01$) or combined NEC/death (12.8% vs 29.5%, respectively; $P = .03$) was significantly less in the SSEF group compared with controls. In infants who survived to discharge, there was no significant difference in the discharge weight or length of stay in PS-adjusted analysis.

Conclusions.—An SSEF protocol significantly reduces the incidence of NEC and combined NEC/death in infants with birth weight <750 g. Despite taking longer to achieve full enteral feeding on this protocol, surviving ELBW infants demonstrated comparable weight gain at discharge without prolonging their hospital stay.

▶ Necrotizing enterocolitis (NEC) is a terrible neonatal illness, especially in extremely low birth weight preterm infants.[1-3] In very low birth weight infants, the mean incidence of NEC ranges from 7% to 9%, with an estimated case fatality rate of 15% to 30% and the greatest mortality in infants requiring surgery for NEC. The authors have noted that significant variations in practice exist as to when feeds are initiated, how they are advanced, and how feeding intolerance is managed in preterm infants. The modifiable risk factors related to enteral feeding for the development of NEC in preterm infants include the timing of introducing the feeds, the duration of trophic feeding and the rate of advancement of feeding, and the type of milk (human milk vs formula feeding). The duration of breast milk feeding has also been an issue as is the rate and individual nutrients supplied. Thus, they sought to utilize a standard slow enteral feeding regimen and compare with current standard of practice.

The overall incidence of NEC (5.6% vs 11.2%) and surgical NEC (1.6% vs 4.8%) were not significantly different between the standardized slow enteral feeding (SSEF) group and controls. However, in infants with birth weight < 750 g, there was a significant reduction in NEC (2% vs 16%) in the SSEF group compared with controls. No infants with birth weight < 750 g in the SSEF group developed surgical NEC compared with 7.8% in controls. Their study demonstrated that an SSEF protocol with maternal human milk/preterm formula reduced the incidence of NEC and combined NEC/death in infants with birth weight < 750 g.

This trial is extremely important because of the devastating nature of the disease process. Reducing or eliminating NEC would be a major breakthrough in pediatric care.

J. M. Daly, MD, FACS, FRCSI (Hon), FRCSG (Hon)

Prevalence of Gallstones Compared in Children With Different Intravenous Lipids

Pichler J, Watson T, McHugh K, et al (Univ Children's Hosp, Vienna, Austria; et al)

J Pediatr Gastroenterol Nutr 61:253-259, 2015

Objective.—The aetiology of biliary liver disease in children with intestinal failure treated with long-term parenteral nutrition (PN) is multifactorial. Risks include the lipid component of PN. The aim of the study was to compare prevalence and outcome of gallstones with different types of intravenous lipids.

Methods.—Liver and biliary tract imaging and relevant clinical details were reviewed in 71 patients (37, 52% boys) treated with PN for >3 months. Types of lipid infused were compared with regard to hepatobiliary abnormalities.

Results.—In total 369 abdominal ultrasounds were performed in 71 patients of age between 3 months and 17 years. Underlying diagnoses were short bowel syndrome in 20 (28%), small intestinal enteropathy in 34 (48%), and motility disorder in 17 (24%). A total of 67 (94%) children had 362/369 scans on lipid-containing PN. Of the total, 15 (21%) patients had gallstones, 8 (11%) had sludge, and both were detected in 7 (10%) children. The gallstones/sludge resolved in 7 patients (10%) and persisted in 10 (13%). In 6 patients, sludge progressed to form discrete gallstones, and in 9 children, gallstones led to biliary duct dilatation. Four (6%) patients underwent cholecystectomy. Fewer children had abnormalities with the newer mixed lipid emulsion ($P = 0.005$). There was a higher prevalence of sludge ($P = 0.01$) on pure soya lipid. Predictors for sludge were young age at PN ($P = 0.001$), lack of enteral feed ($P < 0.001$), and motility disorder with stoma ($P = 0.002$).

Conclusions.—Hepatobiliary pathology is common in children on PN. The use of mixed lipid was associated with less biliary complications and should be the first choice of treatment in children.

▶ Use of long-term total parenteral nutrition in both adults and children is associated with the development of gallstones and/or gallbladder sludge. This retrospective study sought to evaluate the occurrence of such problems in children with intestinal failure who were receiving long-term total parenteral nutrition (TPN) (> 3 months) and were at home. Sludge in the gallbladder, gallstones, or both were found on at least 1 scan in 30 of 71 children. Sludge was seen significantly less frequently in children who were enterally fed in addition to TPN (7%) compared with 20% of children who did not receive enteral feedings along with TPN ($P < .001$). A higher frequency of sludge and/or gallstones was seen with pure soya intravenous lipid emulsions, with sludge in 20% of patients compared with 10% of children who received mixed intravenous lipid emulsions. Results of this retrospective audit are interesting in that they provide some information as to the occurrence of gallbladder sludge or stones in children with intestinal failure receiving TPN. The results emphasize the importance of providing some nutrients enterally if possible in these children.

J. M. Daly, MD, FACS, FRCSI (Hon), FRCSG (Hon)

Early Enteral Nutrition and Aggressive Fluid Resuscitation are Associated with Improved Clinical Outcomes in Acute Pancreatitis

Szabo FK, Fei L, Cruz LA, et al (Cincinnati Children's Hosp Med Ctr, OH)

J Pediatr 167:397-402, 2015

Objectives.—To determine whether recommendations for treatment of acute pancreatitis (AP) in adults impact the outcomes of pediatric AP.

Study Design.—Adult guidelines regarding early management of AP were implemented through an admission order set at Cincinnati Children's Hospital Medical Center at the beginning of the year 2014. Recommendations included administering high rates of intravenous fluid (IVF) within 24 hours of admission and enteral nutrition within 48 hours of admission. A retrospective chart review of AP admissions before and after the implementation of the recommendations was undertaken. Outcomes studied were: hospital length of stay, intensive care unit transfer rates, development of severe AP, pulmonary complications, and readmission rates post discharge from the hospital.

Results.—The study included 201 patients. Children who received feeds within the first 48 hours and received greater than maintenance IVF within 24 hours had a shorter length of stay, less intensive care unit admissions and severe AP rates compared with the patients who remained nil per os during the first 48 hours and received lower rates of IVF.

Conclusion.—Our data support that early enteral nutrition and early aggressive IVF improve outcomes of pediatric AP.

▶ Management of pediatric patients with acute pancreatitis has been traditionally different from that for adults, in part because of the less common incidence of the problem. Given the movement toward evidence-based medicine and the opportunity to standardize care, the authors used specific recommendations regarding the timing of enteral nutrition, as well as timing, type, and rate of intravenous fluid (IVF), that included (1) initiation of enteral feeds on admission (clears with progression to general age-appropriate diet within 6 hours if tolerated) and (2) initiation of IVF at 1.5 to 2 times the maintenance rate of dextrose 5% normal saline on admission.

A retrospective review of admissions of children with acute pancreatitis from 2009 to 2014 was conducted. The authors' study shows that oral feeding in children was safe in mild acute pancreatitis and was associated with shortened hospital length of stay and decreased rate of severe acute pancreatitis and intensive care unit transfer rates. In addition, aggressive fluid management was not associated with increased respiratory or lung complications compared with the group that received lower rates of IVF. The authors are to be commended for initiating a more standard "order set" for the management of acute pancreatitis in children. The next step is for them to perform a prospective trial of the order set's true efficacy perhaps using a multi-institutional approach.

J. M. Daly, MD, FACS, FRCSI (Hon), FRCSG (Hon)

Preoperative Enteral Nutritional Support in Patients Undergoing Hepatectomy for Hepatocellular Carcinoma: A Strengthening the Reporting of Observational Studies in Epidemiology Article

Yao H, Bian X, Mao L, et al (Med School of Nanjing Univ, China; et al)
Medicine (Baltimore) 94:e2006, 2015

To compare the short-term outcomes between hepatocellular carcinoma (HCC) patients with and those without preoperative nutrition on the basis of postoperative enteral nutrition.

HCC patients with postoperative enteral nutrition who underwent liver resection between February 2010 and December 2014 in Nanjing Drum Tower Hospital were considered for the study: 43 patients with and 36 patients without preoperative nutrition. Primary endpoint was the incidence of overall complications. Secondary endpoints were infectious and major complications.

In the preoperative enteral nutrition group, shorter length of postoperative hospital stay (10.5 ± 2.7 versus 13.7 ± 6.3 days, $P = 0.007$), less exogenous albumin infusion (10.2 ± 22.4 versus 47.8 ± 97.7 g, $P = 0.030$), earlier first exhaust time (2.7 ± 0.8 versus 3.0 ± 0.9 days, $P = 0.043$), and first defection time (3.5 ± 0.9 versus 4.4 ± 1.4 days, $P = 0.001$) were observed. No significant differences were observed in the incidence of overall complications (32.6% versus 52.8%, $P = 0.070$), infectious complications (7.0% versus 8.3%, $P = 1$), and major complications (14.0% versus 11.1%, $P = 0.969$) between the preoperative enteral nutrition and control group.

Preoperative enteral nutrition could improve short-term outcomes of HCC patients via accelerating the recovery of gastrointestinal function and shortening the length of postoperative hospital stay.

▶ Use of postoperative enteral nutritional support can significantly improve outcomes in patients who are malnourished preoperatively and who undergo a major procedure that is fraught with potential complications. Patients with substantial liver and kidney abnormalities are susceptible to both postoperative complications and to problems with enteral nutrition.

The retrospective cohort study consisted of 79 HCC patients with postoperative enteral nutrition who underwent curative liver resection over approximately 4 years. Patients in the postoperative enteral nutrition group had a significantly shorter mean postoperative hospital stay than those in the control group (10.5 days vs 13.7 days, $P < .007$). The most common compli-cation was ascites, representing 16% and 42% of the postoperative enteral nutrition group and the control group, respectively ($P < .01$). Morbidity and particularly infectious complications were similar between groups.

This study suffers from its retrospective nature and the small sample size of patients being studied. Clearly, a prospective randomized trial should be conducted before firm conclusions can be made.

J. M. Daly, MD, FACS, FRCSI (Hon), FRCSG (Hon)

Dietary fatty acid content regulates wound repair and the pathogenesis of osteoarthritis following joint injury

Wu C-L, Jain D, McNeill JN, et al (Duke Univ Med Ctr, Durham, NC; et al)

Ann Rheum Dis 74:2076-2083, 2015

Objective.—The mechanisms linking obesity and osteoarthritis (OA) are not fully understood and have been generally attributed to increased weight, rather than metabolic or inflammatory factors. Here, we examined the influence of fatty acids, adipokines, and body weight on OA following joint injury in an obese mouse model.

Methods.—Mice were fed high-fat diets rich in various fatty acids (FA) including saturated FAs (SFAs), ω-6 polyunsaturated FAs (PUFAs), and ω-3 PUFAs. OA was induced by destabilising the medial meniscus. Wound healing was evaluated using an ear punch. OA, synovitis and wound healing were determined histologically, while bone changes were measured using microCT. Activity levels and serum cytokines were measured at various time-points. Multivariate models were performed to elucidate the associations of dietary, metabolic and mechanical factors with OA and wound healing.

Results.—Using weight-matched mice and multivariate models, we found that OA was significantly associated with dietary fatty acid content and serum adipokine levels, but not with body weight. Furthermore, spontaneous activity of the mice was independent of OA development. Small amounts of ω-3 PUFAs (8% by kcal) in a high-fat diet were sufficient to mitigate injury-induced OA, decreasing leptin and resistin levels. ω-3 PUFAs significantly enhanced wound repair, SFAs or ω-6 PUFAs independently increased OA severity, heterotopic ossification and scar tissue formation.

Conclusions.—Our results indicate that with obesity, dietary FA content regulates wound healing and OA severity following joint injury, independent of body weight, supporting the need for further studies of dietary FA supplements as a potential therapeutic approach for OA.

▶ As the authors have noted, the effects of body weight and diet on the occurrence of osteoarthritis (OA) is controversial because arthritic changes occur in non—weight-bearing joints as well as those bearing weight. The findings of this study showed that a small amount of ω-3 polyunsaturated fatty acid (PUFA) supplementation was sufficient to mitigate the effects of obesity on injury-induced OA and to accelerate would repair. Conversely, saturated fatty acids and ω-6 PUFA independently acted as a detrimental factor in OA after joint injury, increasing osteophyte formation, heterotopic ossification, synovitis as well as increasing infiltration of macrophages into synovial tissue. An important aspect of this study was to evaluate the behavioral alterations that occurred with obesity and various fatty acid compositions. Translation of these results to humans suggests, of course, that weight loss would help decrease the occurrence of osteoarthritis. In addition, changes in diet with a greater intake of omega-3 fatty acids should also be helpful in reducing osteoarthritis.

J. M. Daly, MD, FACS, FRCSI (Hon), FRCSG (Hon)

Comparison of short-term mortality and morbidity between parenteral and enteral nutrition for adults without cancer: a propensity-matched analysis using a national inpatient database

Tamiya H, Yasunaga H, Matusi H, et al (Univ of Tokyo, Japan; et al)

Am J Clin Nutr 102:1222-1228, 2015

Background.—Proper artificial nutrition for patients who are unable to eat normally is an ongoing, unresolved concern in geriatric medicine and home medical care. Controversy surrounds prognostic differences between parenteral and enteral nutrition, 2 methods for artificial nutrition.

Objectives.—Short-term outcomes of parenteral and enteral nutrition for patients who are unable to eat normally were compared and analyzed.

Design.—Data were acquired from patients selected from a national inpatient database covering 1057 hospitals in Japan. Participants had received artificial nutrition between April 2012 and March 2013, were aged ≥20 y, and did not have cancer. They were separated into 2 groups: those who received parenteral nutrition and those who received enteral nutrition. We performed one-to-one propensity score matching between the groups. The primary outcome measurements were mortality rates at 30 and 90 d after the start of the procedure. The secondary outcomes were postprocedural complications, pneumonia, and sepsis. We analyzed survival length of stay after the procedure with the use of a Cox proportional hazards model.

Results.—There were 3750 patients in the parenteral group and 22,166 patients in the enteral group. Propensity score matching created 2912 pairs in the 2 groups. Patients with a similar propensity score (probability of being assigned to the enteral group) calculated from the baseline condition were matched. Mortality rates at 30 and 90 d after start of treatment were 7.6% and 5.7% ($P = 0.003$) and 12.3% and 9.9% ($P = 0.002$) in the parenteral and enteral groups, respectively. In Cox regression analysis, the HR for the enteral group relative to the parenteral group was 0.62 (95% CI: 0.54, 0.71; $P < 0.001$). The incidences of postprocedural pneumonia and sepsis were 11.9% and 15.5% ($P < 0.001$) and 4.4% and 3.7% ($P = 0.164$) for the parenteral and enteral groups, respectively.

Conclusion.—The present analysis showed the better survival rate with enteral compared with parenteral nutrition for adults who were not suffering from cancer. This trial was registered at clinicaltrials.gov as NCT02512224.

▶ Controversy continues to exist as to the degree to which parenteral nutrition (TPN) adversely effects individuals versus enteral nutritional support. In most studies, enteral nutrition is associated with better outcomes compared with results in patients who received parenteral nutrition. This large retrospective study used a national database in Japan to evaluate differences in short-term outcomes. There were 3750 patients who had received parenteral nutrition and 22 166 patients who had received enteral nutrition.

Propensity score matching created 2912 pairs in the parenteral and enteral nutrition groups. The area under the curve (AUC) of the receiver operator characteristic (ROC) analysis for goodness-of-fit of the model used for propensity score matching was 0.764 (95% confidence interval: 0.755–0.773; $P < 0.001$). The value of 0.764 indicated a fair level of fit. In this study, patients were generally old, frail patients with chronic diseases.

As the authors noted, several limitations of this study deserve acknowledgment. First, although the study population was large, this investigation was based on a retrospective observational design without randomization. Although a propensity score method was used to adjust for differences in baseline characteristics and severity of conditions, the results may still have been biased by unmeasured confounders, such as the severity of each disease and performance status. The AUC of the ROC analysis for goodness-of-fit of the model used for propensity score matching indicated a fair, but not good, level of fit. Finally, there was tremendous imbalance between the numbers of those that received parenteral versus enteral nutrition support suggesting that the TPN patients were indeed sicker and unable to tolerate enteral nutrition and thus were relegated to TPN. Although a large database analysis can be valuable, it can also provide misleading conclusions.

J. M. Daly, MD, FACS, FRCSI (Hon), FRCSG (Hon)

Gastric vs Small Bowel Feeding in Critically Ill Neurologically Injured Patients: Results of a Multicenter Observational Study

Saran D, Brody RA, Stankorb SM, et al (State Univ of New Jersey, Newark; et al)

JPEN J Parenter Enteral Nutr 39:910-916, 2015

Background.—To evaluate gastric compared with small bowel feeding on nutrition and clinical outcomes in critically ill, neurologically injured patients.

Materials and Methods.—International, prospective observational studies involving 353 intensive care units (ICUs) were included. Eligible patients were critically ill, mechanically ventilated with neurological diagnoses who remained in the ICU and received enteral nutrition (EN) exclusively for at least 3 days. Sites provided data, including patient characteristics, nutrition practices, and 60-day outcomes. Patients receiving gastric or small bowel feeding were compared. Covariates including age, sex, body mass index, and Acute Physiology and Chronic Health Evaluation II score were used in the adjusted analyses.

Results.—Of the 1691 patients who met our inclusion criteria, 1407 (94.1%) received gastric feeding and 88 (5.9%) received small bowel feeding. Adequacy of calories from EN was highest in the gastric group (60.2% and 52.3%, respectively, unadjusted analysis; $P = .001$), but this was not significant in the adjusted model ($P = .428$). The likelihood of EN interruptions due to gastrointestinal (GI) complications was higher for the gastric group (19.6% vs 4.7%, unadjusted model; $P = .015$). There were no significant differences in the rate of discontinuation of mechanical ventilation (hazard ratio [HR], 0.86; 95% confidence interval [CI], 0.66–1.12; $P = .270$) or the rate of being discharged alive from the ICU (HR, 0.94; 95% CI, 0.72–1.23; $P = .641$) and hospital (HR, 1.16; 95% CI, 0.87–1.55; $P = .307$) after adjusting for confounders.

Conclusions.—Despite a higher likelihood of EN interruptions due to GI complications, gastric feeding may be associated with better nutrition adequacy, but neither route is associated with better clinical outcomes.

▶ In the intensive care unit, the preference is to feed patients unable to eat by the enteral route. However, there is controversy as to whether it is better to feed directly into the stomach or into the small intestine. Proponents of gastric feeding note that it is easier and that gastric propulsion and the pyloric sphincter action regulates emptying of nutrients into the small bowel. Proponents of small intestinal feeding note that it may be easier once the catheter tip is in place to feed continuously and to have fewer episodes of esophageal reflux and regurgitation.

This study had an interesting design in that, over a period of 5 (2007–2011) years, intensive care units (ICUs) from around the world collected data on neurologically impaired patients receiving mechanical ventilation and enteral tube feeding. Eligible patients were critically ill adults (≥18 years of age) who were mechanically ventilated within 48 hours of admission to the ICU and who remained in the ICU for a minimum of 72 hours. The PEP uP study (2010) included patients who were ventilated within the first 6 hours of ICU admission, and there was no minimum length of hospital stay. There were few differences in outcomes between gastric feeding and small bowel feeding. Strengths of this study are its real-world approach and the large number of institutions and patients. Next steps would be to perform a prospective randomized trial to investigate these 2 routes of feeding.

J. M. Daly, MD, FACS, FRCSI (Hon), FRCSG (Hon)

Metabolic adaptation to caloric restriction and subsequent refeeding: the Minnesota Starvation Experiment revisited

Müller MJ, Enderle J, Pourhassan M, et al (Christian-Albrechts Univ, Kiel, Germany; et al)

Am J Clin Nutr 102:807-819, 2015

Background.—Adaptive thermogenesis (AT) is the fat-free mass (FFM)–independent reduction of resting energy expenditure (REE) to caloric restriction (CR). AT attenuates weight loss and favors weight regain. Its variance, dynamics, and control remain obscure.

Objectives.—Our aims were to address the variance and kinetics of AT, its associations with body composition in the context of endocrine determinants, and its effect on weight regain.

Design.—Thirty-two nonobese men underwent sequential overfeeding (1 wk at +50% of energy needs), CR (3 wk at −50% of energy needs), and refeeding (2 wk at +50% of energy needs). AT and its determinants were measured together with body composition as assessed with the use of quantitative magnetic resonance, whole-body MRI, isotope dilution, and nitrogen and fluid balances.

Results.—Changes in body weight were +1.8 kg (overfeeding), −6.0 kg (CR), and +3.5 kg (refeeding). CR reduced fat mass and FFM by 114 and 159 g/d, respectively. Within FFM, skeletal muscle (−5%), liver (−13%), and kidneys (−8%) decreased. CR also led to reductions in REE (−266 kcal/d), respiratory quotient (−15%), heart rate (−14%), blood pressure (−7%), creatinine clearance (−12%), energy cost of walking (−22%), activity of the sympathetic nervous system (SNS) (−38%), and plasma leptin (−44%), insulin (−54%), adiponectin (−49%), 3,5,3'-tri-iodo-thyronine (T3) (−39%), and testosterone (−11%). AT was 108 kcal/d or 48% of the decrease in REE. Changes in FFM composition explained 36 kcal, which left 72 kcal/d for true AT. The decrease in AT became significant at ≤3 d of CR and was related to decreases in insulin secretion

($r = 0.92$, $P < 0.001$), heart rate ($r = 0.60$, $P < 0.05$), creatinine clearance ($r = 0.79$, $P < 0.05$), negative fluid balance ($r = 0.51$, $P < 0.01$), and the free water clearance rate ($r = -0.90$, $P < 0.002$). SNS activity and plasma leptin, ghrelin, and T3 and their changes with CR were not related to AT.

Conclusion.—During early weight loss, AT is associated with a fall in insulin secretion and body fluid balance. This trial was registered at clinicaltrials.gov as NCT01737034.

▶ Caloric restriction and weight loss are associated with decreases in resting energy expenditure (REE) and adaptive thermogenesis (AT). AT refers to the decrease in resting energy expenditure beyond those decreases accounted for by changed fat-free mass and fat mass. This effect is seen with diet, exercise, diet and exercise, pharmacologic, and surgical interventions. This adaptation occurs along with changes in the body's physiologic and biochemical pathways, such as decreases in circulation insulin levels and changes in glucose, fatty acid, and ketone production. Ultimately, organs, particularly the central nervous system begin to use ketones as a primary energy source rather than glucose-preserving protein stores.

In this study, 32 nonobese volunteer men underwent sequential overfeeding, caloric restriction, and referring. In the current study, 3 weeks of caloric restriction in these predominantly sedentary individuals decreased fat-free mass by 3.7%, body protein by 2.0%, skeletal muscle mass by 4.7%, and internal organ masses by 7.8% without clinical signs of malnutrition. Adaptive thermogenesis during early weight loss was correlated with a decrease in plasma insulin levels and body water.

This study is important in that it provides a more moderate degree of caloric restriction that is more in keeping with Western world dieting than more severe and extensive malnutrition. This report bears thorough reading to fully appreciate the many variables measured during caloric restriction and referring.

J. M. Daly, MD, FACS, FRCSI (Hon), FRCSG (Hon)

Effect of Critical Illness on Triglyceride Absorption

Ali Abdelhamid Y, Cousins CE, Sim JA, et al (Royal Adelaide Hosp, Australia; Univ of Adelaide, Australia; et al)

JPEN J Parenter Enteral Nutr 39:966-972, 2015

Background.—Adequate nutrition support for critically ill patients optimizes outcome, and enteral feeding is the preferred route of nutrition. Small intestinal glucose absorption is frequently impaired in critical illness. Despite lipid being a major constituent of liquid nutrient administered, there is little information about lipid absorption during critical illness.

Objectives.—To determine small intestinal lipid, as well as glucose, absorption in critical illness compared with health.

Materials and Methods.—Twenty-nine mechanically ventilated critically ill patients and 16 healthy volunteers were studied. Liquid nutrient (60 mL, 1 kcal/mL), containing 200 μL ^{13}C-triolein and 3 g 3-O-methylglucose (3-OMG), was infused directly into the duodenum at a rate of 2 kcal/min. Exhaled $^{13}CO_2$ and serum 3-OMG concentrations were measured at timed intervals over 360 minutes. Lipid absorption was measured as the cumulative percentage dose (cPDR) of $^{13}CO_2$ recovered at 360 minutes. Glucose absorption was measured as the area under the 3-OMG concentration curve. Data are median (range) and analyzed using the Mann-Whitney *U* and Pearson correlation tests.

Results.—Lipid absorption was markedly less in the critically ill (cPDR$^{13}CO_2$: patients, 22.6% [0%−100%] vs healthy participants, 40.7% [5.3%−84.7%]; $P = .018$). While glucose absorption was less at 60 minutes in the critically ill (3-OMG_{60}: 13.2 [3.5−29.5] vs 21.1 [9.3−31.9] mmol/L·min; $P = .003$), this was not apparent at 360 minutes (3- OMG_{360}: 92.7 [54.5−147.9] vs 107.9 [64.0−168.7] mmol/L·min; $P = .126$). There was no relationship between lipid and glucose absorption.

Conclusion.—Small intestinal absorption of lipid is diminished during critical illness.

▶ Enteral feeding is preferred whenever possible in patients requiring nutritional support. However, it is unclear how much of the nutrient solution is actually absorbed.

Data from 29 mechanically ventilated critically ill patients who were receiving enteral nutrition via a nasoduodenal feeding catheter were compared with data from 16 healthy volunteers. Data in the critically ill cohort were derived from the placebo arm of a published study. Healthy participants were recruited as a control group and provided all new data. The major findings of this study are that small intestinal lipid absorption, as measured by the 13C-triolein breath test, is reduced by almost half in critical illness compared with health and appears to be more impaired than glucose absorption. Furthermore, there appears to be no relationship between lipid and glucose absorption in the critically ill.

Results of this study are important in that they provide a basis for limiting the lipids infused in patients who are critically ill, which compounds diarrhea and is frequent in these patients.

J. M. Daly, MD, FACS, FRCSI (Hon), FRCSG (Hon)

Damaging Effects of Total Parenteral Nutrition Formula on Vascular Endothelium

Demircan M, Gurunluoglu K, Karaman A, et al (İnönü Univ Faculty of Medicine, Malatya, Turkey; et al)
J Pediatr Gastroenterol Nutr 61:464-468, 2015

Objectives.—Sepsis in one of the most serious complications that can occur during total parenteral nutrition (TPN) procedures. In this experimental study, we investigated the effects of TPN, with or without lipid emulsion, on vascular endothelial damage.

Methods.—In total, 50 rabbits were used, divided into 5 groups of 10 each. TPN with lipids (group 1), TPN without lipids (group 2), and 0.09% saline (group 3) were given for 10 days via a central venous catheter. Group 4 received no treatment other than placement of a central venous catheter for 10 days. Group 5 was a control group. At the end of day 10, rabbits were sacrificed and tissue samples of liver, kidney, and inferior vena cava were prepared and examined by immunohistochemical methods for vascular cellular adhesion molecule (VCAM)-1 expression.

Results.—In tissue sections of liver, kidney, and inferior vena cava, VCAM-1 activity was increased prominently in TPN with and without lipids compared with the control group. VCAM-1 activity in the TPN with lipids group was decreased versus the TPN without lipids group ($P > 0.05$).

Conclusions.—The TPN procedure results in vascular endothelial cell damage not only in the vein where the solution is introduced but also in other parts of the vascular system. Even if it is not statistically significant, lipids in the TPN formula may decrease this endothelial cell damage, as shown by immunohistochemistry.

▶ It has been argued that the use of total parenteral nutrition (TPN) in patients results in a greater incidence of sepsis than when nutrition is provided enterally. It has been thought that this increase in infection and sepsis is due to gastrointestinal mucosal abnormalities resulting in bacterial translocation. Others have suggested that leaky vascular endothelium results in a greater response to sepsis in those given TPN resulting in a greater degree of ARDS when sepsis occurs.

This animal study showed increased VCAM-1 levels in rabbits given TPN with and without 10% lipid emulsion. Several major questions arise from this study. For example, does this result translate into greater physiologic changes in the vascular endothelium? What are the components of TPN that cause this increase in VCAM-1? Does this result translate into other animal models, and does it result in an altered response to sepsis?

Clearly, more work needs to be done to elucidate both the causes and effects of TPN on vascular endothelium.

J. M. Daly, MD, FACS, FRCSI (Hon), FRCSG (Hon)

Influence of Enteral Nutrition on Occurrences of Necrotizing Enterocolitis in Very-Low-Birth-Weight Infants

Kimak KS, de Castro Antunes MM, Braga TD, et al (Post-Graduate Program in Child and Adolescent Health, Recife, Brazil; Federal Univ of Pernambuco, Recife, Brazil; Instituto de Medicina Integral Prof. Fernando Figueira, Recife, Brazil)

J Pediatr Gastroenterol Nutr 61:445-450, 2015

Objective.—The aim of the present study was to investigate the influence of enteral feeding management on occurrences of necrotizing enterocolitis (NEC) in very-low-birth-weight (VLBW) infants.

Methods.—This was a case-control study conducted in a sample of 1028 VLBW infants (750 to 1499 g) admitted to a neonatal intensive care unit between January 2003 and May 2008. "Cases" were infants born with VLBW and diagnosed with NEC within the first 30 days of life, and "controls" were VLBW infants who did not develop NEC during this period. Occurrences of NEC were defined using the modified Bell criteria (stage ≥2).

Results.—Among the 1028 VLBW infants, 55 (5.4%) developed NEC within the first month of life. Logistic regression analysis showed that breast milk given exclusively for <7 days (odds ratio [OR]=4.02), never achieving full enteral feeding during the first month (OR = 3.50), and parenteral nutrition (OR = 2.70) were factors that increased the chances of NEC occurrence. The use of vasoactive drugs was associated with a lower risk of NEC (OR = 0.15).

Conclusions.—Breast milk should be recommended as a priority for the enteral nutrition of VLBW infants for no <7 days. Enteral nutrition should start early and progress quickly to achieve full enteral feeding; these procedures may help reduce the occurrence of NEC.

▶ There is a higher occurrence (4%–13%) of necrotizing enterocolitis (NEC) in very-low-birth-weight infants. Much research is ongoing to determine the best methods to feed these infants and the best nutrients to obviate NEC. As the authors have noted, "nutritional management for premature infants includes defining the type of food, time when the enteral diet should be started, rate of progression, administration technique, and assessing an infant's food tolerance." Breast milk has been incorporated into feeding regimens, but the question, is how much and for how long?

Logistic regression analysis showed that breast milk given exclusively for < 7 days, never achieving full enteral feeding during the first month, and parenteral nutrition were factors that increased the chances of NEC occurrence. This retrospective, case-control study provides some recommendations regarding the initiation of feeding and the use of breast milk for these very low birth weight infants; however, further prospective trials are necessary to confirm these effects and to intervene to reduce the incidence of this devastating problem.

J. M. Daly, MD, FACS, FRCSI (Hon), FRCSG (Hon)

Outcome Indicators for Home Parenteral Nutrition Care: Point of View From Adult Patients With Benign Disease

Dreesen M, Pironi L, Wanten G, et al (KULeuven and Univ Hosps Leuven, Belgium; Univ of Bologna, Italy; Radboud Univ Nijmegen Med Centre, The Netherlands; et al)

JPEN J Parenter Enteral Nutr 39:828-836, 2015

Background and Aims.—Patients receiving home parenteral nutrition (HPN) deserve a high-quality and patient-centered care. Patient-centered care can be delivered only if the patient's priorities and concerns are known. Therefore, the aim is to identify the top 3 most important outcome indicators according to patients' perspectives and the differences between several centers, HPN regimen, and HPN experience.

Methods.—A questionnaire, based on previously developed outcome indicators, was translated into the mother tongue using forward-backward translation and distributed to adult HPN patients with benign disease in March 2013. To identify differences, a Kruskal-Wallis or Mann-Whitney test was performed with GraphPad Prism (significance level <.05) when applicable.

Results.—Nine centers over 8 countries (300 patients) participated. The top 3 outcome indicators for patients were (1) incidence of catheter-related infection (CRI), (2) survival, and (3) quality of life (QoL). Between the participating centers, significant differences on rating were found for 5 outcome indicators (catheter obstruction, .015; weight, .002; energy, .010; fear, <.001; and independence, .010). The independence outcome indicator (.050) was considered less important for experienced (>2 years HPN) vs less experienced patients. For this outcome indicator, patients' view also differed significantly based on number of HPN days per week (.0103).

Conclusion.—A cohort of HPN patients identified incidence of CRI, survival, and QoL as the most important outcome indicators for their care; however, there were significant differences between the participating centers. For one outcome indicator (independence), there were significant differences based on experience and regimen.

► Home parenteral nutrition is a major industry with new technology, nutritional indicators, and a variety of clinical endpoints measured. Institution of home total parenteral nutrition is lifesaving for the patients who receive it. However, more information is needed to determine the major quality indicators after institution of home parenteral nutrition. This study sought information globally by having a questionnaire completed in an effort to understand the major quality-of-life indicators worldwide.

For the global top 3, the outcome indicator that most strongly contributed to patients' perception of quality of care was the incidence of catheter-related infections. The second ranked indicator was for the incidence of survival followed by individual quality of life.

It is important for us to realize what patients seek when they embark on home total parenteral nutrition and that their individual goals for treatment may be different from those of their treating health care professionals.

J. M. Daly, MD, FACS, FRCSI (Hon), FRCSG (Hon)

Enteral delivery of proteins enhances the expression of proteins involved in the cytoskeleton and protein biosynthesis in human duodenal mucosa

Goichon A, Bertrand J, Chan P, et al (INSERM Unit 1073, Rouen, France; Rouen Univ, France; et al)

Am J Clin Nutr 102:359-367, 2015

Background.—Amino acids are well known to be key effectors of gut protein turnover. We recently reported that enteral delivery of proteins markedly stimulated global duodenal protein synthesis in carbohydrate-fed healthy humans, but specifically affected proteins remain unknown.

Objective.—We aimed to assess the influence of an enteral protein supply on the duodenal mucosal proteome in carbohydrate-fed humans.

Design.—Six healthy volunteers received for 5 h, on 2 occasions and in random order, either an enteral infusion of maltodextrins alone ($0.25\ g \cdot kg^{-1} \cdot h^{-1}$) mimicking the fed state or maltodextrins with a protein powder ($0.14\ g$ proteins $\cdot\ kg^{-1} \cdot h^{-1}$). Endoscopic duodenal biopsy specimens were then collected and frozen until analysis. A 2-dimensional polyacrylamide gel electrophoresis–based comparative proteomics analysis was then performed, and differentially expressed proteins (at least ±1.5-fold change; Student's *t* test, $P < 0.05$) were identified by mass spectrometry. Protein expression changes were confirmed by Western blot analysis.

Results.—Thirty-two protein spots were differentially expressed after protein delivery compared with maltodextrins alone: 28 and 4 spots were up- or downregulated, respectively. Among the 22 identified proteins, 11 upregulated proteins were involved either in the cytoskeleton (ezrin, moesin, plastin 1, lamin B1, vimentin, and β-actin) or in protein biosynthesis (glutamyl-prolyl–transfer RNA synthetase, glutaminyl–transfer RNA synthetase, elongation factor 2, elongation factor 1δ, and eukaryotic translation and initiation factor 3 subunit f).

Conclusions.—Enteral delivery of proteins altered the duodenal mucosal proteome and mainly stimulated the expression of proteins involved in cytoskeleton and protein biosynthesis. These results suggest that protein supply may affect intestinal morphology by stimulating actin cytoskeleton remodeling. This trial was registered at clinicaltrials.-gov as NCT01254110.

▶ Enteral delivery of nutrients is critical to maintaining the function and structure of the gastrointestinal (GI) tract, but the major questions surround the amount and type of proteins that are important to this process.

In the present study, the authors showed in carbohydrate-fed humans that an enteral delivery of proteins modified the duodenal mucosal proteome, particularly by enhancing the expression of several proteins involved in the cytoskeleton and protein synthesis.

Protein supplementation significantly enhanced ezrin, moesin, plastin 1, b-actin, lamin B1, and vimentin expression in human duodenal mucosa, suggesting that enteral protein supply may affect intestinal morphology, particularly the actin cytoskeleton dynamics. Studies such as these are important because they are done under controlled conditions in human volunteers and attempt to decipher the impact of nutrients on the GI tract itself. In addition, these studies showed that the effects of protein were predominantly on intestinal morphology.

J. M. Daly, MD, FACS, FRCSI (Hon), FRCSG (Hon)

Glutamine Improves Innate Immunity and Prevents Bacterial Enteroinvasion During Parenteral Nutrition

Wang X, Pierre JF, Heneghan AF, et al (Univ of Wisconsin School of Medicine and Public Health, Madison; et al)

JPEN J Parenter Enteral Nutr 39:688-697, 2015

Background.—Patients receiving parenteral nutrition (PN) are at increased risk of infectious complications compared with enteral feeding, which is in part explained by impaired mucosal immune function during PN. Adding glutamine (GLN) to PN has improved outcome in some clinical patient groups. Although GLN improves acquired mucosal immunity, its effect on innate mucosal immunity (defensins, mucus, lysozymes) has not been investigated.

Methods.—Forty-eight hours following venous cannulation, male Institute of Cancer Research mice were randomized to chow (n = 10), PN (n = 12), or PN + GLN (n = 13) for 5 days. Small intestine tissue and luminal fluid were collected for mucin 2 (MUC2), lysozyme, cryptdin 4 analysis, and luminal interleukin (IL)-4, IL-10, and IL-13 level measurement. Tissue was also harvested for ex vivo intestinal segment culture to assess tissue susceptibility to enteroinvasive *Escherichia coli.*

Results.—In both luminal and tissue samples, PN reduced MUC2 and lysozyme ($P < .0001$, respectively) compared with chow, whereas GLN addition increased MUC2 and lysozyme (luminal, $P < .05$; tissue, $P < .0001$, respectively) compared with PN alone. PN significantly suppressed cryptdin 4 expression, while GLN supplementation significantly enhanced expression. IL-4, IL-10, and IL-13 decreased significantly with PN compared with chow, whereas GLN significantly increased these cytokines compared with PN. Functionally, bacterial invasion increased with PN compared with chow ($P < .05$), while GLN significantly decreased enteroinvasion to chow levels ($P < .05$).

Conclusions.—GLN supplemented PN improves innate immunity and resistance to bacterial mucosal invasion lost with PN alone. This work confirms a clinical rationale for providing glutamine for the protection of the intestinal mucosa.

▶ The authors have described that innate immunity plays an important role in protecting the gastrointestinal (GI) tract mucosal surfaces. Specialized secretory epithelial cells, specifically goblet cells and Paneth cells within the mucosa, constitute the cellular components of innate mucosal immunity. A mucus layer consisting of glycoproteins released from the goblet cells coats the mucosal surface, concentrates the sIgA produced by the GALT (acquired immunity), and localizes antimicrobial compounds, such cryptdin 4 and lysozymes produced and released by the Paneth cells. The benefit of glutamine is likely in part through modulation of intestinal cytokine levels. Glutamine increases Th2 lymphocyte-derived cytokines—interleukin (IL)-4, IL-10, and IL-13—in small intestinal tissue homogenates compared with parenteral nutrition alone. Parenteral nutrition significantly decreased lysozyme in the intestinal fluid compared with chow. The addition of glutamine to parenteral nutrition significantly increased lysozyme levels in the intestinal fluid compared with parenteral nutrition alone. Compared with chow, the number of invaded *Escherichia coli* recovered from intestinal explants significantly increased following parenteral nutrition. The addition of glutamine to parenteral nutrition significantly reduced the number of invaded *E coli* compared with parenteral nutrition alone.

Many studies have shown that the addition of glutamine to enteral or parenteral diets have been beneficial. Dr Kudsk's lab in particular has done the major new work in this area. Human studies should ultimately be done to corroborate this nice work in mice.

J. M. Daly, MD, FACS, FRCSI (Hon), FRCSG (Hon)

Safety and Efficacy of Parenteral Fish Oil–Containing Lipid Emulsions in Premature Neonates

Zhao Y, Wu Y, Pei J, et al (Sichuan Univ, China; Sichuan Cancer Hosp and Inst, China)

J Pediatr Gastroenterol Nutr 60:708-716, 2015

Objective.—The aim of the study was to evaluate the safety and efficacy of fish oil–containing (FO) lipid emulsions that are rich in ω-3 fatty acids for parenteral nutrition in preterm neonates by using data retrieved from randomized controlled trials.

Methods.—We performed a meta-analysis of 8 randomized controlled trials representing 483 premature neonates to compare FO with control (CO) lipid emulsions.

Results.—This meta-analysis revealed that the levels of ω-3 fatty acids in the form of docosahexaenoic acid, eicosapentaenoic acid, and arachidonic acid (% of total fatty acids) in plasma were statistically higher in FO groups (mean difference [MD] −0.7%, 95% confidence interval [CI] −1.05 to −0.36, $P < 0.001$; MD −1.31%, 95% CI −1.40 to −1.21, $P < 0.001$). The differences were found in red blood cell (RBC) membranes. The levels of arachidonic acid (% of total fatty acids) as ω-6 fatty acid in plasma and red blood cell membranes were significantly lower in FO groups (MD 1.27%, 95% CI 1.12–1.42, $P < 0.001$) (MD 0.92%, 95% CI 0.12–1.72, $P = 0.02$). The mean body weight, serum level of bilirubin, triglycerides or C-reactive protein, all-cause mortality, and rate of lipid emulsion–associated complications were, however, not different between FO and CO groups.

Conclusions.—The level of docosahexaenoic acid is efficiently improved by FO lipid emulsions. The changes observed in eicosapentaenoic acid and arachidonic acid, and the associated safety issue, however, remain to be clarified. Any clinical benefit or detrimental effect of using FO in premature neonates cannot be demonstrated by the present study.

▶ Use of fish oil—based lipid emulsions may be important in the parenteral feeding regimens of premature infants who cannot ingest adequate nutrition or have nutrients administered enterally. However, it is unclear from previous publications whether this hypothesis is true. After searching the literature, the authors found 69 articles, but only eight studies met inclusion criteria of randomized controlled trials and were included in this meta-analysis.

Owing to the limited data, the authors were not able to demonstrate major clinical benefits using the fish oil—containing lipid emulsions. The present study revealed that the docosahexaenoic acid levels could be significantly improved using fish oil—based lipid emulsions, but the safety of the changes observed for eicosapentaenoic acid and arachidonic acid remains to be proven. Sadly, despite a fair number of clinical trials, the efficacy of supplying certain types of lipid emulsions is unclear. This results an indictment on creating small clinical studies that fail to answer important clinical questions.

J. M. Daly, MD, FACS, FRCSI (Hon), FRCSG (Hon)

9 Gastrointestinal

Porcelain Gallbladder: No Longer an Indication for Prophylactic Cholecystectomy

Chen GL, Akmal Y, DiFronzo AL, et al (Kaiser Permanente Los Angeles Med Ctr, CA)

Am Surg 81:936-940, 2015

Porcelain gallbladder (PG) was historically associated with gallbladder cancer (GBC), (range 12–62%, largest series n = 26). Presently, cholecystectomy is still performed in many patients with PG. The objective of this study was to determine the incidence of GBC in patients with radiographic diagnosis of PG. We conducted a retrospective chart review of the Kaiser Permanente southern California electronic medical record database and identified patients with radiographic diagnosis of PG between 2008 and 2013. Extracted were patient demographics, imaging modality, symptoms, surgical and observational outcomes, and pathology results. Out of 192 PG patients, 102 underwent cholecystectomy, and 90 were observed. None of the patients in the surgery group had GBC on pathology review, and none of the observed patients developed GBC during followup (mean 3.5 years). In the surgery group, 82 per cent of the patients were asymptomatic with a perioperative complication rate of 10.7 per cent. Among symptomatic patients, the complication rate was 16.7 per cent. Rate of conversion to open surgery was 5 per cent. Complications led to eight endoscopic or percutaneous interventions and five additional operations. PG is not associated with increased risk of GBC but is associated with high risk of postoperative complications. Cholecystectomy should not be recommended in asymptomatic patients with PG.

► Is porcelain gallbladder by itself an indication for cholecystectomy? Traditionally, this has been the dogma, but evidence over the past decade indicates that the condition may not be as ominous as we once thought. Porcelain gallbladder has been thought to be a risk factor for the development of gallbladder cancer, and these patients have been universally counseled to undergo surgery. This large series of porcelain gallbladders from the Kaiser system suggests that there may not be any risk of cancer. In the patients who underwent cholecystectomy, none had cancer, and those who were followed for an average 3.5 years did not develop cancer. Those patients who had surgery had a 10% complication rate, so this group is recommending that asymptomatic porcelain gallbladders not be removed. The authors recommend an algorithm for the assessment and treatment of these patients (Fig 2 in the original article). Will you change your practice based on this new data set?

O. J. Hines, MD, FACS

Influence of Health Insurance Expansion on Disparities in the Treatment of Acute Cholecystitis

Loehrer AP, Song Z, Auchincloss HG, et al (Massachusetts General Hosp, Boston, MA; et al)
Ann Surg 262:139-145, 2015

Objective.—To evaluate the impact of the 2006 Massachusetts (MA) health reform on disparities in the management of acute cholecystitis (AC).

Background.—Immediate cholecystectomy has been shown to be the optimal treatment for AC, yet variation in care persists depending upon insurance status and patient race. How increased insurance coverage impacts these disparities in surgical care is not known.

Methods.—A cohort study of patients admitted with AC in MA and 3 control states from 2001 through 2009 was performed using the Hospital Cost and Utilization Project State Inpatient Databases. We examined all nonelderly white, black, or Latino patients by insurance type and patient race, evaluating changes in the probability of undergoing immediate cholecystectomy and disparities in receiving immediate cholecystectomy before and after Massachusetts health reform.

Results.—Data from 141,344 patients hospitalized for AC were analyzed. Before the 2006 reform, government-subsidized/self-pay (GS/SP) patients had a 6.6 to 9.9 percentage-point lower ($P < 0.001$) probability of immediate cholecystectomy in both MA control states. The MA insurance expansion was independently associated with a 2.5 percentage-point increased probability of immediate cholecystectomy for all GS/SP patients in MA ($P = 0.049$) and a 5.0 percentage-point increased probability ($P = 0.011$) for nonwhite, GS/SP patients compared to control states. Racial disparities in the probability of immediate cholecystectomy seen before health care reform were no longer statistically significant after reform in MA while persisting in control states.

Conclusions.—The MA health reform was associated with increased probability of undergoing immediate cholecystectomy for AC and reduced disparities in undergoing cholecystectomy by insurance status and patient race (Fig 2).

▶ There is no doubt that as surgeons, we contribute to the disparities in health care often at an unconscious level. There are significant data that patients with insurance have a much higher chance of having emergent/urgent surgery than those who do not. Theoretically, if all patients were insured, this difference should correct. Hutter and colleagues have examined this issue in the state of Massachusetts, which initiated health reform and expanded the insured population in 2006. They found that health reform was associated with increased

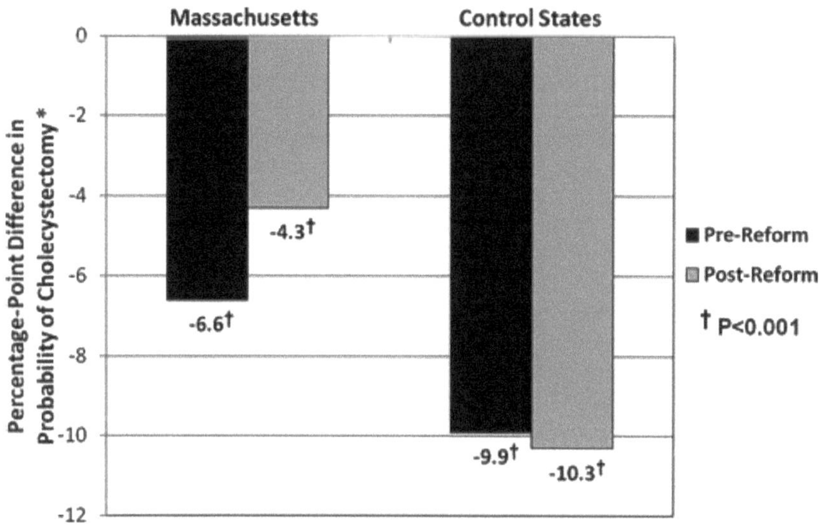

FIGURE 2.—Effect of being GS/SP patient on the probability of receiving immediate cholecystectomy. *Absolute difference in probability of receiving a cholecystectomy between GS/SP and privately insured patients, controlling for patient age, sex, race, comorbidities, hospital type, admission type, and complicated presentation. (Reprinted from Loehrer AP, Song Z, Auchincloss HG, et al. Influence of health insurance expansion on disparities in the treatment of acute cholecystitis. *Ann Surg*. 2015;262:139-145, with permission from Wolters Kluwer Health, Inc.)

probability of undergoing immediate cholecystectomy for acute cholecystitis and reduced disparities in undergoing cholecystectomy by insurance status and patient race (Fig 2). It is clear that early cholecystectomy improves outcomes and decreases hospital cost. When this group looked at the remainder of the country during this time period, disparities increased. These findings suggest that the expansion of insurance, including Medicaid and other government programs, may mitigate disparities in surgical care and serves as a reminder of the role each us play in these issues.

O. J. Hines, MD, FACS

Pain Provocation and Low Gallbladder Ejection Fraction with CCK Cholescintigraphy Are Not Predictive of Chronic Acalculous Gallbladder Disease Symptom Relief After Cholecystectomy

Edwards MA, Mullenbach B, Chamberlain SM (Temple Univ School of Medicine, Philadelphia, PA; Georgia Regents Univ, Augusta)
Dig Dis Sci 59:2773-2778, 2014

Introduction.—Chronic acalculous gallbladder disease (CAGD) falls within the spectrum of diseases associated with gallbladder dysmotility. Cholecystokinin-cholescintigraphy (CCK-CS) has been used to evaluate for CAGD, with a gallbladder ejection fraction (GBEF) of <35 % being indicative of gallbladder dysfunction. The reproduction of biliary colic upon administration of CCK has been cited as indicative of CAGD. Our purpose was to determine whether low GBEF or reproduction of pain during CCK-CS was predictor of surgical outcomes related to resolution of symptoms or as a correlate to gallbladder pathology.

Methods.—A retrospective review of patients was performed to evaluate adults with a diagnosis of CAGD who underwent CCK-CS prior to surgical intervention. CPT and ICD-9 coding queries were used to identify the patient population. Patients with cholelithiasis were excluded.

Results.—Sixty-four patients met inclusion criteria. Two patients were lost to follow-up and were excluded. During CCK-CS, 41 patients (66%) reported symptoms similar to their presenting complaint. Twenty-one patients reported no symptoms with CCK-CS. There was no significant relationship between gallbladder pathology and either GBEF or reproduction of symptoms with CCK-CS ($p = 0.14$). About 81% of patients ($n = 50$) had relief of symptoms following cholecystectomy. Sixty-six percentage of patients ($n = 33$) with long-term symptom relief after cholecystectomy had reproduction of symptoms with CCK-CS. Nineteen percentage of all patients ($n = 12$) had long-term symptom recurrence despite surgery. Eight of these patients (66%) had symptom reproduction with CCK-CS. There was no significant correlation with either the GBEF or symptoms reproduction with CCK-CS as a predictor of postoperative outcome ($p = 0.12$).

Conclusion.—Provocation of pain by CCK-CS and low GBEF are unreliable predictors of postoperative relief of symptoms following cholecystectomy for biliary dyskinesia or chronic acalculous gallbladder disease (Table 3).

▶ It is not uncommon to be faced with a patient who has symptoms suggestive of biliary colic but no evidence of abnormalities on a right upper quadrant ultrasound. These patients may have sludge in the gallbladder that is not identified by ultrasound, acalculous gallbladder disease, or other gastrointestinal conditions responsible for their symptoms. We are then faced with the question of whether a cholecystectomy will address the symptoms. Many have used cholescintigraphy to help guide the decision. An ejection fraction less than 35% suggests gallbladder pathology, and this test can be combined with an injection

TABLE 3.—Long-term (>30 Days After Surgery) CCK-CS Postoperative Symptom Outcomes

	CCK-CS Symptom Provocation	
Long-term Postoperative Symptoms	Positive	Negative
Recurrent symptoms	8 (20 %)	4 (19 %)
Resolved symptoms	33 (80 %)	17 (81 %)

Reprinted from Edwards MA, Mullenbach B, Chamberlain SM. Pain provocation and low gallbladder ejection fraction with CCK cholescintigraphy are not predictive of chronic acalculous gallbladder disease symptom relief after cholecystectomy. *Dig Dis Sci.* 2014;59:2773-2778, with permission from Springer Science+Business Media New York.

of cholecystokinin to see whether this recapitulates the pain and symptoms. This study found that the provocation of pain by cholecystokinin and low ejection fraction were not reliable predictors of pain relief after operation. The good news was that about 80% of the patients had relief of their symptoms after cholecystectomy. The bad news was that pain provocation with cholecystokinin was equally positive or negative between patients who did or did not report relief of symptoms after surgery (Table 3). In the end, we are left with our clinical judgment on whether to recommend cholecystectomy for this challenging group of patients.

O. J. Hines, MD, FACS

Can Laparoscopic Cholecystectomy Prevent Recurrent Idiopathic Acute Pancreatitis? A Prospective Randomized Multicenter Trial

Räty S, Pulkkinen J, Nordback I, et al (Tampere Univ Hosp, Finland; Kuopio Univ Hosp, Finland; et al)

Ann Surg 262:736-741, 2015

Objective.—The aim of the present trial was to ascertain whether laparoscopic cholecystectomy (LCC) can prevent recurrent attacks of idiopathic acute pancreatitis (IAP).

Summary.—Up to 50% to 75% of IAP may be due to microlithiasis, which is undetectable by conventional imaging methods.

Methods.—This randomized, prospective trial included 85 patients (39 in the LCC and 46 in the control group) in 8 hospitals in Finland. We included adult patients (over 18 years) with their first attack of IAP. The diagnosis of IAP was based on the exclusion of common etiological reasons for acute pancreatitis (AP), whereafter the patients were randomized into conservative watchful waiting (controls) or LCC group. The primary end point was the number of patients with recurrent AP during the follow-up. All recurrent attacks of AP after an initial IAP episode were registered.

Results.—During a median follow-up of 36 (5–58) months, the recurrence of IAP was significantly higher in the control group than in LCC group (14/46 vs. 4/39, $P = 0.016$), as was also the number of recurrences (23/46 vs. 8/39, $P = 0.003$). In the subgroup of patients with at least 24 months' follow-up, the recurrence was still higher among controls (14/37 vs. 4/35, $P = 0.008$). In patients with normal liver function, recurrence was also significantly higher in the control than in the LCC group (13/46 vs. 4/39, $P = 0.026$). During surgery, 23/39 (59%) of the gallbladders were found to contain biliary stones or sludge.

Conclusions.—LCC can effectively prevent the recurrence of IAP when all other possible etiologies of pancreatitis are carefully excluded. A total of 5 patients needed to be treated (NNT-value) to prevent 1 IAP.

▶ The cause of acute pancreatitis is never found in as many as 30% of patients. Patients with idiopathic pancreatitis are subject to recurrence and some have advocated the use of cholecystectomy to prevent recurrence, assuming that small stones, sludge, or crystals are responsible for the attacks. This randomized trial attempts to evaluate the efficacy of laparoscopic cholecystectomy for this group of patients. The study found that cholecystectomy was effective at preventing recurrence decreasing the incidence of recurrence by 84% along with the number of recurrences. Interestingly, 59% of the gallbladders removed were found to have stones or sludge, even though 2 preoperative ultrasounds showed no evidence of this. Overall, it took 5 cholecystectomies to prevent 1 episode of recurrent idiopathic pancreatitis. Endoscopic ultrasound is probably more effective at identify gallstones than transabdominal ultrasound, but laparoscopic cholecystectomy seems a viable solution for patients with recurrent idiopathic pancreatitis. However, a clear conversation outlining the utility of this approach should be made with the patient before embarking on this path.

O. J. Hines, MD, FACS

PREOP-Gallstones: A Prognostic Nomogram for the Management of Symptomatic Cholelithiasis in Older Patients

Parmar AD, Sheffield KM, Adhikari D, et al (Univ of Texas Med Branch, Galveston; et al)

Ann Surg 261:1184-1190, 2015

Objective and Background.—The decision regarding elective cholecystectomy in older patients with symptomatic cholelithiasis is complicated. We developed and validated a prognostic nomogram to guide shared decision making for these patients.

Methods.—We used Medicare claims (1996–2005) to identify the first episode of symptomatic cholelithiasis in patients older than 65 years who did not undergo hospitalization or elective cholecystectomy within 2.5 months of the episode. We described current patterns of care and modeled their risk of emergent gallstone-related hospitalization or cholecystectomy at 2 years. Model discrimination and calibration were assessed using a random split sample of patients.

Results.—We identified 92,436 patients who presented to the emergency department (8.3%) or physician's office (91.7%) and who were not immediately admitted. The diagnosis for the initial episode was biliary colic/dyskinesia (65.3%), acute cholecystitis (26.6%), choledocholithiasis (5.7%), or gallstone pancreatitis (2.4%). The 2-year emergent gallstone-related hospitalization rate was 11.1%, with associated in-hospital morbidity andmortality rates of 56.5% and 6.5%. Factors associated with gallstone-related acute hospitalization included male sex, increased age, fewer comorbid conditions, complicated biliary disease on initial presentation, and initial presentation to the emergency department. Our model was well calibrated and identified 51% of patients with a risk less than 10% for 2-year complications and 5.4% with a risk more than 40% (C statistic, 0.69; 95% confidence interval, 0.63–0.75).

Conclusions.—Surgeons can use this prognostic nomogram to accurately provide patients with their 2-year risk of developing

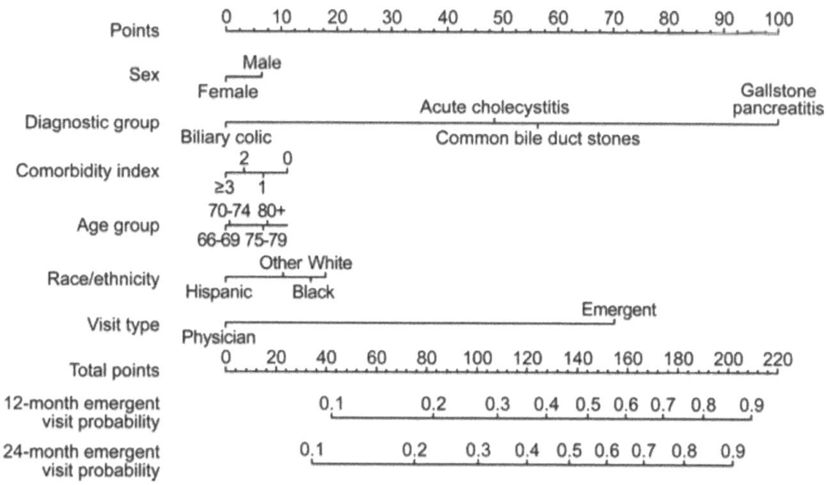

FIGURE 4.—"Predicting risk of complications in older patients with gallstones," PREOP-Gallstones model nomogram. To use the nomogram, a vertical line is drawn from each factor to the corresponding position on the "Points" line. Once the points are tabulated for each factor, the points are then added. A line is drawn from this position on the "Points" line to the "Emergent visit probability" lines to determine a patient's 12-month and 24-month risk for developing emergent gallstone-related complications. HMO indicates Health Maintenance Organization; BC, biliary colic; AC, acute cholecystitis; GP, gallstone pancreatitis; CBDS, common bile duct stones. (Reprinted from Parmar AD, Sheffield KM, Adhikari D, et al. PREOP-gallstones: a prognostic nomogram for the management of symptomatic cholelithiasis in older patients. *Ann Surg*. 2015;261:1184-1190, with permission from Wolters Kluwer Health, Inc.)

gallstone-related complications, allowing patients and physicians to make informed decisions in the context of their symptom severity and its impact on their quality of life (Fig 4).

▶ A Cochrane review indicated that early cholecystectomy for symptomatic cholelithiasis is associated with decreased risk for conversion to open operation, decreased operative time, and decreased length of stay in the hospital when compared with delayed intervention.[1] The decision for cholecystectomy is based on sonographic findings, symptoms, and laboratory values. Often the path is clear, but in older patients, the decision to operate is complicated by the patient's age and other medical conditions. At the same time, older patients are more likely to have complications of gallstone disease. This group has developed a nomogram to help inform this decision by predicting the risk of complications based on symptoms, gender, comorbidity index, age, race, and visit type whether emergent or scheduled (Fig 4). This model is able to predict the risk for complications and therefore allows for a more informed decision for this patient population. They suggest that those with a risk of more than 40% should undergo elective cholecystectomy. This nomogram will help to decrease the morbidity of emergent care and operation while reducing the number of unnecessary cholecystectomies in these patients.

O. J. Hines, MD, FACS

Reference

1. Gurusamy KS, Samraj K, Fusai G, Davidson BR. Early versus delayed laparoscopic cholecystectomy for biliary colic. *Cochrane Database Syst Rev.* 2008;(4): CD007196.

Presentation and Clinical Outcomes of Choledochal Cysts in Children and Adults: A Multi-institutional Analysis

Soares KC, Kim Y, Spolverato G, et al (Johns Hopkins Univ, Baltimore, MD; et al)

JAMA Surg 150:577-584, 2015

Importance.—Choledochal cysts (CCs) are rare, with risk of infection and cancer.

Objective.—To characterize the natural history, management, and long-term implications of CC disease.

Design, Setting, and Participants.—A total of 394 patients who underwent resection of a CC between January 1, 1972, and April 11, 2014, were identified from an international multi-institutional database. Patients were followed up through September 27, 2014. Clinicopathologic characteristics, operative details, and outcome data were analyzed from May 1, 2014, to October 14, 2014.

Intervention.—Resection of CC.

Main Outcomes and Measures.—Management, morbidity, and overall survival.

Results.—Among 394 patients, there were 135 children (34.3%) and 318 women (80.7%). Adults were more likely to present with abdominal pain (71.8% vs 40.7%; $P < .001$) and children were more likely to have jaundice (31.9% vs 11.6%; $P < .001$). Preoperative interventions were more commonly performed in adults (64.5% vs 31.1%; $P < .001$), including endoscopic retrograde pancreatography (55.6% vs 27.4%; $P < .001$), percutaneous transhepatic cholangiography (17.4% vs 5.9%; $P < .001$), and endobiliary stenting (18.1% vs 4.4%; $P < .001$). Type I CCs were more often seen in children vs adults (79.7% vs 64.9%; $P = .003$); type IV CCs predominated in the adult population (23.9% vs 12.0%; $P = .006$). Extrahepatic bile duct resection with hepaticoenterostomy was the most frequently performed procedure in both age groups (80.3%). Perioperative morbidity was higher in adults (35.1% vs 16.3%; $P < .001$). On pathologic examination, 10 patients (2.5%) had cholangiocarcinoma. After a median follow-up of 28 months, 5-year overall survival was 95.5%. On follow-up, 13 patients (3.3%), presented with biliary cancer.

Conclusions and Relevance.—Presentation of CC varied between children and adults, and resection was associated with a degree of morbidity. Although concomitant cancer was uncommon, it occurred in 3.0% of the patients. Long-term surveillance is indicated given the possibility of future development of biliary cancer after CC resection.

▶ The goal of choledochal cyst excision is largely to address the risk for the development of cholangiocarcinoma. Some patients will present with pain or biliary obstruction, however. It is helpful to review the types of choledochal cysts because this informs the planning for the operation. This article reviewed 394 cases from 8 institutions and found that 7 patients had cholangiocarcinoma at the time of operation, and some patients developed cancer later after excision. Most commonly an excision of the extrahepatic bile duct along with a roux-en-Y hepaticojejunostomy was performed. The morbidity from these operations is relatively high (35%) and largely included issues with the hepaticojejunostomy. Sometimes patients will present with this diagnosis and as a child have undergone some type of bypass procedure, usually a side-to-side enterobiliary anastomosis. These patients should undergo operation for formal resection to mitigate the cancer risk. This article enforces the tenant that type 1, 2, and 4 choledochal cysts require excision and lifelong follow-up.

O. J. Hines, MD, FACS

Cost Efficacy of Metal Stents for Palliation of Extrahepatic Bile Duct Obstruction in a Randomized Controlled Trial

Walter D, van Boeckel PGA, Groenen MJ, et al (Univ Med Ctr Utrecht, The Netherlands; Rijnstate Hosp, Arnhem, The Netherlands; et al)

Gastroenterology 149:130-138, 2015

Background & Aims.—Endoscopic stents are placed for palliation of extrahepatic bile duct obstruction. Although selfexpandable metal stents (SEMS) remain patent longer than plastic stents, they are more expensive. We aimed to evaluate which type of stent (plastic, uncovered SEMS [uSEMS], or partially covered SEMS [pcSEMS]) is the most effective and we assessed costs.

Methods.—We performed a multicenter randomized trial in 219 patients at 18 hospitals in The Netherlands from February 2008 through February 2013. Patients were assigned randomly for placement of a plastic stent (n = 73), uSEMS (n = 75), or pcSEMS (n = 71) during endoscopic retrograde cholangiopancreatography. Patients were followed up for up to 1 year. Researchers were not blinded to groups. The main study end points included functional stent time and costs.

Results.—The mean functional stent times were 172 days for plastic stents, 288 days for uSEMS, and 299 days for pcSEMS ($P < .005$ for uSEMS and pcSEMS vs plastic). The initial placement of plastic stents (V1042 or $1106) cost significantly less than placement of SEMS (1973 or $2094) ($P = .001$). However, the total cost per patient at the end of the follow-up period did not differ significantly between plastic stents (7320 or $7770) and SEMS (6932 or $7356) ($P = .61$). Furthermore, in

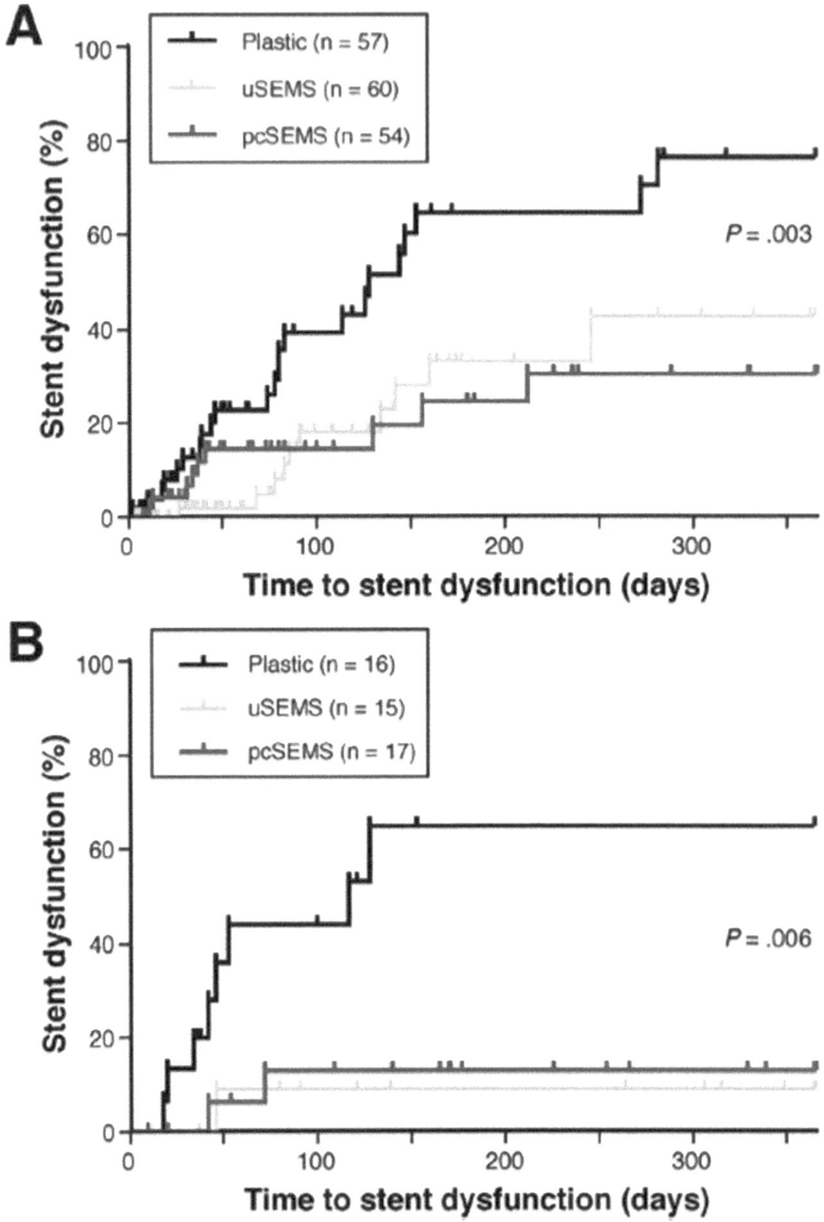

FIGURE 3.—Functional stent time after stent placement for palliation of malignant extrahepatic bile duct obstruction using the Kaplan–Meier method for (*A*) patients with primary stent placement and (*B*) patients with a second stent. (Reprinted from Walter D, van Boeckel PGA, Groenen MJ, et al. Cost efficacy of metal stents for palliation of extrahepatic bile duct obstruction in a randomized controlled trial. *Gastroenterology.* 2015;149:130-138, with permission from AGA Institute.)

patients with short survival times (≤3 mo) or metastatic disease, the total cost per patient did not differ between plastic stents and SEMS. No differences in costs were found between pcSEMS and uSEMS.

Conclusions.—Although placement of SEMS (uncovered or partially covered) for palliation of extrahepatic bile duct obstruction initially is more expensive than placement of plastic stents, SEMS have longer functional time. The total costs after 1 year do not differ significantly with stent type. Dutch Clinical Trial Registration no: NTR1361 (Fig 3).

▶ Biliary obstruction is a common complication of periampullary cancers. Most periampullary cancers are not resectable because of locally advanced or metastatic disease. Endoscopic retrograde cholangiopancreatography and stent placement has largely supplanted operative biliary drainage for many patients with this condition. This randomized study examined the efficacy and costs of using plastic or metal expandable stents. Metal stents are significantly more expensive, and many have argued that because this patient population has a relatively short life expectancy that the plastic stents should be preferred. However, it appears from this work that given the much shorter patency rates of plastic stents and the other costs associated with stent placement, metal stents are more effective and the overall costs equal. The metal stents offered about 100 additional functional days over the plastic stents, and in this patient population, this is meaningful and allows the need for a replacement stent (Fig 3). The group also examined covered metal stents, which offer the potential to protect against tumor ingrowth and reobstruction. The covered stents offered no advantage over the uncovered stents.

O. J. Hines, MD, FACS

A US Multicenter Study of Safety and Efficacy of Fully Covered Self-Expandable Metallic Stents in Benign Extrahepatic Biliary Strictures

Saxena P, Diehl DL, Kumbhari V, et al (The Johns Hopkins Med Institutions, Baltimore, MD; Geisinger Health System, Danville, PA; et al)
Dig Dis Sci 60:3442-3448, 2015

Background.—Endoscopic therapy is considered first line for management of benign biliary strictures (BBSs). Placement of plastic stents has been effective but limited by their short-term patency and need for repeated procedures. Fully covered self-expandable metallic stents (FCSEMSs) offer longer-lasting biliary drainage without the need for frequent exchanges.

Aims.—The aim of this study was to assess the efficacy and safety of FCSEMS in patients with BBS.

Methods.—A retrospective review of all patients who underwent ERCP and FCSEMS placement at five tertiary referral US hospitals was performed. Stricture resolution and adverse events related to ERCP and/or stenting were recorded.

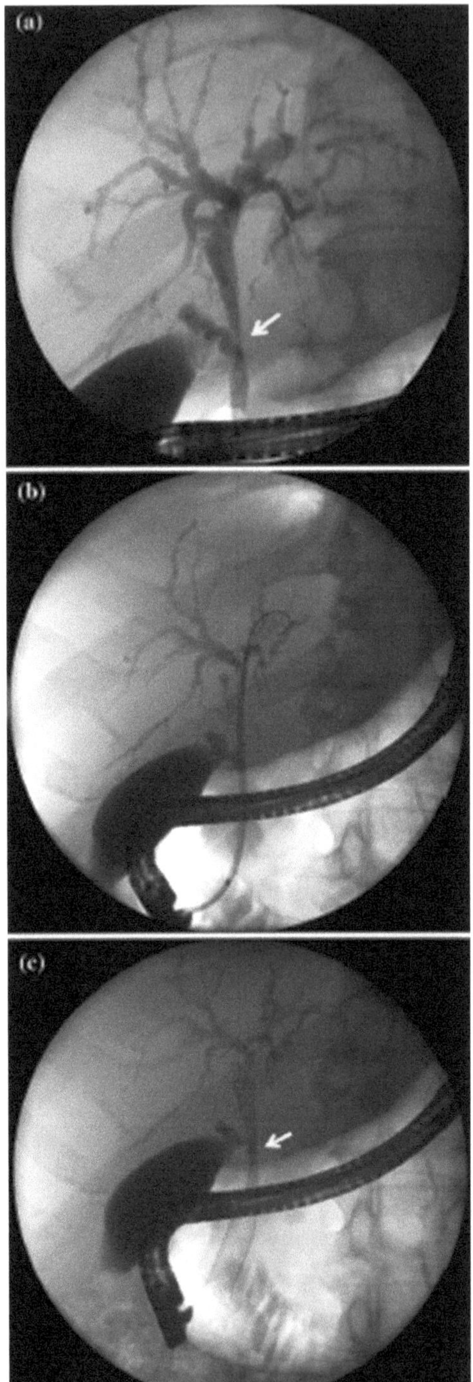

FIGURE 1.—**a** Benign mid-CBD stricture (*yellow arrow*) in a 52-year-old patient with PSC. **b** A wire is advanced through the stricture, and a FCSEMS is advanced over the wire across the stricture. **c** A waist is seen in the center of the stent at the region of the stricture (*yellow arrow*) after deployment. For interpretation of the references to color in this figure legend, the reader is referred to web version of this article. (Reprinted from Saxena P, Diehl DL, Kumbhari V, et al. A US Multicenter Study of Safety and Efficacy of fully covered self-expandable metallic stents in benign extrahepatic biliary strictures. *Dig Dis Sci.* 2015;60:3442-3448, with permission from Springer Science+Business Media New York.)

Results.—A total of 123 patients underwent FCSEMS placement for BBS and 112 underwent a subsequent followup ERCP. The mean age was 62 years (±15.6), and 57% were males. Stricture resolution occurred in 81% of patients after a mean of 1.2 stenting procedures (mean stent dwell time 24.4 ± 2.3 weeks), with a mean follow-up of 18.5 months. Stricture recurrence occurred in 5 patients, and 3 patients required surgery for treatment of refractory strictures. Stent migration (9.7%) was the most common complication, followed by stent occlusion (4.9%), cholangitis (4.1%), and pancreatitis (3.3%). There was one case of stent fracture during removal, and one stent could not be removed. There was one death due to cholangitis.

Conclusions.—Majority of BBS can be successfully managed with 1–2 consecutive FCSEMS with stent dwell time of 6 months (Fig 1).

▶ The management of biliary strictures is largely accomplished with the use of endoscopically placed stents and requires a determination of whether the stricture is benign or malignant. For benign strictures caused by conditions such as primary sclerosing cholangitis, chronic pancreatitis, and stone disease stenting has been very effective. This group investigated the use of metal stents to address these strictures (Fig 1). Stricture resolution was determined by the presence or at least the absence of a waist on cholangiogram, reduction of proximal duct size and improvement of liver function tests, the ability to pass a retrieval balloon through the stricture, or drainage of contrast injected proximal to the stricture. The sustained stricture resolution occurred in 81% of patients, and of these 80% had success after single stent placement; the remaining 20% of patients had success after 2 stents were placed. Most of these stents were in place for 6 to 9 months. These results are impressive. In the entire cohort, only 3 patients required surgery to address the stricture.

O. J. Hines, MD, FACS

A Comparative Study of Laparoscopic vs Open Distal Pancreatectomy for Left-Sided Ductal Adenocarcinoma: A Propensity Score-Matched Analysis

Shin SH, Kim SC, Song KB, et al (Univ of Ulsan College of Medicine, Seoul, South Korea)

J Am Coll Surg 220:177-185, 2015

Background.—Although laparoscopic surgery has many advantages, its application in pancreatic ductal adenocarcinoma has not been sufficiently studied. The objective of this study was to compare the surgical outcomes of laparoscopic distal pancreatectomy (LDP) to those of open distal pancreatectomy (ODP) for left-sided ductal adenocarcinoma.

Study Design.—Among 167 consecutive patients between December 2006 and August 2013, 150 patients were included. Unmatched and propensity score-matched analyses were performed to compare the primary (oncologic adequacy) and secondary outcomes (hospital course and complications) between ODP and LDP groups.

Results.—In unmatched patients, LDP was associated with an earlier return to diet and a shorter hospital stay compared with ODP. The 5-year survival rates were 27.6% in unmatched ODP (n = 80) and 32.5% in unmatched LDP (n = 70). Fifty-one patients from each group were selected by propensity score matching. In this matched patient comparison, LDP was again associated significantly with a shorter median postoperative time to restarting diet and a shorter hospital stay. The 2 groups did not differ significantly in terms of primary outcomes of operative time, number of harvested lymph nodes, resection margin status, and secondary

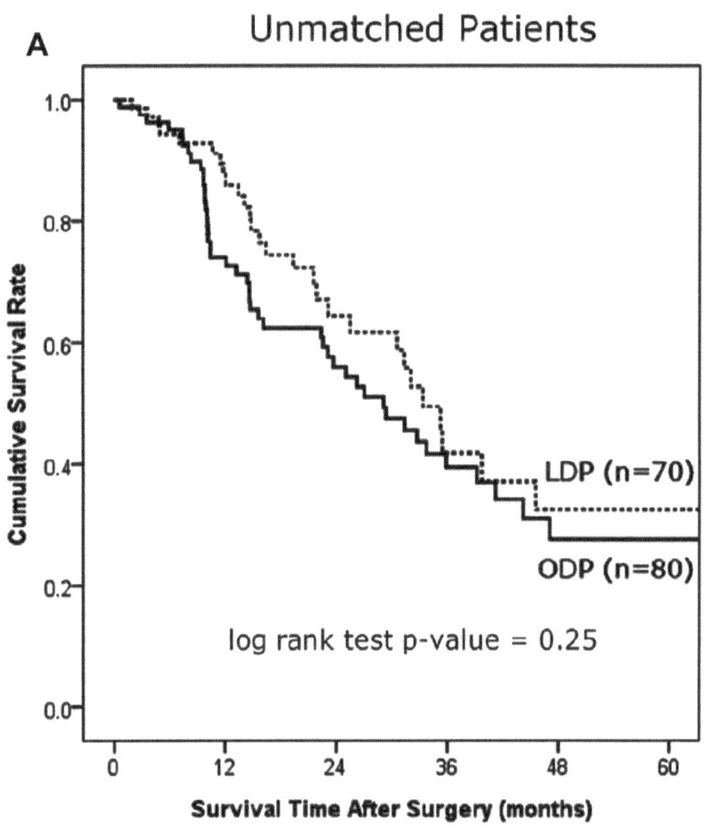

FIGURE 1.—(A) Kaplan-Meier survival curves for survival after surgery for unmatched patients who underwent open distal pancreatectomy (ODP) (n = 80) or laparoscopic distal pancreatectomy (LDP) (n = 70) (p = 0.25). In the ODP group, the median survival was 29.1 months, and estimated 1-, 2-, and 5-year survival rates were 74.0%, 55.9%, and 27.6%, respectively. In the LDP group, the median survival was 33.4 months, and estimated 1-, 2-, and 5-year survival rates were 87.6%, 64.3%, and 32.5%, respectively. (Reprinted from Shin SH, Kim SC, Song KB, et al. A comparative study of laparoscopic vs open distal pancreatectomy for left-sided ductal adenocarcinoma: a propensity score-matched analysis. *J Am Coll Surg*. 2015;220:177-185, with permission from American College of Surgeons.)

outcomes of frequency of pancreatic fistula and complications. The 2 groups also had comparable patient survival ($p = 0.91$).

Conclusions.—This large single-center study of laparoscopic surgery for left-sided pancreatic ductal adenocarcinoma indicated that LDP was safe and more efficacious than OPD after propensity score adjustment for presurgical variables of return to diet and length of stay (Fig 1A).

▶ Pancreatic cancer is a difficult disease to beat, but some progress is being made in the field of chemotherapeutics. Some 10% to 15% of patients will have local disease at the time of diagnosis and are candidates for surgical resection. This study examined their results of open versus laparoscopic distal pancreatectomy for this disease. It is unlikely randomized data like that of colon and rectal cancer evaluating the utility of laparoscopic surgery will ever be available because distal pancreatectomies performed frequently enough for this condition. The results of this study suggest that a laparoscopic approach offers equally good results with regard to morbidity, nodal harvest, and oncologic outcome (Fig 1A). These procedures are not easy and should only be incorporated into your practice if you have extensive experience with the procedure and superb laparoscopic skills. It was curious that this group did not describe a splenectomy as part of this procedure because most would suggest that this be included to provide an adequate lymphadenectomy to properly stage the patient.

O. J. Hines, MD, FACS

Trends in Emergent Hernia Repair in the United States

Beadles CA, Meagher AD, Charles AG (Dept of Veterans Affairs Med Ctr, Durham, NC; Univ of North Carolina at Chapel Hill; et al)

JAMA Surg 150:194-200, 2015

Importance.—Abdominal wall hernia is one of the most common conditions encountered by general surgeons. Rising rates of abdominal wall hernia repair have been described; however, population-based evidence concerning incidence rates of emergent hernia repair and changes with time are unknown.

Objective.—To examine trends in rates of emergent abdominal hernia repair within the United States for inguinal, femoral, ventral, and umbilical hernias from January 1, 2001, to December 31, 2010.

Design, Setting, and Participants.—A retrospective analysis of adults with emergent hernia repair using National Center for Health Statistics data, a nationally representative sample of inpatient hospitalizations in the United States that occurred from January 1, 2001, to December 31, 2010. All emergent hernia repairs were identified during the study period.

Main Outcomes and Measures.—Incidence rates per 100 000 person-years, age, and sex adjusted to the 2010 US census population estimates were calculated for selected subcategories of emergent hernia repairs and time trends were evaluated.

Results.—An estimated 2.3 million inpatient abdominal hernia repairs were performed from 2001 to 2010; of which an estimated 567 000 were performed emergently. A general increase in the rate of total emergent hernias was observed from 16.0 to 19.2 emergent hernia repairs per 100 000 person-years in 2001 and 2010, respectively. In 2010, emergent hernia rates were highest among adults 65 years and older, with 71.3 and 42.0 emergent hernia repairs per 100 000 person-years for men and women, respectively. As expected, femoral hernia rates were higher among women while emergent inguinal hernia rates were higher among men. Rates of emergent incisional hernia repair were high but relatively stable among older women, with 24.9 and 23.5 per 100 000 person-years in 2001 and 2010, respectively. However, rates of emergent incisional hernia repair among older men rose significantly, with 7.8 to 32.0 per 100 000 person-years from 2001 to 2010, respectively.

Conclusions and Relevance.—These increasing rates of emergent incisional hernia repair are troublesome owing to the significantly increased risk morbidity and mortality associated with emergent hernia repair. While this increased mortality risk is multifactorial, it is likely associated with older age and the accompanying serious comorbidities.

▶ Hernias are a common problem for most surgeons, even for the gastrointestinal surgeon. This is because the most common indication for an emergency hernia repair is an intestinal incarceration. This study examined the data from 2001 to 2010 of the National Center for Health Statistics and included 2.3 million hernia repairs. Did you know that 1 in 4 men in the United States will require an inguinal hernia operation and that the incidence of incisional hernia from abdominal operations is 25%? Over the study period, emergency hernia repairs became more common (Fig 3 in the original article), and this trend was particularly isolated to the elderly population. This is a worrisome finding because it is exactly this group that is most likely to have a complication of surgery. No matter what type of specialist you may be, almost all of us who had training in general surgery face these issues. Maximizing outcomes with proper technique, mesh utilization, and patient management is critical to this even "mundane" type of surgery.

O. J. Hines, MD, FACS

Prospective, Randomized Study on the Use of a Prosthetic Mesh for Prevention of Parastomal Hernia of Permanent Colostomy

Vierimaa M, Klintrup K, Biancari F, et al (Oulu Univ Hosp, Oulu, Finland; et al)
Dis Colon Rectum 58:943-949, 2015

Background.—Prophylactic placement of a mesh has been suggested to prevent parastomal hernia, but evidence to support this approach is scarce.

Objective.—The aim of this study was to evaluate whether laparoscopic placement of a prophylactic, dual-component, intraperitoneal onlay mesh around a colostomy is safe and prevents parastomal hernia formation after laparoscopic abdominoperineal resection.

Design.—This is a prospective, multicenter, randomized controlled clinical trial.

Settings.—This study was conducted at 2 university and 3 central Finnish hospitals.

Patients.—From 2010 to 2013, 83 patients undergoing laparoscopic abdominoperineal resection for rectal cancer were recruited. After withdrawals and exclusions, the outcome of 70 patients, 35 patients in each study group, could be examined.

Interventions.—In the intervention group, an end colostomy was created with placement of a intraperitoneal, dual-component onlay mesh and compared with a group with a traditional stoma.

Main Outcome Measures.—The main outcome measures were the incidence of clinically and radiologically detected parastomal hernias and their extent 12 months after surgery. Stoma-related morbidity and the need for surgical repair of parastomal hernia were secondary outcome measures.

Results.—Parastomal hernia was observed by clinical inspection in 5 intervention patients (14.3%) and in 12 control patients (32.3%; p = 0.049). Surgical repair of parastomal hernia was performed in 1 control patient (3.2%) and in none of the patients in the intervention group. CT detected parastomal hernia in 18 intervention patients (51.4%) and in 17 control patients (53.1%; p = 1.00). The extent of hernias was similar according to European Hernia Society classification (p = 0.41). Colostomy-related morbidity (32.3% vs 14.3%; p = 0.140) did not differ between the study groups.

Limitations.—The study was limited by its small size and short follow-up time.

Conclusions.—Prophylactic laparoscopic placement of intraperitoneal onlay mesh does not significantly reduce the overall risk of radiologically detected parastomal hernia after laparoscopic abdominoperineal resection. However, prophylactic mesh repair was associated with significantly lower risk of clinically detected parastomal hernia.

► Parastomal hernias can lead to difficulty in pouch a stoma, pain from the pressure, and, rarely, acute bowel obstruction requiring emergency operation. There has been significant effort to address this problem with prophylactic placement of parastomal mesh, which is a mesh specifically fashioned to be used around a stoma, and some who always advocate for resiting the stoma. This study randomized patients undergoing a laparoscopic abdominoperineal resection to a customary stoma or a stoma with an intraperitoneal dual component onlay mesh. Utilizing clinical evaluation, it seemed that the prophylactic mesh significantly reduced the number of parastomal hernias, but the imaging data showed an equal number of hernias between the 2 groups. The group concluded that placing mesh at the time of a stoma creation was safe and that at least clinically this seemed to decrease hernia rates. Clearly there is still a need in this area, and I have found that your best friend is a well-trained stoma nurse who can offer creative solutions with hernia belts and different stoma appliances. Failing this, sometimes it is necessary to electively repair these hernias.

O. J. Hines, MD, FACS

Association of Postoperative Hyperglycemia With Outcomes Among Patients With Complex Ventral Hernia Repair

Won EJ, Lehman EB, Geletzke AK, et al (Milton S. Hershey Med Ctr, PA; et al)

JAMA Surg 150:433-440, 2015

Importance.—Patients with medically complex conditions undergoing repair of large or recurrent hernia of the abdominal wall are at risk for early postoperative hyperglycemia, which may serve as an early warning for delays in recovery and for adverse outcomes.

Objective.—To evaluate postoperative serum glucose level as a predictor of outcome after open ventral hernia repair in patients with major medical comorbidities.

Design, Setting, and Participants.—We performed a retrospective medical record review of 172 consecutive patients who underwent open ventral hernia repair at Penn State Milton S. Hershey Medical Center, an academic tertiary referral center, from May 1, 2011, through November 30, 2013.We initially identified patients by medical complexity and repair requiring a length of stay of longer than 1 day.

Main Outcomes and Measures.—Postoperative recovery variables, including time to the first solid meal, length of stay, total costs of hospitalization, and surgical site occurrence.

Results.—Postoperative serum glucose values were available for 136 patients (79.1%), with 130 (95.6%) obtained within 48 hours of surgery. Among these patients, Ventral Hernia Working Group grade distributions included 8 patients with grade 1, 79 with grade 2, 41 with grade 3, and 8 with grade 4. Fifty-four patients (39.7%) had a postoperative glucose level of at least 140 mg/dL, and 69 patients (50.7%) required insulin administration. Both outcomes were associated with delays in the interval to the first solid meal (glucose level, ≥140 vs <140 mg/dL: mean [SD] delay, 6.4 [5.3] vs 5.6 [8.2] days; $P = .01$; ≥2 insulin events vs <2: 6.5 [5.5] vs 5.4 [8.4] days; $P = .02$); increased length of stay (glucose level, ≥140 vs <140 mg/dL: mean [SD], 8.0 [6.0] vs 6.9 [8.2] days; $P = .008$; ≥2 insulin events vs <2: 8.3 [6.1] vs 6.5 [8.4] days; $P < .001$); increased costs of hospitalization (glucose level, ≥140 vs <140 mg/dL: mean [SD], $31 307 [$20 875] vs $22 508 [$22 531]; $P < .001$; ≥2 insulin events vs <2: $31 943 [$22 224] vs $20 651 [$20 917]; $P < .001$); and possibly increased likelihood of surgical site occurrence (glucose level, ≥140 vs <140 mg/dL: 37.5% [21 of 56 patients] vs 22.5% [18 of 80 patients]; $P = .06$; ≥2 insulin events vs <2: 36.4%[24 of 66 patients] vs 21.4% [15 of 70 patients]; $P = .06$). Not all patients with diabetes mellitus developed postoperative hyperglycemia or needed more intense insulin therapy; however, 46.4% of the patients who developed postoperative hyperglycemia were not previously known to have diabetes mellitus, although most had at least 1 clinical risk factor for a prediabetic condition.

Conclusions and Relevance.—Postoperative hyperglycemia was associated with outcomes in patients in this study who underwent complex ventral hernia repair and may serve as a suitable target for screening, benchmarking, and intervention in patient groups with major comorbidities.

▶ The outcomes from complex ventral hernia repair remain mixed with relative high rates of recurrence and local complications of infection and, in the worst-case scenario, intestinal fistula. This study examined the influence of hyperglycemia on these occurrences and found some compelling results. If a patient had a glucose ≥140 mg/dL, there was a delay in time to eating, time to discharge, hospital cost, and wound complication (Fig 1A in the original article). In fact, patients had a day longer until a regular diet and length of stay. The wound complication rate in the normoglycemic group was 22.5% and in the hyperglycemic group 37.5%. These are significant findings and should alert you to those patients that need closer medical management postoperatively or are more likely to have a wound infection, seroma, hematoma, nonhealing wound, or hernia recurrence. Whether intervention with tighter glucose control in the perioperative period influences these outcomes is still unknown, however.

O. J. Hines, MD, FACS

Long-term Metabolic Effects of Laparoscopic Sleeve Gastrectomy

Golomb I, Ben David M, Glass A, et al (Beilinson Hosp, Petah Tikva, Israel)

JAMA Surg 150:1051-1057, 2015

Importance.—The prevalence of laparoscopic sleeve gastrectomy (LSG) is increasing, but data on its long-term effect on obesity-related comorbidities are scarce. Because the population of bariatric patients is young, long-term results of those comorbidities are highly relevant.

Objective.—To investigate the long-term effects of LSG on weight loss, diabetes mellitus, hypertension, dyslipidemia, and hyperuricemia.

Design, Setting, and Participants.—Cohort study using a retrospective analysis of a prospective cohort at a university hospital. Data were collected from all patients undergoing LSGs performed by the same team between April 1, 2006, and February 28, 2013, including demographic details, weight follow-up, blood test results, and information on medications and comorbidities.

Main Outcomes and Measures.—Excess weight loss, obesity-related comorbidities, and partial and complete remission at 1, 3, and 5 years of follow-up.

Results.—A total of 443 LSGs were performed. Complete data were available for 241 of the 443 patients (54.4%) at the 1-year follow-up, for 128 of 259 patients (49.4%) at the 3-year follow-up, and for 39 of 56 patients (69.6%) at the 5-year follow-up. The percentage of excess weight loss was 76.8%, 69.7%, and 56.1%, respectively. Complete remission of diabetes was maintained in 50.7%, 38.2%, and 20.0%, respectively, and remission of hypertension was maintained in 46.3%, 48.0%, and 45.5%, respectively. Changes in high-density lipoprotein cholesterol level (mean [SD] level preoperatively and at 1, 3, and 5 years, 46.7 [15.8], 52.8 [13.6], 56.8 [16.0], and 52.4 [13.8] mg/dL, respectively) and triglyceride level (mean [SD] level preoperatively and at 1, 3, and 5 years, 155.2 [86.1], 106.3 [45.3], 107.2 [53.4], and 126.4 [59.7] mg/dL, respectively) were significant compared with preoperative and postoperative measurements ($P < .001$). The decrease of low-density lipoprotein cholesterol level was significant only at 1 year ($P = .04$) and 3 years ($P = .04$) (mean [SD] level preoperatively and at 1, 3, and 5 years, 115.8 [33.2], 110.8 [32.0], 105.7 [25.9], and 110.6 [28.3] mg/dL, respectively). The changes in total cholesterol level did not reach statistical significance (mean [SD] level preoperatively and at 1, 3, and 5 years, 189.5 [38.2], 184.0 [35.4], 183.4 [31.2], and 188.1 [35.7] mg/dL, respectively). No changes in comorbidity status correlated with preoperative excess weight. Hypertriglyceridemia was the only comorbidity whose remission rates at 1 year of follow-up (partial/complete, 80.6%; complete, 72.2%) correlated with percentage of excess weight loss (76.8%) ($P = .005$).

Conclusions and Relevance.—Undergoing LSG induced efficient weight loss and a major improvement in obesity-related comorbidities, with mostly no correlation to percentage of excess weight loss. There was a significant weight regain and a decrease in remission rates of diabetes and, to a lesser extent, other comorbidities over time.

▶ Over the past 3 to 5 years, there has been a large shift to sleeve gastrectomy from roux-en-Y gastric bypass. The longer term outcomes from sleeve gastrectomy have not been fully understood, but this study sheds some light on this. The group followed more than 400 patients and found that excess weight loss was excellent at 1 year (78%) but soon trailed off at 5 years to 56%. Even though the weight was regained in some the group noted that resolution of metabolic syndrome conditions was maintained (Table 2 in the original article). Diabetes and changes in lipid panels were relatively consistent. The group believes that some consideration should be taken into account of the patients comorbidities. For instance, if the patient has a problem with lipids, they suggest a more malabsorptive procedure be offered. Now with 2 new Food and Drug Adminstration–approved drugs for weight loss and the arrival of the gastric balloon, the options and treatment choices are becoming more complex.

O. J. Hines, MD, FACS

Five-Year Outcomes After Laparoscopic Gastric Bypass and Laparoscopic Duodenal Switch in Patients With Body Mass Index of 50 to 60: A Randomized Clinical Trial

Risstad H, Søvik TT, Engström M, et al (Oslo Univ Hosp, Norway; Sahlgrenska Univ Hosp, Gothenburg, Sweden; et al)

JAMA Surg 150:352-361, 2015

Importance.—There is no consensus as to which bariatric procedure is preferred to reduce weight and improve health in patients with a body mass index higher than 50.

Objective.—To compare 5-year outcomes after Roux-en-Y gastric bypass (gastric bypass) and biliopancreatic diversion with duodenal switch (duodenal switch).

Design, Setting, and Participants.—Randomized clinical open-label trial at Oslo University Hospital, Oslo, Norway, and Sahlgrenska University Hospital, Gothenburg, Sweden. Participants were recruited between March 17, 2006, and August 20, 2007, and included 60 patients aged 20 to 50 years with a body mass index of 50 to 60. The current study provides the 5-year follow-up analyses by intent to treat, excluding one participant accepted for inclusion who declined being operated on prior to knowing to what group hewas randomized.

Interventions.—Laparoscopic gastric bypass and laparoscopic duodenal switch.

Main Outcomes and Measures.—Body mass index and secondary outcomes including anthropometric measures, cardiometabolic risk factors, pulmonary function, vitamin status, gastrointestinal symptoms, health-related quality of life, and adverse events.

Results.—Sixty patients were randomly assigned and operated on with gastric bypass (n = 31) and duodenal switch (n = 29). Fifty-five patients (92%) completed the study. Five years after surgery, the mean reductions in body mass index were 13.6 (95% CI, 11.0-16.1) and 22.1 (95% CI, 19.5-24.7) after gastric bypass and duodenal switch, respectively. The mean between-group difference was 8.5 (95% CI, 4.9-12.2; $P < .001$). Remission rates of type 2 diabetes mellitus and metabolic syndrome and changes in blood pressure and lung function were similar between groups. Reductions in total cholesterol, low-density lipoprotein cholesterol, triglycerides, and fasting glucose were significantly greater after duodenal switch compared with gastric bypass. Serum concentrations of vitamin A and 25-hydroxyvitamin D were significantly reduced after duodenal switch compared with gastric bypass. Duodenal switch was associated with more gastrointestinal adverse effects. Health-related quality of life was similar between groups. Patients with duodenal switch underwent more surgical procedures related to the initial procedure (13 [44.8%] vs 3 [9.7%] patients; $P = .002$) and had significantly more hospital admissions compared with patients with gastric bypass.

Conclusions and Relevance.—In patients with a body mass index of 50 to 60, duodenal switch resulted in greater weight loss and greater improvements in low-density lipoprotein cholesterol, triglyceride, and glucose levels 5 years after surgery compared with gastric bypass while improvements in health-related quality of life were similar. However, duodenal switch was associated with more surgical, nutritional, and gastrointestinal adverse effects.

Trial Registration.—clinicaltrials.gov Identifier: NCT00327912.

▶ This randomized study examined the efficacy of a duodenal switch versus a roux-en-Y gastric bypass for super-obese patients. These patients had a body mass index in the 50 to 60 range and had obvious comorbidity from their metabolic syndrome. It has long been recognized that the duodenal switch is an effective bariatric procedure, but issues with excessive weight loss and nutritional problems have limited its application. This group found that the duodenal switch was better than a gastric bypass for weight loss (Fig 1A in the original article) and reductions in serum lipids and glucose. With regard correction of diabetes and hypertension the outcomes were equal, whereas patients who had a duodenal switch did complain of more gastrointestinal issues. The authors suggest that these 2 procedures might be complementary and offered in a staged approach with the gastric bypass as the first procedure followed by the duodenal switch for patients who have not experienced appropriate weight loss. This concept, however, is speculative and not based on any data from this study.

O. J. Hines, MD, FACS

Effect of Mandatory Centers of Excellence Designation on Demographic Characteristics of Patients Who Undergo Bariatric Surgery

Bae J, Shade J, Abraham A, et al (Johns Hopkins School of Public Health, Baltimore, MD; Johns Hopkins Bayview Med Ctr, Baltimore, MD; et al)

JAMA Surg 150:644-648, 2015

Importance.—From February 21, 2006, through September 24, 2013, the Centers for Medicare & Medicaid Services (CMS) required, via the National Coverage Determination manual, that bariatric surgery be performed only in hospitals that had been designated as a Center of Excellence (COE). The effect of this certification requirement on access to bariatric surgery has been reported only anecdotally.

Objective.—To investigate whether the COE certification requirement proved to be a barrier to patients' access to bariatric surgical procedures.

Design, Setting, and Participants.—Using the National Inpatient Sample, we retrospectively identified patients who underwent bariatric surgery from January 1, 2006, through December 31, 2011.

Exposure.—Bariatric surgery.

Main Outcomes and Measures.—Logistic regression and χ^2 tests were used to examine differences in patients' sociodemographic characteristics over time.

Results.—A total of 134 227 bariatric surgical patients were identified. The proportion of the population who were older than 64 years increased from 2.9% in 2006 to 7.0% in 2011 ($P < .001$) and there was a decrease in the proportion of patients who were 49 years and younger ($P < .001$). The percentage of female patients who underwent bariatric surgery decreased from 80.4% to 78.1% ($P < .001$) and the percentage of patients who were classified as black, Hispanic, or Asian or Pacific Islander increased from 12.3% to 15.1% ($P < .001$), 9.7% to 12.5% ($P < .001$), and 0.3% to 0.4% ($P < .001$), respectively. The proportion of patients with Medicare increased from 8.5% to 16.3% ($P < .001$) and those with Medicaid from 6.6% to 11.8% ($P < .001$). The percentage of patients with private insurance declined from 72.4% to 63.3% ($P < .001$). The proportion of patients in the lowest income quartile increased from 20.7% to 22.9% ($P < .001$) while those in the highest income quartile decreased from 25.8% to 23.9% ($P < .001$).

Conclusions and Relevance.—The COE certification requirement by CMS did not appear to limit access to bariatric surgery. Future studies should determine whether CMS's recent (2013) change in policy (ie, removing the mandatory COE certification for bariatric surgical insurance coverage) might sacrifice patient safety without addressing the real cause of limited access to health care.

► Many surgeons across the country perform bariatric procedures and the forecasts are that the volume of these will increase over the coming years. Significant work has been accomplished to improve outcomes, and many studies have documented the durable benefits on health. Until 2013, the Centers for Medicare & Medicaid Services (CMS) required that patients covered by CMS have these procedures performed in only hospitals that had been designated as a center of excellence (COE). Data suggesting that outcomes were better at COE sites supported this program until new findings concluded that the COE designation did not affect patient safety. Many believed that the COE designation block some patients from care requiring them to drive long distances if they want to pursue bariatric surgery. This study suggests that this is not true and documented that more patients in lower incomes and diverse ethnicities were being cared for in the later years of this program. Other insurers, like Blue Cross/Blue Shield, still require COE designation, and this is likely to remain in place. This is clearly another example that across the board surgical volume and infrastructure to support programs affects morbidity and outcome for our patients.

O. J. Hines, MD, FACS

Bariatric Surgery Reduces Features of Nonalcoholic Steatohepatitis in Morbidly Obese Patients

Lassailly G, Caiazzo R, Buob D, et al (Université Lille 2, France)
Gastroenterology 149:379-388, 2015

Background & Aims.—The effects of bariatric surgery in patients with nonalcoholic fatty liver disease (NASH) are not well established. We performed a prospective study to determine the biological and clinical effects of bariatric surgery in patients with NASH.

Methods.—From May 1994 through May 2013, one hundred and nine morbidly obese patients with biopsy-proven NASH underwent bariatric surgery at the University Hospital of Lille, France (the Lille Bariatric Cohort). Clinical, biological, and histologic data were collected before and 1 year after surgery.

Results.—One year after surgery, NASH had disappeared from 85% of the patients (95% confidence interval [CI]: 75.8%–92.2%). Compared with before surgery, patients had significant reductions in mean ± SD body mass index (BMI, from 49.3 ± 8.2 to 37.4 ± 7) and level of alanine aminotransferase (from 52.1 ± 25.7 IU/L to 25.1 ± 20 IU/L); mean levels of γ-glutamyltransferases were reduced from 51 IU/L before surgery (interquartile range [IQR], 34–87 IU/L) to 23 IU/L afterward (IQR, 14–33 IU/L) and mean insulin resistance index values were reduced from 3.6 ± 0.5 to 2.9 ± 0.5 ($P < .01$ for each comparison). NASH disappeared from a higher proportion of patients with mild NASH before surgery (94%) than severe NASH (70%) ($P < .05$) according to Brunt score. In histologic analysis, steatosis was detected in 60% of the tissue before surgery (IQR, 40%–80%) but only 10% 1 year after surgery (IQR, 2.5%–21.3%); the mean nonalcoholic fatty liver disease score was reduced from 5 (IQR, 4–5) to 1 (IQR, 1–2) (each $P < .001$). Hepatocellular ballooning was reduced in 84.2% of samples (n = 69; 95% CI: 74.4–91.3) and lobular inflammation in 67.1% (n = 55; 95% CI: 55.8–77.1). According to Metavir scores, fibrosis was reduced in 33.8% of patients (95% CI: 23.6%–45.2%). Patients whose NASH persisted 1 year after surgery (n = 12) had lost significantly less weight (change in BMI, 9.1 ± 1.5) than those without NASH (change in BMI, 12.3 ± 0.6) ($P = .005$). Patients who underwent laparoscopic gastric banding lost less weight (change in BMI, 6.4 ± 0.7) than thosewho underwent gastric bypass (change in BMI, 14.0 ± 0.5) ($P < .0001$), and a higher proportion had persistent NASH (30.4% vs 7.6% of those with gastric bypass; $P = .015$).

Conclusions.—Bariatric surgery induced the disappearance of NASH from nearly 85% of patients and reduced the pathologic features of the disease after 1 year of follow-up. It could be a therapeutic option for appropriate morbidly obese patients with NASH who do not respond to lifestyle modifications. More studies are needed to determine the long-term effects of bariatric surgery in morbidly obese patients with NASH.

▶ The benefits of bariatric surgery have clearly been documented, but the impact of these surgeries on nonalcoholic steatohepatitis (NASH) is not clear. Traditional medical therapies for this have included treatment with vitamin E or thiazolidinediones, but these can increase the risk of bladder and prostate cancers. This study examined histologic changes of liver parenchyma a year following surgery. NASH had disappeared from 85% of patients, and this was accompanied by a normalization of liver function tests. Steatosis was found in only 10% of patients after surgery. A subset analysis found that of those patients undergoing a gastric banding NASH was persistent in 30% of patients. Add these findings to the long list of benefits of bariatric surgery including correction of diabetes and hypertension, decreased incidence of cancer, and overall reduced death rate. It is unclear whether this impact on NASH is durable for years following the surgery. Several studies have documented a defined rate of recurrence for the manifestations of metabolic syndrome.

O. J. Hines, MD, FACS

Inferior Vena Cava Filters for Prevention of Venous Thromboembolism in Obese Patients Undergoing Bariatric Surgery: A Systematic Review

Rowland SP, Dharmarajah B, Moore HM, et al (Charing Cross Hosp, London, United Kingdom)

Ann Surg 261:35-45, 2015

Objective.—The use of inferior vena cava (IVC) filters for prevention of venous thromboembolism (VTE) in bariatric surgery is a contentious issue. We aim to review the evidence for the use of IVC filters in bariatric surgical patients, describe trends in practice, and discuss challenges in developing evidence-based guidelines.

Background.—The incidence of VTE in modern bariatric procedures with traditional methods of thromboprophylaxis, such as sequential calf compression devices and perioperative low molecular weight heparin, is approximately 2%.

Methods.—A systematic review of the literature was conducted according to PRISMA guidelines. We searched Medline up until July 2013 with the terms "bariatric filter" and "gastric bypass filter." Two investigators independently screened search results according to an agreed list of eligibility criteria.

Results.—Eighteen studies were included. There were no randomized controlled trials. Data from controlled cohort studies suggest that those who undergo IVC filter insertion preoperatively may be at higher risk of developing deep vein thrombosis (DVT) and pulmonary embolism (PE). A small cohort of patients with multiple risk factors for VTE benefitted from reduced PE-related mortality after preoperative IVC filter insertion. Data from 12 case series reporting VTE outcomes from a total of 497 patients who underwent preoperative IVC filter insertion demonstrated DVT rates of 0% to 20.8% and PE rates ranging from 0% to 6.4%.

Conclusions.—Published data reporting the safety and efficacy of IVC filter use in bariatric surgical patients is highly heterogeneous. There is no evidence to suggest that the potential benefits of IVC filters outweigh the significant risks of therapy.

▶ There is no doubt that patients undergoing bariatric surgery are at higher risk for deep venous thrombosis (DVT) and pulmonary embolism (PE). These patients require perioperative thromboprophylaxis, but the proper prophylaxis is sometimes not clear given the patient's risk factors. Some bariatric surgeons have advocated the use of inferior vena cave filters to prevent pulmonary embolus for this population. This article attempted to collate the available data on this topic. Unfortunately, the data available are not great. Some studies have actually observed higher rates of DVT and PE in patients who had a filter placed. Patients with a prior history of venous thromboembolism or DVT, pulmonary hypertension, history of coagulopathy, chronic severe immobility, and evidence of lower limb venous stasis should be considered for a filter. We should always aim to have these filters removed in 4 to 6 weeks when the risk of thromboembolism has dropped. Leaving these in place can lead to complications, including inferior vena cava thrombosis and PE from clot propagated by the filter.

O. J. Hines, MD, FACS

A systematic review and meta-analysis of mesh vs suture cruroplasty in laparoscopic large hiatal hernia repair

Tam V, Winger DG, Nason KS (Dept of Cardiothoracic Surgery, Pittsburgh, PA; Univ of Pittsburgh, PA)

Am J Surg 211:226-238, 2016

Background.—Equipoise exists regarding whether mesh cruroplasty during laparoscopic large hiatal hernia repair improves symptomatic outcomes compared with suture repair.

Data Source.—Systematic literature review (MEDLINE and EMBASE) identified 13 studies (1,194 patients; 521 suture and 673 mesh) comparing mesh versus suture cruroplasty during laparoscopic repair of large hiatal hernia. We abstracted data regarding symptom assessment, objective recurrence, and reoperation and performed meta-analysis.

Conclusions.—The majority of studies reported significant symptom improvement. Data were insufficient to evaluate symptomatic versus asymptomatic recurrence. Time to evaluation was skewed toward longer follow-up after suture cruroplasty. Odds of recurrence (odds ratio .51, 95% confidence interval .30 to .87; overall $P = .014$) but not need for reoperation (odds ratio .42, 95% confidence interval .13 to 1.37; overall $P = .149$) were less after mesh cruroplasty. Quality of evidence supporting routine use of mesh cruroplasty is low. Mesh should be used at surgeon discretion until additional studies evaluating symptomatic outcomes, quality of life, and long-term recurrence are available (Fig 2).

▶ Whether to use mesh at the time of first operation or at reoperation for large hiatal hernias remains controversial. Many have advocated for mesh, but

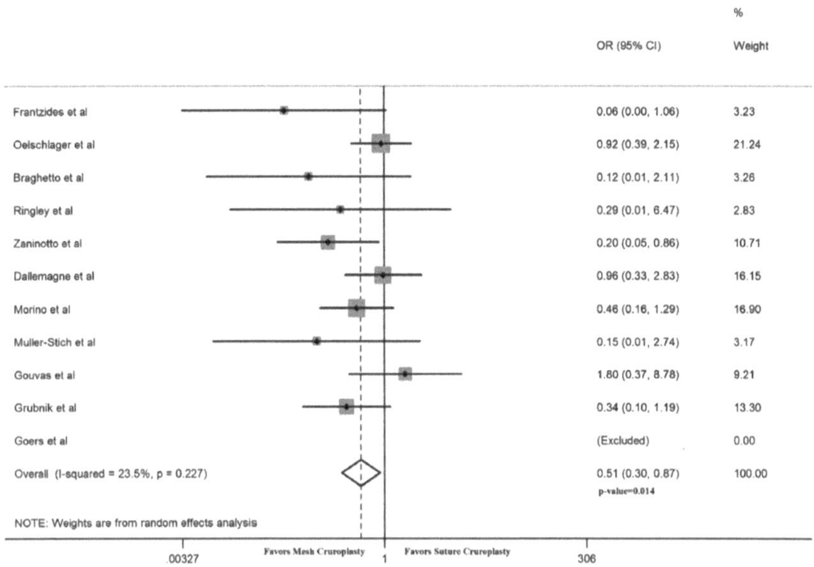

FIGURE 2.—Meta-analysis of recurrence after laparoscopic large hiatal hernia repair. (Reprinted from Tam V, Winger DG, Nason KS. A systematic review and meta-analysis of mesh vs suture cruroplasty in laparoscopic large hiatal hernia repair. *Am J Surg*. 2016;211:226-238, with permission from Elsevier Inc.)

complications including erosion and death have been described. This article attempts to collate all the data on the issue to reach a final conclusion. Unfortunately, the data are not great, so the authors hedge; but overall, the data suggest that the odds of a recurrence are lower with mesh but the need for reoperation is not affected by the use of mesh (Fig 2). Although rare, some have reported the need for esophagectomy or partial or total gastrectomy because of mesh complications. My approach has been to use permanent suture if the crura hold the stitches well without tearing and reinforce with mesh when these do not hold or in the case of a reoperation. We know that as many as 25% to 50% recur, but most of these are asymptomatic and do not require surgery.

O. J. Hines, MD, FACS

Repair of Paraesophageal Hiatal Hernias—Is a Fundoplication Needed? A Randomized Controlled Pilot Trial

Müller-Stich BP, Achtstätter V, Diener MK, et al (Univ of Heidelberg, Germany; et al)

J Am Coll Surg 221:602-610, 2015

Background.—The need for a fundoplication during repair of paraesophageal hiatal hernias (PEH) remains unclear. Prevention of gastroesophageal reflux represents a trade-off against the risk of fundoplication-related side effects. The aim of this trial was to compare laparoscopic mesh-augmented hiatoplasty with simple cardiophrenicopexy (LMAH-C) with laparoscopic mesh-augmented hiatoplasty with fundoplication (LMAH-F) in patients with PEH.

Study Design.—The study was designed as a patient- and assessor-blinded randomized controlled pilot trial, registration number: DRKS00004492 (www.germanctr.de/). Patients with symptomatic PEH were eligible and assigned by central randomization to LMAH-C or LMAH-F. Endpoints were postoperative gastroesophageal reflux, complications, and quality of life 12 months postoperatively.

Results.—Forty patients (9 male, 31 female) were randomized. Patients were well matched for baseline characteristics. At 3 months, the DeMeester score was higher after LMAH-C compared with LMAH-F (40.9 ± 39.9 vs. 9.6 ± 17; $p = 0.048$). At 12 months, the reflux syndrome score was higher after LMAH-C compared with LMAH-F (1.9 ± 1.2 vs. 1.1 ± 0.4; $p = 0.020$). In 53% of LMAH-C patients and 17% of LMAH-F patients, postoperative esophagitis was present ($p = 0.026$). Values of dysphagia (2.1 ± 1.6 vs 1.9 ± 1.4; $p = 0.737$), gas bloating (2.6 ± 1.4 vs 2.8 ± 1.4; $p = 0.782$), and quality of life (116.0 ± 16.2 vs 115.9 ± 15.8; $p = 0.992$) were similar. Relevant postoperative complications occurred in 4 (10%) patients and did not differ between the groups.

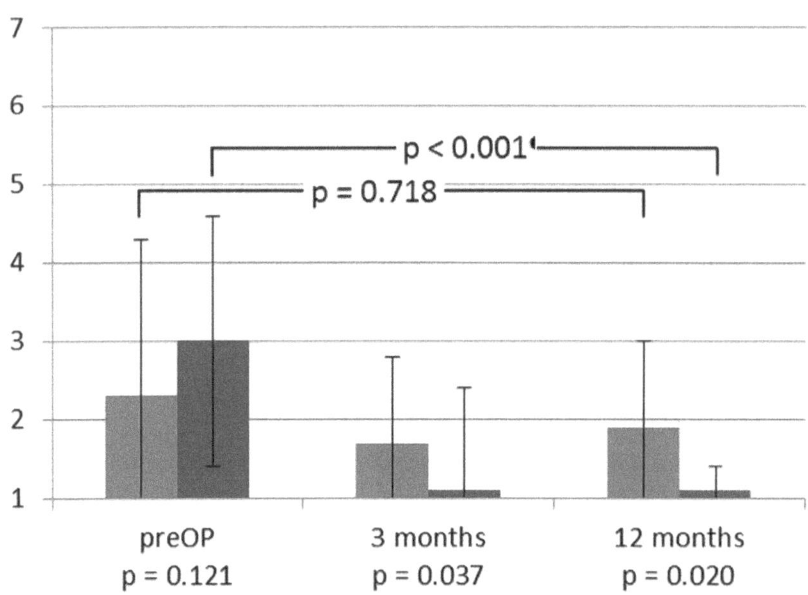

FIGURE 2.—Reflux syndrome score. Light gray bar, laparoscopic mesh-augmented hiatoplasty with cardiophrenicopexy; dark gray bar, laparoscopic mesh-augmented hiatoplasty with fundoplication. For interpretation of the refernces to colour in this figure legend, the reader in referred to web vision of this article. (Reprinted from Müller-Stich BP, Achtstätter V, Diener MK, et al. Repair of paraesophageal hiatal hernias—is a fundoplication needed? A randomized controlled pilot trial. *J Am Coll Surg.* 2015;221:602-610, with permission from American College of Surgeons.)

Conclusions.—Laparoscopic repair of PEH should be combined with a fundoplication to avoid postoperative gastroesophageal reflux and resulting esophagitis. Fundoplication-related side effects do not appear to be clinically relevant. Multicenter randomized trials are required to confirm these findings (Figs 2 and 5).

▶ Do you perform a fundoplication when repairing a paraesophageal hernia? For some time many have advocated a fundoplication to prevent reflux, and there has been some thought that the fundoplication helps to prevent recurrence of the hernia. This randomized study examined the utility of the Nissen fundoplication after paraesophageal hernia repair with mesh. Patients who received a fundoplication had less reflux after surgery than those who did not without difference in postoperative gastrointestinal complaints (Figs 2 and 5). What's more, the patients who did not have a fundoplication had more frequent occurrence of esophagitis on endoscopy (53% vs 17%), and issues of gas bloat were equal between groups. The impact of the fundoplication on recurrence was not completely addressed by this trial but was not significantly different at 33% in the repair only group and 21% in the Nissen group. It seems that the current tenet favoring fundoplication for patients undergoing

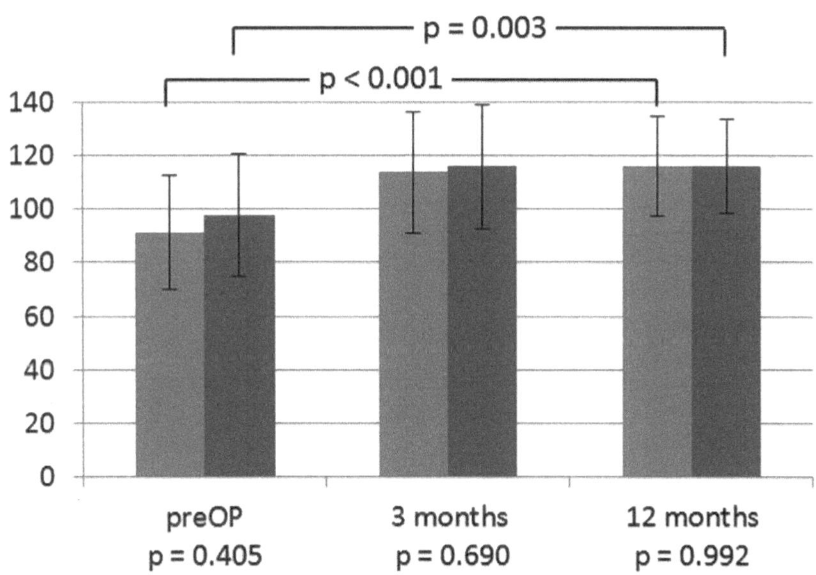

FIGURE 5.—Gastrointestinal Quality of Life Index (GIQLI). Light gray bar, laparoscopic mesh-augmented hiatoplasty with cardiophrenicopexy; Dark gray bar, laparoscopic mesh-augmented hiatoplasty with fundoplication. For interpretation of the refernces to colour in this figure legend, the reader in referred to web vision of this article. (Reprinted from Müller-Stich BP, Achtstätter V, Diener MK, et al. Repair of paraesophageal hiatal hernias–is a fundoplication needed? A randomized controlled pilot trial. *J Am Coll Surg*. 2015;221:602-610, with permission from American College of Surgeons.)

paraesophageal repair is borne out by this trial and should remain a part of your approach.

O. J. Hines, MD, FACS

Laparoscopic Repair of Very Large Hiatus Hernia With Sutures Versus Absorbable Mesh Versus Nonabsorbable Mesh: A Randomized Controlled Trial

Watson DI, Thompson SK, Devitt PG, et al (Flinders Univ, Bedford Park, South Australia, Australia; Univ of Adelaide, South Australia, Australia; et al)

Ann Surg 261:282-289, 2015

Objective.—Determine whether absorbable or nonabsorbable mesh in repair of large hiatus hernias reduces the risk of recurrence, compared with suture repair.

Background.—Repair of large hiatus hernia is associated with radiological recurrence rates of up to 30%, and to improve outcomes mesh repair has been recommended. Previous trials have shown less short-term recurrence with mesh, but adverse outcomes limit mesh use.

Methods.—Multicentre prospective double blind randomized controlled trial of 3 methods of repair: sutures versus absorbable mesh versus nonabsorbable mesh. Primary outcome—hernia recurrence assessed by barium meal radiology and endoscopy at 6 months. Secondary outcomes—clinical symptom scores at 1, 3, 6, and 12 months.

Results.—A total of 126 patients enrolled: 43 sutures, 41 absorbable mesh, and 42 nonabsorbable mesh. Among them, 96.0% were followed up to 12 months, with objective follow-up data in 92.9%. A recurrent hernia (any size) was identified in 23.1% after suture repair, 30.8% after absorbable mesh, and 12.8% after nonabsorbable mesh ($P = 0.161$). Clinical outcomes were similar, except less heartburn at 3 and 6 months and less bloating at 12 months with nonabsorbable mesh; more heartburn at 3 months, odynophagia at 1 month, nausea at 3 and 12 months, wheezing at 6 months; and inability to belch at 12 months after absorbable mesh. The magnitudes of the clinical differences were small.

Conclusions.—No significant differences were seen for recurrent hiatus hernia, and the clinical differences were unlikely to be clinically significant. Overall outcomes after sutured repair were similar to mesh repair.

▶ Recurrence after hiatal hernia repair is common, ranging from 25% to 50%. The majority of these patients do not have symptoms from the recurrence, so most surgeons do not routinely study patients postoperatively. This study performed a randomized trial of patients undergoing laparoscopic hiatal hernia repair to determine whether suture, biologic mesh reinforcement, or permanent mesh reinforcement is more effective at preventing recurrence. The mesh was laid over the suture repair and posterior to the esophagus and fixed with a tacking device. Although not statistically significant, the permanent mesh group had half the number of recurrences at 12 months. These patients had also less heartburn and other gastrointestinal complaints long term. The biologic mesh group had the same recurrence rate as the suture group and more issues with gastrointestinal complaints. From this study, we can surmise that biologic mesh reinforcement offers no advantage over suture repair alone and that permanent mesh may help reduce issues of recurrence.

O. J. Hines, MD, FACS

Thoracic Esophageal Diverticula: A 15-Year Experience of Minimally Invasive Surgical Management

Macke RA, Luketich JD, Pennathur A, et al (Univ of Pittsburgh School of Medicine, PA; et al)

Ann Thorac Surg 100:1795-1802, 2015

Background.—Thoracic esophageal diverticula are uncommon, and controversies exist regarding their management. The objective of this study was to evaluate the outcomes of a relatively large cohort of patients with thoracic esophageal diverticula treated with minimally invasive surgical techniques.

Methods.—We conducted a retrospective review of patients who underwent minimally invasive surgical treatment for symptomatic esophageal diverticula during a 15-year period. The primary end point was 30-day mortality. In addition, we evaluated the morbidity, improvement in dysphagia (score: 1, best to 5, worst), and quality of life (Gastroesophageal Reflux Disease–Health-Related Quality of Life score: 0, best to 50, most symptoms).

Results.—Fifty-seven patients underwent minimally invasive surgical treatment of symptomatic thoracic esophageal diverticula. The most common symptom was dysphagia (45 of 57; 79%). A motility disorder or distal mechanical obstruction was identified in 49 patients (86%). Approaches used included video-assisted thoracoscopic surgery (n = 33), laparoscopy (n = 18), and combined video-assisted thoracoscopic surgery and laparoscopy (n = 6). The most common procedure performed was diverticulectomy and myotomy (47 of 57 patients; 82.5%). The 30-day mortality was 0%. There were 4 patients (7%) with postoperative leaks requiring reoperation. During follow-up, the median dysphagia score improved from 3 to 1 ($p < 0.001$). The median Gastroesophageal Reflux Disease–Health-Related Quality of Life score after surgery was 5 (excellent).

Conclusions.—A minimally invasive surgical approach for the management of thoracic esophageal diverticula is safe and effective during intermediate-term follow-up when performed by surgeons experienced in esophageal surgery and minimally invasive techniques. Further follow-up is required to assess the durability of these results. The optimal

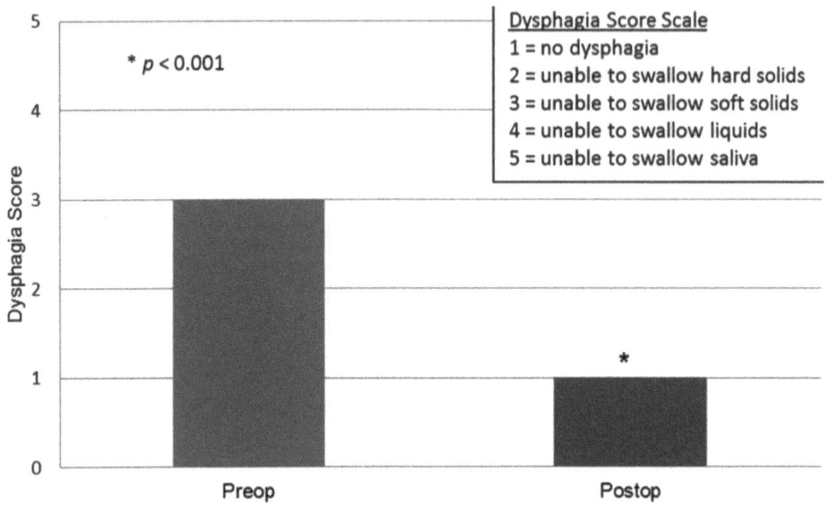

FIGURE 6.—Median preoperative (preop) and postoperative (postop) dysphagia scores. The median postoperative score was significantly decreased (improved; $p < 0.001$).(Reprinted from Macke RA, Luketich JD, Pennathur A, et al. Thoracic esophageal diverticula: a 15-year experience of minimally invasive surgical management. *Ann Thorac Surg*. 2015;100:1795-1802, with permission from The Society of Thoracic Surgeons.)

approach and procedures performed should be determined on an individualized basis after a thorough investigation (Fig 6).

▶ Mid and lower esophageal diverticula are uncommon but can be the source of significant functional difficulty for patients. These are usually caused by esophageal dysmotility resulting in a pulsion diverticulum that involves only the mucosa. This article is the largest reported series of thoracic esophageal diverticula, and the group is reporting the results. These 57 cases were nearly all completed either thoracoscopically or laparoscopically and usually included a myotomy that extended from the level of the diverticulum to the gastroesophageal junction. On occasion, the group performed a partial fundoplication. Postoperatively the outcomes were excellent with significant decreases in dysphagia (Fig 6). Four patients did have an esophageal leak requiring reoperation. These cases are fascinating, and usually the diverticulectomy not quite as difficult as one might imagine. However, the laparoscopic skill required to complete these along with the long myotomy is significant. The article is a good reminder of the pathophysiology and treatment of this uncommon condition.

O. J. Hines, MD, FACS

Per-Oral Endoscopic Myotomy: A Series of 500 Patients

Inoue H, Sato H, Ikeda H, et al (Northern Yokohama Hosp, Yokohama, Japan; et al)

J Am Coll Surg 221:256-264, 2015

Background.—After the first case of per-oral endoscopic myotomy (POEM) at our institution in 2008, the procedure was quickly accepted as an alternative to surgical myotomy and is now established as an excellent treatment option for achalasia. This study aimed to examine the safety and outcomes of POEM at our institution.

Study Design.—Per-oral endoscopic myotomy was performed on 500 consecutive achalasia patients at our institution between September 2008 and November 2013. A review of prospectively collected data was conducted, including procedure time, myotomy location and length, adverse events, and patient data with short- (2 months) and long-term (1 and 3 years) follow-up.

Results.—Per-oral endoscopic myotomy was successfully completed in all patients, with adverse events observed in 3.2%. Two months post-POEM, significant reductions in symptom scores (Eckardt score 6.0 ± 3.0 vs 1.0 ± 2.0, $p < 0.0001$) and lower esophageal sphincter (LES) pressures (25.4 ± 17.1 vs 13.4 ± 5.9 mm Hg, $p < 0.0001$) were achieved, and this persisted at 3 years post-POEM. Gastroesophageal reflux was seen in 16.8% of patients at 2 months and 21.3% at 3-year follow-up.

Conclusions.—Per-oral endoscopic myotomy was successfully completed in all cases, even when extended indications (extremes of age, previous interventions, or sigmoid esophagus) were used. Adverse events were rare (3.2%), and there were no mortalities. Significant improvements in Eckardt scores and LES pressures were seen at 2 months, 1 year, and 3 years post-POEM. Based on our large series, POEM is a safe and effective treatment for achalasia; there are relatively few contraindications, and the procedure may be used as either first- or second-line therapy (Fig 1).

▶ Per-oral endoscopic myotomy for achalasia is taking off with more reports expanding the indications. Many have advocated strict selection criteria for this procedure, but as experience grows, doctors are becoming more comfortable with the outcomes. This publication is the largest to date with 500 procedures and a 3-year follow-up. The procedure involves making a myotomy and tunneling along the length to be addressed and incising the inner circular layer with an endoscopic spray coagulation device (Fig 1). The reported success rate with this series was 91% and 88% at 1 and 3 years with regard to symptom improvement. Manometric analysis postprocedure showed normalization of lower esophageal sphincter pressures. Twenty percent of the patients complained of heartburn. One criticism of this article is that the follow-up data were only available for 77% of patients at 3 years, so it is possible the reported

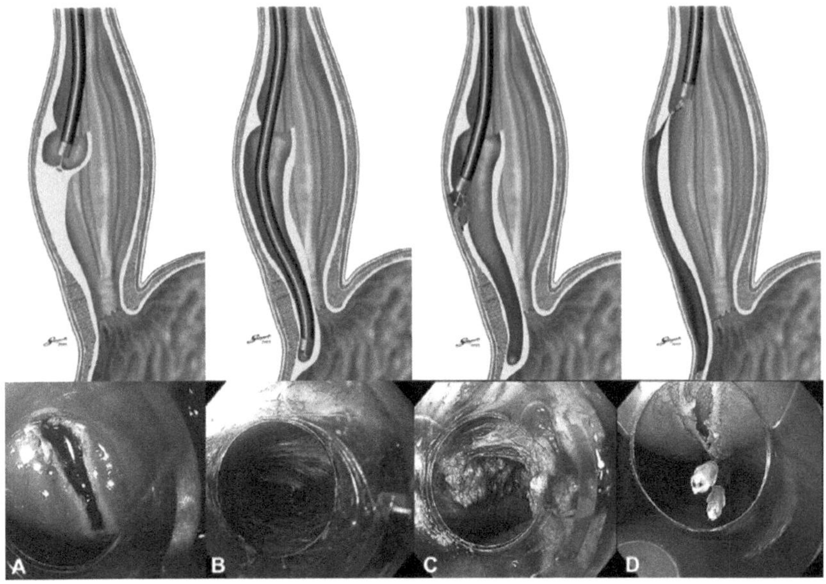

FIGURE 1.—Steps in per-oral endoscopic myotomy. (A) Entry to the submucosal space is made after submucosal injection with saline. (B) The submucosa is progressively dissected distally along the muscular layer, using spray coagulation at 50 W (ERBE VIO300D), creating a submucosal tunnel extending beyond the gastroesophageal junction. (C) Myotomy of the circular esophageal and gastric muscle bundles is performed under direct vision. (D) After myotomy has been successfully completed, the mucosal entry site is closed with hemostatic clips from the distal to the proximal end of the mucosal fenestration. (Reprinted from Inoue H, Sato H, Ikeda H, et al. Per-oral endoscopic myotomy: a series of 500 patients. *J Am Coll Surg*. 2015;221:256-264, with permission from the American College of Surgeons.)

success was not as great. The conclusion is, this procedure is here to stay and worth learning about for your patients with achalasia.

O. J. Hines, MD, FACS

Long-Term Outcome of the Treatment of Zenker's Diverticulum

Greene CL, McFadden PM, Oh DS, et al (Keck School of Medicine of the Univ of Southern California, Los Angeles)
Ann Thorac Surg 100:975-978, 2015

Background.—Treatment of Zenker's diverticulum can be accomplished by use of a transcervical myotomy (TCM) with diverticulopexy/diverticulectomy or by the transoral endoscopic stapling (TOS) approach. Our aim was to evaluate the short-term and long-term outcomes of these two techniques.

Methods.—A retrospective review was performed to identify all patients who had received either treatment for Zenker's diverticulum from July 1998 to August 2013. Telephone interviews were attempted of all surviving patients to assess long-term outcome.

Results.—There were 77 patients, with a median age of 71 years (range, 37 to 97 years). All patients had dysphagia, and 33 (43%) had regurgitation. TCM was performed in 68 patients, and TOS was done in nine. The median size of the diverticulum was 2.5 cm in the TCM group and 4 cm in the TOS group ($p = 0.13$). The operation was primary in 66 patients (86%) and a reoperation in 11 patients. The median hospital stay was 1 day for TOS and 3 for TCM ($p = 0.0005$). The median time to oral intake for both groups was 1 day. There were three adverse events in the TCM group and none in the TOS group. Early outcome was assessed in all 77 patients at a median of 4 months (interquartile range [IQR], 1 to 13.5 months). Symptomatic improvement occurred in all patients, with 55 patients (71%) reporting complete resolution. Long-term symptoms were assessed at a median of 54 months (IQR, 34 to 77 months) in 38 of 59 (64%) surviving patients.

Conclusions.—Cricopharyngeal myotomy with diverticulopexy/diverticulectomy and TOS are both safe and effective treatments for Zenker's diverticulum. All patients reported improvement in symptoms, with complete resolution in the majority of patients (Table 2).

▶ Zenker diverticulum can be a real nuisance for patients, and these patients are usually older. The outcomes from cricopharyngeal myotomy are excellent, and this is usually accompanied by either a diverticulopexy or excision of the diverticulum. Over the past 2 decades, transoral techniques have been developed with staplers and lasers that aim to create a common channel between the diverticulum and the esophagus. This cases series examines the outcomes of both approaches and finds excellent symptom relief in both. The transoral approach seemed to offer more consistent symptom relief and at the same time limited the complications of bleeding, esophageal leak, and recurrent nerve injury (Table 2). Success with the transoral approach appears higher when the diverticulum is larger than 3 centimeters because this will allow for the entire cricopharyngeal muscle to be incised and obviously in patients who have reasonable neck mobility. Neck mobility can obviously be a limitation in this patient population. If you treat Zenker diverticulum, it is probably a good

TABLE 2.—Early Symptomatic Outcome

Outcome	Transcervical Myotomy n = 68	Transoral Endoscopic Stapling n = 9	*p*
Median follow-up, mo (range)	4 (1–16)	3 (1–7)	0.46
Complete resolution of symptoms	47 (69%)	9 (100%)	0.10
Residual symptoms			
Dysphagia	11 (16%)	0	0.34
Regurgitation	8 (12%)	0	0.58
Belching	4 (6%)	0	1.0
Aspiration	0	0	1.0

Reprinted from Greene CL, McFadden PM, Oh DS, et al. Long-term outcome of the treatment of Zenker's diverticulum. *Ann Thorac Surg.* 2015;100:975-978, with permission from The Society of Thoracic Surgeons.

idea to add the transoral approach to your armamentarium. Patients know about this and almost always request a less invasive approach if it is available.

O. J. Hines, MD, FACS

An Assessment of the Optimal Time for Removal of Esophageal Stents Used in the Treatment of an Esophageal Anastomotic Leak or Perforation

Freeman RK, Ascioti AJ, Dake M, et al (St. Vincent Hosp, Indianapolis, IN)

Ann Thorac Surg 100:422-428, 2015

Background.—Esophageal stent for the treatment of a perforation or anastomotic leak has been shown to be effective and safe. However, the optimal timing for stent removal is in question. This purpose of this investigation was to identify a time for stent removal in patients treated for an acute perforation or anastomotic leak that resulted in sealing of the leak while minimizing the incidence of stent-related complications.

Methods.—Patients undergoing esophageal stent placement for the treatment of an acute perforation or intrathoracic anastomotic leak were identified from a single institution's prospectively collected database. Patient outcomes were recorded and analyzed. Complications were segregated by stent dwell time.

Results.—During the study period, 162 patients underwent esophageal stent placement for an acute perforation (n = 117) or anastomotic leak (n = 45). Patients whose stent was removed in less than 28 days after placement for an acute perforation realized a stent complication rate that was independently reduced by 39% (odds ratio, 0.61; 95% confidence interval, 0.54 to 0.78; $p < 0.01$), whereas patients whose stent was removed in less than 14 days after placement for an acute perforation realized a stent complication rate that was independently reduced by 56% (odds ratio, 0.44; 95% confidence interval, 0.38 to 0.69; $p < 0.001$).

Conclusions.—Endoluminal esophageal stent placement is a safe and effective treatment for patients with an acute esophageal perforation or intrathoracic anastomotic leak after esophagectomy. Removal of stents at 2 weeks for anastomotic leak or 4 weeks for perforation has the potential to significantly decrease the incidence of complications associated with stent use (Table 2).

▶ Esophageal leaks from acute perforation or after esophagectomy are a real problem, with an extremely high morbidity and mortality rate. The tenants have been closure for early acute perforations and wide drainage otherwise. These patients often go on to experience severe sepsis and prolonged hospitalizations. The arrival of esophageal stents has provided a real solution to this problem that is extremely effective and simpler than operative repair. When a leak is identified by esophagram, these stents can be placed quickly and often result in closure within a matter of days. These stents are not immune to complication, however, and this can include migration, vascular fistulization from erosion, stent fracture, and severe dysphagia. This large series of more than

TABLE 2.—Results After Esophageal Stent Placement

Variable	Anastomotic Leak	Perforation
Resolution of leak	43 (96%)	111 (95%)
Stent removal, days (mean ± SD)	12 ± 11	19 ± 16
Range	6–39	7–51
Hospital length of stay, days (mean ± SD)	9 ± 6	8 ± 11
Range	3–29	5–31

SD = standard deviation.

Reprinted from Freeman RK, Ascioti AJ, Dake M, et al. An assessment of the optimal time for removal of esophageal stents used in the treatment of an esophageal anastomotic leak or perforation. *Ann Thorac Surg*. 2015;100:422-428, with permission from The Society of Thoracic Surgeons.

162 patients examined these complications and concluded that stent removal within 14 to 28 days can significantly limit these outcomes and provides plenty of time for the perforation to heal (Table 2). This new approach to esophageal leak provides a real opportunity to quickly salvage these patients and limit the subsequent convalescence.

O. J. Hines, MD, FACS

Laparoscopic pyloroplasty is a safe and effective first-line surgical therapy for refractory gastroparesis

Shada AL, Dunst CM, Pescarus R, et al (The Oregon Clinic, Portland)
Surg Endosc 2015 [Epub ahead of print]

Introduction.—Surgical options for symptomatic delayed gastric emptying include gastric stimulator implantation, subtotal gastrectomy, and pyloroplasty. Pyloroplasty has been shown to improve gastric emptying yet is seldom described as a primary treatment for gastroparesis. We present a single-institution experience of laparoscopic Heineke–Mikulicz pyloroplasty (LP) as treatment for gastroparesis.

Methods and Procedures.—A prospective foregut surgery database was queried for LP over a 5-year period. Charts were reviewed for indications, complications, symptom score, and outcomes. Gastroparesis was defined by (1) abnormal gastric emptying study, (2) endoscopic visualization of retained food after prolonged NPO status, or (3) clinical symptoms suspicious of vagal nerve injury following complex re-operative foregut surgery. Results were analyzed using a paired *T* test and single-factor ANOVA.

Results.—One hundred and seventy-seven LP patients were identified and reviewed. One hundred and five had a concurrent fundoplication for objective reflux. There were no intraoperative complications or conversions to laparotomy. Overall morbidity rate was 6.8% with four return to OR and two confirmed leaks (1.1% leak rate). Average length of stay was 3.5 days, and readmission rate was 7%. Eighty-six percent had

TABLE 3.—Gastric Emptying Scintigraphy (GES) Results

GES Results	Preoperative	Postoperative	*P* Value
% 4-h retained	32 (23)	3.3 (2.8)	0.001
T1/2 (min)	167 (97)	74 (26)	0.001

T1/2: time to allow 50 % of material to leave the stomach

Reprinted from Shada AL, Dunst CM, Pescarus R, et al. Laparoscopic pyloroplasty is a safe and effective first-line surgical therapy for refractory gastroparesis. *Surg Endosc.* 2015 [Epub ahead of print], with permission from Springer Science+Business Media.

improvement in GES with normalization in 77%. Gastric emptying half-time decreased from 175 ± 94 to 91 ± 45 min. Nineteen patients (10.7%) had subsequent surgical interventions: gastric stimulator implantation (12), feeding jejunostomy and/or gastrostomy tube (6), or subtotal gastrectomy (4). Symptom severity scores for nausea, vomiting, bloating, abdominal pain, and early satiety decreased significantly at 3 months.

Conclusion.—Laparoscopic pyloroplasty improves or normalizes gastric emptying in nearly 90% of gastroparesis patients with very low morbidity. It significantly improves symptoms of nausea, vomiting, bloating, and abdominal pain. Some patients may go on to another surgical treatment for GP, but it remains a safe and less invasive alternative to a subtotal gastrectomy in these clinically challenging patients (Table 3).

▶ Gastroparesis can be a vexing problem, and the solutions are limited. The causes of this condition are both medical (often diabetes) and surgical after upper gastrointestinal (GI) surgery and vagal nerve injury. Options include pro-motility agents, gastric stimulators, feeding tubes, pyloroplasty, gastrojejunostomy, and total gastrectomy. This study examined a large case series of patients with gastroparesis who underwent laparoscopic pyloroplasty. The outcomes were superb with 86% having improvement in gastric emptying with average emptying times cut more than half from 167 minutes to 76 minutes (Table 3). Patients underwent a Heineke-Mikulicz pyloroplasty with a single layer running closure tested for leakage with an intraoperative endoscopy. Postoperatively, patients had an upper GI test, and drain fluid amylase was checked to confirm no leak. Patients were discharged on average 3.5 days postoperatively on a pureed diet for 2 weeks. The results of this study are quite promising and may be an important offering for patients with this difficult condition. Coordinated care with a gastroenterologist is critical to fully understanding and treating this patient population.

O. J. Hines, MD, FACS

Small bowel obstruction: A practical step-by-step evidence-based approach to evaluation, decision making, and management

Azagury D, Liu RC, Morgan A, et al (Stanford Univ School of Medicine, CA; Kaiser Diablo Service Area, Livermore, CA; Univ of California San Francisco East Bay, Hayward)

J Trauma Acute Care Surg 79:661-668, 2015

The initial goal of evaluating a patient with SBO is to immediately identify strangulation and need for urgent operative intervention, concurrent with rapid resuscitation. This relies on a combination of traditional clinical signs and CT findings. In patients without signs of strangulation, a protocol for administration of Gastrografin immediately in the emergency department efficiently sorts patients into those who will resolve their obstructions and those who will fail nonoperative management. Furthermore, because of the unique ability of Gastrografin to drawwater into the bowel lumen, it expedites resolution of partial obstructions, shortening time to removal of nasogastric tube liberalization of diet, and discharge from the hospital. Implementation of such a protocol is a complex, multidisciplinary, and time-consuming endeavor. As such, we cannot overemphasize the importance of clear, open communication with everyone involved.

If surgical management is warranted, we encourage an initial laparoscopic approach with open access. Even if this results in immediate conversion to laparotomy after assessment of the intra-abdominal status, we encourage this approach with a goal of 30% conversion rate or higher. This will attest that patients will have been given the highest likelihood of a successful laparoscopic LOA.

▶ The decision to operate in the face of a small bowel obstruction can be difficult because nearly 80% of those due to adhesions will resolve without surgery. Clearly, signs of sepsis, peritonitis, or significantly abnormal laboratory values necessitate exploration early on after the patient presents. For the remainder of patients, this study attempted to identify clinical and CT findings that predicted the need for operation. Twenty-six percent of the patients required operation, and operations were usually performed by day 1.5. The group found no flatus (3.28 odds ratio), presence of free fluid on CT (2.59 odds ratio), and high-grade obstruction by CT (2.44 odds ratio) to be predictors of the need for surgery. The group examined the sensitivity and specificity of several other CT finding. Interestingly a closed loop obstruction on CT was not a sensitive finding. This patient population is a difficult group to manage because a wrong decision can be catastrophic leading to massive bowel resection or enteric fistulas. A careful, measured approach using data like these can help.

O. J. Hines, MD, FACS

A multi-institution prospective observational study of small bowel obstruction: Clinical and computerized tomography predictors of which patients may require early surgery

Kulvatunyou N, Pandit V, Moutamn S, et al (Univ of Arizona, Tucson; et al)

J Trauma Acute Care Surg 79:393-398, 2015

Background.—For patients with adhesive small bowel obstruction (ASBO), early surgery after a failed trial of nonoperative treatment can improve outcome. However, deciding which patients require early surgery is difficult, given the lack of specific clinical or radiographic signs. The study goals were to identify clinical and computed tomography (CT) predictors of which patients may need early surgery and to evaluate the utility of the common CT findings.

Methods.—This was a multi-institution prospective observational study for patients who were admitted with ASBO. Patients were excluded if their SBO were not managed conservative initially; were within 30 days postoperatively; were caused by external hernias, small bowel tumor, or intussusception; and were related to Crohn's disease. Clinical and laboratory variables were collected prospectively. CT findings were interpreted by a blinded designated radiologist. To identify significant predictors, we performed a multivariable regression analysis.

Results.—During 22 months, we enrolled 200 patients with ASBO. Patients' mean (SD) age was 60 (18) years; 50% were male. Fifty-two patients (26%) underwent surgery. Of those who underwent surgery, the median duration of nonoperative treatment was 1.5 days (interquartile range, 1–2.5 days). In the regression model, we identified no flatus (odds ratio [OR], 3.28; 95% confidence interval [CI], 1.51–7.12; $p = 0.003$), presence of free fluid on CT (OR, 2.59; 95% CI, 1.13–5.90; $p = 0.023$), and high-grade obstruction by CT (OR, 2.44; 95% CI, 1.10–5.43; $p = 0.028$) to be significant predictors for ASBO patients who may need early surgery.

Conclusion.—In this study, we prospectively derived one clinical and two CT predictors which ASBO patients may benefit from an early surgical intervention. However, a future study to validate these predictors is needed.

Level of Evidence.—Therapeutic study, level III; prognostic study, level II (Table 5).

▶ The decision to operate in the face of a small bowel obstruction can be difficult because nearly 80% of those due to adhesions will resolve without surgery. Clearly signs of sepsis, peritonitis, or significantly abnormal laboratory values necessitate exploration early on after the patient presents. For the remainder of patients this study attempted to identify clinical and CT findings that predicted the need for operation. Twenty-six percent of the patients required operation, and the operation was usually performed by day 1.5. The group found no flatus (odds ratio [OR] 3.28), presence of free fluid on CT

TABLE 5. Utility of CT Signs

	Sensitivity %	Specificity %	PPV %	NPV %	Accuracy %
Transition point	94	10	27	82	32
Free fluid	73	53	36	85	58
Multiple fluid locations	24	81	41	66	61
Small bowel fecalization	35	54	21	70	49
Mesenteric edema	51	68	36	80	64
Closed loop	8	94	31	74	71
High-grade obstruction	59	70	40	84	67

NPV, negative predictive value.

Reprinted from Kulvatunyou N, Pandit V, Moutamn S, et al. A multi-institution prospective observational study of small bowel obstruction: clinical and computerized tomography predictors of which patients may require early surgery. *J Trauma Acute Care Surg*. 2015;79:393-398, with permission from Wolters Kluwer Health, Inc.

(OR 2.59), and high-grade obstruction by CT (OR 2.44) to be predictors of the need for surgery. The group examined the sensitivity and specificity of several other CT findings (Table 5). Interestingly, a closed loop obstruction on CT was not a sensitive finding. This patient population is a difficult group to manage because a wrong decision can be catastrophic, leading to massive bowel resection or enteric fistulas. A careful measured approach using data like these can help.

O. J. Hines, MD, FACS

Small Bowel Obstruction Is a Surgical Disease: Patients with Adhesive Small Bowel Obstruction Requiring Operation Have More Cost-Effective Care When Admitted to a Surgical Service

Bilderback PA, Massman JD III, Smith RK, et al (Virginia Mason Med Ctr, Seattle, WA)

J Am Coll Surg 221:7-13, 2015

Background.—Adhesive small bowel obstruction (ASBO), although a potential surgical emergency, is increasingly being managed by medical hospitalists due to the likelihood these patients will not require operation. However, the value of care delivered by medical hospitalists to patients with ASBO has not been reported.

Study Design.—We hypothesized that patients admitted to the medical hospitalist service (MHS) for presumed ASBO have increased length of stay (LOS) and charges compared with patients admitted to the surgical service (SS). There were 555 consecutive admissions with presumed ASBO from 2008 to 2012; these were reviewed and grouped according to admitting service and whether an operation was performed. Group medians were compared and multivariate analysis was performed to identify variables independently associated with increased LOS, time to operation (TTO), and charges.

TABLE 2.—Main Outcomes Variables

	Operation			No Operation		
Variables	MHS (n = 79)	SS (n = 51)	*p* Value	MHS (n = 381)	SS (n = 44)	*p* Value
LOS, d, median, (IQR)	9.57 (7.36, 13.91)	6.99 (5.02, 9.98)	0.002	2.98 (2.03, 4.99)	2.85 (1.69, 4.75)	0.494
Time to operation, h, median, (IQR)	51.72 (19.91, 98.25)	8.40 (5.21, 50.19)	<0.001			
Charges, $, median, (IQR)*	38.8 (28.1, 51.9)	30.1 (23.4, 43.4)	0.025	9.2 (6.3, 14.2)	8.4 (5.2, 13.4)	0.228
Intestinal resection, n (%)	14 (17.7)	3 (5.9)	0.063			
Complications, n (%)	24 (30.4)	14 (27.5)	0.872	5 (1.3)	0 (0.0)	1.000
30-d readmission, n (%)	4 (5.1)	7 (13.7)	0.109	47 (12.3)	10 (22.7)	0.093

IQR, interquartile range; LOS, length of stay; MHS, medical hospitalist service; SS, surgical service.

*Units of $1,000.

Reprinted from Bilderback PA, Massman JD III, Smith RK, et al. Small bowel obstruction is a surgical disease: patients with adhesive small bowel obstruction requiring operation have more cost-effective care when admitted to a surgical service. *J Am Coll Surg.* 2015;221:7-13, with permission from the American College of Surgeons.

Results.—Median LOS among patients whose ASBO resolved nonoperatively was similar for those on SS and MHS (2.85 days vs 2.98 days; $p = 0.49$). In patients without nonoperative resolution of ASBO, those admitted to MHS had longer median LOS when compared with those admitted to SS (9.57 days vs 6.99 days; $p = 0.002$) and higher median charges ($38,800 vs $30,100; $p = 0.025$). Patients admitted to MHS who had an operation, had a greater median TTO than operative patients on SS (51.72 hours vs 8.4 hours; $p < 0.001$). Multivariate analysis did not identify factors independently predictive of increased LOS, TTO, or charges.

Conclusions.—Adhesive small bowel obstruction patients are treated in a heterogeneous fashion in our hospital, causing disparate outcomes depending on admitting service when patients undergo operation. Admitting all suspected ASBO patients to SS has the potential to dramatically decrease LOS and reduce waste in those requiring operation, thereby reducing health care expenditures (Table 2).

▶ Small bowel obstruction due to adhesive disease is a common and sometimes recurrent problem for patients that have undergone abdominal surgery. The management of these patients has evolved toward one of more conservative management because a fair percentage of these will resolve without operation. Who is best to manage these patients, a medical doctor or a surgeon? This study investigates this issue and clearly concludes that patients with a small bowel obstruction are better managed by a surgeon. They found that patients had shorter hospital stays, fewer radiographs, and less expensive hospital stays (Table 2). What was maybe more concerning was that patients on the medical service were more likely to have a bowel resection presumably from ischemic compromise. The authors suggest that this observation occurred because there were delays in the decision to operate on the medical service. This is a highly biased report, but the information is compelling. It probably makes sense to standardize the treatment of these patients in your facility across all service lines.

O. J. Hines, MD, FACS

Laparoscopic Surgery or Conservative Treatment for Appendiceal Abscess in Adults? A Randomized Controlled Trial

Mentula P, Sammalkorpi H, Leppäniemi A (Helsinki Univ Central Hosp, Finland)

Ann Surg 262:237-242, 2015

Objective.—We hypothesized that immediate laparoscopic surgery for appendiceal abscess would result in faster recovery than conservative treatment.

Background.—On the basis of the retrospective studies, conservative management of appendiceal abscess is recommended as a first line treatment, but some controversy exists.

Methods.—Sixty adult patients diagnosed with appendiceal abscess were randomly assigned to either laparoscopic surgery (n = 30) or conservative treatment (n = 30). Hospital stay, recurrences, additional interventions, and complications within 60 days from randomization were recorded.

Results.—There was no difference in hospital stay: 4 days (interquartile range: 3–5 days) in the laparoscopy group versus 5 days (3–8) in the conservative group, $P = 0.105$. Patients in the laparoscopy group had 10% risk for bowel resection and 13% risk for incomplete appendectomy. There were significantly fewer patients with unplanned readmissions in the laparoscopy group: 1 (3%) versus 8 (27%), $P = 0.026$. Additional interventions were required in 2 (7%) patients in the laparoscopy group (percutaneous drainage) and in 9 (30%) patients in the conservative group (surgery), $P = 0.042$. Recurrent abscesses and failure to respond to conservative treatment were the main reasons for additional interventions. Open surgery was required in 3 (10%) patients in the laparoscopy group and in 4 (13%) patients in the conservative group. Postoperative complications occurred in 3 patients in laparoscopic group versus 2 patients in the conservative group. The rate of uneventful recovery was 90% in the laparoscopy group versus 50% in the conservative group, $P = 0.002$.

Conclusions.—Laparoscopic surgery in experienced hands is safe and feasible first-line treatment for appendiceal abscess. It is associated with fewer readmissions and fewer additional interventions than conservative treatment with comparable hospital stay (Table 3).

▶ Globally there has been a trend toward conservative management of all conditions related to appendicitis. Many have advocated the use of percutaneous drainage and antibiotics for patients who present late with an appendiceal

TABLE 3.—Outcome Within 60 Days From Randomization

	Laparoscopy Group	Conservative Group	*P*
Attempted procedure failed,* n	4 (13%)	9 (30%)	0.209
Length of stay (primary), d	3 (3–5)	3 (2–4)	0.228
Length of stay (60 day),† d	4 (3–5)	5 (3–8)	0.105
Readmission, n	1 (3%)	8 (27%)	**0.026**
Recurrent or residual abscess between day 7–60	3 (10%)	8 (27%)	0.181
Additional intervention, n	2 (7%)	9 (30%)	**0.042**
Unplanned operation	0 (0%)	9 (30%)	**0.002**
Repeated CT scan	3 (10%)	13 (43%)	**0.007**
Uneventful recovery	27 (90%)	15 (50%)	**0.002**

Bold values indicate statistically significant.

*Appendectomy failed (no appendectomy or subtotal appendectomy performed) in the laparoscopy group or attempted drainage of abscess failed in the conservative group.

†T test for normally distributed data used.

Reprinted from Mentula P, Sammalkorpi H, Leppäniemi A. Laparoscopic surgery or conservative treatment for appendiceal abscess in adults? A randomized controlled trial. *Ann Surg.* 2015;262:237-242, with permission from Wolters Kluwer Health, Inc.

abscess. This randomized study suggests that early laparoscopy with drainage and appendectomy may be a better approach, limiting the need for subsequent procedures and readmissions (Table 3). Only half of the patients who were randomized to percutaneous drainage had an uneventful recovery, whereas 90% of those who underwent laparoscopic surgery first recovered without incident. Patients who had surgery first were more likely to have an incomplete appendectomy or require ileocecostomy. The authors also point out that in the case of an underlying malignancy as a cause of the presentation, surgery first makes sense, diagnosing these patients earlier so that definitive treatment can be established. This well-designed study appears to be pushing the pendulum back toward surgery for complex appendicitis.

O. J. Hines, MD, FACS

Clinical Health Service Research on the Surgical Therapy of Acute Appendicitis: Comparison of Outcomes Based on 3 German Multicenter Quality Assurance Studies Over 21 Years

Sahm M, Pross M, Otto R, et al (Otto von Guericke Univ, Magdeburg, Germany; DRK Kliniken Berlin Köpenick, Germany)

Ann Surg 262:338-346, 2015

Objective.—The treatment of acute appendicitis has seen changes in diagnosis and therapy in Germany. The objective of this analysis was to assess changes in therapy and outcome after open appendectomy (OA) and laparoscopic appendectomy (LA) over the last 21 years.

Background.—The analysis was based on 3 prospective multicenter quality assurance studies conducted by the Institute for Quality Control in Operative Medicine of the University of Magdeburg.

Methods.—All inpatients with a diagnosis of appendicitis in these studies (1988/1989, 1996/1997, 2008/2009) were included. Multiple linear and logistic regression analyses were performed. Statistical significance was set at $P < 0.05$.

Results.—Data from 17,732 treatments of patients diagnosed with appendicitis were collected. The average age of patients increased between the 3 studies from 25.7 to 34.6 years ($P < 0.001$). The preoperative selection of LA or OA was based on American Society of Anesthesiologists' classification ($P < 0.001$). Between 1996/1997 and 2008/2009, the share of LA climbed from 33.1% to 85.8% ($P < 0.001$). In the study from 2008 to 2009, LA showed a significant advantage over the conventional technique in wound healing disturbances ($P < 0.001$) and the clinical duration of stay ($P < 0.001$). At no stage of appendix inflammation did LA significantly increase intra-abdominal abscesses. The use of a stapler is currently the most common method of appendiceal stump closure (83.6%).

Conclusions.—Changes in patient data reflected demographic changes. Preoperative selection leads to 2 clearly defined groups. LA is the most dominant method of current operative therapy. The negative selection in OA group has influenced the worse outcome of that group.

▶ Appendectomy remains one of the most common surgical procedures worldwide despite recent trends to address this condition with antibiotics alone. Over the past decade, there has been a shift from open to laparoscopic appendectomy, and this article details this change in Germany. The study confirms that the postoperative abscess rate and bowel obstruction, along with hospital stay, is lower with laparoscopic surgery. Incidences of bleeding were higher in the laparoscopic group. An interesting finding focused on the method of closure/transection of the appendiceal stump. Postoperative abscess was equal between the use of endoloops or staplers, but the use of a clip resulted in higher rates of postoperative abscesses. The authors conclude that laparoscopic appendectomy is the standard of care for this disease, while open appendectomy remains a feature of treatment. However, it looks as though Germany has some ways to go with regard to length of stay after this procedure because most patients required a minimum of 5 days of hospitalization after laparoscopic surgery.

O. J. Hines, MD, FACS

Ketorolac Use and Postoperative Complications in Gastrointestinal Surgery

Kotagal M, Hakkarainen TW, Simianu VV, et al (Univ of Washington, Seattle; et al)

Ann Surg 263:71-75, 2016

Objective.—To study the association between ketorolac use and postoperative complications.

Background.—Nonsteroidal anti-inflammatory drugs may impair wound healing and increase the risk of anastomotic leak in colon surgery. Studies to date have been limited by sample size, inability to identify confounding, and a focus limited to colon surgery.

Methods.—Ketorolac use, reinterventions, emergency department (ED) visits, and readmissions in adults (≥18 years) undergoing gastrointestinal (GI) operations was assessed in a nationwide cohort using the MarketScan Database (2008–2012).

Results.—Among 398,752 patients (median age 52, 45% male), 55% underwent colorectal surgery, whereas 45% had noncolorectal GI surgery. Five percent of patients received ketorolac. Adjusting for demographic characteristics, comorbidities, surgery type/indication, and preoperative medications, patients receiving ketorolac had higher odds of reintervention (odds ratio [OR] 1.20, 95% confidence interval [CI] 1.08–1.32), ED visit (OR 1.44, 95% CI 1.37–1.51), and readmission within 30 days (OR 1.11, 95% CI 1.05–1.18) compared to those who did not receive ketorolac. Ketorolac use was associated with readmissions related to anastomotic complications (OR 1.20, 95% CI 1.06−1.36). Evaluating only admissions with ≤3 days duration to exclude cases where ketorolac might have been used for complication-related pain relief, the odds of complications associated with ketorolac were even greater.

Conclusions.—Use of intravenous ketorolac was associated with greater odds of reintervention, ED visit, and readmission in both colorectal and noncolorectal GI surgery. Given this confirmatory evaluation of other reports of a negative association and the large size of this cohort, clinicians should exercise caution when using ketorolac in patients undergoing GI surgery (Fig 1).

▶ Perioperative pain control is an important factor in determining length of stay, readmission, and patient satisfaction. In addition, significant data now exist suggesting that a meaningful number of patients become addicted to narcotics in the postoperative period. Nonsteroidal anti-inflammatory drugs (NSAIDs) offer an important adjunct to pain control. This study examined a large database from insurance claims and included an analysis of patients undergoing gastrointestinal surgery. The aim was to determine the outcomes of those who received ketorolac. Patients who received this drug where 44% more likely to have an emergency department visit within 30 days of the operation, 11% more likely to require readmission, and 20% more likely to require a reintervention (Fig 1). NSAIDs do have the potential to inhibit wound healing

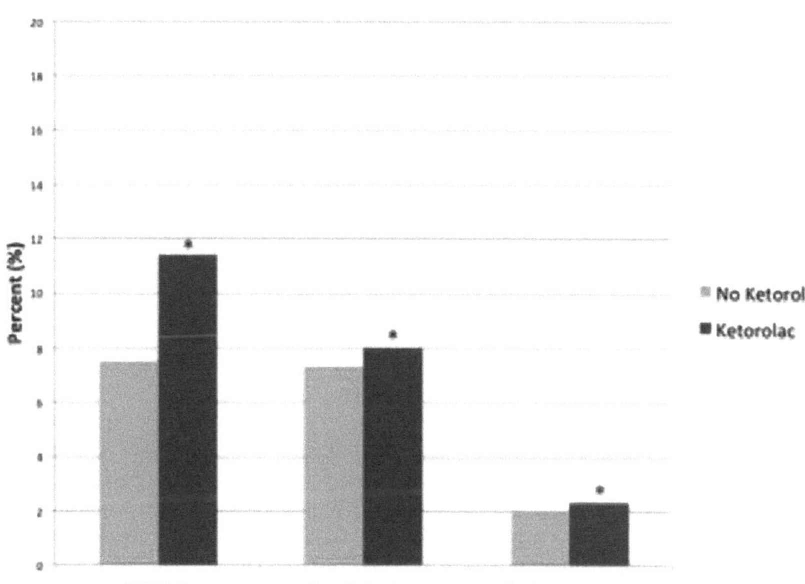

FIGURE 1.—Unadjusted rate of ED visit, readmission, and reintervention within 30 days by ketorolac use.(Reprinted from Kotagal M, Hakkarainen TW, Simianu VV, et al. Ketorolac use and postoperative complications in gastrointestinal surgery. *Ann Surg.* 2016;263:71-75, with permission from Wolters Kluwer Health, Inc.)

through the inhibition of cyclo-oxygenase attenuating granulocyte function, epithelial cell migration, and intestinal restitution. These factors are critical components for proper healing of an intestinal anastomosis. Where the findings of this study are causal or correlative cannot be answered by this analysis, but the implications are important.

O. J. Hines, MD, FACS

Thromboembolic Complications and Prophylaxis Patterns in Colorectal Surgery

Colorectal Writing Group for the Surgical Care and Outcomes Assessment Program—Comparative Effectiveness Research Translation Network (SCOAP-CERTAIN) Collaborative (Madigan Army Med Ctr, Fort Lewis, Washington; et al)

JAMA Surg 150:712-720, 2015

Importance.—Venous thromboembolism (VTE) is an important complication of colorectal surgery, but its incidence is unclear in the era of VTE prophylaxis.

Objective.—To describe the incidence of and risk factors associated with thromboembolic complications and contemporary VTE prophylaxis patterns following colorectal surgery.

Design, Setting, and Participants.—Prospective data from the Washington State Surgical Care and Outcomes Assessment Program (SCOAP) linked to a statewide hospital discharge database. At 52 Washington State SCOAP hospitals, participants included consecutive patients undergoing colorectal surgery between January 1, 2006, and December 31, 2011.

Main Outcomes and Measures.—Venous thromboembolism complications in-hospital and up to 90 days after surgery.

Results.—Among 16 120 patients (mean age, 61.4 years; 54.5% female), the use of perioperative and in-hospital VTE chemoprophylaxis increased significantly from 31.6% to 86.4% and from 59.6% to 91.4%, respectively, by 2011 ($P < .001$ for trend for both). Overall, 10.6% (1399 of 13 230) were discharged on a chemoprophylaxis regimen. The incidence of VTE was 2.2% (360 of 16 120). Patients undergoing abdominal operations had higher rates of 90-day VTE compared with patients having pelvic operations (2.5% [246 of 9702] vs 1.8% [114 of 6413], $P = .001$). Those having an operation for cancer had a similar incidence of 90-day VTE compared with those having an operation for nonmalignant processes (2.1% [128 of 6213] vs 2.3% [232 of 9902], $P = .24$). On adjusted analysis, older age, nonelective surgery, history of VTE, and operations for inflammatory disease were associated with increased risk of 90-day VTE ($P < .05$ for all). There was no significant decrease in VTE over time.

Conclusions and Relevance.—Venous thromboembolism rates are low and largely unchanged despite increases in perioperative and postoperative prophylaxis. These data should be considered in developing future guidelines.

▶ Are you using venous thromboembolism (VTE) prophylaxis in your patients who are undergoing colon and rectal surgery. Many publications suggest that this is an imperative, and the American College of Chest Physicians' guidelines set the standard.[1] This article documents the trends in VTE prophylaxis in the state of Washington (Fig 1 in the original article). A couple of interesting points are made. The incidence of perioperative VTE (2.2%) did not change over the study period despite a steady rise in the use of prophylaxis. About 40% of VTEs occurred after discharge suggesting that an area for improvement may be to increase the use of prophylaxis for 90 days postoperatively as many have suggested. Finally, the patients who received chemoprophylaxis did have a higher rate of postoperative blood transfusion, but not reoperation for bleeding. Specific guidelines regarding VTE prophylaxis for colorectal surgery are largely based on a Cochrane review,[2] which concluded that the optimal prophylaxis in colorectal surgery is the combination of graduated compression stockings and low molecular weight heparin. Clearly the ultimate recommendations for this area have not yet been established, and we will need to keep abreast of the latest updates.

O. J. Hines, MD, FACS

References

1. Pannucci CJ, Laird S, Dimick JB, Campbell DA, Henke PK. A validated risk model to predict 90-day VTE events in postsurgical patients. *Chest.* 2014;145:567-573.
2. Wille-Jørgensen P, Rasmussen MS, Andersen BR, Borly L. Heparins and mechanical methods for thromboprophylaxis in colorectal surgery. *Cochrane Database Syst Rev.* 2003;(4):CD001217.

Treatment options for chylous ascites after major abdominal surgery: a systematic review

Weniger M, D'Haese JG, Angele MK, et al (Ludwig-Maximilians-Univ, Munich, Germany)

Am J Surg 211:206-213, 2016

Background.—Chylous leakage is a relevant clinical problem after major abdominal surgery leading to an increased length of stay.

Data Sources.—A systematic search of MEDLINE/PubMed and the Cochrane Library was performed according to the PRISMA statement. The search for the MeSH terms "chylous ascites" and/ or "lymphatic fistula" retrieved a total of 2,348 articles, of which 36 full-text articles were reviewed by 2 independent investigators.

Results.—Chylous ascites is described with an incidence of up to 11%, especially after pancreatic surgery. The incidence is increasing with the number of lymph nodes harvested. In patients treated with total parenteral nutrition, conservative treatment is demonstrated to be effective in up to 100% of cases.

Conclusions.—The extent of abdominal surgery mainly predicts the risk of chylous ascites. Conservative treatment has been shown to be effective in almost all cases and is the treatment of choice.

▶ Postoperative chylous ascites is rare, but when it occurs, it can be difficult to resolve and, on occasion, it can be life threatening. The literature regarding this problem is limited because of the infrequent nature of the condition. This article performed a systematic review of the available data and provides some important clues to evaluation and management. Overall this is a rare condition, but predispose to this include a concomitant vascular resection, extensive nodal dissection, manipulation of the paraaortic area, retroperitoneal tumor invasion, and higher blood loss. The diagnosis is made by the assessment of the fluid with low levels of amylase and bilirubin and high levels of chylomicrons and triglyceride concentrations above 110 mg/dL. Total parenteral nutrition and strict nothing by mouth feeding appears to be particularly effective, with reported rates of resolution approaching 100% in 10 to 15 days. Others report a resolution rate of 75% with a medium chain triglyceride diet and this can be increase to 100% with the addition of somatostatin. For those cases in which the ascites does not resolve, a peritoneovenous shunt has been reported, although with high complication rates. Small cases series have advocated lymphangiography with embolization of the lymphatics or cisterna chyli.

O. J. Hines, MD, FACS

The effect of mechanical bowel preparation on anastomotic leaks in elective left-sided colorectal resections

Elnahas A, Urbach D, Lebovic G, et al (Univ of Toronto, Ontario, Canada; St. Michael's Hosp, Toronto, Ontario, Canada)

Am J Surg 210:793-798, 2015

Background.—Routine preoperative mechanical bowel preparation (MBP) for left-sided colorectal resections remains controversial. This study aims to evaluate the association between MBP and 30-day anastomotic leaks.

Methods.—A retrospective cohort study was conducted using data from the National Surgical Quality Improvement Program from 2011 to 2012. Multiple imputation was used for missing data, and a multivariable logistic regression was performed to adjust for clinically relevant variables. A propensity score–adjusted model was performed as a sensitivity analysis.

Results.—A total of 2,581 patients (57%) received preoperative MBP, whereas 1,935 (43%) did not. The 30-day anastomotic leak rate with and without preoperative MBP was 3.1% and 5.1%, respectively. After covariate adjustment, MBP omission was significantly associated with a

40% increased odds of 30-day anastomotic leaks (odds ratio 1.41, $P = .04$, 95% confidence interval 1.01 to 1.93).

Conclusions.—MBP omission was associated with a higher rate of 30-day anastomotic leaks. A large, well-designed, randomized controlled trial is needed to further evaluate this relationship.

▶ For years, it was routine to prep patients before colon surgery with oral antibiotics and a mechanical preparation. Then about 10 years ago, data came forward to suggest that there was no advantage to this with regard to anastomotic leak rates and overall complications. A Cochrane review on this subject concluded that mechanical bowel preparation elective colorectal surgery has no effect on lowering anastomotic leakage rates.[1] This study, however, has found the opposite. The analysis of National Surgical Quality Improvement Program data including nearly 5500 patients found that patients who underwent a mechanical bowel preparation were 40% less likely to have an anastomotic leak (odds ratio [OR] 1.40; $P = .04$, 95% confidence interval [CI] 1.01-1.93). In addition to this, the authors found that patients on chronic steroids had a much higher leak rate (OR 2.58; $P < .01$; 95% CI, 1.31-5.08). Finally patients who had received chemotherapy tended to have a higher leak rate. I have always used a mechanical bowel prep with either Golytely or magnesium citrate along with neomycin and erythromycin base the day before operation as long as the patient was not obstructed. Funny how practices ebb and flow through the arc of one's career in surgery.

O. J. Hines, MD, FACS

Reference

1. Guenaga KF, Matos D, Wille-Jørgensen P. Mechanical bowel preparation for elective colorectal surgery. *Cochrane Database Syst Rev.* 2011;(9):CD001544.

Nonsteroidal Anti-inflammatory Drugs: Do They Increase the Risk of Anastomotic Leaks Following Colorectal Operations?

Paulasir S, Kaoutzanis C, Welch KB, et al (Saint Joseph Mercy Health System, Ann Arbor, MI; Univ of Michigan, Ann Arbor; et al)
Dis Colon Rectum 58:870-877, 2015

Background.—Nonsteroidal anti-inflammatory drugs have become an important component of narcotic-sparing postoperative pain management protocols. However, conflicting evidence exists regarding the adverse association of nonsteroidal anti-inflammatory drug use with intestinal anastomotic healing in colorectal surgery.

Objective.—This study compares patients receiving nonsteroidal anti-inflammatory drugs on postoperative day 1 with patients who did not receive nonsteroidal anti-inflammatory drugs with regard to the occurrence of anastomotic leaks.

Design.—This is a retrospective study from a protocol-driven prospectively collected statewide database. A propensity score model was used to adjust for differences between the groups in patient demographics, characteristics, comorbidities, and laboratory values.

Settings.—The multicenter data set used in this analysis represents a variety of academic and community hospitals within the state of Michigan from July 2012 through February 2014.

Patients.—Nonpregnant patients over the age of 18 who underwent colon and rectal surgery with bowel anastomosis were selected.

Main Outcome Measures.—Occurrence of anastomotic leak, composite surgical site infection, sepsis, and death within 30 days of surgery were the primary outcomes measured.

Results.—A total of 4360 patients met inclusion criteria, of which 1297 (29.7%) received nonsteroidal anti-inflammatory drugs and 3063 (70.3%) did not receive nonsteroidal anti-inflammatory drugs. There was no statistically significant difference between the 2 groups in the proportion of cases with anastomotic leak (OR, 1.33; CI, 0.86–2.05; $p = 0.20$), composite surgical site infection (OR, 1.26; CI, 0.96–1.66; $p = 0.09$), or death within 30 days (OR, 0.58; CI, 0.28–1.19; $p = 0.14$). There was a significantly greater risk of sepsis for patients given nonsteroidal anti-inflammatory drugs than for those patients not given nonsteroidal anti-inflammatory drugs (OR, 1.47; CI, 1.05–2.06; $p = 0.03$).

Limitations.—This is a nonrandomized study performed retrospectively, and it is based on data collected only within a subset of hospitals in the state of Michigan.

Conclusions.—No statistically significant increase in the proportion of patients with anastomotic leak was observed when prescribing nonsteroidal anti-inflammatory drugs for analgesia in the early postoperative period for patients undergoing elective colorectal surgery. Unexpectedly, there was an increased risk of sepsis that warrants further investigation (see video, Supplemental Digital Content 1, http://links.lww.com/DCR/A192, for a synopsis of this study) (Table 3).

▶ Do you prescribe nonsteroidal anti-inflammatory drugs (NSAIDs) to your patients postoperatively to manage pain? Many of us do, and this is a very effective way to provide pain relief without the negative effects of narcotics. NSAIDs do have other effects but primarily work as inhibitors of prostanoids. This group examined the impact of anastomotic in patients receiving NSAIDs. They used the statewide Michigan database and the study included more than 4000 patients who were undergoing largely colonic procedures. Luckily they found no difference in the rate of leak, surgical site infection, or death in patients using NSAIDS (Table 3). There was an increased rate of sepsis though in the patients taking NSAIDS. The data regarding anastomosis healed true when different sites/levels of anastomoses were analyzed. Many have postulated that NSAIDs would have an impact because of the potential inhibitory influence these may have on the wound healing process. This does not appear to be the case for the anastomosis, but these drugs may have other effects that the

TABLE 3.—Comparison of the Outcomes of Interest Between NSAID and Non-NSAID Groups

Outcomes of Interest	NSAID n (%)	Non-NSAID n (%)	Unadjusted OR[a] (95% CI)	*p*	Adjusted OR[b] (95% CI)	*p*
Anastomotic leak	37 (2.9)	79 (2.6)	1.17 (0.75–1.66)	0.61	1.33 (0.86–2.05)	0.20
Any SSI	108 (8.3)	279 (9.1)	0.91 (0.72–1.15)	0.41	1.26 (0.96–1.66)	0.09
Sepsis	68 (5.2)	165 (5.4)	0.98 (0.73–1.3)	0.85	1.47 (1.05–2.06)	0.03
Death within 30 days	10 (0.8)	74 (2.4)	0.33 (0.17–0.63)	<0.01	0.58 (0.28–1.19)	0.14
Total number of subjects	1297	3063				

NSAID = nonsteroidal anti-inflammatory drug; SSI = surgical site infection.
[a]Unadjusted OR: odds ratio for NSAID versus non-NSAID groups.
[b]Adjusted OR: odds ratio for NSAID versus non-NSAID groups based on a generalized linear mixed model, after adjusting for significant predictors of each outcome and propensity score quintile, and including hospital as a random effect.
Reprinted from Paulasir S, Kaoutzanis C, Welch KB, et al. Nonsteroidal anti-inflammatory drugs: do they increase the risk of anastomotic leaks following colorectal operations? *Dis Colon Rectum.* 201558:870-877, with permission from The American Society of Colon & Rectal Surgeons, Inc.

surgeon will need to consider when prescribing NSAIDS in the postoperative period.

O. J. Hines, MD, FACS

High-Dose Barium Impaction Therapy for the Recurrence of Colonic Diverticular Bleeding: A Randomized Controlled Trial

Nagata N, Niikura R, Shimbo T, et al (International Clinical Res Ctr Res Inst, Tokyo, Japan; et al)
Ann Surg 261:269-275, 2015

Objective.—We compared the clinical efficacy of barium therapy and conservative therapy in preventing recurrence in patients with diverticular bleeding.

Background.—Previous case reports have indicated that barium impaction therapy provides initial hemostasis for diverticular bleeding and prevention against rebleeding.

Methods.—After spontaneous cessation of bleeding, patients were randomly assigned to conservative treatment (n = 27) or high-dose barium impaction therapy (n = 27). Patients were followed up for 1 year after enrollment of the last patient. The main outcome measure was rebleeding.

Results.—Median follow-up period was 584.5 days. The probability of rebleeding at 30-day, 180-day, 1-year, and 2-year follow-up in all patients was 3.7%, 14.8%, 28.4%, and 32.7%, respectively. By group, probability at 1 year was 42.5% in the conservative group and 14.8% in the barium group (log-rank test, $P = 0.04$). After adjustment for a history of hypertension, the hazard ratio of rebleeding in the barium group was 0.34 (95% confidence interval, 0.12–0.98). No complications or laboratory abnormalities due to barium therapy were observed. Compared with the conservative group, the barium group had significantly ($P < 0.05$) fewer hospitalizations per patient (1.7 vs 1.2), units of blood transfused (1.9 vs 0.7), colonoscopies (1.4 times vs 1.1 times), and hospital stay days (15 days vs 11 days) during the follow-up period. No patients died and none required angiographic or surgical procedures in either group.

Conclusions.—High-dose barium impaction therapy was effective in the long-term prevention of recurrent bleeding, and reduced the frequency of rehospitalization and need for blood transfusion and colonoscopic examination. ClinicalTrials.gov Identifier, UMIN 000002832 (Figs 1 and 3B).

▶ Lower gastrointestinal (GI) bleeding remains a vexing problem characterized by difficulty in identifying the source, controlling the vessel, and preventing rebleeding. Sometimes surgeons are called in to consider a colectomy, but the risk is high and the outcome unpredictable if the source has not been definitively established. The majority of lower GI bleeding is due to colonic diverticula and an arterial source. This study used high-pressure barium enema to fill diverticula with barium and prevent rebleeding. This intervention was extremely effective cutting the rate of rebleeding from 42.5% to 14.8% at 1 year (Fig 3B). The authors used a high concentration enema with tap water placing the bag at 3 to 4 feet above the patient. The patient was then asked to rotate in a stepwise fashion from prone, left lateral, supine, to right lateral position to ensure filling of each diverticulum (Fig 1). There were no complications in the group that

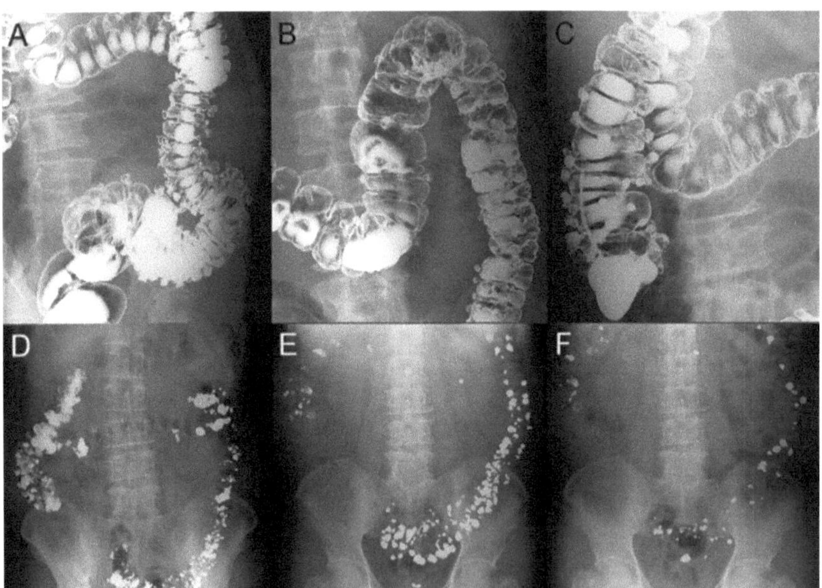

FIGURE 1.—X-ray findings of colonic diverticula. X-ray revealing multiple diverticula in the sigmoid colon (A), descending and transverse colon (B), and ascending colon at (C) 1 day (D), 2 months (E), and 6 months (F) after barium impaction therapy. (Reprinted from Nagata N, Niikura R, Shimbo T, et al. High-dose barium impaction therapy for the recurrence of colonic diverticular bleeding: a randomized controlled trial. *Ann Surg*. 2015;261:269-275, with permission from Wolters Kluwer Health, Inc.)

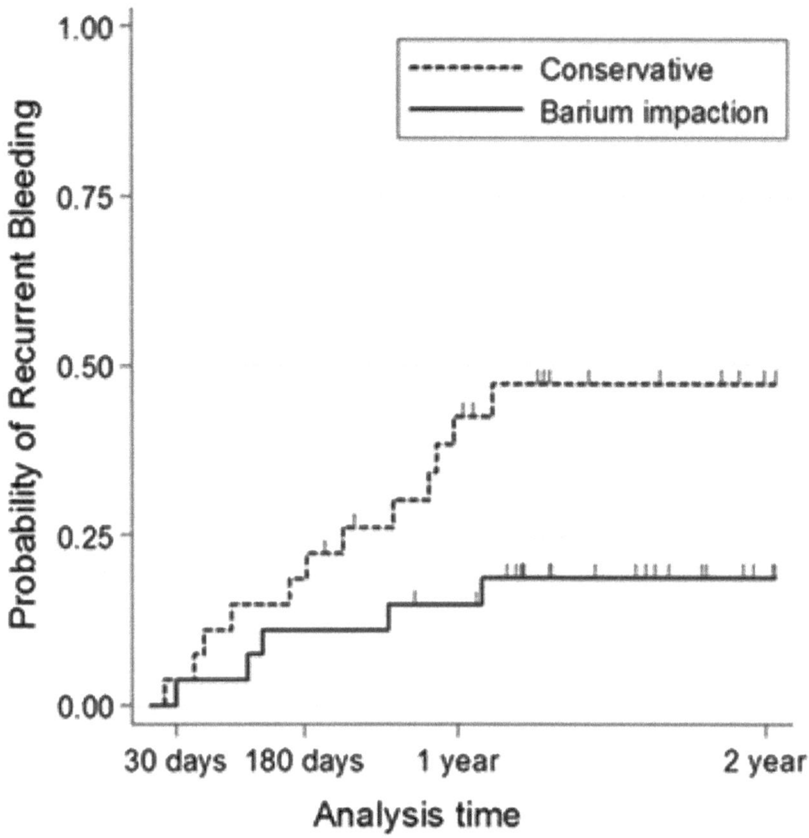

FIGURE 3.—Probability of recurrent bleeding. (B) Probability of rebleeding was significantly higher in the barium group than in the conservative group ($P = 0.04$). (Reprinted from Nagata N, Niikura R, Shimbo T, et al. High-dose barium impaction therapy for the recurrence of colonic diverticular bleeding: a randomized controlled trial. *Ann Surg*. 2015;261:269-275, with permission from Wolters Kluwer Health, Inc.)

received the impaction therapy. The authors propose that this method works by tamponade of the bleeding vessel, a direct hemostatic effect of the barium, and protection of the diverticulum from colonic fluids. This approach is an interesting concept and another option for this difficult condition.

O. J. Hines, MD, FACS

Cost-effectiveness of Enhanced Recovery Versus Conventional Perioperative Management for Colorectal Surgery

Lee L, Mata J, Ghitulescu GA, et al (McGill Univ Health Centre, Montreal, Quebec, Canada; Sir Mortimer B. Davis Jewish General Hosp, Montreal, Quebec, Canada; et al)

Ann Surg 262:1026-1033, 2015

Objective.—To determine the cost-effectiveness of enhanced recovery pathways (ERPs) versus conventional care for patients undergoing elective colorectal surgery.

Background.—ERPs for colorectal surgery are clinically effective, but their cost-effectiveness is unknown.

Methods.—A multi-institutional prospective cohort cost-effectiveness analysis was performed. Adult patients undergoing elective colorectal resection at 2 university-affiliated institutions from October 2012 to October 2013 were enrolled. One center used an ERP, whereas the other did not. Postoperative outcomes were recorded up to 60 days. Total costs were reported in 2013 Canadian dollars. Effectiveness was measured using the SF-6D, a health utility measure validated for postoperative recovery. Uncertainty was expressed using bootstrapped estimates (10,000 repetitions).

Results.—A total of 190 patients were included (conventional care: n = 95; ERP: n = 95). There were no differences in patient characteristics except for a higher proportion of laparoscopy in the ERP group. Mean length of stay was shorter in the ERP group (6.5 vs 9.8 days; $P = 0.017$), but there were no differences in complications or readmissions. Patients in the ERP group returned to work quicker and had less caregiver burden. There was no difference in quality of life between the 2 groups. The cost of the ERP program was $153 per patient. Overall societal costs were lower in the ERP group (mean difference = −2985; 95% confidence interval, −5753 to −373). The ERP had a greater than 99% probability of cost-effectiveness. The results were insensitive to a range of assumptions and subgroups.

Conclusions.—Enhanced recovery is cost-effective compared with conventional perioperative management for elective colorectal resection (Table 1).

▶ Early recovery pathways have been discussed and championed for some time, but these have not made it to prime time for many surgical patients. The protocolization of these programs usually results in much improved outcomes and shorter hospital stay.[1] This group examined an early recovery pathway for colorectal patients included preoperative patient education and preparation for surgery; attenuation of the surgical stress response, pain, and postoperative nausea and vomiting through anesthetic, analgesic, and surgical techniques; and aggressive early postoperative mobilization, enteral feeding, and avoidance or early removal of drains and tubes (Table 1). Patients who received this pathway had a decrease in hospital stay by more than 3 days, and this did not result

TABLE 1.—Comparison of Perioperative Management Between CC and ERP

CC	ERP
Preoperative management	
Medical optimization of risk factors	Medical optimization of risk factors
No formal patient education	Psychological preparation for surgery and postoperative recovery: oral and written explanation of perioperative pathway, diet and ambulation plan, presence of drains, expectation about duration of hospital stay (3–4 d)
No instructions for preoperative exercise given	Physical preparation with exercises at home: anaerobic and resistance 1–2 hr/d, gradual increase from 50% to 80% of maximum capacity, breathing exercises
Nil per os starting midnight before surgery	Carbohydrate loading drink the night before and the morning of surgery. Clear fluids allowed until 2 hr before general anesthesia
Variable use of oral bowel preparation	Oral bowel preparation only if diverting ileostomy or intraoperative colonoscopy planned
Variable use of sedation routine	No preoperative sedation
Intraoperative management	
Antibiotic and DVT prophylaxis	Antibiotic and DVT prophylaxis
Maintain normothermia	Maintain normothermia
IV infusion as per anesthesia	Avoid overhydration (6 mL/kg/hr)
Insert an epidural catheter at the discretion of the anesthetist	Insert an epidural catheter routinely for open or laparoscopic rectal procedures, and local anesthetic infiltration of surgical incision
No routine nasogastric or abdominal drainage	No routine nasogastric or abdominal drainage
No routine prophylactic antiemetics	Routine prophylactic antiemetics
Postoperative management	
Clear fluids starting after flatus, daily progression to diet as tolerated	Fluids (including 2 cans of Ensure) on POD0, diet as tolerated starting POD1
No structured mobilization plan	Structured mobilization: Patient encouraged to sit in a chair on POD0. Mobilization goal of at least 6 hr starting POD1
Urinary drainage catheter kept until epidural analgesia removed	Urinary drainage catheter removed on POD1
IV fluids discontinued only after resumption of oral intake	IV fluids discontinued upon arrival onto surgical ward on POD0
Thoracic epidural analgesia or patient-controlled analgesia until resumption of oral intake and then transition to oral analgesia (opioids).	Thoracic epidural analgesia or patient-controlled analgesia until POD2 and then transition to multimodal analgesia (minimizing opioids)

DVT indicates deep vein thrombosis; IV, intravenous; POD, postoperative day.

Reprinted from Lee L, Mata J, Ghitulescu GA, et al. Cost-effectiveness of enhanced recovery versus conventional perioperative management for colorectal surgery. *Ann Surg*. 2015;262:1026-1033, with permission from Wolters Kluwer Health, Inc.

in a higher complication or readmission rate. Those patients on the early recovery pathway returned to work sooner, and the total cost to implement this pathway was $153 per patient. Choosing a bundle of items that can be used in your practice or inpatient facility can be tailored to the local issues, but almost always results in improved outcomes.

O. J. Hines, MD, FACS

Reference

1. Feldman LS, Baldini G, Lee L, et al. *Enhanced Recovery Pathways: Organization of Evidence-Based, Fast-Track Perioperative Care. ACS Surgery: Principles and Practices.* Hamilton, Canada: Decker Intellectual Properties; 2013.

Randomized clinical trial investigating the stress response from two different methods of analgesia after laparoscopic colorectal surgery

Day AR, Smith RVP, Scott MJP, et al (Univ of Surrey, Guildford, United Kingdom; et al)
Br J Surg 102:1473-1479, 2015

Background.—One of the key elements of managed recovery is thought to be suppression of the neuroendocrine response using regional analgesics. This may be superfluous in laparoscopic colorectal surgery with small wounds. This trial assessed the effects of spinal analgesia *versus* intravenous patient-controlled analgesia (PCA) on neuroendocrine responses in that setting.

Methods.—A randomized clinical trial was conducted with participation of patients undergoing laparoscopic colorectal surgery within a managed recovery programme. Consenting patients were allocated randomly to spinal analgesia or morphine PCA as primary postoperative analgesia. The primary outcome was interleukin (IL) 6 levels; secondary outcomes were levels of cortisol, glucose, insulin and other cytokines, pain scores, morphine use and length of hospital stay. Stress response analysis was conducted before operation, and 3, 6, 12, 24 and 48 h after surgery.

Results.—Of 143 eligible patients, 133 were randomized and 120 completed the study. Baseline patient characteristics were similar in the two groups. There were no significant differences in median levels of insulin, IL-2, IL-4, IL-6, IL-8, IL-10, IL-12, interferon γ, tumour necrosis factor α or vascular endothelial growth factor between the spinal analgesia and PCA groups at any time point. Three hours after surgery (but at no other time point) median (i.q.r.) levels of cortisol (468 (329–678) *versus* 701 (429–820) nmol/l; $P = 0.004$) and glucose (6.1 (5.4–7.5) *versus* 7.0 (6.0–7.7) mmol/l; $P = 0.012$) were lower in the spinal analgesia group than in the PCA group. Median (i.q.r.) levels of total intravenous morphine were lower in the spinal analgesia group (10.0 (3.3–15.8) *versus* 45.5 (34.0–60.5) mg; $P < 0.001$).

Conclusion.—Spinal analgesia reduced early neuroendocrine responses and overall parenteral morphine use. Registration number: NCT01128088 (http://www.clinicaltrials.gov).

▶ Many surgeons have adopted measures to limit intravenous narcotic use postoperatively with alternative methods to address pain in order to reduce complications and length of stay. This study examined the use of spinal anesthesia to inhibit the inflammatory response induced by surgery and improve outcomes in patients undergoing laparoscopic colorectal surgery. Patients either received a spinal injection or intravenous patient-controlled analgesia. A variety of serum inflammatory markers were checked, and no differences were observed, but patients who had spinal analgesia had lower cortisol levels postoperatively, less need for narcotic usage, and about a third of the complications of those patients who used the intravenous narcotics. This difference in complications was largely due to decreases in ileus. Whether this is an option in your practice or if you are able to adopt alternate methods of pain control depends on the setting, but there is little doubt that your outcomes will improve by addressing pain in a systematic fashion.

O. J. Hines, MD, FACS

Effect of Coffee on the Length of Postoperative Ileus After Elective Laparoscopic Left-Sided Colectomy: A Randomized, Prospective Single-Center Study

Dulskas A, Klimovskij M, Vitkauskiene M, et al (Natl Cancer Inst, Vilnius, Lithuania)

Dis Colon Rectum 58:1064-1069, 2015

Background.—Postoperative ileus is common problem after colorectal surgery. A positive effect of coffee to bowel movement has been described. It is still unclear whether coffee decreases the risk of postoperative ileus.

Objective.—The purpose of this study was to determine whether consuming a 100-mL cup of coffee is effective in preventing or reducing postoperative ileus.

Design.—This was a prospective, single-center, randomized controlled study.

Settings.—The study was conducted at a university teaching hospital.

Patients.—All of the patients who were scheduled for elective laparoscopic left-sided colectomy at our hospital after the detection of malignant disease in a preoperative biopsy between January 2013 and December 2014 entered the study. The patients were assigned randomly before surgery to receive coffee with caffeine (first group), coffee without caffeine (second group), or water (third group) after the procedure (100 mL 3 times daily).

Main Outcome Measures.—The primary end point was time to first bowel movement; secondary end points were time to first flatus and time to tolerance of solid food.

Results.—A total of 105 patients were randomly assigned, 35 to each group. Fifteen patients were excluded. Patient demographic characteristics were similar in the groups. The time until the first bowel movement (measured in days) was significantly ($p < 0.05$) shorter in the decaffeinated coffee group (3.00 ± 1.50) versus the coffee with caffeine (3.75 ± 1.53) and water groups (4.14 ± 1.14). The time until tolerance of solid food was significantly shorter in decaffeinated group versus coffee with caffeine and water groups (1.85 versus 2.60 and 2.80; $p < 0.05$). Time until the first flatus (1.47 versus 1.57 and 1.77 for decaffeinated coffee versus coffee with caffeine and water; $p > 0.05$) did not show statistical significance. Postoperative hospital stay was similar in all 3 of the groups.

Limitations.—This is a single-center study with a relatively small sample size.

Conclusions.—Coffee consumption after colectomy was safe and in the decaffeinated group associated with a reduced time to first bowel action. Caffeine is not a main ingredient affecting the length of postoperative ileus (Fig 2).

▶ Coffee to speed bowel activity after colon surgery? Yes—this is a randomized trial examining the use of coffee, decaffeinated coffee, or water to stimulate bowel activity. Many studies have been conducted to find a means to reverse postoperative ileus including early feeding, intravenous fluid restriction, chewing gum, early ambulation, carbohydrate-rich liquids, epidural analgesia, laparoscopic surgery, and new drugs. We all know though that coffee has a tendency to stimulate a bowel movement. The results of this study found that

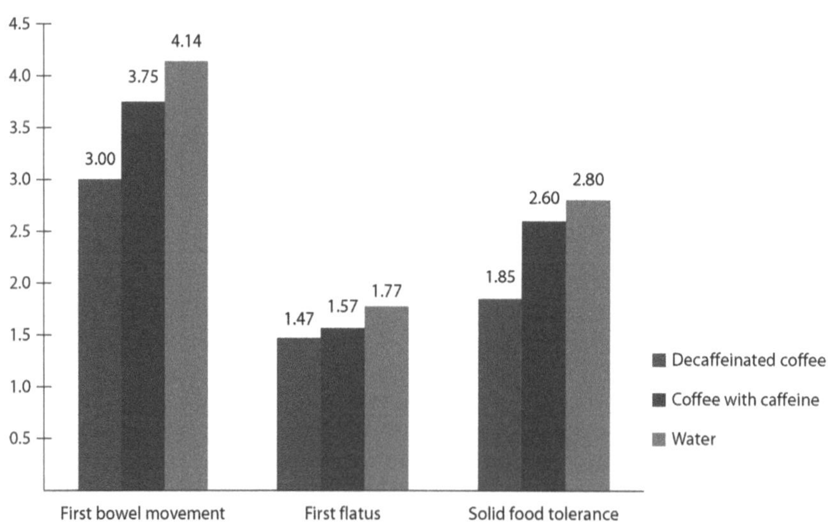

FIGURE 2.—Postoperative day for the selected criteria, $p < 0.05$. (Reprinted from Dulskas A, Klimovskij M, Vitkauskiene M, et al. Effect of coffee on the length of postoperative ileus after elective laparoscopic left-sided colectomy: a randomized, prospective single-center study. *Dis Colon Rectum.* 2015;58:1064-1069, with permission from The American Society of Colon & Rectal Surgeons, Inc.)

the time to first bowel movement with decaffeinated coffee was 3 days versus 3.75 days for coffee and 4.14 days in the water group (Fig 2). These differences were significantly significant. Each group drank 3 cups spread throughout the day (100 mL at 8:00 AM, 12:00 PM, and 4:00 PM starting the first morning after surgery). With efforts to decrease length of stay and efforts at fast tracking, this may be a very simple and likely very safe addition for your patients.

O. J. Hines, MD, FACS

International, Expert-Based, Consensus Statement Regarding the Management of Acute Diverticulitis

O'Leary DP, Lynch N, Clancy C, et al (Galway Univ Hosp, Ireland)
JAMA Surg 150:899-904, 2015

Importance.—This Delphi study provides consensus related to many aspects of acute diverticulitis and identifies other areas in need of research.

Objective.—To generate an international, expert-based, consensus statement to address controversies in the management of acute diverticulitis.

Design, Setting, and Participants.—This study was conducted using the Delphi technique from April 3 through October 21, 2014. A survey website was used and a panel of acute diverticulitis experts was formed via the snowball method. The top 5 acute diverticulitis experts in 5 international geographic regions were identified based on their number of publications related to acute diverticulitis.

Interventions.—The Delphi study used 3 rounds of questions, after which the consensus statement was collated.

Main Outcomes and Measures.—A consensus statement related to the management of acute diverticulitis.

Results.—Twenty items were selected for inclusion in the consensus statement following 3 rounds of questioning. A clear definition of uncomplicated and complicated diverticulitis is provided. In uncomplicated diverticulitis, consensus was reached regarding appropriate laboratory and radiological evaluation of patients as well as nonsurgical, surgical, and follow-up strategies. A number of important topics, including antibiotic treatment, failed to reach consensus. In addition, consensus was reached regarding many nonsurgical and surgical treatment strategies in complicated diverticulitis.

Conclusions and Relevance.—Controversy continues internationally regarding the management of acute diverticulitis. This study demonstrates that there is more nonconsensus among experts than consensus regarding most issues, even in the same region. It also provides insight into the status quo regarding the treatment of acute diverticulitis and provides important direction for future research (Table 4).

► The management of acute diverticulitis has rapidly evolved to include a more nonoperative approach for patients with uncomplicated disease. Recent

TABLE 4.—Uncomplicated Diverticulitis Consensus Statements

Uncomplicated Diverticulitis
Definition
Is defined radiologically
Investigation
Laboratory
White blood cell count is a useful laboratory marker
Neutrophil count is a useful laboratory marker
C-reactive protein a useful laboratory marker
Radiology
An erect CR is not required where a CT abdomen and pelvis is planned
CT abdomen and pelvis should be part of the workup
Intravenous contrast should be part of the CT protocol
An ultrasound of the abdomen should be considered in a pregnant patient
Management
Nonsurgical
Can be managed safely in the outpatient setting
Surgical
Primary resection and anastomosis is the gold standard approach in the elective setting
Elective resections should be performed laparoscopically where appropriate
The decision to perform an elective resection is multifactorial
Follow-up
There is insufficient evidence available to support the role of a high-fiber diet to prevent recurrence
Mandatory colonoscopy is required with persistent symptoms with or without equivocal CT scan

Abbreviations: CR, chest radiograph; CT, computed tomographic scan.
Reprinted from O'Leary DP, Lynch N, Clancy C, et al. International, expert-based, consensus statement regarding the management of acute diverticulitis. *JAMA Surg*. 2015;150:899-904; with permission from American Medical Association.

evidence supports that patients with mild attacks may not even need antibiotics, suggesting that this disease may be a form of inflammatory bowel disease.[1] Clearly the rule that patients with 2 episodes of diverticulitis require surgical resection is no longer a tenant that most gastroenterologists and surgeons uphold. This article has attempted to provide international consensus on the current management of acute diverticulitis and propose 20 items that should be used to guide management decisions (Table 4). The consensus is to use CT scan, white blood cell count, neutrophil count, and C-reactive protein to establish the diagnosis and determine the level of severity. Whether antibiotics should be used for uncomplicated diverticulitis is still open to debate. The surgical management of uncomplicated diverticulitis is multifactorial and not based solely on the number of episodes. When surgery is recommended, a laparoscopic approach should be used, but in the setting of feculent peritonitis, a Hartmann procedure is recommended. Overall, there remains a significant variation in care for diverticulitis, and it will be important to stay up to date on this changing field.

O. J. Hines, MD, FACS

Reference

1. Chabok A, Påhlman L, Hjern F, Haapaniemi S, Smedh K, AVOD Study Group. Randomized clinical trial of antibiotics in acute uncomplicated diverticulitis. *Br J Surg*. 2012;99:532-539.

Laparoscopic Lavage vs Primary Resection for Acute Perforated Diverticulitis: The SCANDIV Randomized Clinical Trial

Schultz JK, for the SCANDIV Study Group (Akershus Univ Hosp, Lørenskog, Norway; et al)

JAMA 314:1364-1375, 2015

Importance.—Perforated colonic diverticulitis usually requires surgical resection, which is associated with significant morbidity. Cohort studies have suggested that laparoscopic lavage may treat perforated diverticulitis with less morbidity than resection procedures.

Objective.—To compare the outcomes from laparoscopic lavage with those for colon resection for perforated diverticulitis.

Design, Setting, and Participants.—Multicenter, randomized clinical superiority trial recruiting participants from 21 centers in Sweden and Norway from February 2010 to June 2014. The last patient follow-up was in December 2014 and final review and verification of the medical records was assessed in March 2015. Patients with suspected perforated diverticulitis, a clinical indication for emergency surgery, and free air on an abdominal computed tomography scan were eligible. Of 509 patients screened, 415 were eligible and 199 were enrolled.

Interventions.—Patients were assigned to undergo laparoscopic peritoneal lavage (n = 101) or colon resection (n = 98) based on a computer-generated, center-stratified block randomization. All patients with fecal peritonitis (15 patients in the laparoscopic peritoneal lavage group vs 13 in the colon resection group) underwent colon resection. Patients with a pathology requiring treatment beyond that necessary for perforated diverticulitis (12 in the laparoscopic lavage group vs 13 in the colon resection group) were also excluded from the protocol operations and treated as required for the pathology encountered.

Main Outcomes and Measures.—The primary outcome was severe postoperative complications (Clavien-Dindo score >IIIa) within 90 days. Secondary outcomes included other postoperative complications, reoperations, length of operating time, length of postoperative hospital stay, and quality of life.

Results.—The primary outcome was observed in 31 of 101 patients (30.7%) in the laparoscopic lavage group and 25 of 96 patients (26.0%) in the colon resection group (difference, 4.7% [95% CI, −7.9% to 17.0%]; *P* = .53). Mortality at 90 days did not significantly differ between the laparoscopic lavage group (14 patients [13.9%]) and the colon resection group (11 patients [11.5%]; difference, 2.4% [95% CI, −7.2% to 11.9%]; *P* = .67). The reoperation rate was significantly higher in the laparoscopic lavage group (15 of 74 patients [20.3%]) than in the colon resection group (4 of 70 patients [5.7%]; difference, 14.6% [95% CI, 3.5% to 25.6%]; *P* = .01) for patients who did not have fecal peritonitis. The length of operating time was significantly shorter in the laparoscopic lavage group; whereas, length of postoperative hospital stay and quality of life did not differ significantly between groups. Four sigmoid carcinomas were missed with laparoscopic lavage.

Conclusions and Relevance.—Among patients with likely perforated diverticulitis and undergoing emergency surgery, the use of laparoscopic lavage vs primary resection did not reduce severe postoperative complications and led to worse outcomes in secondary end points. These findings do not support laparoscopic lavage for treatment of perforated diverticulitis.

Trial Registration.—clinicaltrials.gov Identifier: NCT01047462.

▶ Diverticulitis is a complex disease to manage these days, with lots of different options. One can treat with probiotics, antibiotics, percutaneous drainage, laparoscopic lavage, laparoscopic or open resection with or without primary anastomosis, and with or without a diverting proximal stoma. Over the past few years, some have advocated the use of lavage alone, stating that this is all that is needed for patients without fecal peritonitis and that this avoids to possibility of a stoma and the complications that can come from resection. This randomized trial from the Netherlands suggests that this approach may not be a useful option and in some cases may lead to worse outcomes. Laparoscopic surgery did not reduce severe complications compared with the resection group, and length of stay was equal. What was most alarming was the finding that 4 carcinomas were missed in the lavage group. It seems like the pendulum has swung too far back to a time when 3-stage procedures were in vogue. We learned that the offending perforated colon required resection, and this approach was abandoned.

O. J. Hines, MD, FACS

A comparison of outcomes of emergent, urgent, and elective surgical treatment of diverticulitis

Moghadamyeghaneh Z, Carmichael JC, Smith BR, et al (Univ of California, Irvine)

Am J Surg 210:838-845, 2015

Background.—There is a controversy regarding the best urgent surgical treatment of colonic diverticulitis. We sought to compare outcomes of patients who underwent surgery for diverticulitis by the type of admission.

Methods.—The National Surgical Quality Improvement Program databases were used to examine the clinical data of patients who underwent colorectal resection for diverticulitis during 2012 to 2013. Multivariate regression analysis was performed to identify outcomes of patients.

Results.—We sampled a total of 13,510 patients admitted for diverticulitis who underwent colorectal resection, of which 7.8% had emergent and 19.7% had urgent operation. Patients with perforation (adjusted odds ratio [AOR] 188.56, $P < .01$) and preoperative sepsis (AOR 28.17,

$P < .01$) had significantly higher rates of emergent surgery. Patients who underwent emergent operation had higher mortality (AOR 4.08, $P = .04$) and morbidity (AOR 2.14, $P < .01$). Emergent operations had a significantly higher risk of anastomosis leakage compared with elective operation (AOR 3.92, $P = .02$).

Conclusions.—Emergent treatment of diverticulitis is associated with a high morbidity and mortality. In the setting of emergent treatment of diverticulitis, colonic anastomosis without a stoma has a high risk of anastomosis leakage (Table 5).

▶ Over the past decade, there has been significant discussion regarding the use of 1-stage operations for emergent rejections for diverticulitis. Many have published data that this is feasible with relative good outcomes. In addition the chance of a stoma being reversed is about 50%. This study examined the American College of Surgeons National Surgical Quality

TABLE 5.—Risk-Adjusted Analysis of Outcomes of Emergent, Urgent, and Elective Surgical Treatment of Diverticulitis in Laparoscopic Approach Compared with Open Approach

	Elective Surgery		Urgent Surgery		Emergent Surgery	
Complication	AOR and 95% CI	*P* Value	AOR and 95% CI	*P* Value	AOR and 95% CI	*P* Value
Mortality	1.13 (.27–4.79)	<.86	.15 (.05–.42)	<.01	.91 (.89–.93)	<.01
Overall morbidity	.43 (.37–.50)	<.01	.62 (.43–.90)	.01	.62 (.38–.99)	.04
Prolonged ileus	.41 (.33–.52)	<.01	.63 (.39–1.01)	.05	.85 (.49–1.48)	.57
Hemorrhagic complications	.59 (.42–.84)	<.01	.45 (.22–.91)	.02	.19 (.05–.66)	<.01
Return to operation room	.63 (.46–.86)	<.01	.58 (.24–1.36)	.21	.42 (.13–1.27)	.12
Wound disruption	.23 (.11–.48)	<.01	.20 (.02–1.69)	.14	.82 (.20–3.34)	.78
Deep vein thrombosis	.33 (.15–.73)	<.01	3.33 (.66–16.8)	.14	.68 (.08–5.46)	.71
Superficial SSI	.37 (.29–.47)	<.01	.99 (.48–2.02)	.98	.60 (.19–1.87)	.38
Deep incisional SSI	.30 (.16–.57)	<.01	.55 (.12–2.48)	.44	1.04 (.20–5.31)	.95
Unplanned readmission	.71 (.56–.91)	<.01	.80 (.45–1.41)	.44	.91 (.41–2)	.82
Hospitalization > 30 days	.34 (.14–.82)	.01	.54 (.14–2.07)	.37	.95 (.93–.96)	.03
Organ space SSI	.70 (.50–.99)	.04	.81 (.35–1.87)	.62	.97 (.41–2.29)	.94
Ventilator dependency	1.16 (.43–3.12)	.76	.47 (.08–2.56)	.38	.89 (.87–.91)	<.01
Acute renal failure	.26 (.05–1.33)	.10	.26 (.06–1.12)	.05	.91 (.90–.93)	.14
Myocardial infarction	.70 (.19–2.59)	.60	.99 (.98–.99)	.02	.99 (.98–1)	.43
Septic shock	.87 (.36–2.06)	.75	.37 (.06–2.24)	.28	.13 (.01–1.02)	.05
Unplanned intubation	.77 (.26–2.25)	.63	.23 (.02–2.04)	.19	.27 (.03–2.15)	.21
Pneumonia	.46 (.20–1.03)	.06	.23 (.02–2.51)	.23	1.35 (.44–4.12)	.58
Central vascular accident	.09 (.08–1.04)	.05	.99 (.99–1)	.13	.99 (.99–1)	.60
Anastomosis leakage*	.74 (.50–1.09)	.13	.27 (.06–1.13)	.07	1.14 (.11–11.59)	.91
Pulmonary embolism	.73 (.25–2.11)	.56	.45 (.03–5.98)	.54	.95 (.11–8.07)	.96
Cardiac arrest	.97 (.18–5.01)	.97	.22 (.03–1.71)	.11	.98 (.97–1)	.28
Urinary tract infection	.68 (.43–1.08)	.10	.37 (.10–1.39)	.14	.38 (.03–4)	.42

AOR = adjusted odds ratio; CI = confidence Interval; SSI = surgical site infection.

*Subanalysis of data in patients who had anastomosis without colostomy.

Reprinted from Moghadamyeghaneh Z, Carmichael JC, Smith BR, et al. A comparison of outcomes of emergent, urgent, and elective surgical treatment of diverticulitis. *Am J Surg*. 2015;210:838-845, with permission from Elsevier Inc.

Improvement Program database detailing the differences in outcomes between urgent, emergent, and elective colectomy for diverticulitis with some sobering findings. The mortality rate for emergent procedures was 6.9% and 0.2% for emergent and elective operations, respectively. The morbidity of an emergent operation was 61%, and for these patients who underwent a resection with primary anastomosis, the risk of leakage was higher with an odds ratio of 3.92 compared with patients undergoing elective resection. Of the patients who leaked, 64.3% required reoperation. Risk factors for a complication included American Society of Anesthesiologists class, renal failure, preoperative sepsis, perforation of the colon, and ascites (Table 5). The authors recommend that in the face of an emergent operation, if a primary anastomosis is performed, this may be best coupled with a diverting ileostomy.

O. J. Hines, MD, FACS

Effect of Laparoscopic-Assisted Resection vs Open Resection on Pathological Outcomes in Rectal Cancer: The ALaCaRT Randomized Clinical Trial

Stevenson ARL, for the ALaCaRT Investigators (Univ of Queensland, Brisbane, Australia; et al)

JAMA 314:1356-1363, 2015

Importance.—Laparoscopic procedures are generally thought to have better outcomes than open procedures. Because of anatomical constraints, laparoscopic rectal resection may not be better because of limitations in performing an adequate cancer resection.

Objective.—To determine whether laparoscopic resection is noninferior to open rectal cancer resection for adequacy of cancer clearance.

Design, Setting, and Participants.—Randomized, noninferiority, phase 3 trial (Australasian Laparoscopic Cancer of the Rectum; ALaCaRT) conducted between March 2010 and November 2014. Twenty-six accredited surgeons from 24 sites in Australia and New Zealand randomized 475 patients with T1-T3 rectal adenocarcinoma less than 15 cm from the anal verge.

Interventions.—Open laparotomy and rectal resection (n = 237) or laparoscopic rectal resection (n = 238).

Main Outcomes and Measures.—The primary end point was a composite of oncological factors indicating an adequate surgical resection, with a noninferiority boundary of $\Delta = -8\%$. Successful resection was defined as meeting all the following criteria: (1) complete total mesorectal excision, (2) a clear circumferential margin (≥1 mm), and (3) a clear distal resection margin (≥1 mm). Pathologists used standardized reporting and were blinded to the method of surgery.

Results.—A successful resection was achieved in 194 patients (82%) in the laparoscopic surgery group and 208 patients (89%) in the open surgery group (risk difference of −7.0% [95% CI, −12.4% to ∞]; $P = .38$ for noninferiority). The circumferential resection margin was clear in 222 patients (93%) in the laparoscopic surgery group and in 228 patients (97%) in the open surgery group (risk difference of −3.7% [95% CI, −7.6% to 0.1%]; *P* =.06), the distal margin was clear in 236 patients (99%) in the laparoscopic surgery group and in 234 patients (99%) in the open surgery group (risk difference of −0.4% [95% CI, −1.8% to 1.0%]; *P* =.67), and total mesorectal excision was complete in 206 patients (87%) in the laparoscopic surgery group and 216 patients (92%) in the open surgery group (risk difference of −5.4% [95% CI, −10.9% to 0.2%]; *P* =.06). The conversion rate from laparoscopic to open surgery was 9%.

Conclusions and Relevance.—Among patients with T1-T3 rectal tumors, noninferiority of laparoscopic surgery compared with open surgery for successful resection was not established. Although the overall quality of surgery was high, these findings do not provide sufficient evidence for the routine use of laparoscopic surgery. Longer follow-up of recurrence and survival is currently being acquired.

	Total No. of Patients		Successful Resection, No. (%)				
	Laparoscopic Rectal Resection (n=238)	Open Laparotomy and Rectal Resection (n=235)	Laparoscopic Rectal Resection	Open Laparotomy and Rectal Resection	Risk Difference, % (95% CI)	Favors Open Resection / Favors Laparoscopic Resection	P Value for Interaction
Preoperative radiotherapy							
No	119	119	105 (88)	105 (88)	0 (-9.0 to 9.0)		.07
Yes	119	116	89 (75)	103 (89)	-14.0 (-24.5 to -3.5)		
Body mass index[a]							
<30	182	181	149 (82)	157 (87)	-4.9 (-12.9 to 3.1)		.16
≥30	56	54	45 (80)	51 (94)	-14.1 (-28.0 to -0.2)		
Planned procedure							
Lower anterior resection	220	218	183 (83)	194 (89)	-5.8 (-12.7 to 1.1)		.48
Abdominoperineal resection	18	17	11 (61)	14 (82)	-21.2 (-55.9 to 13.4)		
Tumor location[b]							
High	53	50	48 (91)	49 (98)	-7.4 (-18.2 to 3.3)		.35[c]
Middle	103	102	85 (83)	90 (88)	-5.7 (-16.3 to 4.9)		
Low	82	83	61 (74)	69 (83)	-8.7 (-22.4 to 4.9)		
Nodal status							
N0	107	125	87 (81)	108 (86)	-5.1(-15.5 to 5.3)		.38[c]
N1	92	80	81 (88)	75 (94)	-5.7 (-15.4 to 4.0)		
N2	37	30	24 (65)	25 (83)	-18.5 (-41.8 to 4.9)		
T stage							
T1 or T2	86	79	74 (86)	68 (86)	0 (-11.8 to 11.8)		.13
T3	151	155	119 (79)	139 (90)	-10.9 (-19.6 to -2.1)		
Tumor size, cm							
≥0-3.0	79	66	67 (85)	57 (87)	-1.6 (-14.4 to 11.3)		.29[c]
3.1-4.9	67	77	53 (79)	68 (88)	-9.2 (-22.7 to 4.3)		
≥5.0	81	78	67 (83)	72 (92)	-9.6 (-21.0 to 1.8)		
All patients	238	235	194 (82)	208 (89)	-7.0 (-12.4 to ∞)		

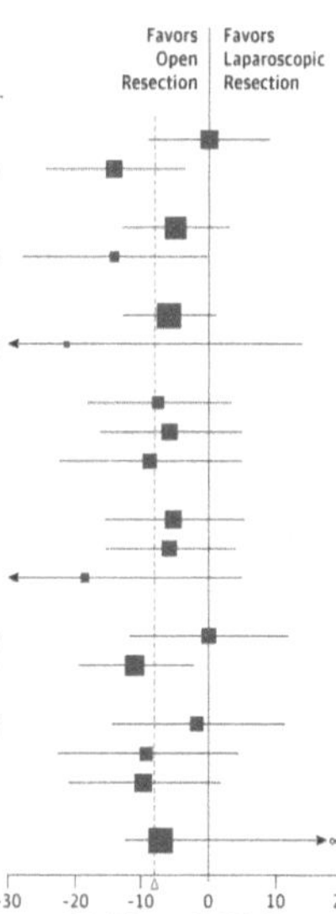

FIGURE 2.—Resection rate for all patients and major subgroups in the ALaCaRT trial. Successful resection defined as negative circumferential and distal margins and complete total mesorectal excision. The 2-sided confidence limits are 95% CIs for each subgroup. The noninferiority boundary (dashed line, Δ = −8%) lies above the lower bound of the 95% CI for the group, all patients, so noninferiority has not been established. ALaCaRT indicates Australasian Laparoscopic Cancer of the Rectum. [a]Calculated as weight in kilograms divided by height in meters squared. [b]High defined as 10-15 cm from the anal verge; middle, 5-10 cm; and low, less than 5 cm. [c]Test for linear trend used. (Reprinted from Stevenson ARL, for the ALaCaRT Investigators. Effect of laparoscopic-assisted resection vs open resection on pathological outcomes in rectal cancer: the ALaCaRT randomized clinical trial. *JAMA*. 2015;314:1356-1363, with permission from American Medical Association.)

Trial Registration.—anzctr.org Identifier: ACTRN12609000663257 (Fig 2).

▶ The data regarding the use of laparoscopic surgery for colon and rectal cancer are relatively strong, with several randomized trials demonstrating at least equal outcomes to open surgery and in some cases better outcomes.[1-3] This randomized trial from Australia calls this into question. The study randomized more than 400 rectal cancer patients to either laparoscopic or open resection. The outcomes were good with a leak rate of 7%, and nearly all patients received a coloanal anastomosis. The primary outcome was to look at the pathological data, and they found that the laparoscopic group was more likely to have a positively circumferential margin and less likely to undergo a complete mesorectal excision. Analysis suggested that patients with a higher body mass index, larger T3 tumors, or who had received neoadjuvant treatment may be better served by an open operation (Fig 2). This study did not evaluate robotic resection, which may offer some advantages that could address these findings.

O. J. Hines, MD, FACS

References

1. Guillou PJ, Quirke P, Thorpe H, et al. Short-term endpoints of conventional versus laparoscopic-assisted surgery in patients with colorectal cancer (MRC CLASICC trial). *Lancet.* 2005;365:1718-1726.
2. Fleshman J, Sargent DJ, Green E, et al. Laparoscopic colectomy for cancer is not inferior to open surgery based on 5-year data from the COST Study Group trial. *Ann Surg.* 2007;246:655-662.
3. Jeong SY, Park JW, Nam BH, et al. Open versus laparoscopic surgery for mid-rectal or low-rectal cancer after neoadjuvant chemoradiotherapy (COREAN trial). *Lancet Oncol.* 2014;15:767-774.

Is a diverting ostomy needed in mid-high rectal cancer patients undergoing a low anterior resection after neoadjuvant chemoradiation? An NSQIP analysis

Messaris E, Connelly TM, Kulaylat AN, et al (The Pennsylvania State Univ, College of Medicine, Hershey)
Surgery 158:686-691, 2015

Introduction.—A diverting stoma is often performed at the time of low anterior resection (LAR) for rectal cancer after neoadjuvant chemoradiation (nCRT) to protect the anastomosis. The aim of this study was to compare surgical outcomes in large cohorts of mid-high rectal cancer patients undergoing LAR after nCRT with and without a diverting stoma.

Methods.—Patients undergoing LAR for rectal cancer (ICD-9 diagnosis code 154.1) after nCRT were identified from the American College of Surgeons National Surgical Quality Improvement Program database records from 2005 to 2012. Using Current Procedural Terminology (CPT) codes for LAR for mid-high rectal tumors, patients were stratified into diverting stoma (CPT: 44146, 44208) or no diverting stoma (CPT: 44145, 44207) cohorts. Emergency resection, stage IV disease, and permanent end colostomy patients were excluded.

Results.—We included 1,406 patients in the analysis. All patients received nCRT; 607 (43%) received a diverting stoma and 799 (57%) were not diverted. The diverted group was more likely to have a higher body mass index (28.3 vs 27.4 kg/m^2; $P = .02$) and hypertension (46% vs 39%; $P = .002$). Otherwise, the group demographics and comorbidities were comparable. Overall morbidity was 28% for the entire cohort with no differences in deep organ space infection, sepsis and septic shock, unplanned reoperation, duration of stay, or overall mortality between the groups.

Conclusion.—Diverting stoma does not decrease mortality or infectious complications in mid-high rectal cancer patients undergoing LAR after nCRT. The decision to construct a protective stoma should not be driven solely on the receipt of nCRT.

▶ Do you divert when performing a colorectal anastomosis? Over the past decade, there has clearly been a shift toward diverting, and the rationale has been that if the anastomosis leaks, then the severity of this complication can be mitigated with the stoma in place. Of course, a second procedure is then required to reverse the stoma, and this carries with it risk of complication and need for readmission. Most would agree that for very/ultra low colorectal anastomosis, a stoma makes sense; this may make even more sense if the patient has undergone neoadjuvant chemoradiation for a rectal cancer. This study examined National Surgical Quality Improvement Program data of patients undergoing mid to high colorectal anastomosis after neoadjuvant treatment. They found no difference in the need for return to surgery, superficial or deep infection, or other complications between those patients who had a diverting stoma and those that did not. The patients who were diverted had a higher body mass index and incidence of hypertension, suggesting that surgeons were diverting those at higher risk for complication. Although one of many studies examining this issue, this report provides evidence that not all patients should be diverted, and this approach will save our patients a second operation.

O. J. Hines, MD, FACS

Clinical Outcomes of Surgery Versus Endoscopic Balloon Dilation for Stricturing Crohn's Disease

Greener T, Shapiro R, Klang E, et al (Tel Aviv Univ, Israel)

Dis Colon Rectum 58:1151-1157, 2015

Background.—Endoscopic balloon dilation and surgery are commonly practiced in stricturing Crohn's disease. Nonetheless, there are still scant data directly comparing these 2 strategies.

Objective.—The aim of this study was to compare the short- and long-term outcomes of endoscopic balloon dilation versus surgical resection in symptomatic Crohn's strictures.

Design.—This was a retrospective cohort study.

Settings.—The study was conducted at a single tertiary center.

Patients.—Seventy-nine patients were identified, 40 in the surgical group and 39 in the endoscopic balloon dilation group (mean age 42.8 ± 13.9 versus 38.5 ± 12.2 years).

Main Outcome Measures.—The outcomes of all patients referred for endoscopic balloon dilation were compared with patients referred to surgery because of stricturing disease between the years 2006 and 2013. The primary outcome was the need for reintervention (either endoscopic balloon dilation or surgery) for symptomatic Crohn's disease during follow-up.

Results.—The proportion of patients who required any reintervention during follow-up was significantly lower in the surgical group versus the endoscopic balloon dilation group (OR = 5.62 (95% CI, 1.66–19.01); $p = 0.005$). The need for surgery/resurgery during follow-up was also significantly lower in the surgically treated group (OR = 3.53 (95% CI, 1.01–12.29); $p = 0.047$). Reintervention-free survival and surgery-free survival were both significantly shorter in the endoscopically treated group in a Kaplan-Mayer analysis. The rate of major complications was similar in the endoscopically and surgically treated groups (7.6% versus 7.5%; $p = 0.7$).

Limitations.—The small cohort and the retrospective data collection were limitations of this study.

Conclusions.—In our cohort of patients with fibrostenotic Crohn's disease, a direct comparison showed reduced need for reinterventions with a similar rate of immediate major complications after surgery compared with endoscopic balloon dilation (Table 4).

▶ Traditional approaches to strictures from Crohn disease have been with medical management and surgical stricturoplasty or resection. About a third of patients will form new strictures after surgery. Because of the frequency of stricture formation and the general opinion to keep Crohn patients out of the

TABLE 4.—Complications in the Endoscopic Balloon Dilation Cohort

Total Complications	N = 7 (17%)
Major complications, n (%)	3 (8)
Major bleeding, n (%)	2 (5)
Prolonged hospitalization, n (%)	2 (5)
Fever and abdominal pain (without perforation), n (%)	3 (7)

Reprinted from Greener T, Shapiro R, Klang E, et al. Clinical outcomes of surgery versus endoscopic balloon dilation for stricturing Crohn's disease. *Dis Colon Rectum.* 2015;58:1151-1157, with permission from The American Society of Colon & Rectal Surgeons, Inc.

operating room, there has been interest in performing endoscopic balloon dilation of strictures. This study evaluated a cohort of patients who underwent surgery and compared these with patients who had endoscopic dilation. The need for reintervention was significantly lower in the patients who had surgery and the major complication rate we virtually equal between the 2 groups (Table 4). In the endoscopic group, nearly 40% of the patients required reintervention, and about 30% required surgery, whereas only 10% of patients in the surgery group required reintervention. But what's more concerning was that the survival was significantly shorter in the patients who had endoscopic intervention. This may have been explained by a selection bias pushing more poor operative candidates into an endoscopic treatment approach. Endoscopic dilation likely offers some advantages for subgroup of patients who are malnourished and may have a higher risk of anastomotic leak. Endoscopic dilation may also be used as a bridging procedure to surgery.

O. J. Hines, MD, FACS

Long-term impact of full-thickness rectal prolapse treatment on fecal incontinence

Wallenhorst T, Bouguen G, Brochard C, et al (Univ Hosp of Rennes, Pontchaillou, France; et al)
Surgery 158:104-111, 2015

Background.—Fecal incontinence is frequently associated with rectal prolapse, but little is known about recovery after treatment of the prolapse.

Objective.—We therefore aimed to investigate the long-term outcome of fecal incontinence in a cohort of patients suffering from full-thickness rectal prolapse.

Design.—A database of 145 patients diagnosed with full-thickness rectal prolapse was compiled prospectively over a 7-year period (2003–2010).

Main Outcome Measures.—Patients were referred to a single institution and assessed by standardized questionnaires, anorectal manometry, endosonography, and evacuation proctography. Fecal incontinence was evaluated according to the Cleveland Clinic Score; continence improvement was defined by ≥50% improvement of the Cleveland Clinic Score.

Results.—Among the population studied (134 women, 11 men; median follow-up, 38.9 months [range, 21.2–67.2]), 103 patients (71%) underwent operation for their prolapse and 42 (29%) did not. According to the Cleveland Clinic Score, 139 patients (96%) suffered from fecal incontinence before treatment and 64 (46%) reported improvement at the end of the follow-up. Pretreatment history of incontinence symptoms for >2 years (hazard ratio [HR], 1.99; 95% CI, 1.14–3.46; $P = .015$) and ventral rectopexy (HR, 1.86; 95% CI, 1.026–3.326; $P = .04$) were associated with continence improvement. Patients who underwent an operative procedure other than ventral rectopexy had similar outcome as compared with nonoperated patients. Conversely, chronic pelvic pain precluded fecal incontinence improvement (HR, 0.32; 95% CI, 0.135–0.668; P =.0017).

Limitations.—Follow-up, returned questionnaires, and the heterogeneous reasons put forth for declining surgery may introduce some methodologic bias.

Conclusion.—Fecal incontinence in patients suffering from rectal prolapse is improved when ventral rectopexy is performed compared with other operative or medical therapies (Fig 3B).

▶ Rectal prolapse resulting in pelvic pain and fecal incontinence is a complex entity often presenting in patients with significant risk factors for surgery. There is no doubt that the evaluation of these patients requires particular expertise and studies including functional assessment and physiologic testing. These patients often undergo endosonography, defecating proctogram, and anal manometry to fully understand the etiology for their symptoms. Because these patients may be older and not the best of operative candidates, some have tried to improve symptoms with biofeedback. The surgical options are many, including perineal approaches, laparoscopic techniques, and open

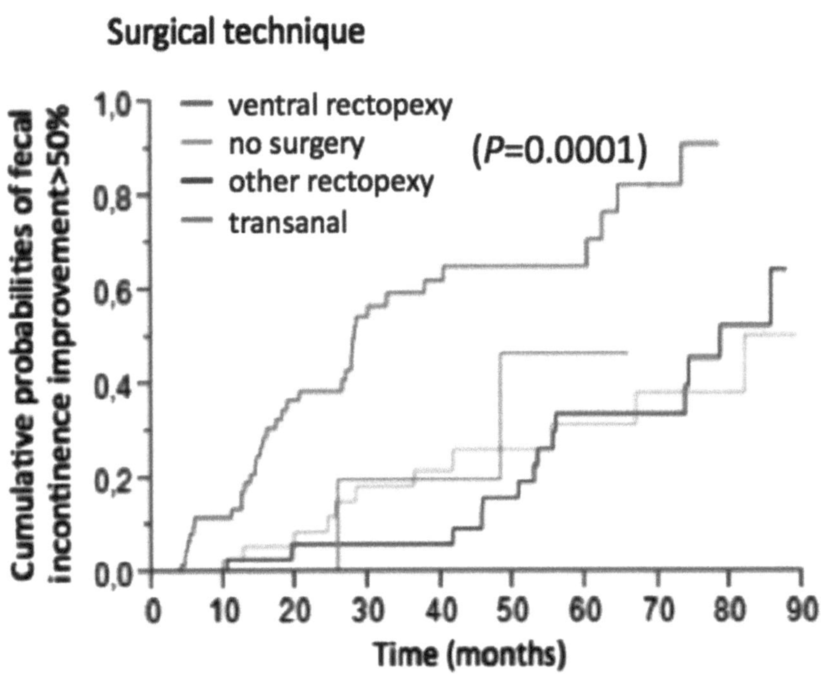

FIGURE 3.—Cumulative probabilities of significant fecal incontinence score improvement according to 3 main factors (Kaplan–Meier). (*B*) Operative technique. Earlier and greater incontinence improvements were observed in patients who underwent ventral rectopexy compared with those treated with other operative methods or a nonoperative approach (P =.0001). (Reprinted from Wallenhorst T, Bouguen G, Brochard C, et al. Long-term impact of full-thickness rectal prolapse treatment on fecal incontinence. *Surgery.* 2015;158:104-111, with permission from Elsevier Inc.)

operation. This study examined the use of ventral rectopexy, which may have some advantages because the colon/rectum is left intact and the innervation undisturbed. Overall, ventral rectopexy offered superior control of incontinence over other procedures (Fig 3B). Still, however, some patients are not able to tolerate an abdominal operation, and the recommendation needs to be tailored to address these issues.

O. J. Hines, MD, FACS

Lateral internal sphincterotomy for surgically recurrent chronic anal fissure

Liang J, Church JM (Digestive Diseases Inst, Cleveland, OH)

Am J Surg 210:715-719, 2015

Background.—Lateral internal sphincterotomy cures chronic anal fissure by preventing internal sphincter hypertonia. However, cutting sphincter predisposes to sphincter dysfunction, manifests as incontinence of gas, liquid, or stool. Surgeons, therefore, can be too cautious in its use, making ineffective superficial incisions or avoiding the operation altogether. This study is designed to confirm the role of redo lateral internal sphincterotomy in the treatment of surgically recurrent chronic anal fissure.

Methods.—Patients undergoing repeat lateral internal sphincterotomy for surgically recurrent chronic anal fissure were accessed from a prospectively maintained database. Chronicity was defined by symptoms persisting more than 3 weeks. Contralateral sphincterotomy was performed with electrocautery through a stab incision over the intersphincteric plane. The length of sphincter division was the same as the length of the fissure. Phone questionnaire was administered and fecal continence was assessed by modified Cleveland Clinic Incontinence Score. Patients were asked to rank their overall satisfaction with the operation, and pre- and postoperative quality of life.

Results.—There were 57 patients, 24 women and 33 men; mean age was 47.9 ± 14.8 years. Mean follow-up was 12.5 ± 4.2 years (range 6.2 to 25.2 years). Presenting symptoms included pain (100%), bleeding (80%), pruritus ani (39%), constipation (26%), and diarrhea. Fifty patients (90%) presented with 1 fissure, and 40 were posterior. Most procedures were performed on an outpatient basis. Fissure healing rate was 98%, and 2 patients (4%) developed minor incontinence postoperatively (one of gas, the other, gas and seepage). Overall satisfaction was 9.7 ± .9 out of 10 with a significant improvement in the quality of life from 5.7 ± 2.4 out of 10 to 9.3 ± 1.4 out of 10 ($P < .001$).

Conclusion.—Judicious repeat lateral sphincterotomy cures recurrent chronic fissures with minimal risk of incontinence.

▶ Many treatment options are now available for anal fissures including both "chemical" and surgical sphincterotomy. Hydrocortisone, zylocaine, glyceril trinitrate, isosorbide dinitrate, and botox all have reported high healing rates. However, a recent meta-analysis suggests that these approaches have similar rates of healing to placebo.[1] New attention to surgical sphincterotomy is now occurring given the very high cure rate. Internal sphincterotomy decreases sphincter tone improving blood flow and tissue oxygenation resulting in healing. However, sphincterotomy can lead to issues of incontinence. This article reviews the experience with open lateral internal sphincterotomy. This approach allows for a more limited sphincterotomy up to the level of the apex of the fissure theoretically reducing issues of incontinence. The authors report a healing rate of 98% and a minor incontinence rate of 4%. One last pointer is to remember that nearly all patients will have a single fissure, and usually this is posterior. For patients with multiple concurrent fissure issues as is the case with Crohn disease, ulcerative colitis, HIV, syphilis, and tuberculosis, should be considered.

O. J. Hines, MD, FACS

Reference

1. Nelson R. A systematic review of medical therapy for anal fissure. *Dis Colon Rectum*. 2004;47:422-431.

A Randomized Trial Comparing Stapled Rectal Mucosectomy Versus Open and Semiclosed Hemorrhoidectomy

Ripetti V, La Vaccara V, Greco S, et al (Campus Bio-Medico Univ, Rome, Italy)
Dis Colon Rectum 58:1083-1090, 2015

Background.—Different results have been reported concerning the postoperative outcomes of different surgical approaches for hemorrhoids.

Objective.—We aimed to determine the postoperative outcome following 3 main surgical techniques.

Design.—A prospective, randomized trial was designed with 180 patients in 3 arms of 60 patients each.

Settings.—The study was conducted from April 1999 to January 2007 at the University Hospital "Campus Bio- Medico di Roma."

Patients.—All of the patients who were referred for hemorrhoid surgery were enrolled according to inclusion and exclusion criteria (ISRCTN12040297).

Interventions.—Treatments according to the open, semiclosed, and stapled techniques were compared.

Main Outcome Measures.—Sample size was calculated to determine a difference in terms of the intensity of postoperative pain at the first week and the days required for return to work activity.

Results.—After 1 week, patients who underwent semiclosed hemorrhoidectomy reported significantly less pain ($p < 0.01$) and a significant decrease in analgesic intake from the third postoperative day ($p < 0.01$) than after the other 2 techniques. The patients resumed work ≈11 days after semiclosed and stapled techniques (11.8 and 11.6 days), which was earlier compared with 21.3 days in the open group ($p < 0.05$).

TABLE 4.—Complication

Complication	SCH, n (%)	OH, n (%)	SRM, n (%)	p^a
Incontinence	0	0	1 (1.8)	0.38
Bleeding	1 (2.0)	3 (5.3)	2 (3.6)	0.66
Stenosis	0	9 (15.8)	3 (5.4)	0.004
Thrombosis	1 (2.0)	1 (1.8)	3 (5.4)	0.47
Fissure	1 (2.0)	4 (7.0)	0	0.08
Fistula	0	1 (1.8)	0	0.39
Urinary retention	2 (4.0)	7 (12.3)	3 (5.4)	0.20
Proctitis	0	0	2 (3.6)	0.14

SCH = semiclosed hemorrhoidectomy; OH = open hemorrhoidectomy; SRM = stapled rectal mucosectomy.
[a]Data were calculated with the Pearson χ^2 test.
Reprinted from Ripetti V, La Vaccara V, Greco S, et al. A randomized trial comparing stapled rectal mucosectomy versus open and semiclosed hemorrhoidectomy. *Dis Colon Rectum*. 2015;58:1083-1090, with permission from The American Society of Colon & Rectal Surgeons, Inc.

Limitations.—The high number of patients excluded might be considered a limitation of the study, but our selection criteria including patients living within 50 km of the hospital allowed for a low rate (9.4%) of patients lost to follow-up.

Conclusions.—This study found an earlier resumption of work and less pain in patients who underwent the stapled and semiclosed procedures rather than open, which was associated with more complications, particularly because of a higher rate of stenosis (**see Video, Supplemental Digital Content 1,** http://links.lww.com/DCR/A196) (Table 4).

▶ Hemorrhoids are common and a great source of disability. Alternate approaches to managing hemorrhoids have evolved, and this study aims to determine the efficacy between a traditional open approach, semiopen approach, and a stapled hemorrhoidectomy. Overall, the semiopen approach won out, with patients recording less pain and decreased use of pain medication. The open technique performed the worse with regard to returning to work with this group returning after 3 weeks while the other 2 groups after 11 days. The open group also had a higher complication rate largely attributable to stenosis, and the semiclosed approach clearly had the lowest rate of complication (Table 4). Four months after surgery, a third of the open group was still suffering from pain and experienced pain with defecation. The options are many now for the treatment of hemorrhoids, including sclerotherapy, banding, photodynamic ablation, and cryotherapy. Other studies suggest the stapled approach may be associated with significant complications. This study suggests that the semiclosed technique may be the best approach for your patients requiring operative intervention of hemorrhoids.

O. J. Hines, MD, FACS

10 Oncology

Breast

Axillary Ultrasound After Neoadjuvant Chemotherapy and Its Impact on Sentinel Lymph Node Surgery: Results From the American College of Surgeons Oncology Group Z1071 Trial (Alliance)

Boughey JC, Ballman KV, Hunt KK, et al (Mayo Clinic, Rochester, MN; The Univ of Texas MD Anderson Cancer Ctr, Houston; et al)

J Clin Oncol 33:3386-3393, 2015

Purpose.—The American College of Surgeons Oncology Group Z1071 trial reported a 12.6% false-negative rate (FNR) for sentinel lymph node (SLN) surgery after neoadjuvant chemotherapy (NAC) in cN1 disease. Patients were not selected for surgery based on response, but a secondary end point was to determine whether axillary ultrasound (AUS) after NAC after fine-needle aspiration cytology can identify abnormal nodes and guide patient selection for SLN surgery.

Patients and Methods.—Patients with T0-4, N1-2, M0 breast cancer underwent AUS after neoadjuvant chemotherapy. AUS images were centrally reviewed and classified as normal or suspicious lymph nodes. AUS findings were tested for association with pathologic nodal status and SLN FNR. The impact of AUS results to select patients for SLN surgery to reduce the FNR was assessed.

Results.—Postchemotherapy AUS images were reviewed for 611 patients. One hundred thirty (71.8%) of 181 AUS-suspicious patients were node positive at surgery compared with 243 (56.5%) of 430 AUS-normal patients ($P < .001$). Patients with AUS-suspicious nodes had a greater number of positive nodes and greater metastasis size ($P < .001$). The SLN FNR was not different based on AUS results; however, using a strategy where only patients with normal AUS undergo SLN surgery would potentially reduce the FNR in Z1071 patients with ≥ two SLNs removed from 12.6% to 9.8% when preoperative AUS results are considered as part of SLN surgery.

Conclusion.—AUS is recommended after chemotherapy to guide axillary surgery. An FNR of 9.8% with the combination of AUS and SLN

surgery would be acceptable for the adoption of SLN surgery for women with node-positive breast cancer treated with neoadjuvant chemotherapy.

▶ It has been shown that patients with early-stage breast cancer and clinically negative nodes do not require axillary dissection if sentinel nodes are negative and they are to receive chemotherapy. This question is not as clear in patients with clinically positive nodes undergoing neoadjuvant chemotherapy. In the ACOSOG Z1071 trial, patients with clinically positive nodes and T0-4 breast cancer underwent neoadjuvant chemotherapy and had a fine-needle aspiration or core biopsies to confirm positive axillary nodes. These patients then had a sentinel lymph node biopsy with axillary dissection performed at the time of breast surgery, and the majority also had axillary ultrasound to evaluate the lymph nodes. This study set out to look at whether the adjunct of axillary ultrasound (AUS) can decrease the false-negative rate of sentinel lymph node biopsy after neoadjuvant treatment, which was 12.6% in this trial. If the false-negative rate could be improved, some patients with negative sentinel lymph node biopsies might benefit from the omission of axillary dissection.

In the Z1071 trial, there were 470 patients who had AUS that could be reviewed for quality assurance metrics. In those 470 patients, 138 (30%) had normal lymph nodes observed on AUS and 70% had suspicious nodes seen. The judgment of normal versus suspicious is made by looking at the cortex and the hilum of the lymph node, with normal lymph nodes having a thin, < 3 mm thick and hypoechoic cortex, and a fatty hilum. When the cortex is focally or diffusely thickened, or if the hilum is deformed or absent, this is considered suspicious. Of patients with normal lymph nodes as assessed by AUS, 57% were found to have positive lymph nodes on final pathology, and 72% of those with suspicious lymph nodes had node-positive disease. The overall rate of complete pathologic response was 39%. In patients with suspicious lymph nodes on AUS versus those with normal lymph nodes, there were generally more sentinel lymph nodes found, more additionally positive axillary lymph nodes, more macrometastases, and a higher metastasis size (Table 3 in the original article). For the calculation of the false-negative rate, only patients who had 2 or more sentinel lymph nodes removed were considered. Of 470 patients in this group, 286 had residual nodal disease, with 250 having positive and 36 having negative sentinel lymph nodes (but residual nodal disease in nonsentinel nodes), for an overall false-negative rate of 12.6%. In patients with suspicious nodes, post-neoadjuvant residual nodal disease was found in 99 of 138 (72%), and no residual nodal disease was found in 39 of 138 patients (28%). In the 334 patients with normal lymph nodes seen on AUS, 159 had positive sentinel lymph nodes, whereas 175 had negative sentinel lymph nodes, but 28 of these 175 had residual nodal disease. The overall false-negative rate in the group of patients with normal nodes by AUS was therefore 9.8%, which was slightly less than the 12.6% seen overall. Therefore, the authors conclude that the addition of axillary ultrasound improves the false-negative rate to below 10%, which is considered a reasonable cutoff for sentinel lymph node biopsy as a diagnostic test. However, it should be noted that the 90% confidence interval in this group included the 12.6%, and therefore it is possible that AUS does not add much to sentinel lymph node biopsy alone. The authors feel that the utility of this test could be used to select patients who have normal appearing nodes to have sentinel lymph node biopsy alone and not undergo axillary dissection. Patients with suspicious nodes would continue to have axillary dissection performed as was done previously. Currently, the option of treating the axilla of patients with positive sentinel lymph nodes having neoadjuvant chemotherapy with radiation is being evaluated in the Alliance A11202 randomized trial, which compares axillary radiation to axillary dissection in these patients.

J. R. Howe, MD

Adjuvant Ovarian Suppression in Premenopausal Breast Cancer

Francis PA, for the SOFT Investigators and the International Breast Cancer Study Group (Univ of Melbourne, Victoria, Australia)

N Engl J Med 372:436-446, 2015

Background.—Suppression of ovarian estrogen production reduces the recurrence of hormone-receptor–positive early breast cancer in premenopausal women, but its value when added to tamoxifen is uncertain.

Methods.—We randomly assigned 3066 premenopausal women, stratified according to prior receipt or nonreceipt of chemotherapy, to receive 5 years of tamoxifen, tamoxifen plus ovarian suppression, or exemestane plus ovarian suppression. The primary analysis tested the hypothesis that tamoxifen plus ovarian suppression would improve disease-free survival, as compared with tamoxifen alone. In the primary analysis, 46.7% of the patients had not received chemotherapy previously, and 53.3% had received chemotherapy and remained premenopausal.

Results.—After a median follow-up of 67 months, the estimated disease-free survival rate at 5 years was 86.6% in the tamoxifen–ovarian suppression group and 84.7% in the tamoxifen group (hazard ratio for disease recurrence, second invasive cancer, or death, 0.83; 95% confidence interval [CI], 0.66 to 1.04; $P = 0.10$). Multivariable allowance for prognostic factors suggested a greater treatment effect with tamoxifen plus ovarian suppression than with tamoxifen alone (hazard ratio, 0.78; 95% CI, 0.62 to 0.98). Most recurrences occurred in patients who had received prior chemotherapy, among whom the rate of freedom from breast cancer at 5 years was 82.5% in the tamoxifen–ovarian suppression group and 78.0% in the tamoxifen group (hazard ratio for recurrence, 0.78; 95% CI, 0.60 to 1.02). At 5 years, the rate of freedom from breast cancer was 85.7% in the exemestane–ovarian suppression group (hazard ratio for recurrence vs. tamoxifen, 0.65; 95% CI, 0.49 to 0.87).

Conclusions.—Adding ovarian suppression to tamoxifen did not provide a significant benefit in the overall study population. However, for women who were at sufficient risk for recurrence to warrant adjuvant chemotherapy and who remained premenopausal, the addition of ovarian suppression improved disease outcomes. Further improvement was seen with the use of exemestane plus ovarian suppression. (Funded by Pfizer and others; SOFT ClinicalTrials.gov number, NCT00066690.)

▶ Premenopausal women with estrogen and progesterone (ER/PR)-positive breast cancers benefit from antiestrogen therapy. Since the ovaries can continue to produce estrogen, the question of whether the addition of ovarian suppression therapy would lead to benefits in terms of recurrence or survival rates in these patients is unknown. In 2003, an international consortium initiated the suppression of ovarian function trial (SOFT), in which premenopausal women with operable breast cancer having the following were included: >10% of cells ER/PR positive; having mastectomy or breast-conserving surgery; with either sentinel lymph node biopsy or axillary dissection. Patients were randomized to receive tamoxifen alone, tamoxifen and ovarian suppression, or the aromatase inhibitor exemestane plus ovarian suppression. Ovarian suppression consisted of triptorelin depot (a gonadotrophin-releasing hormone agonist that reduces pituitary LH and FSH levels) every 28 days, bilateral oophorectomy, or ovarian irradiation. The main end point of the study was disease-free survival (DFS), with secondary end points being overall survival, and interval without recurrent breast cancer. The three randomized groups in this study included 3066 patients; two-thirds of the patients had prior adjuvant or neoadjuvant chemotherapy. This study had a median follow-up of 67 months, and the DFS rates were similar among the 3 groups, and more than half of recurrences were in distant sites. Most recurrences were seen in patients who had received chemotherapy, most likely because of their more advanced stage of disease; patients rendered amenorrheic by chemotherapy were not included in the trial. Women younger than age 35 also appeared to benefit from ovarian suppression, with a rate of freedom from breast cancer of 68% for tamoxifen alone, 79% for tamoxifen and ovarian suppression, and 83% for exemestane and ovarian suppression. There was no improvement in survival of patients who did not receive chemotherapy or in overall survival of the 3 groups. Adverse effects occurred in 31% of patients with tamoxifen and ovarian suppression versus 24% of those receiving tamoxifen alone. This trial showed that adding ovarian suppression to adjuvant tamoxifen did not improve DFS overall but did show a DFS benefit in those who had had chemotherapy, especially those younger than 35 years of age (Fig 2A, 2B in the original article). Therefore, there may be a role for ovarian suppression, but this difference is only on the order of 2% overall and 4.5% for the patients receiving chemotherapy. Limitations of the study were the 67-month follow-up, and surely there will be more recurrences after this time. From this well-conducted randomized trial, it appears that the ovarian suppression does add something to tamoxifen alone, and that exemestane plus ovarian suppression may be superior to tamoxifen and ovarian suppression for reducing breast cancer recurrence.

J. R. Howe, MD

A Randomized, Controlled Trial of Cavity Shave Margins in Breast Cancer

Chagpar AB, Killelea BK, Tsangaris TN, et al (Yale Univ School of Medicine, New Haven, CT; Thomas Jefferson Univ, Philadelphia, PA)

N Engl J Med 373:503-510, 2015

Background.—Routine resection of cavity shave margins (additional tissue circumferentially around the cavity left by partial mastectomy) may reduce the rates of positive margins (margins positive for tumor) and reexcision among patients undergoing partial mastectomy for breast cancer.

Methods.—In this randomized, controlled trial, we assigned, in a 1:1 ratio, 235 patients with breast cancer of stage 0 to III who were undergoing partial mastectomy, with or without resection of selective margins, to have further cavity shave margins resected (shave group) or not to have further cavity shave margins resected (no-shave group). Randomization occurred intraoperatively after surgeons had completed standard partial mastectomy. Positive margins were defined as tumor touching the edge of the specimen that was removed in the case of invasive cancer and tumor that was within 1 mm of the edge of the specimen removed in the case of ductal carcinoma in situ. The rate of positive margins was the primary outcome measure; secondary outcome measures included cosmesis and the volume of tissue resected.

Results.—The median age of the patients was 61 years (range, 33 to 94). On final pathological testing, 54 patients (23%) had invasive cancer, 45 (19%) had ductal carcinoma in situ, and 125 (53%) had both; 11 patients had no further disease. The median size of the tumor in the greatest diameter was 1.1 cm (range, 0 to 6.5) in patients with invasive carcinoma and 1.0 cm (range, 0 to 9.3) in patients with ductal carcinoma in situ. Groups were well matched at baseline with respect to demographic and clinicopathological characteristics. The rate of positive margins after partial mastectomy (before randomization) was similar in the shave group and the no-shave group (36% and 34%, respectively; $P = 0.69$). After randomization, patients in the shave group had a significantly lower rate of positive margins than did those in the no-shave group (19% vs. 34%, $P = 0.01$), as well as a lower rate of second surgery for margin clearance (10% vs. 21%, $P = 0.02$). There was no significant difference in complications between the two groups.

Conclusions.—Cavity shaving halved the rates of positive margins and reexcision among patients with partial mastectomy. (Funded by the Yale Cancer Center; ClinicalTrials.gov number, NCT01452399.)

▶ Partial mastectomy is associated with an approximately 20% to 40% rate of positive margins. This increases the rate of local recurrence, the need for second procedures for reexcision, and potentially reduced cosmesis. This study sets out to evaluate the effect of performing circumferential shave margins after partial mastectomy at reducing margin positivity, reexcision rates, and cosmetic outcome as determined by patients. They randomized patients 1:1 with stage I to III breast carcinoma to taking an additional circumferential shave margin or not. They defined positive margins in cases of invasive ductal cancer as tumor at the edge of the specimen or, in cases of ductal carcinoma in situ, tumor within 1 mm of the margin. Four surgeons took part in this single institutional study, and each performed excision with an additional margin taken closest to the margin thought to most likely be positive. During surgery, randomization was carried out, and surgeons then removed additional tissue from the excision cavity with the idea of encompassing the entire cavity with these shave margins. Patients randomized to no shave margins were then closed. Patients were given a 4-point Likert scale to rate cosmesis at their first postoperative visit. This study revealed that the rate of margin positivity decreased from 34% down to 19% in those having the additional shave margins, which was statistically significantly improved. Thirty-six percent of the patients in the shave margin group had positive margins before randomization, and 53% of these patients had margins deemed negative after shave margins. Interestingly, of 76 patients in the shave margin group who had negative margins on the initial excision, 12% were found to have cancer in the shave margins. Multivariate analysis revealed that the size of the DCIS was significantly associated with margin positivity, and not performing shave margins approached significance ($P = .06$; Table 3 in the original article). The cosmesis was deemed by patients to be similar between the 2 groups. This was a well-conducted study showing that routine performance of circumferential shave margins will reduce the margin positivity rate by about half, which resulted in fewer patients undergoing reexcision (10% vs 21% in the no shave group). The median follow-up of this study was 22 months, and therefore recurrence rates were not assessed in this study.

J. R. Howe, MD

Bilateral Risk-Reduction Mastectomy in BRCA1 and BRCA2 Mutation Carriers: A Meta-analysis

De Felice F, Marchetti C, Musella A, et al (Policlinico Umberto I "Sapienza" Univ of Rome, Italy; "Sapienza" Univ of Rome, Italy)

Ann Surg Oncol 22:2876-2880, 2015

Background.—Women with BRCA1 and BRCA2 mutations have substantially elevated risk of developing breast cancer. The aim of this study was to clarify the role of bilateral risk-reducing mastectomy (BRRM) in reducing breast cancer risk in women carriers of BRCA1 and BRCA2 mutations.

Methods.—The Pubmed, MEDLINE and Scopus databases were searched to retrieve articles written in the English language. Two investigators independently extracted the characteristics and results of the selected studies. Only prospective trials with available absolute numbers of breast cancer and death events were included. Pooled hazard ratio (HR) with 95 % confidence interval (CI) was calculated using fixed or random effects model.

Results.—Meta-analysis of four prospective studies, including 2635 patients, demonstrated a significant risk reduction of breast cancer incidence in BRCA1 and BRCA2 mutation carriers receiving BRRM (HR 0.07; 95 % CI 0.01–0.44; $p = 0.004$). Among patients without previous risk-reducing salpingo-oophorectomy, a significant benefit was similarly recorded (HR 0.06; 95 % CI 0.01–0.41; $p = 0.005$).

Conclusions.—Performing BRRM may lead to highly significant risk reduction of breast cancer in BRCA1 and BRCA2 mutation carriers. These data allow clinicians to discuss more in-depth with patients all the available options in order to design better management strategies (Fig 2).

▶ Patients with *BRCA1* and *BRCA2* mutations have a 65% to 85% risk of breast cancer, and 25% to 65% risk of ovarian cancer. Women diagnosed with these mutations have a difficult decision to make: whether to undergo bilateral, risk-reducing mastectomy (BRRM) and risk-reducing salpingo-oophorectomy (RRSO). Although reducing the risk of cancer, these procedures can impair one's body image and reduce reproductive choices. There are no prospective, randomized trials of BRRM in *BRCA1* and *BRCA2* mutation carriers to definitively know the benefit versus careful screening. This study performed a meta-analysis of articles in the literature relating to this topic. Of 210 potential articles, only 11 fulfilled the criteria of this study, which demanded that articles were prospective, in the English language, and were not review articles. Seven additional articles were eliminated because they did not have the desired end-point of the risk of developing breast cancer. Two of the remaining 4 articles also had information regarding RRSO. The studies selected were deemed to be at low-risk for bias and included 2635 patients, 24% who underwent BRRM and 76% who had regular surveillance. Results showed a significant benefit of BRRM in reducing the risk of breast cancer (Fig 2), with an overall risk ratio of 0.07 (confidence interval 0.01-0.44), equating to a 93% risk reduction in BRRM patients. A subgroup analysis was also performed to see what the difference was in risk reduction for patients who had BRRM with or without RRSO. Both groups appeared to benefit, with a risk ratio of 0.06 in those without RRSO and 0.11 in those with RRSO. Interestingly, previous studies have shown that having RRSO alone can reduce the risk of breast cancer by 46%. This study showed that having RRSO provided benefit, but not as much benefit was seen in patients having BRRM without RRSO. Overall, in these studies, RRSO was performed with the frequency of 38% to 82% in the control groups

Study or Subgroup	log[Risk Ratio]	SE	Weight	Risk Ratio IV, Random, 95% CI	Year
Meijers–Heijboer 2001	–3.0181	1.4453	20.9%	0.05 [0.00, 0.83]	2001
Domchek 2010	–3.5719	1.4161	21.4%	0.03 [0.00, 0.45]	2010
Skytte 2011	–0.8865	0.617	36.3%	0.41 [0.12, 1.38]	2011
Hemskerk–Gerritsen 2013	–4.2229	1.4177	21.4%	0.01 [0.00, 0.24]	2013
Total (95% CI)			**100.0%**	**0.07 [0.01, 0.44]**	

Heterogeneity. $Tau^2 = 1.95$; $Chi^2 = 7.37$, df = 3 (P = 0.06); $I^2 = 59\%$
Test for overall effect: Z = 2.85 (P = 0.004)

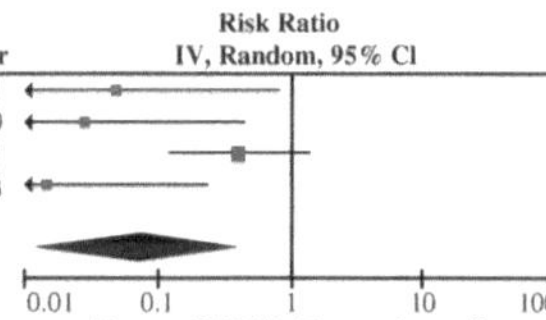

FIGURE 2.—Relative risk estimates for risk reduction of breast cancer associated with BRRM in the overall population of BRCA1 and BRCA2 mutation carriers. *BRRM* bilateral risk-reducing mastectomy, *CI* confidence interval, *df* degrees of freedom, *IV* inverse variance, *SE* standard error. (Reprinted from De Felice F, Marchetti C, Musella A, et al. Bilateral risk-reduction mastectomy in BRCA1 and BRCA2 mutation carriers: a meta-analysis. *Ann Surg Oncol.* 2015;22:2876-2880, with permission from Society of Surgical Oncology.)

and 18% to 69% of those who underwent BRRM. This study was limited by relatively short follow-up in the studies examined, which did not allow for evaluation of the survival benefit. Nevertheless, it did show convincing benefit to BRRM in *BRCA1* and *BRCA2* mutation carriers. Ideally, a randomized prospective trial would be performed but is unlikely to be performed because this would be unethical given the clear benefit of the procedure.

J. R. Howe, MD

Survival is Better After Breast Conserving Therapy than Mastectomy for Early Stage Breast Cancer: A Registry-Based Follow-up Study of Norwegian Women Primary Operated Between 1998 and 2008

Hartmann-Johnsen OJ, Kåresen R, Schlichting E, et al (Cancer Registry of Norway, Oslo; Univ of Oslo, Norway; Oslo Univ Hosp, Norway)
Ann Surg Oncol 22:3836-3845, 2015

Background.—Breast-conserving therapy (BCT) and mastectomy (MTX) has been considered to have a similar long-time survival. However, better survival in women undergoing BCT compared with MTX is found in two recent register studies from the United States. The purpose of this study was to compare survival after BCT and MTX for women with early-stage breast cancer in Norway.

Methods.—Women with invasive, early-stage breast cancer (1998–2008) where BCT and MTX were considered as equally beneficial treatments were included for a total of 13,015 women. Surgery was divided in two main cohorts (primary BCT, primary MTX) and five subcohorts. Analyses were stratified into T1N0M0, T2N0M0, T1N1M0, T2N1M0, and age groups (<50, 50–69, ≥70). Overall survival and breast cancer-specific survival (BCSS) were calculated in life tables, hazard ratios by Cox regression, and sensitivity analyses.

Results.—Five-year BCSS for women who underwent primary BCT or primary MTX was 97 and 88%, respectively. Women who underwent primary MTX had a hazard ratio of 1.64 (95% confidence interval 1.43–1.88) for breast cancer death compared with women who underwent primary BCT after adjusting for the year of diagnosis, age at diagnosis, stage, histology, and grade.

Conclusions.—Survival was better or equal after breast-conserving therapy than mastectomy in all early stages, surgical subcohorts, and age groups. This advantage could not only be attributed to differences in tumor biology (Fig 1).

▶ Previous randomized controlled trials for early-stage breast cancer have revealed no significant differences in survival for patients undergoing mastectomy versus breast-conserving therapy (BCT) with radiation. However, 2 recent studies have revealed that there might be a survival advantage in patients undergoing BCT over mastectomy (MTX), which had been thought to be due to either differences in tumor biology or differences in compliance for

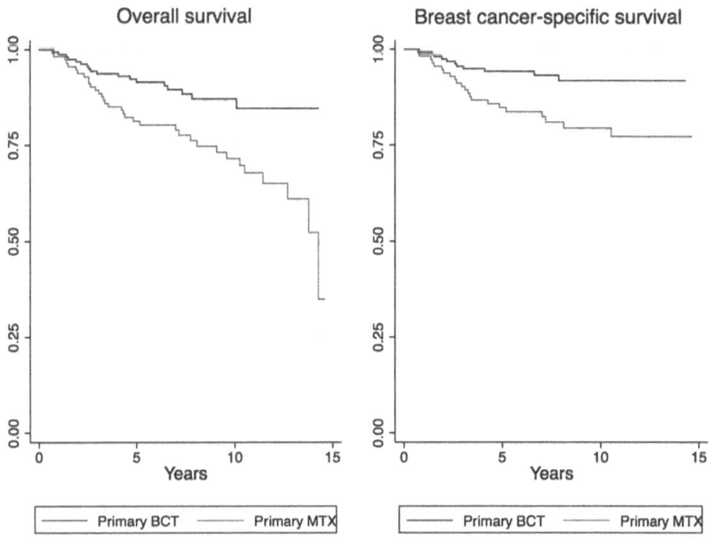

FIGURE 1.—Kaplan–Meier, surgical main cohorts stratified in T1N1M0, grade 3, ductal carcinoma, and age 50–69. (Hartmann-Johnsen OJ, Kåresen R, Schlichting E, et al. Survival is better after breast conserving therapy than mastectomy for early stage breast cancer: a registry-based follow-up study of Norwegian women primary operated between 1998 and 2008. *Ann Surg Oncol.* 2015;22:3836-3845, with permission from The Author(s).)

adjuvant therapy.[1,2] This study set out to look at differences in survival in Norway for patients receiving BCT and MTX to determine whether there were differences in long term survival.

To do this, they selected women with early-stage breast cancer (T1-T2, N0-N1, M0) and excluded women with previous breast cancer, multiple tumors, and those who did not undergo surgery. All women undergoing BCT were recommended to have radiation therapy (RT), and patients undergoing MTX with positive axillary lymph nodes were also recommended to have RT, as were women with positive margins. In general, neoadjuvant treatment was not recommended, and this database did not contain information regarding adjuvant treatment. The study included 13015 women with early stage breast cancer, of whom 62% had BCT and 38% had MTX. A higher proportion of women over 70 years of age had MTX over BCT, and those with T2 versus T1 tumors. The overall 5-year survival was 95% in patients undergoing BCT versus 80% in those undergoing MTX (Fig 1), and breast cancer-specific survival was 97% and 88%, respectively. In examining patients over 70 years of age who more commonly had MTX performed, the 5-year overall survival was 87% for those undergoing BCT and 69% for those undergoing MTX, and the 5-year breast cancer-specific survival was 94 and 86%, respectively. The overall hazard ratio for patients undergoing MTX was 1.65 versus BCT; by different age groups was 1.43 for women <50 years of age, 1.74 for women 50 to 69 years of age, and 1.56 for women >70 years of age. In none of the T1-2N0-1 substages was there a benefit of MTX over BCT, and even patients with node-positive disease did not have improved survival with MTX. Limitations of this study were that there might have been selection bias in patients receiving MTX over BCT, which could have been based on tumor biology; however, stage-for-stage, there did not appear to be a benefit to MTX. How axillary nodes were managed in the study was also not discussed. The Norwegian database also does not have information on comorbidities influencing selection of operation, nor does it have information based on *BRCA1* or *2* status, where carriers are more likely to have MTX performed; approximately 2.5% of patients in Norway are mutation carriers. Other patients requested MTX over BCT in up to 14% of cases. Furthermore, there is no information on chemotherapy or anti-estrogen therapy in this database. On the positive side, complete information is available in the registry for most patients, and all patients have access to the same health care system. This study is significant in that it goes farther than previous randomized trials showing equal survival in BCT versus MTX groups and even shows an improvement in survival in the BCT group over MTX. In today's era of increasing use of chemotherapy and hormonal therapy, the need for MTX seems to be decreasing, and this study suggests a survival advantage of choosing BCT over MTX for most women with early-stage breast cancer.

J. R. Howe, MD

References

1. Hwang ES, Lichtensztajn DY, Gomez SL, Fowble B, Clarke CA. Survival after lumpectomy and mastectomy for early stage invasive breastcancer: the effect of age and hormone receptor status. *Cancer.* 2013;119:1402-1411.
2. Agarwal S, Pappas L, Neumayer L, Kokeny K, Agarwal J. Effect of breast conservation therapy vs mastectomy on disease-specific survival for early-stage breast cancer. *JAMA Surg.* 2014;149:267-274.

Impact of Neoadjuvant Chemotherapy in Stage II–III Triple Negative Breast Cancer on Eligibility for Breast-conserving Surgery and Breast Conservation Rates: Surgical Results from CALGB 40603 (Alliance)

Golshan M, on behalf of the Alliance for Clinical Trials in Oncology (Brigham and Women's Hospital, Boston, MA; et al)
Ann Surg 262:434-438, 2015

Objective.—To assess the efficacy of neoadjuvant systemic therapy (NST) at increasing the rate of successful breast-conserving therapy (BCT) in triple negative breast cancer.

Background.—Inducing tumor regression to permit BCT is often cited to support administration of NST. To quantify this benefit, we conducted a surgical companion study to CALGB40603, a randomized phase II, 2 × 2 factorial trial of neoadjuvant paclitaxel ± carboplatin ± bevacizumab (B) followed by doxorubicin plus cyclophosphamide ± B in stage II–III triple negative breast cancer.

Methods.—Before and after NST, treating surgeons evaluated BCT candidacy by clinico-radiographic criteria; surgery performed was at surgeon and patient discretion. We measured (1) conversion rates from BCT-ineligible to BCT-eligible, (2) surgical choices in BCT candidates, and (3) rates of successful BCT with tumor-free margins.

Results.—Four hundred four patients were assessable for surgical outcomes. Two hundred nineteen (54%) were BCT candidates before NST. One hundred ninety-seven (90%) remained BCT candidates after NST, of whom 138 (70%) chose BCT, which was successful in 130 (94%). Of 185 (46%) who were not BCT candidates before NST, 78 (42%) converted to candidates with NST. Of these, 53 (68%) chose BCT with a 91% (48/53) success rate. The overall BCT-eligibility rate rose from 54% to 68% (275/404) with NST. Addition of carboplatin, B, or both increased conversion rates.

Conclusions.—This is the first study to document prospectively a 42% conversion rate from BCT-ineligible to BCT-eligible, resulting in a 14% absolute increase in BCT eligibility. BCT was successful in 93% of patients who opted for it, but 31% of BCT-eligible patients still chose mastectomy.

▶ Several trials have demonstrated the utility of neoadjuvant systemic therapy (NST) at increasing the rates of breast conservation therapy (BCT), including the National Surgical Adjuvant Breast and Bowel Project B18 trial. The majority of these trials, however, have been nonprospective. In this CALGB 40603 trial, patients with triple negative breast cancer were randomly allocated to 4 treatment arms, including Adriamycin and cyclophosphamide (with or without paclitaxel, carboplatin, and/or bevacizumab), and then the rates of patients who were eligible for BCT were determined before and after treatment. Patients all had clinical stage 2 and stage 3 breast cancer and all were estrogen receptor/progesterone receptor negative and *HER2* negative. Patients had baseline mammography with or without ultrasound, and surgeons determined whether the patients were eligible for BCT or not based on physical examination, breast size, and imaging. The primary focus of the study was to determine how many patients that were deemed ineligible for BCT converted to eligibility after NST. The secondary end points were the number of people who were candidates for BCT before and after treatment, the proportion of patients who actually underwent BCT, the incidence of success, and the final surgical procedures performed. There were 404 women who had complete surgical data, and of those, 54% were deemed to be candidates for BCT pre-NST, and 46% were deemed not to be candidates. Of those who were candidates for BCT preoperatively, 90% remained so after NST, and of those who were deemed to be ineligible for BCT, after NST 42% of those patients converted to eligibility. Overall, BCT was attempted in 70% of pre-NST eligible and 68% of those who converted to eligibility after NST. BCT was successful in more than 90% of patients, as deemed by no ink on tumor. Overall, only 47% of patients underwent BCT whereas 53% underwent mastectomy (Table 2 in the original article). BCT ineligibility was most commonly for the tumor being too large, the likelihood of poor cosmetic outcome, diffuse microcalcifications, or multicentric disease. The differences in BCT were not significant among chemotherapy groups, and the difference was only 33% for patients with paclitaxel only (in addition to

Adriamycin and cyclophosphamide), 38% with paclitaxel plus bevacizumab, 45% with paclitaxel plus carboplatin, and up to 50% with paclitaxel, carboplatin, and bevacizumab.

The main conclusion from this study was that 42% of women were converted to eligibility for BCT after neoadjuvant treatment, and only 10% became ineligible after treatment. This study is somewhat confused by the different treatment arms, which all included and there appeared to be improvement with more aggressive regimens. However, toxicity in patients receiving these treatments was not discussed. This study is unique in that surgeons determine eligibility pre- and post-NST, but there was a high rate of mastectomy; the authors state that this might have been due to the strong recommendation that MRI be performed, which appears to increase the rate of mastectomy. It is also not clear how the decision for the surgical procedure was made, although it was presumably based on patient preference, and patients were not randomized to receive particular operations.

J. R. Howe, MD

Applicability of the ACOSOG Z0011 Criteria in Women with High-Risk Node-Positive Breast Cancer Undergoing Breast Conserving Surgery

Chung A, Gangi A, Mirocha J, et al (Cedars Sinai Med Ctr, Los Angeles, CA)

Ann Surg Oncol 22:1128-1132, 2015

Background.—The relevance of the American College of Surgeons Oncology Group (ACOSOG) Z0011 trial in patients with high-risk breast cancer has been questioned. We hypothesize that Z0011 applies to women with HER2-positive disease (HER2+), triple-negative breast cancer (TNBC), and/or age <50 years at diagnosis (YA).

Methods.—Women with node-positive HER2+, TNBC, or YA were identified from a prospectively maintained database. Patients were grouped based on Z0011 trial eligibility criteria into those meeting criteria (eligible) and those who did not (ineligible). Patient and tumor characteristics were compared survival of those meeting Z0011 criteria was determined.

Results.—We identified 186 node-positive women undergoing lumpectomy/radiation for high-risk breast cancer: 57 of 186 (31 %) HER2+, 55 of 186 (30 %) TNBC, 74 of 186 (40 %) YA. Overall, 125 of 186 (67 %) met Z0011 criteria. HER2 positivity was associated with the lowest rate of ineligibility compared with TNBC and YA (16 vs. 53 and 31 %, respectively, $p < 0.01$). Larger tumor size, high grade, extranodal extension, and high Ki67 were associated with Z0011 ineligibility. Among those who were eligible, 105 of 125 (84 %) had ALND and 48 of 125 (38 %) had involvement of nonsentinel nodes (NSLN) median number of NSLNs involved was one (range 1–3). With median follow-up of 5.5 years, there was no difference in survival between those who had ALND and those who did not. After patients with clinically palpable nodes were excluded, 125 of 149 (84 %) met criteria.

Conclusions.—The Z0011 trial eligibility requirements apply to a significant proportion of patients with HER2+, TNBC, and YA. ALND can be avoided in 67 % node-positive cases and in 84 % of those with clinically negative nodes (Table 2).

▶ The American College of Surgeons Oncology Group Z0011 trial randomized patients with clinical T1-T2N0 invasive breast cancer found to have 1 or 2 positive sentinel lymph nodes to axillary dissection or no dissection. The study revealed that there was no survival difference in these 2 groups, which has led to a significant change in the practice of breast surgery, with patients no longer receiving routine axillary dissection when there is a positive sentinel lymph node. In this retrospective study by Chung et al, the authors look specifically at a group of high-risk women with breast cancer who might have been eligible for this trial to see whether the findings of Z0011 would apply to them as well. High-risk breast cancer was defined by 1 of 3 criteria: HER2-positive disease, triple-negative breast cancer (ER-/PR-/HER2-), or age of diagnosis < 50 years of age. These patients had to have clinical T1-T2N0 lesions as seen in the Z0011 trial. Patients were excluded if they had T3 lesions, clinically palpable nodes, had neoadjuvant therapy, never had sentinel lymph node biopsy, or had 3 or more positive sentinel lymph nodes. They retrospectively

TABLE 2.—Comparison of Patient and Tumor Characteristics Between Group That Met Z0011 Eligibility Criteria and Group That Did Not Meet Z0011 Criteria

Characteristic	Did Not Met Z0011 Criteria ($N = 61$)	Met Z0011 Criteria ($N = 125$)	p Value	Test
Histology, % (n/N)			0.15	Fisher
Ductal	93 (57/61)	86 (107/125)		
Lobular	0 (0/61)	6 (7/125)		
Mixed	7 (4/61)	9 (11/125)		
Tumor grade, % (n/N)			**0.02**	**Fisher**
Low	**2 (1/61)**	**6 (7/124)**		
Intermediate	**18 (11/61)**	**34 (42/124)**		
High	**80 (49/61)**	**61 (75/124)**		
Multifocality, % (n/N)	16 (9/53)	23 (29/124)	0.33	Fisher
Lymphovascular invasion, % (n/N)	59 (31/53)	63 (77/123)	0.62	Fisher
Extranodal extension, % (n/N)	53 (30/57)	29 (35/123)	**<0.01**	**Fisher**
Tumor size, median (IQR)	**26.5 (18.5–38) N = 60**	**21.5 (14.5–29.5) N = 124**	**<0.01**	**WRST**
Tumor size, % (n/N)			**0.05**	**Fisher**
<2 cm	27 (16/60)	44 (55/124)		
2–5 cm	65 (39/60)	51 (63/124)		
≥5 cm	8 (5/60)	5 (6/124)		
Ki67, median (IQR)	**40 (22–52) N = 54**	**22 (14–39) N = 117**	**<0.01**	**WRST**
Ki67 level, % (n/N)			**<0.01**	**Fisher**
Low	6 (3/54)	15 (17/117)		
Intermediate	**24 (13/54)**	**40 (47/117)**		
High	**70 (38/54)**	**45 (53/117)**		
Age, mean (SD)	54 (15)	48 (12)	0.01	*t* test

Bold values indicate the results that had a significant p value

IQR interquartile range, *SD* standard deviation, *WRST* Wilcoxon rank-sum test

Reprinted from Chung A, Gangi A, Mirocha J, et al. Applicability of the ACOSOG Z0011 criteria in women with high-risk node-positive breast cancer undergoing breast conserving surgery. *Ann Surg Oncol.* 2015;22:1128-1132, with permission from Society of Surgical Oncology.

reviewed their patients between 2000 and 2011 and found 516 patients defined to be at high risk. Of these, 299 patients were excluded because they had mastectomy, and others were excluded for insufficient pathology and nodal disease only found by immunohistochemistry (and not by hematoxylin and eosin). This left 186 patients with high-risk tumors over this time period. Of these 186 patients, another one-third were ineligible because they had T3 tumors, neoadjuvant therapy, failed sentinel lymph node mapping, or had 3 or more positive sentinel lymph nodes. They then compared the groups of patients who were deemed ineligible versus eligible for the different high-risk factors. Significant factors between patients meeting and not meeting the Z0011 criteria include higher incidence of higher tumor grade, extranodal extension, increased tumor size, and higher Ki67 rate in those found to be ineligible for Z0011 (Table 2).

They found that patients with HER2+ tumors had the lowest rate of ineligibility, and the highest rate of ineligibility was seen in patients with triple negative breast cancers. Fifty-three percent of patients with triple-negative breast cancer were ineligible mostly because of clinically involved nodes at presentation. When removing these patients within clinically N1 and T3 tumors, 85% would have been eligible. Eighty percent of patients with young-onset breast cancer would have been eligible for the Z0011 trial. Most importantly, of those patients who would have been eligible for Z0011, 84% had axillary lymph node dissection, while 16% did not have axillary lymph node dissection. Interestingly, of those who had axillary dissection, 38% had involvement of a nonsentinel lymph node with a median number of nodes involved being 1. However, their survival was not different from the group not having axillary node dissection, with a mean survival of 5.5 years. In both groups, there was no local recurrence. The final conclusion of this study was that patients with high-risk features such as HER2 positivity, triple-negative breast cancer, and early age of onset have similar results when they do not have axillary nodal dissection for T1-T2N0 breast cancers. Therefore, they conclude that the findings of Z0011 can be applied to these high-risk patients if they meet eligibility criteria.

J. R. Howe, MD

Marking Axillary Lymph Nodes With Radioactive Iodine Seeds for Axillary Staging After Neoadjuvant Systemic Treatment in Breast Cancer Patients: The MARI Procedure

Donker M, Straver ME, Wesseling J, et al (Netherlands Cancer Inst-Antoni van Leeuwenhoek Hosp, Amsterdam)

Ann Surg 261:378-382, 2015

Objective.—The MARI procedure [marking the axillary lymph node with radioactive iodine (^{125}I) seeds] is a new minimal invasive method to assess the pathological response of nodal metastases after neoadjuvant systemic treatment (NST) in patients with breast cancer. This method allows axilla-conserving surgery in patients responding well to NST.

Methods.—Prior to NST, proven tumor-positive axillary lymph nodes were marked with a ^{125}I seed. This marked lymph node is the so-called MARI-node. After NST, the MARI node was selectively removed using a γ-detection probe. A complementary axillary lymph node dissection was performed in all patients to assess whether pathological response in the MARI node was indicative for the pathological response in the additional lymph nodes.

Results.—A tumor-positive axillary lymph node was marked with a ^{125}I seed in 100 patients. The MARI node was successfully identified in 97 of these 100 patients (identification rate 97%). Two patients did not undergo subsequent axillary lymph node dissection, leaving 95 patients for further analysis. The MARI node contained residual tumor cells in 65 of these 95 patients. In the other 30 patients, the MARI node was free of tumor, but additional positive lymph nodes were found in 5 patients. Thus, the MARI procedure correctly identified 65 of 70 patients with residual axillary tumor activity (false negative rate 5/70 = 7%).

Conclusions.—This study shows that marking and selectively removing metastatic lymph nodes after neoadjuvant systemic treatment has a high identification rate and a low false negative rate. The tumor response in the marked lymph node may be used to tailor further axillary treatment after NST (Table 2).

▶ Neoadjuvant treatment is being given with increasing frequency in patients with breast cancer. This may lead to complete pathologic responses in the breast in up to half of patients and in the axilla in 20% to 40% of patients. If there were a means of identifying whether an involved lymph node had a complete pathologic response, then nonsurgical therapy of the axilla might be a viable option. Studies looking at sentinel lymph node biopsy (SLNB) after chemotherapy, such as the ACOSOG Z1071 trial, revealed a false-negative rate of 13%, and overall accuracy rate of 84%, which was especially difficult when patients have clinically node-positive disease and converted to clinically node-negative disease.

TABLE 2.—Pathologic Results of the MARI Node and Additional Axillary Lymph Nodes in Patients in Whom the MARI Node Was Identified (n = 95)*

	Outcome Additional Lymph Nodes		
	Positive	Negative	Total
Outcome MARI node			
Positive	46	19	65
Negative	5	25	30
Total	51	44	95

*False negative rate: 5/70 = 7% (95% CI: 2–16); overall accuracy: 90/95 = 95% (95% CI: 88–95); negative predicting value: 25/30 = 83% (95% CI: 65–94); positive predicting value: 100% (by definition); sensitivity: 46/51 = 90% (95% CI: 79–97); specificity: 100% (by definition).

Reprinted from Donker M, Straver ME, Wesseling J, et al. Marking axillary lymph nodes with radioactive iodine seeds for axillary staging after neoadjuvant systemic treatment in breast cancer patients: the MARI procedure. *Ann Surg.* 2015;261:378-382, with permission from Wolters Kluwer Health, Inc.

This group from the Netherlands attempted to develop a procedure in which an involved lymph node identified preoperatively could be found again after neoadjuvant chemotherapy. They looked at 100 patients in whom an I-125 seed had been placed in the breast and into an axillary lymph node that had been previously identified as being histologically positive. These I-125 seeds had an activity between 1 and 7 MBq and a half-life of 60 days. All patients in the study had clinically positive lymph nodes, with 60% being N1, 13% being N2, and 27% being N3. Chemotherapy was given based on the histologic subtype, including triple-negative breast cancer, ER positive/HER2 negative, and HER2 positive. After receiving neoadjuvant chemotherapy, the lymph node in which the iodine seed had been placed was sought out using a gamma probe with the incision made over the area of greatest activity. This node, designated as the MARI node (marking axillary node with radioactive iodine), was then removed, and an axillary lymph node dissection was performed in addition to the breast surgery. These MARI lymph nodes were examined under 3 sections with hematoxylin and eosin (H + E), and if negative, immunohistochemistry was done for keratin. Subsequent axillary lymph nodes from the dissection were all examined by H + E. In these 100 patients, the MARI procedure was carried out, and the MARI node was identified in 97%. In 95 patients in whom axillary node dissection was performed, the MARI node showed residual tumor in 65 patients versus no tumor or complete pathologic response in 30 patients. In 3 patients, the MARI node could not be identified because the seed was not in the lymph node, giving an overall identification rate of 97%. In the 65 patients of whom the MARI node was positive, there was an additional positive node found in 46 patients, with a median number of 3 additional positive nodes. In those 30 patients who had a negative MARI node, residual disease was found in 5 patients, and 2 of these patients had just micro-metastatic disease. Therefore, the overall accuracy in these patients was 90 of 95 (95% rate), and the false-negative rate was 7% (5 of 70 patients) (Table 2).

This study revealed that the MARI procedure is effective in identifying the node found preoperatively to be histologically involved, which appeared to be an improvement over SLNB after neoadjuvant chemotherapy. The surgeons found this relatively easy to perform and perhaps even easier than SLNB because there is no background radiation. One of the challenges of the procedure is that it requires a preprocedural biopsy of the lymph node showing positivity and then a separate procedure where the iodine seeds are placed, and therefore the authors stress the importance of good documentation of the location of this lymph node to put the seed in the correct lymph node. This procedure can be performed up to several months after iodine seed placement, and here this was performed at a median of 17 weeks, with a range of 9 to 31 weeks. The radiation dose from this iodine seed is minimal, and therefore there is little hazard to the patient, but it does require strict monitoring as does any radioactive protocol. The important question raised by this study is how this will alter treatment. If patients are found to have a pathologic complete response in the MARI node, because the false-negative rate is only 7%, then these patients can be considered to just have radiotherapy of the axilla rather than axillary lymph node dissection. If future trials demonstrated no survival difference, perhaps axillary treatment could be omitted all together. This trial did establish that this procedure is feasible, is surgeon friendly, safe, and has a low false-negative rate.

J. R. Howe, MD

Rectal

A Randomized Trial of Laparoscopic versus Open Surgery for Rectal Cancer

Bonjer HJ, for the COLOR II Study Group (VU Univ Med Ctr, Amsterdam, the Netherlands)

N Engl J Med 372:1324-1332, 2015

Background.—Laparoscopic resection of colorectal cancer is widely used. However, robust evidence to conclude that laparoscopic surgery and open surgery have similar outcomes in rectal cancer is lacking. A trial was designed to compare 3-year rates of cancer recurrence in the pelvic or perineal area (locoregional recurrence) and survival after laparoscopic and open resection of rectal cancer.

Methods.—In this international trial conducted in 30 hospitals, we randomly assigned patients with a solitary adenocarcinoma of the rectum within 15 cm of the anal verge, not invading adjacent tissues, and without distant metastases to undergo either laparoscopic or open surgery in a 2:1 ratio. The primary end point was locoregional recurrence 3 years after the index surgery. Secondary end points included disease-free and overall survival.

Results.—A total of 1044 patients were included (699 in the laparoscopic-surgery group and 345 in the open-surgery group). At 3 years, the locoregional recurrence rate was 5.0% in the two groups (difference, 0 percentage points; 90% confidence interval [CI], −2.6 to 2.6). Disease-free survival rates were 74.8% in the laparoscopic-surgery group and 70.8% in the open-surgery group (difference, 4.0 percentage points; 95% CI, −1.9 to 9.9). Overall survival rates were 86.7% in the laparoscopic-surgery group and 83.6% in the open-surgery group (difference, 3.1 percentage points; 95% CI, −1.6 to 7.8).

Conclusions.—Laparoscopic surgery in patients with rectal cancer was associated with rates of locoregional recurrence and disease-free and overall survival similar to those for open surgery. (Funded by Ethicon Endo-Surgery Europe and others; COLOR II ClinicalTrials.gov number, NCT00297791.)

▶ In 1994 the first results of the clinical outcomes of surgical therapy study group (COST) revealed similar recurrence rates in those patients having laparoscopically assisted versus open colectomies, and the same 3-year survival.[1] The follow-up study in 2007 revealed that 5-year disease-free and overall survival were not significantly different between the 2 groups.[2] This trial specifically excluded patients with rectal cancer, and therefore the current study performed a multi-institutional, international, randomized trial of laparoscopic versus open rectal cancer resection. This was a large study including 1044 patients randomized 2:1 to the laparoscopic versus open groups. Tumors had to be within 15 cm of the anal verge, and T4 tumors or T3 tumors within 2 mm of the endopelvic fascia were excluded from the study. Neoadjuvant therapy was administered per individual institutional tumor board recommendations, and there was no stratification for this. Surgeons had to comply with the principles of total mesorectal excision and were required to submit 5 videos of laparoscopic mesorectal excisions to recruit patients. Patients had annual clinical examinations and had CT or MRI of the pelvis performed 3 years after the initial surgery with imaging of the liver and chest. The majority of patients had 3-year follow-up data, which revealed that similar numbers of patients had received preoperative chemotherapy (32%-34%) and radiotherapy (58%-59%). The final pathologic stages were very similar in both groups, and complete resection was achieved in 84% of patients having laparoscopic versus 88% of those having open surgery. The median lymph nodes harvested were 13 in the laparoscopic and 14 in the open surgery group. Interestingly, there was a lower recurrence rate in patients having laparoscopic surgery for lower rectal lesions, which was 9% in the laparoscopic group versus 22% in the open surgery group. Also, in patients with positive lymph nodes, the 3-year disease-free survival was higher in patients having laparoscopic surgery (65%) versus those after open surgery (52%). Overall 3-year disease-free survival rates were similar at 75% versus 71% in laparoscopic versus open groups and overall survival was 87% versus 84%, respectively. The locoregional recurrence rate was 5% in both groups (Table 2 in the original article). This study demonstrated that laparoscopic surgery is as safe and effective as open surgery if total mesorectal excision is performed with similar rates of local recurrence, disease-free and overall survival. Some subgroups appeared to have an advantage with the laparoscopic approach, including those with lower third rectal tumors as well as patients who were found to have node-positive disease. Although the reasons for this are unclear, one possibility is that reduced surgical trauma may reduce the rate of tumor recurrence.

J. R. Howe, MD

References

1. Clinical Outcomes of Surgical Therapy Study Group. A comparison of laparoscopically assisted and open colectomy for colon cancer. *N Engl J Med.* 2004; 350:2050-2059.
2. Fleshman J, Sargent DJ, Green E, et al. Laparoscopic colectomy for cancer is not inferior to open surgery based on 5-year data from the COST Study Group trial. *Ann Surg.* 2007;246:655-662.

Comparative Effectiveness of Sphincter-Sparing Surgery Versus Abdominoperineal Resection in Rectal Cancer: Patient-Reported Outcomes in National Surgical Adjuvant Breast and Bowel Project Randomized Trial R-04

Russell MM, Ganz PA, Lopa S, et al (Operations and Biostatistical Ctrs, Pittsburgh, PA; et al)

Ann Surg 261:144-148, 2015

Objective.—National Surgical Adjuvant Breast and Bowel Project (NSABP) R-04 was a randomized controlled trial of neoadjuvant chemoradiotherapy in patients with resectable stage II-III rectal cancer. We hypothesized that patients who underwent abdominoperineal resection (APR) would have a poorer quality of life than those who underwent sphincter-sparing surgery (SSS).

Methods.—To obtain patient-reported outcomes (PROs) we administered two symptom scales at baseline and 1 year postoperatively: the Functional Assessment of Cancer Therapy-Colorectal (FACT-C) and the European Organization for the Research and Treatment of Cancer module for patients with Colorectal Cancer Quality of Life Questionnaire (EORTC QLQ-CR38). Scoring was stratified by nonrandomly assigned definitive surgery (APR vs SSS). Analyses controlled for baseline scores and stratification factors: age, sex, stage, intended surgery, and randomly assigned chemoradiotherapy.

Results.—Of 1,608 randomly assigned patients, 987 had data for planned analyses; 62% underwent SSS; 38% underwent APR. FACT-C total and subscale scores were not statistically different by surgery at 1 year. For the EORTC QLQ-CR38 functional scales, APR patients reported worse body image (70.3 vs 77.0, $P = 0.0005$) at 1 year than did SSS patients. Males undergoing APR reported worse sexual enjoyment (43.7 vs 54.7, $P = 0.02$) at 1 year than did those undergoing SSS. For the EORTC QLQ-CR38 symptom scale scores, APR patients reported worse micturition symptoms than the SSS group at 1 year (26.9 vs 21.5, $P = 0.03$). SSS patients reported worse gastrointestinal tract symptoms than did the APR patients (18.9 vs 15.2, $P < 0.0001$), as well as weight loss (10.1 vs 6.0, $P = 0.002$).

Conclusions.—Symptoms and functional problems were detected at 1 year by EORTC QLQ-CR38, reflecting different symptom profiles in patients who underwent APR than those who underwent SSS. Information from these PROs may be useful in counseling patients anticipating surgery for rectal cancer (Table).

► Patients with rectal cancer are generally treated by low anterior resection (LAR) or abdominal peritoneal resection (APR), often in conjunction with neoadjuvant chemoradiation. With this strategy, 5-year survival has been improving to approximately 68%. The National Surgical Adjuvant Breast and Bowel Project R04 trial randomized patients with rectal cancer to receive 1 of 4 potential chemoradiotherapy treatments before surgery, including (1) 5-fluorouracil

TABLE.—Patient Characteristics Stratified by Surgical Treatment: NSABP R-04

Characteristic, %	Abdominoperineal Resection (N = 372)	Sphincter-Saving Surgery (N = 615)	Total (N = 987)	P*
Age group, yr				
≤59	53.5	60.3	57.8	0.04
≥60	46.5	39.7	42.3	
Sex				
Male	66.4	66.7	66.6	0.94
Female	33.6	33.3	33.4	
Stage				
II	57.8	63.7	61.5	0.07
III	42.2	36.3	38.5	
Intended surgery				
Abdominoperineal resection	56.7	8.9	27	<0.0001
Sphincter saving	43.3	91.1	73.1	
Adjuvant chemotherapy				
5-FU	10.8	9.6	10	0.72
Capecitabine	14.5	15.5	15.1	
Irinotecan	0	0.3	0.2	
5-FU/Leucovorin	10	8	8.7	
5-FU/Leucovorin/Irinotecan	1.1	1.3	1.2	
Other/none	63.7	65.4	64.7	
Location of tumor	N = 356	N = 571	N = 927	
Upper	1.1	10.7	7	<0.0001
Middle	20.8	50.6	39.2	
Lower	78.1	38.7	53.8	
Tumor size	N = 311	N = 483	N = 794	
0.0–3.0	75.9	81	79	0.23
3.1–6.0	21.9	17.4	19.1	
6.1–10.0	2.3	1.7	1.9	

*χ^2 test for difference between surgical treatment groups.

Reprinted from Russell MM, Ganz PA, Lopa S, et al. Comparative effectiveness of sphincter-sparing surgery versus abdominoperineal resection in rectal cancer: patient-reported outcomes in national surgical adjuvant breast and bowel project randomized trial R-04. *Ann Surg.* 2015;261:144-148, with permission from Lippincott Williams & Wilkins.

(FU) with radiation, (2) 5-FU/oxaliplatin and radiation, (3) capecitabine and radiation, and (4) capecitabine/oxaliplatin and radiation. Patients received chemoradiation and then surgery 6 to 8 weeks later. During this study, quality-of-life assessments were performed at baseline, after chemoradiotherapy, and then 1 year after surgery. The aim of this study was to see whether there were any significant differences in quality-of-life issues in patients who receive LAR vs APR. The operations performed were not randomized and were at the surgeon's discretion. Quality of life was assessed through 2 questionnaires, the first being the Functional Assessment of Cancer Therapy (FACT-C), and the second the European Organization for Research and Treatment of Cancer (EORTC QLQ-CR38). The former includes information on physical, social, emotional, and functional well-being, as well as colorectal cancer-specific concerns. The second consists of 38 questions that cover 4 functional scales, including body image, sexual function, sexual enjoyment, and future perspective, as well as 8 symptoms, involving micturition, gastrointestinal (GI) chemotherapeutic side effects, defecation problems, stomach problems, sexual problems, and weight loss.

Of 1502 patients randomized, 926 (62%) had LAR and 576 (38%) had APR. The majority of patients filled out the questionnaires (90%) at baseline, and approximately 73% complied at 1 year. Patients who underwent LAR vs APR were similar, with the exception (not surprisingly) that 78% of patients undergoing APR had lower third rectal tumors versus 39% in the LAR group; there were more older patients in the APR group, and 43% of the patients undergoing APR were originally planned to have an LAR (Table). There was no statistically significant difference with respect to type of surgery in the FACT-C score or for any of the subscales. On the other hand, in the EORTC functional scale, patients who had APR had a worse body image, decreased male sexual enjoyment, and were less sexually active. Patients who had APR had a baseline of worse symptoms of sexual function and GI tract, possibly due to having more tumors of the lower third of the rectum. After 1 year, there was no difference in sexual function between patients undergoing APR and LAR, but patients who had LAR had worse GI symptoms and higher weight loss than patients who had APR. Patients who had APR had a worse body image, micturition, and sexual enjoyment after 1 year. Conclusions of this study were that there were some procedure-specific differences in quality of life 1 year after surgery, as described. Limitations of this study were that the study was not randomized for surgical procedure, some people did not fill out the quality-of-life questionnaires, and patients who had stage 3 disease often did not fill out the questionnaire because of recurrent disease. There were also a high proportion of patients who were intended to have an LAR but ended up with an APR. This study is significant because of its large numbers and its identification of procedure-specific differences in quality of life that will help with preoperative counseling for patients with rectal cancer.

J. R. Howe, MD

Melanoma

Pooled Analysis of Long-Term Survival Data From Phase II and Phase III Trials of Ipilimumab in Unresectable or Metastatic Melanoma

Schadendorf D, Hodi FS, Robert C, et al (Univ Hosp Essen, Germany; Dana-Farber Cancer Inst, Boston, MA; Inst Gustave Roussy, Villejuif, France; et al)
J Clin Oncol 33:1889-1894, 2015

Purpose.—To provide a more precise estimate of long-term survival observed for ipilimumab-treated patients with advanced melanoma, we performed a pooled analysis of overall survival (OS) data from multiple studies.

Methods.—The primary analysis pooled OS data for 1,861 patients from 10 prospective and two retrospective studies of ipilimumab, including two phase III trials. Patients were previously treated (n = 1,257) or treatment naive (n = 604), and the majority of patients received ipilimumab 3 mg/kg (n = 965) or 10 mg/kg (n = 706). We also conducted a secondary analysis of OS data (n = 4,846) with an additional 2,985 patients from an expanded access program. OS rates were estimated using the Kaplan-Meier method.

Results.—Among 1,861 patients, median OS was 11.4 months (95% CI, 10.7 to 12.1 months), which included 254 patients with at least 3 years of survival follow-up. The survival curve began to plateau around year 3, with follow-up of up to 10 years. Three-year survival rates were 22%, 26%, and 20% for all patients, treatment-naive patients, and previously treated patients, respectively. Including data from the expanded access program, median OS was 9.5 months (95% CI, 9.0 to 10.0 months), with a plateau at 21% in the survival curve beginning around year 3.

Conclusion.—To our knowledge, this is the largest analysis of OS to date for ipilimumab-treated patients with advanced melanoma. We observed a plateau in the survival curve, beginning at approximately 3 years, which was independent of prior therapy or ipilimumab dose. These data add to the evidence supporting the durability of long-term survival in ipilimumab-treated patients with advanced melanoma.

▶ Patients with stage 4 melanoma have poor survival, and until recently, high dose interleukin (IL)-2 was the preferred form of therapy in patients with this disease. However, in 2011, it was shown that 2 new agents have had significant activity. These included vemurafenib, which inhibits BRAF kinase in patients with V600 mutation, and ipilimumab, an antibody to CTLA-4. Multiple trials have been conducted using ipilimumab to augment T-cell killing, and this study set out to do a pooled analysis of trials using this drug and examine its effect on long-term survival. This authors search for trials in which there were data on overall survival and in which ipilimumab was given every 3 weeks for at least 4 doses. They selected 10 prospective and 2 retrospective studies, which varied significantly from treatment of naive patients to those being treated with other agents, such as gp100 melanoma peptide vaccine, dacarbazine, or budesonide. Some of these trials also compared different doses of ipilimumab in phase 2 trials, and some included patients with brain metastasis. From these 12 trials, there were 1861 patients, that included 1257 that had been previously treated and the remainder were treatment-naive. In 965 patients ipilimumab was given at 3 mg/kg, in 706 at 10 mg/kg, and the remainder had a variety of different doses. Some patients were only treated up front with ipilimumab for at least 4 doses, others could receive maintenance therapy thereafter or were retreated when disease progression was found. With a median follow-up of approximately 11 months (10% of patients for at least 50 months), the median overall survival was 11.4 months and the 3-year survival was 22%. What was most interesting about this study was that there was a plateau in the survival curve at approximately 3 years (Fig 1 in the original article). This means that patients who survive for 3 years were likely to have a durable response, and many survived up to 10 years. Survival was also evaluated by whether there was previous therapy, and patients who were treatment-naive appeared to do slightly better than those who were previously treated. Also, patients receiving the higher dose at 10 mg/kg had a slightly improved survival over those who received 3 mg/kg. Similar effects of durable long-term survival have been seen in patients treated with IL-2, although the proportion of patients was lower. This has raised the question of whether a subset of patients with melanoma could be cured by these therapies, but these studies were not designed to see whether patients were completely free of disease or might be alive with disease. In some of these studies, the finding of an objective complete or partial response was not necessary for long-term survival. This study is limited by the fact that results from multiple studies with different treatment arms were included, and therefore results could have been affected by some of the other treatments received. However, it is the largest collection of patients in whom overall survival data are available who have been treated with ipilimumab. There were also no consistent control groups. The salient finding is that approximately 20% of patients will survive 3 years, and in those patients, these responses appear to be durable, giving hope to patients with this lethal disease.

J. R. Howe, MD

Pembrolizumab versus Ipilimumab in Advanced Melanoma

Robert C, for the KEYNOTE-006 investigators (Service de Dermatologie, Villejuif, France; et al)

N Engl J Med 372:2521-2532, 2015

Background.—The immune checkpoint inhibitor ipilimumab is the standard-of-care treatment for patients with advanced melanoma. Pembrolizumab inhibits the programmed cell death 1 (PD-1) immune checkpoint and has antitumor activity in patients with advanced melanoma.

Methods.—In this randomized, controlled, phase 3 study, we assigned 834 patients with advanced melanoma in a 1:1:1 ratio to receive pembrolizumab (at a dose of 10 mg per kilogram of body weight) every 2 weeks or every 3 weeks or four doses of ipilimumab (at 3 mg per kilogram) every 3 weeks. Primary end points were progression-free and overall survival.

Results.—The estimated 6-month progression-free-survival rates were 47.3% for pembrolizumab every 2 weeks, 46.4% for pembrolizumab every 3 weeks, and 26.5% for ipilimumab (hazard ratio for disease progression, 0.58; $P < 0.001$ for both pembrolizumab regimens versus ipilimumab; 95% confidence intervals [CIs], 0.46 to 0.72 and 0.47 to 0.72, respectively). Estimated 12-month survival rates were 74.1%, 68.4%, and 58.2%, respectively (hazard ratio for death for pembrolizumab every 2 weeks, 0.63; 95% CI, 0.47 to 0.83; $P = 0.0005$; hazard ratio for pembrolizumab every 3 weeks, 0.69; 95% CI, 0.52 to 0.90; $P = 0.0036$). The response rate was improved with pembrolizumab administered every 2 weeks (33.7%) and every 3 weeks (32.9%), as compared with ipilimumab (11.9%) ($P < 0.001$ for both comparisons). Responses were ongoing in 89.4%, 96.7%, and 87.9% of patients, respectively, after a median follow-up of 7.9 months. Efficacy was similar in the two pembrolizumab groups. Rates of treatment-related adverse events of grade 3 to 5 severity were lower in the pembrolizumab groups (13.3% and 10.1%) than in the ipilimumab group (19.9%).

Conclusions.—The anti–PD-1 antibody pembrolizumab prolonged progression-free survival and overall survival and had less high-grade toxicity than did ipilimumab in patients with advanced melanoma. (Funded by Merck Sharp & Dohme; KEYNOTE-006 ClinicalTrials.gov number, NCT01866319.)

▶ The outlook for patients with stage 3 and 4 melanoma has generally been very poor, but new developments in medical therapy for patients with advanced melanoma have significantly changed the landscape. These include inhibitors for the approximately 50% of patients with *BRAF* mutations, and more recently, immunotherapy for melanoma. These immunotherapeutic approaches have targeted 2 pathways. One is blockade of the CTLA-4T lymphocyte associated protein, which is an inhibitory molecule expressed on T cells that inhibits the development of immune responses. The drug ipilimumab works in this way. Another new class is the PD-1 inhibitors. PD-1 is a receptor on T cells where binding of its ligand (PD-L1) causes programmed cell death. Cancers have evolved to producing PD-1, which represents another mechanism for their escape from immune surveillance. Drugs targeted at PD-1 include pembrolizumab and nivolumab. Ipilimumab has been shown to result in survival benefit for patients with advanced melanoma, and the current study set out to compare the value of the PD-1 inhibitor pembrolizumab to that of ipilimumab at 2 doses, and specifically, for progression-free (PFS) and overall survival, as well as adverse effects.

This was a randomized trial that assigned patients to receive pembrolizumab every 2 weeks or 3 weeks and ipilimumab every 3 weeks. In total, 834 patients were randomized and were well balanced for various factors, including PD-L1 positive tumors, *BRAF* mutations (approximately 35%), brain metastases, and stage. This trial included patients with unresectable stage 3 or 4 melanoma and allowed for previous treatment with *BRAF* inhibitors but excluded those with previous treatment using CTLA-4, PD-1, or PD-L1 inhibitors and those who with ocular melanoma or a history of serious auto-immune disease. The median follow-up was 7.9 months, and over the study period, 289 deaths were recorded. Both treatment regimens with pembrolizumab showed an improvement in PFS versus ipilimumab, with a 6-month PFS of 47% for pembrolizumab every 2 weeks, 46% every 3 weeks, and 27% for ipilimumab (Fig 1 in the original article). Median PFS for the pembrolizumab arms were 5.5 months versus 2.8 months for ipilimumab, and the hazard ratio was 0.58 for those receiving pembrolizumab. Overall survival also showed an advantage, with 74% of patients receiving pembrolizumab every 2 weeks being alive at 1 year, 68% in the every 3 week dosage, versus 58% in those receiving ipilimumab. All patient subgroups showed a benefit with pembrolizumab except those whose tumor cells were PD-L1 negative. Overall response rates were 34% for pembrolizumab given every 2 weeks, 33% every 3 weeks, and 12% for ipilimumab. Complete responses were seen infrequently, with approximately 5% with pembrolizumab versus 1.4% with ipilimumab. However, when responses did occur, they were durable, and approximately 90% of each group who responded continued to have response at the time of analysis, which was 12 months. The frequency of adverse events was 10% to 13% in the pembrolizumab groups versus 20% in the ipilimumab group. The most common adverse events were fatigue, diarrhea, rash, and pruritis. Autoimmune effects seen with pembrolizumab included hypothyroidism, hyperthyroidism, colitis, and hepatitis. In summary, this large randomized trial showed that response rates, PFS, and overall survival were improved with both dosages of pembrolizumab versus ipilimumab in patients with advanced melanoma. The frequency of adverse events were less, and the only subgroup not benefiting were those who had tumors which were PD-L1 negative. The limitations of this study were short follow-up and relatively low response rates. However, from this study it appears that PD-1 blockade immunotherapy represent improvement over that of CTLA-4 blockade and should be offered to patients with stage 3 and 4 melanoma.

J. R. Howe, MD

Sentinel Lymph Node Biopsy Is Indicated for Patients With Thick Clinically Lymph Node-Negative Melanoma

Yamamoto M, Fisher KJ, Wong JY, et al (Univ of California at Irvine Med Ctr, Orange; H. Lee Moffitt Cancer Ctr and Res Inst, Tampa, FL; Penn State Hershey Med Ctr, PA; et al)
Cancer 121:1628-1636, 2015

Background.—Sentinel lymph node biopsy (SLNB) is indicated for the staging of clinically lymph node-negative melanoma of intermediate thickness, but its use is controversial in patients with thick melanoma.

Methods.—From 2002 to 2012, patients with melanoma measuring ≥4 mm in thickness were evaluated at a single institution. Associations between survival and clinicopathologic characteristics were explored.

Results.—Of 571 patients with melanomas measuring ≥4 mm in thickness and no distant metastases, the median age was 66 years and 401 patients (70.2%) were male. The median Breslow thickness was 6.2 mm; the predominant subtype was nodular (45.4%). SLNB was performed in 412 patients (72%) whereas 46 patients (8.1%) presented with clinically lymph node-positive disease and 113 patients (20%) did not undergo SLNB. A positive SLN was found in 161 of 412 patients (39.1%). For SLNB performed at the study institution, 14 patients with a negative SLNB developed disease recurrence in the mapped lymph node basin (false-negative rate, 12.3%). The median disease-specific survival (DSS), overall survival (OS), and recurrence-free survival (RFS) for the entire cohort were 62.1 months, 42.5 months, and 21.2 months, respectively. The DSS and OS for patients with a negative SLNB were 82.4 months and 53.4 months, respectively; 41.2 months and 34.7 months, respectively, for patients with positive SLNB; and 26.8 months and 22 months, respectively, for patients with clinically lymph node-positive disease ($P < .0001$). The median RFS was 32.4 months for patients who were

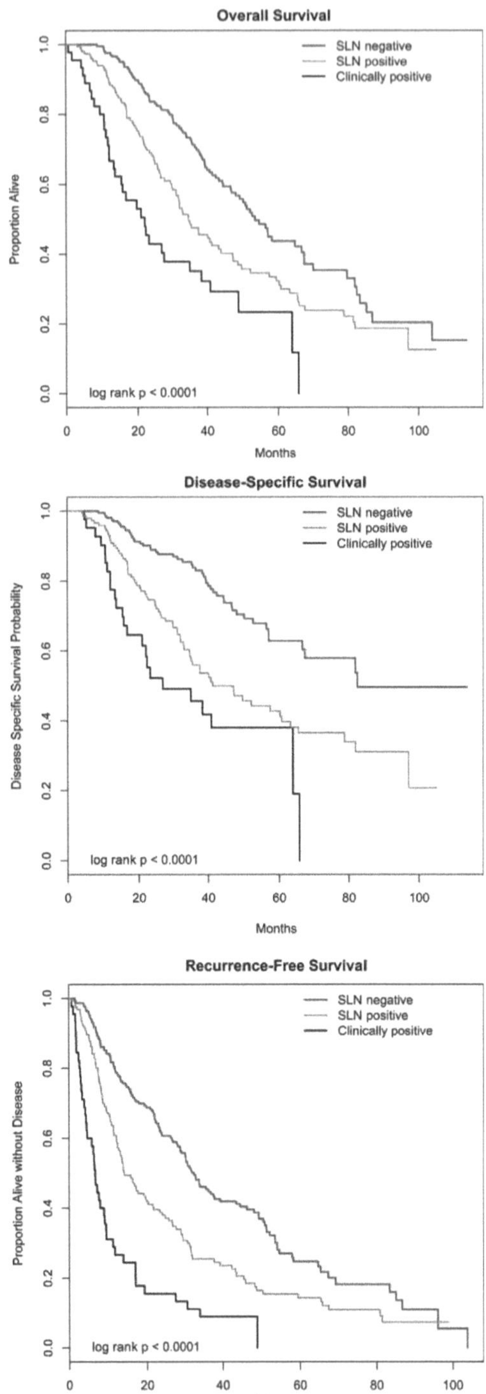

FIGURE 2.—Kaplan-Meier curves are shown for (*Top*) overall survival, (*Middle*) disease-specific survival, and (*Bottom*) recurrence-free survival. Clinically positive indicates patients with clinically positive regional disease at the time of presentation who underwent therapeutic lymph node dissection; SLN, sentinel lymph node. (Reprinted from Yamamoto M, Fisher KJ, Wong JY, et al. Sentinel lymph node biopsy is indicated for patients with thick clinically lymph node-negative melanoma. *Cancer.* 2015;121:1628-1636, with permission from American Cancer Society.)

SLNB negative, 14.3 months for patients who were SLNB positive, and 6.8 months for patients with clinically lymph node-positive disease ($P < .0001$).

Conclusions.—With an acceptably low false-negative rate, patients with thick melanoma and a negative SLNB appear to have significantly prolonged RFS, DSS, and OS compared with those with a positive SLNB. Therefore, SLNB should be considered as indicated for patients with thick, clinically lymph node-negative melanoma (Fig 2).

▶ The prognostic value of sentinel lymph node biopsy (SLNB) in patients with intermediate thickness melanoma has been well established. However, the utility of SLNB in patients in thick melanomas is unclear. Arguments against performing SLNB in thick melanoma are the increased risk of distant metastases in these patients and a lack of survival advantage. The reasons to perform it are to improve staging and prognostication so that adjuvant therapy can be administered and to avoid progression to clinically node-positive disease. This was a single-institutional retrospective series with patients collected from 2002 to 2012, including those with tumors >4 mm in Breslow thickness and absence of distant metastasis. It included 571 patients, 46 of whom were clinically node-positive and 525 with clinically node-negative disease. SLNB was performed in 419 patients and was not attempted in others because of medical comorbidities, patient preference, or other reasons. Of those having SNLB, it was successful in 412, and in 7 there was a failure to find the sentinel node. About one-third of patients had their SLNB performed at an outside hospital, and on examination of the subset of SLNB performed at this institution, 197 (66%) had negative sentinel nodes and 100 patients had a positive sentinel nodes (34%). Fourteen patients in the negative SLNB group developed nodal recurrence, and therefore the false-negative rate was 12.3%. There was a statistically significant increase in positive SLNB on multivariate analysis in patients with trunk or extremity sites versus head and neck, in patients with superficial spreading versus desmoplastic melanoma, and in those patients with satellitosis. Survival analysis revealed a significantly improved overall survival in patients with negative SLNB (53.4 months) versus those with positive SLNB (34.7 months) or clinically node-positive disease (22 months, $P < .001$; Fig 2). A similar trend was found for disease-free survival, which was 32.4 months for SLNB negative, 14.3 for SLNB positive, and 6.8 months for those with clinically node-positive disease ($P < .001$). On multivariate analysis, positive SLNB status and >5 mitoses/mm^2 were statistically significantly associated with reduced survival. This is the largest series reporting on SLNB in patients with thick melanomas, and the authors concluded that this could be done with a high success rate (99%), low false-negative rate (12.3%), and the finding of an overall SLNB positive rate of approximately 34%. They suggest that this is a valuable prognostic procedure and will better select patients for adjuvant therapy (interferon and/or radiation in this study), which was given to 34% of patients.

J. R. Howe, MD

Detailed Pathological Examination of Completion Node Dissection Specimens and Outcome in Melanoma Patients with Minimal (<0.1 mm) Sentinel Lymph Node Metastases

Holtkamp LHJ, Wang S, Wilmott JS, et al (Melanoma Inst Australia, Sydney, New South Wales; et al)

Ann Surg Oncol 22:2972-2977, 2015

Background.—Nonsentinel lymph nodes (NSLNs) are rarely involved in patients with minimal volume melanoma metastases in sentinel lymph nodes (SLNs). Therefore, it has been suggested that completion lymph node dissection (CLND) is not required. However, the lack of routine immunohistochemical staining and multiple sectioning may have led to failure to identify additional positive nodes. The present study sought to more reliably determine the tumor status of NSLNs in patients with minimally involved SLNs and their clinical outcome.

Methods.—A total of 21 tumor-negative CLND specimens from 20 patients with SLN metastases of <0.1 mm in diameter treated between 1991 and 2013 were examined with a more detailed pathologic protocol (five new sections stained with/for H&E, S-100, HMB45, Melan-A, and H&E). Clinical follow-up data were also obtained.

Results.—Of the 343 examined NSLNs, 1 was found to harbor a 0.18-mm subcapsular sinus metastasis. No metastases were identified in the other NSLNs. Median follow-up was 48 months (range 17–130 months). Six patients (30 %) developed a recurrence. At the end of followup, 15 patients (75 %) were alive without sign of melanoma recurrence and 5 patients (25 %) had died of melanoma. Estimated 5-year melanoma-specific survival was 64 %. The patient with the additional positive NSLN remains without recurrence after 130 months follow-up.

Conclusions.—Although the risk of additional nodal involvement is low, detailed pathologic examination may identify NSLN metastases not identified using routine protocols. Therefore, nodal clearance appears to be the safest option for these patients, pending the results of prospective trials.

▶ Sentinel lymph node biopsy in patients with melanoma is an accurate way of staging regional nodal involvement. When a positive sentinel node is found, at lymphadenectomy the nonsentinel lymph nodes (NSLN) are negative in 67% to 93% of cases. Therefore, many patients with a positive sentinel lymph node could potentially be spared from completion lymph node dissection, which is being explored in the Multicenter Selective Lymphadenectomy Trial II (MSLT-2) trial. However, the majority of NSLNs are not examined in detail pathologically, and rarely is immunohistochemistry (IHC) employed for them, potentially underestimating their rate of involvement.

This study set out to examine NSLNs in patients who had microscopically positive sentinel lymph nodes to determine their frequency of involvement and the outcome in these patients. They selected 20 patients treated over a 22-year period at a single institution in Australia, all of whom had a sentinel lymph node metastases with a maximum tumor diameter of <0.1 mm; the Breslow depth of primary melanomas ranged from 0.40 to 6.00. They took lymph nodes from completion lymph node dissection specimens and examined 5 consecutive 4-micron sections from each node and stained these with hematoxylin and eosin, and in the first and last sections also used IHC for S-100, HMB45, and later Melan-A. These lymph nodes were assessed by 2 pathologists, and a total of 343 NSLNs were examined from these 20 patients. In only 1 patient was a metastasis found, and this was a subcapsular sinus deposit 0.18 mm in size. There were no metastases identified in 342 other lymph nodes, although 3 patients had subcapsular nevus found within a node. Median follow-up was 48 months, and in this group of 20 patients with minimal sentinel lymph node disease, 6 developed recurrence and 5 died of melanoma (all had Breslow depth lesions >2.5 mm). The patient with a positive NSLN had not recurred after 130 months of follow-up. This study also found that the prognosis for patients with minimally involved sentinel lymph node was not as good as previously estimated, which was 64% for a 5-year melanoma specific survival, in contrast to other studies reporting anywhere between 83% and 100% melanoma specific survival. The authors believe that some of the differences between this and these other studies was a 1-year-longer follow-up interval, the possibility of lead-time bias, or perhaps random effects due to small sample sizes in all of these studies. The authors continue to recommend completion lymph node dissection in patients with positive sentinel lymph nodes despite the low incidence of finding additional involved nodes. Furthermore, the number of sections taken from each NSLN was only 5, and therefore further pathologic examination could have revealed additional nodal involvement. However, the yield of this procedure seemed quite low, in that more than 1500 sections were taken to find 1 positive node. This study did highlight that even a minimally involved sentinel lymph node is a risk factor for long-term survival. The true answer to the question of whether completion lymph node dissection is required after a positive sentinel node should come from the MSLT-II and European Organisation for Research and Treatment of Cancer studies.

J. R. Howe, MD

Pancreatic

Treatment of 200 Locally Advanced (Stage III) Pancreatic Adenocarcinoma Patients With Irreversible Electroporation: Safety and Efficacy

Martin RCG II, Kwon D, Chalikonda S, et al (Univ of Louisville School of Medicine, KY; Henry Ford Hosp, Detroit, MI; Cleveland Clinic, OH; et al)
Ann Surg 262:486-494, 2015

Objectives.—Ablative therapies have been increasingly utilized in the treatment of locally advanced pancreatic cancer (LAPC). Irreversible electroporation (IRE) is an energy delivery system, effective in ablating tumors by inducing irreversible membrane destruction of cells. We aimed to demonstrate efficacy of treatment with IRE as part of multimodal treatment of LAPC.

Methods.—From July 2010 to October 2014, patients with radiographic stage III LAPC were treated with IRE and monitored under a multicenter, prospective institutional review board–approved registry. Perioperative 90-day outcomes, local failure, and overall survival were recorded.

Results.—A total of 200 patients with LAPC underwent IRE alone (n = 150) or pancreatic resection plus IRE for margin enhancement (n = 50). All patients underwent induction chemotherapy, and 52% received chemoradiation therapy as well for a median of 6 months (range, 5–13 months) before IRE. IRE was successfully performed in all patients. Thirty-seven percent of patients sustained complications, with a median grade of 2 (range, 1–5). Median length of stay was 6 days (range, 4–36 days). With a median follow-up of 29 months, 6 patients (3%) have experienced local recurrence. Median overall survival was 24.9 months (range: 4.9–85 months).

Conclusions.—For patients with LAPC (stage III), the addition of IRE to conventional chemotherapy and radiation therapy results in substantially prolonged survival compared with historical controls. These results suggest that ablative control of the primary tumor may prolong survival.

▶ Locally advanced pancreatic cancer (LAPC) is a difficult problem that is usually treated with neoadjuvant chemotherapy with or without radiation, then reassessment for resectability. The problem is, many patients do not have a radiologic response, and therefore the decision to attempt resection may be difficult. If there were a way to explore these patients and resect them if possible, or if unresectable, to instead treat them with some form of local therapy that would improve their long-term survival, that would be helpful to patients.

In this study, Martin et al evaluated using irreversible electroporation (IRE) as a means of treating tumors in patients with locally advanced pancreatic cancer. It was a multi-institutional study in which patients were preoperatively staged with triple-phase CT, and patients were defined as LAPC when they had >180 degree encasement of the SMA or celiac artery, unreconstructible venous involvement, and no evidence of distant metastasis. Patients were treated with neoadjuvant chemotherapy and/or chemoradiation, and after the completion of therapy, they were restaged with triple-phase CT. Patients without evidence of tumor progression or development of metastases were deemed suitable for inclusion in this study. Patients were then explored, and if deemed to be resectable, had the pancreatic neck transected, then electroporation was carried out with the placement of 2 or 3 probes. For patients not deemed to be resectable, the pancreatic tumor was left in place, and electroporation was carried out in situ. This is a technically challenging procedure that requires intraoperative ultrasound and very precise placement of the IRE probes. Successful electroporation was defined as the planned therapy being delivered to the site of the tumor on a 3-month postoperative CT scan, with no evidence of residual tumor on cross-sectional imaging. Recurrence was defined as viable or persistent tumor on the postoperative CT. Two hundred patients were included in their study, of whom 50 had resection plus IRE and 150 had IRE performed in situ without resection. Three-quarters of the resected lesions were in the body or neck with only 25% in the head, and for those treated with IRE alone, 63% were in the head and 37% in the body and neck. The tumor sizes were similar, and resection was more likely if only the celiac axis was involved. All patients received chemotherapy, and approximately 50% in each of the resection plus IRE and IRE-only groups had radiation. The median time of delivery of IRE was 21 minutes with a maximum time of 125 minutes. Fifty-four of 150 patients having IRE alone had 100 complications, and 20 who had IRE plus resection had 49 complications. There were 3 mortalities in the IRE-only group and none in the resection group; the mortalities resulted from bleeding from an ulcerated tumor, liver failure, and portal venous thrombosis and pulmonary embolism in 1 patient. The median follow-up was 29 months, and 3 of 150 having IRE alone had failure at 3 months and 6 had local recurrence after initial success. The median progression-free survival was 12.4 months, and the most common site of recurrence was the liver. The median overall survival was 24.9 months, with 28.3 months for the resection plus IRE group versus 23.2 months for IRE alone. These numbers suggested a doubling of survival compared with historical results achieved with chemotherapy and chemoradiotherapy. The authors also make the point that patients with unresectable tumors treated with chemotherapy have similar complication rates as seen for these patients having IRE. They conclude that the morbidity of IRE seems worthwhile based on the survival advantage. They do caution that this procedure takes technical expertise for placement of the probes and that there was selection bias in their study. Patients who progressed during chemotherapy were eligible for IRE, and patients who had metal stents placed had to have these removed for IRE.

The authors suggest that percutaneous IRE would be difficult to perform and is not advisable at this time. This study is important in that it describes another option for patients with LAPC who are unresectable at exploration that appears to have a survival benefit. This procedure is only available in a few centers currently and requires the purchase of an expensive piece of equipment (the generator for IRE). Further studies are needed to more clearly define the role of IRE in patients with LAPC.

J. R. Howe, MD

Radiological and Surgical Implications of Neoadjuvant Treatment With FOLFIRINOX for Locally Advanced and Borderline Resectable Pancreatic Cancer

Ferrone CR, Marchegiani G, Hong TS, et al (Harvard Med School, Boston, MA; et al)

Ann Surg 261:12-17, 2015

Purpose.—On the basis of the ACCORD trial, FOLFIRINOX is effective in metastatic pancreatic adenocarcinoma (PDAC), making it a rational choice for locally advanced PDAC(LA). Aims of this study are to evaluate the accuracy of imaging in determining the resectability of

PDAC and to determine the surgical and clinicopathologic outcomes of pancreatic resections after neoadjuvant FOLFIRINOX therapy.

Patients and Methods.—Clinicopathologic data were retrospectively collected for surgical PDAC patients receiving neoadjuvant FOLFIRINOX or no neoadjuvant therapy between April 2011 and February 2014. Americas Hepato-Pancreato-Biliary Association/Society of Surgical Oncology/Society for Surgery of the Alimentary Tract consensus guidelines defined LA and borderline. Imaging was reviewed by a blinded senior pancreatic surgeon.

Results.—Of 188 patients undergoing resection for PDAC, 40 LA/borderline received FOLFIRINOX and 87 received no neoadjuvant therapy. FOLFIRINOX resulted in a significant decrease in tumor size, yet 19 patients were still classified as LA and 9 as borderline. Despite post-FOLFIRINOX imaging suggesting continued unresectability, 92% had an R0 resection. When compared with no neoadjuvant therapy, FOLFIRINOX resulted in significantly longer operative times (393 vs 300 minutes) and blood loss (600 vs 400 mL), but significantly lower operative morbidity (36% vs 63%) and no postoperative pancreatic fistulas. Length of stay (6 vs 7 days), readmissions (20% vs 30%), and mortality were equivalent (1% vs 0%). On final pathology, the FOLFIRINOX group had a significant decrease in lymph node positivity (35% vs 79%) and perineural invasion (72% vs 95%). Median follow-up was 11 months with a significant increase in overall survival with FOLFIRINOX.

Conclusions.—After neoadjuvant FOLFIRINOX imaging no longer predicts unresectability. Traditional pathologic predictors of survival are improved, and morbidity is decreased in comparison to patients with clearly resectable cancers at the time of presentation (Fig 3, Table 3).

▶ Despite several decades of clinical trials in pancreatic ductal adenocarcinoma (PDA), the value of neoadjuvant chemotherapy is still ambiguous. The recent ACCORD trial from 2011 showed that there was a survival advantage for patients with metastatic PDA receiving FOLFIRINOX versus gemcitabine, with median survival rates of 11.1 versus 6.8 months, respectively. Therefore, many have suggested that with the improved activity of this regimen in metastatic PDA, it makes sense to use it in patients who have locally advanced or borderline resectable lesions. In this single-institution, retrospective study the authors looked at patients who had resection for PDA between 2011 and 2014 and divided them into 2 groups: those who had resectable disease at presentation and who were not treated with neoadjuvant therapy, and those patients with locally advanced disease or borderline resectable disease who were treated with neoadjuvant therapy. The primary aim was to see what kind of imaging response occurred in these latter patients, and the second was to look at surgical outcomes. One hundred eighty-eight patients underwent pancreatic resections during this interval. Locally advanced tumors were defined as long-segment occlusion of the superior mesenteric vein (SMV) or portal vein (PV), >180 degrees involvement of the superior mesenteric artery (SMA) or involvement of the hepatic artery or celiac trunk. Borderline resectable lesions were when there was tumor abutment or

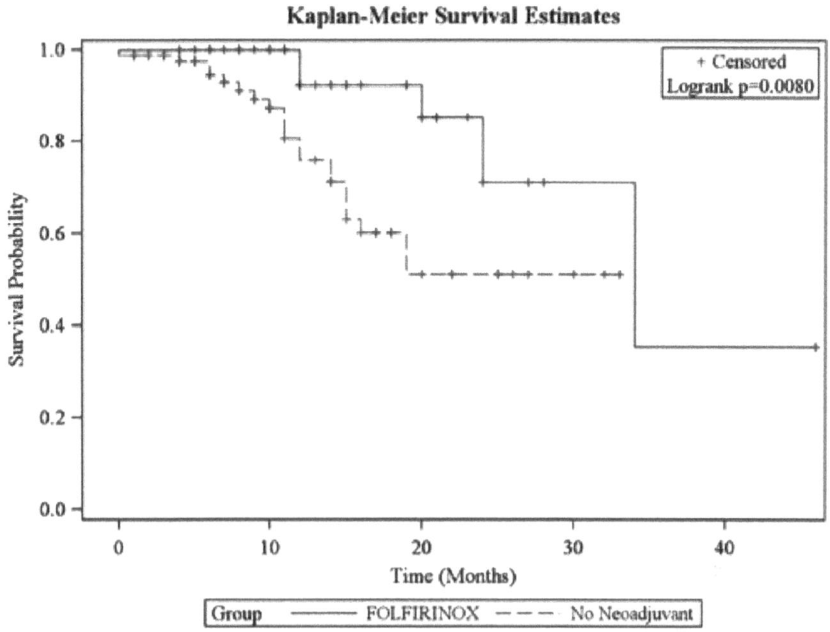

FIGURE 3.—Overall survival curves for patients who were treated with neoadjuvant FOLFIRINOX versus no neoadjuvant chemotherapy. (Reprinted from Ferrone CR, Marchegiani G, Hong TS, et al. Radiological and surgical implications of neoadjuvant treatment with FOLFIRINOX for locally advanced and borderline resectable pancreatic cancer. *Ann Surg.* 2015;261:12-17, with permission from Lippincott Williams & Wilkins.)

short segment occlusion on the SMV or PV, gastroduodenal artery encasement up to the hepatic artery, or < 180 degrees of abutment of the SMA. A senior surgeon blinded to patient identity reviewed the pretreatment and posttreatment CT scans for assessment of response to FOLFIRINOX. Over this time period, 87 patients underwent surgical resection without neoadjuvant therapy because they presented with resectable disease, and 40 were resected who were treated with neoadjuvant FOLFIRINOX. Of these 40, 5 had FOLFIRINOX alone, 30 had some combination of FOLFIRINOX and radiation therapy, and another 5 had FOLFIRINOX and other treatment. A total 47 patients were treated with FOLFIRINOX, of whom 40 were resected but 7 were not ultimately resected (3 who had metastatic disease and 4 who remained locally advanced and unresectable). Of the 40 who were resected, 25 were considered preoperatively to be locally advanced, and 15 borderline resectable; posttreatment CT review demonstrated that 6 had a complete response, 30 a partial response, and stable disease was seen in 4. Posttreatment, 19 patients were classified as locally advanced, 9 as borderline, and 12 as resectable.

The majority of patients in each group had pancreaticoduodenectomy (Table 3), including 85% in the FOLFIRINOX group and 73% in the no neoadjuvant treatment group. The most significant differences between the 2 groups were that the operating room time was longer in those patients receiving

TABLE 3.—Operative Outcomes

	No Neoadjuvant (N = 87)	FOLFIRINOX (N = 40)	*P*
Operation			0.276
Whipple	63 (73%)	34 (85%)	
Distal pancreatectomy	23 (26%)	6 (15%)	
Total pancreatectomy	1 (1%)	0	
OR time (min)	300 (60–600)	393.5 (180–890)	<0.001
Blood loss (mL)	400 (100–1800)	600 (200–7800)	0.007
Postoperative complications	55 (63%)	14 (36%)	0.006
Pancreatic Fistula	19 (22%)	0	<0.001
LOS (median)	7 (4–54)	6 (4–35)	0.145
Readmission (90 d)	26 (30%)	8 (20%)	0.286
Postoperative death (within 90 d)	1(1.1%)	0	0.999
Median FU (from diagnosis)	10 (0–33)	13.5 (4–46)	0.003
Progression	43 (49.4%)	15 (37.5%)	0.252
Progression pattern	(N = 40)	(N = 15)	0.481
Local			
Pancreas bed	7 (17.5%)	4 (26.7%)	
Regional nodes	4 (10%)	0	
Distant			
Multiple metastases	3 (7.5%)	3 (20%)	
Lungs	4 (10%)	1 (6.7%)	
Liver	17 (42.5%)	4 (26.7%)	
Peritoneum	5 (12.5%)	3 (20%)	
Dead of disease	21 (24%)	5 (12.5%)	0.160

Reprinted from Ferrone CR, Marchegiani G, Hong TS, et al. Radiological and surgical implications of neoadjuvant treatment with FOLFIRINOX for locally advanced and borderline resectable pancreatic cancer. *Ann Surg*. 2015;261:12-17, with permission from Lippincott Williams & Wilkins.

FOLFIRINOX, most likely because they had more advanced disease. Postoperative complications were decreased from 63% in the no treatment group down to 36% in the neoadjuvant group, and remarkably there were no pancreatic fistulas in the group receiving FOLFIRINOX. Postoperative mortality and readmission rates were similar in the 2 groups. Remarkably, only 35% of patient's receiving FOLFIRINOX had positive lymph nodes versus 79% in the no neoadjuvant treatment group, and the size of the tumors were smaller in the neoadjuvant group (mean of 2.5 cm vs 3.2 cm for no treatment group). An R0 resection could be performed in 92% of patients in the neoadjuvant group versus 86% of patients without neoadjuvant treatment. Two patients receiving FOLFIRINOX had had no evidence of cancer in pathologic examination, and 4 had <1-mm tumors. The follow-up was 11 months, and the median overall survival significantly improved in those receiving neoadjuvant therapy over resectable lesions not receiving therapy (Fig 3). Important conclusions from this study were that the radiologic findings are not useful for assessing patients resectability rate after FOLFIRINOX treatment. The vast majority had R0 resections (92%) and many of these patients had tumors that just showed fibrosis at the vascular margins. Therefore, these authors suggest that patients with locally advanced or borderline resectable lesions should have resection attempted and frozen sections performed along these vessels before proceeding with resection. If these biopsies are positive, resection should not be carried out; if they are negative, then patients should have resection performed. This is an important study, although retrospective and prone to selection bias, but hopefully it will lead to randomized trials to answer the question as to whether neoadjuvant FOLFIRINOX will improve survival and outcomes in patients with PDA in the locally advanced or borderline resectable situation. Another important, unanswered question is whether neoadjuvant treatment would improve survival even in patients with disease that looks resectable at presentation.

J. R. Howe, MD

FOLFIRINOX Induction Therapy for Stage 3 Pancreatic Adenocarcinoma

Sadot E, Doussot A, O'Reilly EM, et al (Memorial Sloan Kettering Cancer Ctr, New York)

Ann Surg Oncol 22:3512-3521, 2015

Background.—Reports show that FOLFIRINOX therapy for pancreatic ductal adenocarcinoma (PDAC) results in objective response rates two to threefold higher than those of other regimens. This study aimed to assess response and resection rates for locally unresectable (stage 3) patients initially treated with induction FOLFIRINOX.

Methods.—The institutional cancer database was queried for patients treated with induction FOLFIRINOX therapy between 2010 and 2013. Patients were included in the study if they were treated at the authors' institution for stage 3 PDAC (locally unresectable) that had been adjudicated at a weekly multidisciplinary tumor board.

Results.—The study identified 101 patients. The median age was 64 years (range 37–81 years), and the median follow-up period was 12 months (range 3–37 months). The patients received a median of six cycles (range 1–20 cycles) of induction FOLFIRINOX. No grade 4 or 5 toxicity was recorded. At the initial restaging (median of 3 months after diagnosis), 23 patients (23 %) had developed distant metastases, 15 patients (15 %) had undergone resection, and 63 patients (63 %) had proceeded to chemoradiation. In the group of 63 patients who had proceeded to chemoradiation (median of 9 months after diagnosis), an additional 16 patients (16 %) had undergone resection, and 5 patients (5 %) had developed metastases. A partial radiographic response was observed in 29 %of all the patients, which was associated with ability to perform resection ($p = 0.004$). The median overall survival time was 11 months for the group that progressed with FOLFIRINOX and 26 months for the group that did not progress.

Conclusion.—Nearly one third of the patients who had been initially identified as having stage 3 pancreatic carcinoma and had been treated with FOLFIRINOX responded radiographically and underwent tumor resection (Table 2).

▶ The outlook for patients with pancreatic adenocarcinoma (PDAC) may be improving. The ACCORD trial revealed that patients with metastatic PDAC

TABLE 2.—Outcome After Completed Protocol

Characteristic	All Patients ($n = 101$) n (%)	Resected ($n = 31$) n (%)	Unresectable ($n = 70$) n (%)	p Value
Size: cm (range)[a]	2.9 (1.1–8)	2.5 (1.1–4.7)	3.3 (1.6–8)	**<0.001**
Size reduction: % (range)[a]	−16 (−67 to 44)	−29 (−63 to 14)	−10 (−67 to 44)	**0.001**
Size reduction>30 %[a]	29 (29)	15 (48)	14 (20)	**0.004**
Primay tumor (T)[a]				**<0.001**
ycT2	2 (2)	2 (6)	0	
ycT3	33 (33)	25 (81)	8 (11)	
ycT4	66 (65)	4 (13)[b]	62 (89)	
ycN0[a]	86 (85)	23 (74)	63 (90)	**0.04**
CA19-9: U/ml (range)[c]	52 (0–2921)	41 (0–670)	63 (1–2921)	0.3
CA19-9 reduction>50 %[c]	45 (50)	18 (78)	27 (40)	**0.001**
CEA: ng/ml (range)[c]	4.1 (0.8–84.9)	3.6 (0.8–29.6)	4.1 (0.9–84.9)	0.5
Surgical exploration[a]	35 (35)	31 (100)	4 (6)	–
Resection rate[a]	31 (31)	–	–	–
R0 resection rate	–	16 (55)[d]	–	–

Induction FOLFIRINOX therapy with or without subsequent chemoradiation therapy. Continuous variables are expressed as median (range); categorical variables are expressed as n (%); p value refers to the comparison of the resected and unresectable groups

Bold values are statistically significant ($p < 0.05$)

[a]After protocol

[b]Four patients were classified as ycT4 and underwent Appleby operation ($n = 3$) and hepatic artery resection ($n = 1$)

[c]After FOLFIRINOX

[d]Calculated for 29 patients (pathology report is pending for 2 patients)

Reprinted from Sadot E, Doussot A, O'Reilly EM, et al. FOLFIRINOX induction therapy for stage 3 pancreatic adenocarcinoma. *Ann Surg Oncol.* 2015;22:3512-3521, with permission from Society of Surgical Oncology.

had a 32% response rate with FOLFIRINOX versus 9% with gemcitabine. Therefore, multiple groups have begun looking at the regimen of FOLFIRINOX for patients with borderline resectable or locally advanced PDAC. There have been no randomized trials and few prospective studies evaluating these patients, however, previous regimens employing mostly gemcitabine-based regimens for patients with locally unresectable PDAC have converted to respectability in 7% to 19% of patients. This single-institutional study retrospectively identified patients with locally advanced PDAC who had received FOLFIRINOX between 2010 and 2013. Patients with T4, N0 or N1, and M0 disease were included, and locally advanced was defined as >180 degrees encasement of the SMA, celiac abutment, inferior vena cava or unreconstructable superior mesenteric vein/portal vein occlusion, or aortic involvement. Patients needed to have a clinic note affirming their locally advanced status and radiology review. Patients were given FOLFIRINOX for 4 cycles then a CT scan was performed to reevaluate resectability. Patients with stable disease then underwent chemoradiotherapy.

One hundred and one patients were identified who met these criteria, and the median number of cycles was 6, lasting for 13 weeks, with no grade 4 or 5 toxicities. Forty-five percent of patients had a dose reduction or delay. After the initial 4 cycles, 16 patients underwent exploration, of which 15 could be resected, and 23 patients during this interval developed distant disease. Sixty-three others then underwent chemoradiation, and during this period, 5 developed metastasis and 16 ultimately underwent resection, and 42 patients had stable, unresectable disease. Of those patients undergoing resection versus those who were not resected, there was a higher reduction in median tumor size; 48% of patients had a reduction >30%, reduction in nodal status, and decrease in CA19-9 levels. The overall objective response rate was 29%, which was 20% when chemoradiation was not used, and 50% of patients who had a partial response (defined as >30% size reduction) were resected. Thirty-one percent of patients ultimately had resection, and of these, 55% had an R0 resection (Table 2). Mean duration of therapy was 7 months, and when patients received chemoradiation, there was a higher rate of vascular resection, pathologic node-negative disease, and of >50% pathologic response. The median follow-up in this study was 12 months with a progression-free survival of 16 months and overall survival of 25 months. Overall survival was not reached in patients who had resection and was 26 months in those with stable disease after treatment. The main findings of this study were an objective response rate of 29%, which was similar to recent series from the Massachusetts General Hospital (MGH) and France. The recent study by Ferrone et al[1] from MGH suggested that imaging did not necessarily predict resectability, but this study points out that that study included only patients who were taken to the operating room, and therefore there may have been selection bias. The response rates were higher than historical controls using gemcitabine therapy alone and toxicity was acceptable. However, limitations included the fact that some patients got chemoradiotherapy but others did not. We can conclude that FOLFIRINOX does appear to have activity in the neoadjuvant setting and currently is likely the most effective regimen for this purpose; however, in the metastatic setting, similar activity was seen with regimens with gemcitabine and nab-paclitaxel. It would be difficult to do randomized studies evaluating FOLFIRINOX versus no treatment for patients with locally advanced or borderline resectable disease to fully answer this question. However, a neoadjuvant trial of FOLFIRINOX versus gemcitabine nab-paclitaxel could be useful and interesting.

J. R. Howe, MD

Reference

1. Ferrone CR, Marchegiani G, Hong TS, et al. Radiological and surgical implications of neoadjuvant treatment with FOLFIRINOX for locally advanced and borderline resectable pancreatic cancer. *Ann Surg*. 2015;261:12-17.

Approach to Patients With Pancreatic Cancer Without Detectable Metastases

Heestand GM, Murphy JD, Lowy AM (Univ of California at San Diego, La Jolla)

J Clin Oncol 33:1770-1778, 2015

The poors outcomes associated with pancreatic cancer clearly reflect the advanced stage of disease at diagnosis for most patients. Through this lens, it is easy to lose sight of the fact that roughly 50% of patients with pancreatic cancer have no clinically detectable metastases at presentation. Herein, we discuss how patients with localized pancreatic cancer are currently managed. The primary goal of care for patients with resectable and borderline-resectable tumors is cure, facilitated by achieving margin-negative resection of the primary disease and delivering effective adjuvant and/or neoadjuvant therapy. For patients with locally advanced disease, the focus is on limiting local progression and outgrowth of metastatic disease and maintaining quality of life. Although it was once a centerpiece of therapy for localized pancreatic cancer, the value and place of radiation therapy in the treatment algorithm is now under increased scrutiny. In contrast, given its value as demonstrated in multiple prospective trials, chemotherapy is an established part of the treatment paradigm for all patients. With the demonstration that cytotoxic combinations such as fluorouracil, leucovorin, irinotecan, and oxaliplatin as well as gemcitabine/nab-paclitaxel are active in the metastatic setting, these agents are now being studied in patients with localized disease. The neoadjuvant setting provides a particularly favorable setting for evaluating new systemic strategies. Given the array of new targets, including immunomodulatory approaches, there is reason for optimism that we can markedly improve survival for all patients with pancreatic cancer and enter an era in which surgery with curative intent actually fulfills this goal on a much more regular basis.

▶ This is an excellent review article discussing the trials that have been performed for borderline resectable and locally advanced pancreatic adenocarcinoma, reviewing previous studies, trials in progress, and investigations in the planning stage. The article states that 20% of newly diagnosed patients may have resectable disease, and 70% of these the patients will have locally advanced pancreatic cancer. The definitions of locally advanced are important and have varied from study to study, confounding comparison of some trials. Currently acceptable definitions for resectable are as follows: a clear plane between the tumor and the celiac axis, hepatic artery, superior mesenteric artery (SMA); no contact with the superior mesenteric vein (SMV), or <180 degrees of contact without deformity, with a patent SMV-portal vein. For patients that are resectable based on these criteria, several studies have looked at the benefits of adjuvant therapy. The CONKO-001 trial randomized patients who had resection of pancreatic ductal adenocarcinoma (PDA) to gemcitabine chemotherapy versus observation and found a doubling of 5-year survival from 10% to 21% in the gemcitabine arm. However, the median survival was only slightly improved from 20 to 23 months, but patients who were in the observation arm could be switched to gemcitabine if they showed progression (Table 1 in the original article). Another valuable study was the ESPAC3 trial, where patients were randomized after PDA resection to have 6 months of 5-fluorouracil (FU) and leucovorin or gemcitabine. The survival was equivalent in both arms, but it was found that gemcitabine was better tolerated. The JASPAC-01 trial from Japan randomized patients who had PDA resection to either gemcitabine or the oral fluoropyrimidine S1 and found that there was a survival benefit in those patients receiving S1, with a 70% 2-year survival versus 53% for gemcitabine. This agent was well tolerated. The article highlights the uncertain benefit of adjuvant chemoradiation because most clinical trials have given conflicting results or had issues with their design. There are several other adjuvant trials accruing patients currently, one looking at adjuvant gemcitabine versus FOLFIRINOX (5-FU, leucovorin, irinotecan, and oxaliplatin) after resection, and 2 immunotherapy trials using vaccines from pancreatic cancer cell lines in addition to chemotherapy.

A major philosophic change for many surgeons has been to give neoadjuvant chemotherapy to patients with PDA with the idea that there could be improvement in the R0 resection rate, giving time for selection of patients who might develop metastatic disease and, hypothetically, to eliminate micrometastatic disease. The 2 most active regimens in metastatic disease are FOLFIRINOX and gemcitabine/NAB paclitaxel. An adjuvant trial is underway looking at these 2 regimens given before radiation and surgery in the adjuvant setting. For patients with borderline resectable pancreatic cancer, which is defined as tumor interface >180 degrees on the SMV or portal vein; occlusion of the SMV or portal vein with a normal vein above and below; abutment between the tumor and the hepatic artery, SMA, or celiac axis with <180 degree abutment. The benefit of neoadjuvant treatment here is that patients may be rendered resectable by shrinking of the tumor or potentially killing the edge of the tumor along the vessels. There have been multiple single-institution trials with various neoadjuvant therapy regimens (mostly chemotherapy based but some with chemoradiation) showing rates of resectability from 50% to 100% of patients. Surprisingly, in the majority of these patients, negative margins could be achieved, and median overall survival has been in the approximately 2-year range. These studies are generally retrospective and the definitions of borderline resectable have differed. The article makes the point that a minority of patients, perhaps as low as 12%, will have response evaluation criteria for solid tumors (RECIST) criteria of response, yet approximately 60% of patients may successfully have a R0 resection. Therefore, one cannot count on radiologic response to determine whether a patient should undergo attempted resection after neoadjuvant therapy. Randomized clinical trials are clearly needed in this area. For locally advanced disease, in which the tumor is unresectable by virtue of circumferential involvement of major arteries or unresectable SMV-portal vein disease, the goal of therapy should be to maximize survival and maintain quality of life, and it is unlikely that these patients will be rendered resectable. Chemotherapy has typically been the approach, although some studies have also combined it with chemoradiotherapy, and there are several ongoing trials to look at various combinations of chemotherapy with or without radiation. It seems as if little progress has been made over several decades, but the improved activity of FOLFIRINOX as well as the gemcitabine/NAB paclitaxel regimen give us improved hope for both neoadjuvant and adjuvant treatment of patients with PDA. These treatments show promise for extending the lives of patients with this deadly cancer, and perhaps new vaccine therapies will add to our armamentarium, and new biomarkers may be found that will better select patients for therapy.

J. R. Howe, MD

Early Drain Removal—The Middle Ground Between the Drain Versus No Drain Debate in Patients Undergoing Pancreaticoduodenectomy: A Prospective Validation Study

Ven Fong Z, Correa-Gallego C, Ferrone CR, et al (Massachusetts General Hosp, Boston)

Ann Surg 262:378-383, 2015

Objective.—To perform an unbiased assessment of first postoperative day (POD 1) drain amylase level and pancreatic fistula (PF) after pancreaticoduodenectomy (PD).

Background.—Recent evidence demonstrated that drain abandonment in PD is unsafe. Early drain amylase levels have been proposed as predictors of PF after PD, allowing for selection of patients for early drain removal.

Methods.—Daily drain amylase levels were correlated with the development of PF in 2 independent cohorts of patients undergoing PD: training cohort (n = 126; year 2008) and validation cohort (n = 369; years 2009–2012).

Results.—POD 1 drain amylase level had the highest predictive ability (concordance index: 0.911) for PF in the training cohort. An amylase level of 612 U/L or higher showed the best accuracy (86%), sensitivity (93%), and specificity (79%). Thus, a cutoff value of 600 U/L was utilized. In the validation cohort, 229 (62.1%) patients had a POD 1 drain amylase level of lower than 600 U/L, and PF developed in only 2 (0.9%) cases; whereas in patients with POD 1 drain amylase level of 600 U/L or higher (n = 140) the PF rate was 31.4% (odds ratio [OR] = 52, $P < 0.0001$). On multivariate analysis, POD 1 drain amylase level of lower than 600 U/L (OR = 0.0192, $P < 0.0001$) was a stronger predictor of the absence of PF than pancreatic gland texture (OR = 0.193, $P = 0.002$) and duct diameter (OR = 0.861, $P = 0.835$).

Conclusions.—After PD, the risk of PF is less than 1% if POD 1 drain amylase level is lower than 600 U/L. We propose that in this group, which comprise more than 60% of patients, drains should be removed on POD 1 (Table 1).

▶ Pancreatic fistula is a common complication of pancreaticoduodenectomy, affecting approximately 20% to 35% of patients. For this reason, most surgeons in the past have left intra-abdominal drains in proximity to the pancreatic anastomosis to reduce the potential complications of amylase rich fluid in the abdomen. This has been shown to lead to gastroparesis, intra-abdominal abscess, and erosion into mesenteric vessels. Several trials have revealed no difference in complication rates with placement versus no placement of intra-abdominal

TABLE 1.—Demographics and Preoperative Variables of Patients Undergoing PD Dichotomized According to POD1 Drain Amylase Value

	All Patients (n = 369),%	POD 1 Drain Amylase <600 U/L (n = 229),%	POD 1 Drain Amylase ≥600 U/L (n = 140),%	*P*
Male	50.4	51.9	47.9	0.444
Age, yr	66 ± 12.1	66 ± 12.2	65.6 ± 11.9	0.409
Body mass index	25.7 ± 5.9	25.0 ± 5.2	27.4 ± 6.5	0.0001*
ASA ≥3	41.3	42.0	38.5	0.689
Age-adjusted Charlson index	5 ± 2.3	5 ± 2.3	4 ± 2.1	0.001*
Surgeon volume				
High (>25 cases/yr)	72.6	68.9	78.6	0.06
Intermediate (5–25 cases/yr)	21.4	23.1	18.6	
Low (<5 cases/yr)	6.0	8.0	2.9	
Pathology				
Pancreatic adenocarcinoma	52.0	64.6	31.4	<0.001*
Cholangiocarcinoma	4.1	3.9	4.3	0.867
Ampullary adenocarcinoma	7.1	6.9	7.1	0.955
Duodenal adenocarcinoma	1.9	0.9	3.6	0.065
Chronic pancreatitis	3.5	3.5	3.6	0.969
Intraductal papillary mucinous neoplasm	13.3	9.2	20.0	0.003*
Pancreatic neuroendocrine tumor	5.7	4.4	7.9	0.160

*Statistical significance was achieved at the $P < 0.05$ level.

Reprinted from Ven Fong Z, Correa-Gallego C, Ferrone CR, et al. Early drain removal—the middle ground between the drain versus no drain debate in patients undergoing pancreaticoduodenectomy: a prospective validation study. *Ann Surg.* 2015;262:378-383, with permission from Wolters Kluwer Health, Inc.

drains, and one argument against drain placement is that suction may actually induce fistula formation. Other studies have shown that early drain removal may lead to fewer complications than later drain removal.

This study from a single institution attempted to determine whether amylase values on postoperative days 1 or 2 could select which patients would benefit from early drain removal and whether this would potentially lead to fewer complications. This study looked at patients undergoing pancreaticoduodenectomy (PD) in 2008 to determine a cutoff for drain amylase, and then applied this to patients undergoing PD between 2009 and 2012. It should be noted that at this institution, routine placement of 2 drains was performed, and 90% of patients had an external pancreatic duct stent, which was commonly removed at 3 weeks after patient follow-up. In the training set of patients operated on in 2008, it was determined that an amylase value of 612 units per liter was the cutoff point with the highest accuracy, sensitivity, and specificity for prediction of pancreatic fistula. Therefore, they examined the 369 patients undergoing PD between 2009 and 2012 and found that 62% had an amylase level of < 600 on the first postoperative day, and in these patients, a pancreatic fistula only developed in 1% of cases. In the 38% of patients who had an amylase > 600, 31% developed a pancreatic fistula. In those patients with amylase greater than 600, the BMA was slightly higher, the Charlson comorbidity index was lower, as was the incidence of pancreatic adenocarcinoma versus IPMN, the surgery was shorter, the pancreatic duct was smaller, and the glands were softer (Table 1). The complication rates between those patients with high and low amylase were similar despite the lower pancreatic fistula rate in the low amylase group. Patients with low amylase levels had a higher rate of ileus and the length of hospital stay was similar, but the readmission rate was significantly lower in the low amylase group. Furthermore, the mortality in the high amylase group was 2-fold higher, but this difference was not statistically significant. On multivariate analysis, the only statistically significant factor for prediction of pancreatic fistula formation was the amylase level on postoperative day 1. Although gland texture, duct size, whether vessels were resected or not, estimated blood loss, and blood transfusion were significant by univariate analysis, they dropped out on multivariate analysis. The authors conclude that measurement of amylase on postoperative day 1 after PD can help predict those patients who will develop pancreatic fistula, and in those where this is < 600 there is a very low likelihood of pancreatic fistula. In these patients, a strategy of early drain removal can be employed, which may further reduce complication rates. In patients with higher amylase levels, it may be better to leave these drains because the pancreatic fistula rate was 31%. The limitations of this study were that the practice of external pancreatic duct drainage is not practiced in most institutions, and this may be one reason why the overall pancreatic fistula rate was relatively low at 12.5%. This study is helpful for those performing PD because it provides a coherent strategy for management of drains and early removal of drains in patients unlikely to develop pancreatic fistula.

J. R. Howe, MD

Morbidity Among Long-Term Survivors After Pancreatoduodenectomy for Pancreatic Adenocarcinoma

Chen KT, Devarajan K, Hoffman JP (Southcoast Health System, New Bedford, MA; Fox Chase Cancer Ctr, Philadelphia, PA)

Ann Surg Oncol 22:1185-1189, 2015

Background.—Because pancreatoduodenectomy for pancreatic adenocarcinoma is focused on disease-free and overall survival, morbidity among long-term survivors is not well described. This study sought to evaluate outcomes for long-term survivors of pancreatic cancer after pancreatoduodenectomy.

Methods.—The authors identified 29 patients from their prospectively collected database of patients with pancreatic adenocarcinoma who had undergone pancreatoduodenectomy and were without evidence of disease during at least 3 years of follow-up evaluation. Demographics, treatment, and pathologic characteristics were collected for review. Data with regard to long-term sequelae also were collected, focusing on those complications requiring additional procedures and on the development of metachronous cancers.

Results.—The median follow-up period was 83 months, with 62% of patients still alive. All patients received an R0 resection, and 34% of the patients had N1 disease. For 42% of the patients, no significant subsequent sequelae occurred. In the four remaining patients (14%), ascites developed, requiring repeated paracentesis or Denver shunt, with a median time to development (MTD) of 63 months. Six patients (21%) experienced a biliary stricture requiring stent placement (MTD, 56 months). One patient experienced portal venous thrombosis requiring a venous stent (MTD, 52 months), and four patients (14%) experienced clinically significant ulcers (MTD, 52 months). With regard to metachronous cancers, two patients experienced subsequent lymphomas (MTD, 92 months).

Conclusions.—Long-term survivors among patients who undergo pancreatoduodenectomy for pancreatic adenocarcinoma can experience significant late sequelae, which often manifest more than 3 years after surgery. As such, continued follow-up evaluation and counseling are warranted.

▶ Long-term survivors of pancreatic cancer are few, and most studies have focused on both disease-free and overall survival. However, patients surviving pancreaticoduodenectomy have a number of late sequela, and studies examining these have been limited. This report examined a single-institutional experience with pancreaticoduodenectomy for pancreatic adenocarcinoma and looked specifically for patients who survived at least 3 years without evidence of disease recurrence. They identified 29 patients in their series of 280 total patients who had follow-up with serum CA19-9, CT, MRI, or other diagnostic procedures. They looked specifically for late-term complications, which were defined as occurring at least 1 year after the initial operation, and then they examined variables that might be associated with these sequela, including type of procedure, pathologic stage, the receipt of neoadjuvant or adjuvant chemotherapy and/or radiation, and immediate postoperative complications.

Eighty-two percent of their patients received chemoradiation, half in the neoadjuvant setting and the other half in the adjuvant setting. This was generally gemcitabine or Fluorouracil (5FU) with 50.4 Gy of radiation. Seventy-two percent of patients had a classic Whipple procedure with antrectomy, and 28% had pylorus-preserving pancreaticoduodenectomy. All patients ultimately had an R0 resection and 6 patients had a pathologic complete response to neoadjuvant therapy. Sixty-seven percent of patients were node-negative. Eight patients had immediate postoperative complications, 3 requiring reoperations, and 3 patients had postoperative pancreatic fistula. Delayed complications included the need for medication for diabetes in 34% and pancreatic enzyme supplements in 73%. Forty-two percent of patients had no delayed adverse events. Five patients (17%) had ascites with the mean development at 63 months, and these were treated by multiple paracenteses, and 2 had Denver shunt placement, but none of these patients were found to have positive cytology; 4 of these 5 patients were thought to have cryptogenetic cirrhosis. Six patients developed biliary strictures requiring multiple procedures, most presenting with cholangitis, managed by stent placement usually requiring multiple procedures for dilatation and stent exchange; only 1 patient was able to remain stent free long term. Four or 14% of patients developed ulcer disease, 2 with perforated gastrojejunal anastomotic ulcers. All patients were treated long-term with proton pump inhibitors after surgery. Both patients with perforation had classic Whipple with antrectomy. Two patients developed incisional hernias; 1 had significant bile reflux gastritis, another had radiation enteritis (with repeated bowel obstructions and development of jejuno-colic fistula), 1 with portal vein thrombosis. Two patients developed lymphoma, and 1 patient was diagnosed with colon cancer 3 months after pancreatic cancer resection. In univariate analysis, none of the demographic, pathologic, or treatment factors appeared to be significantly associated with these complications. However, the sample size was limited, making such associations difficult.

This is an interesting study showing that even if patients receiving pancreaticoduodenectomy are fortunate enough to be 3-year survivors, 58% would still have late adverse events, most commonly ascites or biliary stricture. It is unclear whether radiation therapy is associated with biliary stricture, and a large study from the Mayo Clinic showed that in patients with benign disease, the probability of biliary stricture was 8% and 13% at 5 and 10 years, respectively. These patients have not generally received radiation, and thus it is thought that stricture is due to ischemia or reflux into the biliary system. Whether ulcer disease is also related to the ischemia provoked by radiation is unclear, but this can also happen after gastrojejunostomy for benign conditions. The author suggests that patients remain on long-term antiulcer therapy because of the 2 gastrojejunal perforations seen in their study. The incidence of secondary malignancy was low, but with longer follow-up, it is possible that these numbers would increase. Limitations of this study include that it is from a single institution and has low numbers and that patients received a variety of neoadjuvant and adjuvant therapies. This study shows what problems develop late after pancreaticoduodenectomy so that one can anticipate them in patients returning for long-term follow-up.

J. R. Howe, MD

A Prospective, Randomized, Double-Blind, Placebo Controlled Trial on the Efficacy of Ethanol Celiac Plexus Neurolysis in Patients with Operable Pancreatic and Periampullary Adenocarcinoma

Lavu H, Lengel HB, Sell NM, et al (Thomas Jefferson Univ, Philadelphia, PA; et al)

J Am Coll Surg 220:497-508, 2015

Background.—Ethanol celiac plexus neurolysis (ECPN) has been shown to be effective in reducing cancer-related pain in patients with locally advanced pancreatic and periampullary adenocarcinoma (PPA). This study examined its efficacy in patients undergoing PPA resection.

Study Design.—There were 485 patients who participated in this prospective, randomized, double-blind placebo controlled trial. Patients were stratified by preoperative pain and disease resectability. They received either ECPN (50% ethanol) or 0.9% normal saline placebo control. The primary endpoint was short- and long-term pain and secondary endpoints included postoperative morbidity, quality of life, and overall survival.

Results.—Data from 467 patients were analyzed. The primary endpoint, the percentage of PPA patients experiencing a worsening of pain compared with preoperative baseline for resectable patients, was not different between the ethanol and saline groups in either the resectable/pain stratum (22% vs 18%, relative risk [RR] 1.23 [0.34, 4.46]), or the resectable/no pain stratum (37% vs 34%, RR 1.10 [0.67, 1.81]). In multivariable analysis of resected pancreatic ductal adenocarcinoma (PDA) patients, there was a significant reduction in pain in the resectable/pain group, suggesting that surgical resection of the malignancy alone (independent of ECPN) decreases pain to a significant degree.

Conclusions.—In this study, we demonstrated a significant reduction in pain after surgical resection of PPA. However, the addition of ECPN did not synergize to result in a further reduction in pain, and in fact, its effect may have been masked by surgical resection. Given this, we cannot recommend the use of ECPN to mitigate cancer-related pain in resectable PPA patients (Fig 1).

▶ Patients with pancreatic and periampullary adenocarcinomas often have significant epigastric pain. In previous studies of unresectable patients, celiac plexus neurolysis was found to be effective at reducing this pain. One previous study[1] randomly assigned patients with unresectable disease to saline injection around the celiac axis versus ethanol neurolysis, and there was a significant improvement in pain relief in the latter group. Another study[2] randomly assigned patients with unresectable disease to endoscopic ethanol nerve block versus systemic analgesia alone, with a significant reduction in pain in the nerve block group. Because of the usefulness of the celiac plexus block in patients with unresectable periampullary tumors, this study randomly assigned patients with resectable periampullary adenocarcinomas to ethanol celiac plexus neurolysis (ECPN) versus placebo injection with saline. Patients were randomly selected in the operating room to receive either 50% ethanol or saline; syringes were supplied by the pharmacy with the surgeon blinded, and 20 mL were injected on both sides of the aorta at the level of the celiac axis (Fig 1). Patients were further stratified regarding whether they had pain or no pain preoperatively. Unresectable patients were also included in the study, but the numbers of these patients were low. This was a large study, with 485 total patients, of whom, 404 had resectable disease. The primary outcome being measured was a change in pain scores over baseline, with secondary endpoints being morbidity, mortality, quality of life, and overall survival. This study was plagued by a low return rate of surveys; therefore, the numbers of patients had to be increased over the study. The return rate was 44% within the first year, and the most significant finding was that there was no difference in pain levels seen between patients with resectable disease receiving ECPN versus saline. The median survival rates between groups were also similar. Patients who were resected did have a significant reduction in pain at the 3-month time point, which continued to 9 months postsurgery. However, this

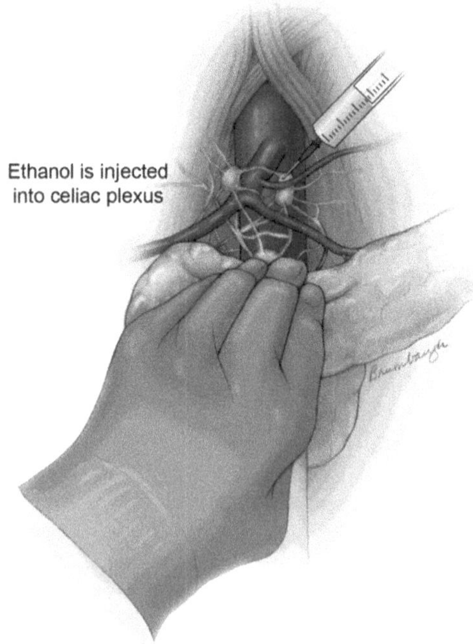

FIG. 1.—Intraoperative ethanol celiac plexus neurolysis procedure with injection of 50% ethanol into the celiac nerve plexus. A 20-mL volume injection was performed on each side of the aorta. (Reprinted from Lavu H, Lengel HB, Sell NM, et al. A prospective, randomized, double-blind, placebo controlled trial on the efficacy of ethanol celiac plexus neurolysis in patients with operable pancreatic and periampullary adenocarcinoma. *J Am Coll Surg.* 2015;220:497-508, with permission from American College of Surgeons.)

finding was the same in both ECPN and saline groups, suggesting that resection of the tumor was what improved the pain. Secondary measures such as quality of life and survival were similar among groups; therefore, the conclusion of this study was that ECPN is not helpful in reducing pain levels in patients with resectable periampullary malignancies. This was a very large study, well-conducted, and performed in a randomized, prospective fashion with blinding of the surgeon to the modality of the plexus injection. The biggest shortcoming was a poor return rate of surveys and not having information on the amount of narcotics used by patients or knowledge of their adjuvant treatment. We conclude that the adjunct of celiac plexus neurolysis in patients undergoing resection is not helpful.

J. R. Howe, MD

References

1. Lillemoe KD, Cameron JL, Kaufman HS, Yeo CJ, Pitt HA, Sauter PK. Chemical splanchnicectomy in patients with unresectable pancreatic cancer. A prospective randomized trial. *Ann Surg.* 1993;217:447-457.

2. Wong GY, Schroeder DR, Carns PE, et al. Effect of neurolytic celiac plexus block on pain relief, quality of life, and survival in patients with unresectable pancreatic cancer: a randomized controlled trial. *JAMA*. 2004;291:1092-1099.

Gastric

Laparoscopic Versus Open Gastrectomy for Gastric Adenocarcinoma in the West: A Case–Control Study

Kelly KJ, Selby L, Chou JF, et al (Memorial Sloan-Kettering Cancer Ctr, New York)

Ann Surg Oncol 22:3590-3596, 2015

Introduction.—Data on laparoscopic gastrectomy in patients with gastric cancer in the Western hemisphere are lacking. This study aimed to compare outcomes following laparoscopic versus open gastrectomy for gastric adenocarcinoma at a Western center.

Methods.—Eighty-seven consecutive patients who underwent laparoscopic gastrectomy from November 2005 to April 2013 were compared with 87 patients undergoing open resection during the same time period. Patients were matched for age, stage, body mass index, and procedure (distal subtotal vs. total gastrectomy). Endpoints were short- and long-term perioperative outcomes.

Results.—Overall, 65 patients (37 %) had locally advanced disease, and 40 (23 %) had proximal tumors. The laparoscopic approach was associated with longer operative time (median 240 vs. 165 min; $p < 0.01$), less blood loss (100 vs. 150 mL; $p < 0.01$), higher rate of microscopic margin positivity (9 vs. 1 %; $p = 0.04$), decreased duration of narcotic and epidural use (2 vs. 4 days, $p = 0.04$, and 3 vs. 4 days, $p = 0.02$, respectively), decreased minor complications in the early (27 vs. 16 %) and late (17 vs. 7 %) postoperative periods ($p < 0.01$), decreased length of stay (5 vs. 7 days; $p = 0.01$), and increased likelihood of receiving adjuvant therapy (82 vs. 51 %; $p < 0.01$). There was no difference in the number of lymph nodes retrieved (median 20 in both groups), major morbidity, or 30-day mortality.

Conclusions.—Laparoscopic gastrectomy for gastric adenocarcinoma is safe and effective for select patients in the West (Fig 1).

▶ Minimally invasive gastrectomy has been established as a reasonable alternative to open gastrectomy in patients with adenocarcinoma in series from Asia. However, patients with gastric cancer from the East differ from Western patients in that they have generally earlier stage tumors and more distal tumors. This study set out to determine whether laparoscopic gastrectomy is a feasible option in patients from the West with adenocarcinoma of the stomach. This study was retrospective and included all patients having laparoscopic gastrectomy for curative intent between 2005 and 2013 at Memorial Sloan-Kettering Cancer Center. The patients who were converted to open procedures were excluded. Laparoscopic cases were then matched to open cases over the same period based on having similar age, body mass index (BMI), tumor

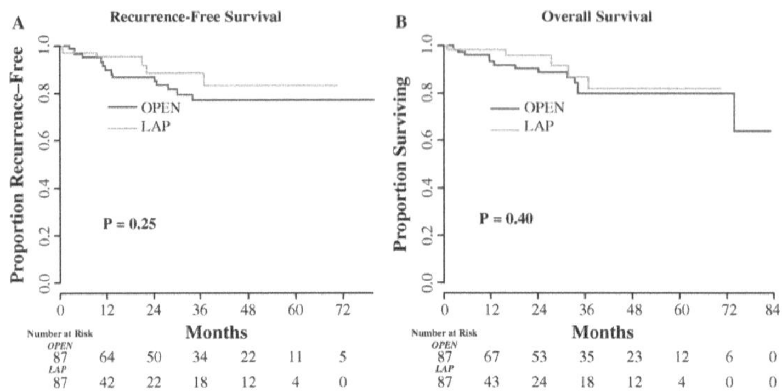

FIGURE 1.—**a** Recurrence-free survival and **b** overall survival for patients undergoing laparoscopic versus open gastrectomy for gastric adenocarcinoma. The median follow-up for survivors was 19.2 months (31.1 for open, 11.0 for laparoscopic). *LAP* laparoscopic. (Reprinted from Kelly KJ, Selby L, Chou JF, et al. Laparoscopic versus open gastrectomy for gastric adenocarcinoma in the west: a case—control study. *Ann Surg Oncol.* 2015;22:3590-3596, with permission from Society of Surgical Oncology.)

stage, and distal versus total gastrectomy. The 2 groups were similar in terms of percentages of patients with stage 2 and 3 disease, race, and BMI but there was an increased incidence of female patients in the laparoscopic group. A similar number of patients received neoadjuvant therapy. Patients having a laparoscopic approach had a longer operative time at 240 versus 165 minutes for the open procedure, commonly lost less blood (100 vs 150 ml), less intravenous narcotic use, and had decreased length of stay (median 5 vs 7 days). Minor complications were more common in the open group at 27% versus 16% for the laparoscopic group, and major complications were similar between both groups. The median number of lymph nodes removed in each group was 20, and there was a significant difference in patients with microscopically positive margins, which was 9% in the laparoscopic versus 1% in the open group. Forty percent of patients received adjuvant treatment in the laparoscopic group versus only 25% in the open group. The median length of follow-up was 19 months, and the 5-year recurrence-free survival and overall survival were not significantly different between groups (Fig 1). This study showed that a laparoscopic approach to gastrectomy is feasible and comparable to an open approach in patients from the West with gastric adenocarcinoma. Patients having a laparoscopic approach had better outcomes in terms of postoperative pain, blood loss, and length of stay. Negatives in this group were a slightly longer operative time and a higher rate of positive margins. Another important advantage of the laparoscopic approach was that a higher percentage of patients could receive adjuvant therapy, which has been shown to improve survival in patients with gastric adenocarcinoma. However, in this study with short follow-up times, no significant differences in recurrence-free survival or overall survival were seen, but these might become evident with a longer follow-up period.

J. R. Howe, MD

Comparison of Gastric Cancer Survival Between Caucasian and Asian Patients Treated in the United States: Results from the Surveillance Epidemiology and End Results (SEER) Database

Wang J, Sun Y, Bertagnolli MM (Brigham and Women's Hosp, Boston, MA; Fudan Univ, Shanghai, China; Harvard Med School, Boston, MA)

Ann Surg Oncol 22:2965-2971, 2015

Background.—The prognosis for gastric cancer is better for Asian than for Caucasian patients. The primary driver of this difference is unknown. This study determined whether the survival advantage of Asian ethnicity continued to hold after control was used for other well-known prognostic factors.

Methods.—In this study, 12,773 patients who underwent gastrectomy for treatment of adenocarcinoma of the stomach were identified from the Surveillance, Epidemiology, and End Results cancer registry. Patients with cardia tumor were excluded from the study. The independent prognostic effect of ethnicity was evaluated by adjusting for other known factors.

Results.—The Asian patients tended to have a diagnosis at an earlier age (66.8 vs. 68.5 years), more lymph nodes examined (16 vs. 13), and more positive lymph nodes (5.1 vs. 4.8). Survival was better for the Asian patients than for the Caucasian patients, with a 12 % 5-year survival difference. Among the patients with IB, IIA, and IIB disease, the Asian patients had 37, 72, and 13 months longer median survival time than the corresponding Caucasian patients. The multivariate Cox model showed persistence of this result after adjustment for imbalances of age, gender, tumor grade, and number of examined and positive lymph nodes. The largest risk reduction was observed for the stage IA patients (31 %) and the smallest for the stage IIIC patients (9 %).

Conclusion.—After excluding proximal gastric cancers, controlling for the imbalance of known prognostic factors, and decreasing in the influence of D2 lymphadenectomy, stage migration, and chemo/radiation therapy by including only patients treated in the United States, this study found that the survival advantage of Asian ethnicity continued to be present (Fig 1).

▶ The incidence of gastric cancer is 4- to 10-fold higher in Asian countries than it is in Western countries. It has also been well established that Asian patients have improved survival compared with Western patients with gastric cancer. This is due in part to the fact that Asian patients present with more distal rather than proximal tumors, a younger age of diagnosis, an earlier overall stage disease, and possibly because some of these patients receive more extended lymphadenectomies. There may also be a difference in adjuvant and neoadjuvant treatment, which is more commonly administered in the west. With all these differences between Asian and Western cultures, an important question is whether there is something intrinsic to the Asian race that results in better prognosis, as opposed to cultural or societal factors.

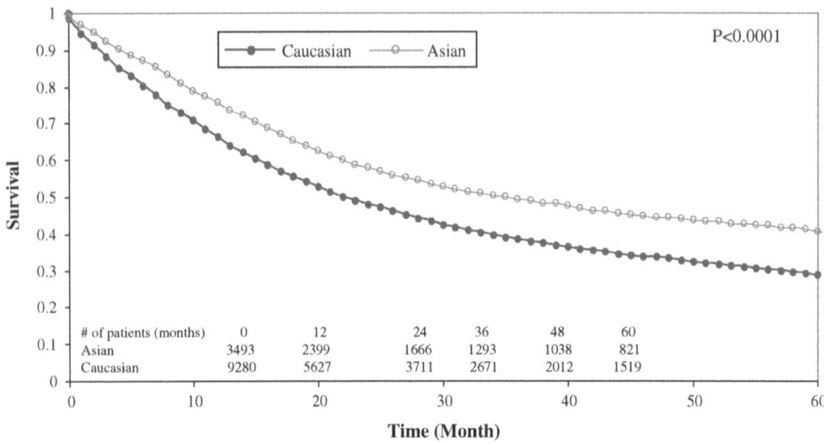

FIGURE 1.—Survival comparison between Caucasian and Asian gastric cancer patients. (Reprinted from Wang J, Sun Y, Bertagnolli MM. Comparison of gastric cancer survival between Caucasian and Asian patients treated in the United States: results from the surveillance epidemiology and end results (SEER) database. *Ann Surg Oncol.* 2015;22:2965-2971, with permission from Society of Surgical Oncology.)

This study tries to address this question by looking at patients with gastric cancer in the Surveillance Epidemiology and End Results database between 1988 and 2007. They examined patients being classified as white versus those of Asian ethnicity in terms of a variety of different clinicopathologic factors. They excluded patients with tumors in the gastric cardia or the gastroesophageal junction. The study included 12 773 patients, of whom 27% were Asian and the remainder were white. Significant differences seen between these 2 groups were that the mean age of Asian patients was 2 years younger, the mean tumor size was slightly smaller, the mean number of nodes was increased, and the mean number of positive nodes was slightly increased. Asian patients had more tumors in the antrum (40% vs 32% in white patients), a higher frequency of T1A tumors (16% vs 9% in whites), and fewer stage 2A tumors. The median survival of Asian patients was 35 months versus 23 months in white patients, and 5-year overall survival was 41% versus 29%, respectively, both being statistically significant (Fig 1). When Asian and white patients were compared across different TNM stages, the statistically significantly improved survival persisted for all categories in Asian patients. A multivariate analysis within each stage was performed, which revealed that Asian race was a significant factor for improved survival. This paper confirms the fact that Asian patients with gastric cancer do better than their Western counterparts, even if they were raised in the United States and were subject to similar operations and chemotherapeutic treatments as white patients. A limitation of this study is that the actual operations performed, and additional chemotherapy or radiation received was not part of this analysis; therefore there could have been differences between these groups. Either way, it appears that Asians with gastric cancer do better, which may be due to having more distal tumors, younger age, and probably something intrinsic to Asian ethnicity, not as yet determined.

J. R. Howe, MD

Hepatic Colorectal

Resection Margin and Survival in 2368 Patients Undergoing Hepatic Resection for Metastatic Colorectal Cancer: Surgical Technique or Biologic Surrogate?

Sadot E, Groot Koerkamp B, Leal JN, et al (Memorial Sloan Kettering Cancer Ctr, New York)

Ann Surg 262:476-485, 2015

Objectives.—The impact of margin width on overall survival (OS) in the context of other prognostic factors after resection for colorectal liver metastases is unclear. We evaluated the relationship between resection margin and OS utilizing high-resolution histologic distance measurements.

Methods.—A single-institution prospectively maintained database was queried for all patients who underwent an initial complete resection of colorectal liver metastases between 1992 and 2012. R1 resection was defined as tumor cells at the resection margin (0 mm). R0 resection was further divided into 3 groups: 0.1 to 0.9 mm, 1 to 9 mm, and 10 mm or greater.

Results.—A total of 4915 liver resections were performed at Memorial Sloan Kettering Cancer Center between 1992 and 2012, from which 2368 patients were included in the current study. Half of the patients presented with synchronous disease, 43% had solitary metastasis, and the median tumor size was 3.4 cm. With a median follow-up for survivors of 55 months, the median OS of the R1, 0.1 to 0.9 mm, 1 to 9 mm, and 10 mm or more groups was 32, 40, 53, and 56 months, respectively ($P < 0.001$). Compared with R1 resection, all margin widths, including submillimeter margins correlated with prolonged OS ($P < 0.05$). The association between the margin width and OS remained significant when adjusted for all other clinicopathologic prognostic factors.

Conclusions.—Resection margin width is independently associated with OS. Wide margins should be attempted whenever possible. However, resection should not be precluded if narrow margins are anticipated, as submillimeter margin clearance is associated with improved survival. The prolonged OS observed with submillimeter margins is likely a microscopic surrogate for the biologic behavior of a tumor rather than the result of surgical technique (Fig 2).

▶ Studies of resection of hepatic colorectal liver metastasis (CRLM) have previously indicated that 1-cm margins should be obtained to improve patient survival because the vast majority of microsatellite lesions will be located within 1 cm. Questions have arisen more recently because of the advent of oxaliplatin and irinotecan based chemotherapy regimens as to whether a 1-cm margin is actually necessary, as opposed to just having a microscopically negative

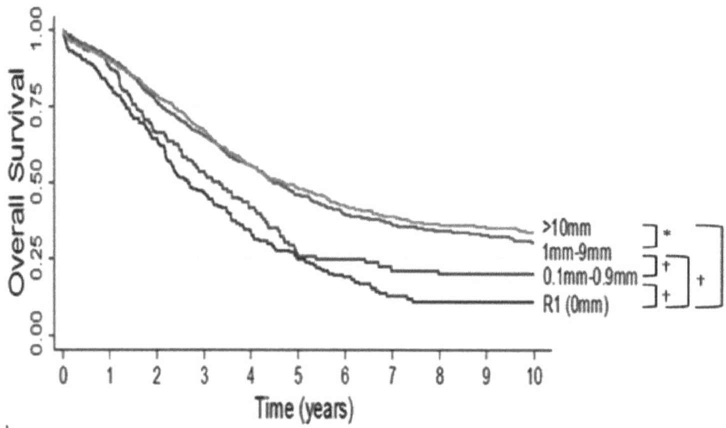

Number at risk

R1	245	39	9
0.1 - 0.9 mm	160	27	10
1 - 9 mm	1191	353	86
>10 mm	765	262	111

FIGURE 2.—Overall survival curves stratified according to 4 categories of resection margin width. *P = not significant; †$P < 0.05$. (Reprinted from Sadot E, Groot Koerkamp B, Leal JN, et al. Resection margin and survival in 2368 patients undergoing hepatic resection for metastatic colorectal cancer: surgical technique or biologic surrogate? *Ann Surg*. 2015;262:476-485, with permission from Wolters Kluwer Health, Inc.)

margin. This large, single-institutional study evaluated all patients having resection for CRLM between 1992 and 2012. Pathologists looked at margins using high-resolution, correcting for total magnification within the microscopic field to determine actual width of margins in all patients. They included 2368 patients, half of whom had synchronous disease and the other half had metachronous disease. Forty-three percent of patients had solitary metastases, with a mean tumor size of 3.4 cm and median follow-up of 55 months. When margin width was looked at as a continuous variable, there was an inflection point at 3 to 4 mm for median overall survival. The authors then categorized margins into R1 with tumor present at the margin versus 3 subcategories: 0.1 to 0.9 mm, 1 to 9 mm, and 10 mm or more.

Interestingly, median survivals in these 4 groups were 32, 40, 53, and 56 months, respectively. Therefore, there was improved survival even with a margin <1 mm, but the survival was further improved by having margins >1 mm. There was no difference in overall survival between 1- and 9-mm margins and 10 mm or more (Fig 2). Independent predictors of margin width <1 mm included >3 lesions, size >5 cm, carcinoembryonic antigen >200, and ablation status.

This was a very large study with excellent statistical power that demonstrated an independent association between improved survival and margins of 1 cm, 1 mm, or submillimeter, and the authors concluded that liver resection should still be performed in patients who may have a close margin. Even in the narrow margin group, 5% of patients were 10-year survivors, and in the R1 group, 4% were 10-year survivors, showing that long-term survival is still possible with positive or close margins. They felt that surgical technique was not the most important factor for improved survival, but that, more likely, the margin width was a microscopic surrogate for the biologic behavior of the tumor. Limitations to this study were that it was retrospective, may have been subject to temporal bias, the rate of local recurrence was not reported, and that these results may not be generalized well to centers that are not high volume. The positive aspects of the study were the very large number of patients, a consistent surgical technique using the Kelly clamp for liver transection, and multivariate analysis to look for independent associations. This is the largest study to date looking at the relationship of resection margin and survival.

J. R. Howe, MD

Chemotherapy for Patients with Colorectal Liver Metastases Who Underwent Curative Resection Improves Long-Term Outcomes: Systematic Review and Meta-analysis

Araujo RLC, Gönen M, Herman P (Univ of São Paulo Med School, Brazil; Memorial Sloan-Kettering Cancer Ctr, New York)

Ann Surg Oncol 22:3070-3078, 2015

Background.—Hepatic resection is considered the standard of care for patients with resectable colorectal liver metastases (CRLM), but the benefits of using systemic chemotherapy for these patients have not been completely proven. Although systemic chemotherapy is likely to improve recurrence-free survival (RFS), no differences in overall survival (OS) have been demonstrated to date. This study aimed to compare surgery plus systemic chemotherapy, regardless timing of administration, with surgery alone, analyzing long-term outcomes for patients with CRLM who underwent liver resection with curative intent.

Methods.—Systematic review and meta-analysis of studies published from January 1991 to December 2013 were used to compare surgery alone and surgery plus chemotherapy for patients with CRLM who underwent liver resection with curative intent. All randomized clinical trials (RCTs) were included in the study. Selection of high-quality observational comparative studies (OCSs) was based on a validated tool, the Methodological Index for Nonrandomized Studies. Comparison of RFS and OS was performed using a fixed-effects model and the hazard ratio (HR).

Results.—Concerning OS, 5 studies (3 RCTs and 2 OCSs) comprising 2,475 patients were analyzed, and chemotherapy (1,024 patients) relatively improved OS rates for 23 % of the patients versus surgery alone (HR, 0.77; 95 % confidence interval [CI] 0.67–0.88; $p < 0.001$). Four studies, totaling 1,592 patients, reported RFS (3 using RCTs and 1 using OCSs), showing that chemotherapy (702 patients) relatively improved RFS for 29 % of the patients (HR, 0.71; 95 % CI 0.61–0.83; $p < 0.001$).

Conclusion.—This meta-analysis demonstrated that the use of chemotherapy for patients with CRLM who underwent resection with curative intent is a worthwhile strategy for improving both RFS and OS (Fig 3).

▶ Resection is the treatment most likely to yield long-term survival in patients with colorectal liver metastases. Although chemotherapy is routinely administered preoperatively or in the adjuvant setting, randomized controlled trials have not demonstrated whether there is a survival benefit to these strategies. Randomized controlled trials are an excellent way to answer important clinical questions, but they can take a long time to perform, may be limited in statistical power due to patient recruitment issues, and the literature is biased toward publications showing a positive result.

The authors of this study set out to perform a meta-analysis of trials looking at any chemotherapy either pre- or postoperatively in association with resection of hepatic metastases versus those undergoing resection alone. They searched

A

Study	Year	Hazard Ratio	Upper Limit	Lower Limit
Langer[21]	2002	0.77	0.42	1.4
Portier[12]	2006	0.73	0.48	1.1
Parks[7]	2007	0.75	0.62	0.91
Nordlinger[10]	2008	0.87	0.66	1.14
Adam[8]	2010	0.68	0.47	0.99
Fixed Effect		**0.77**	**0.67**	**0.88**

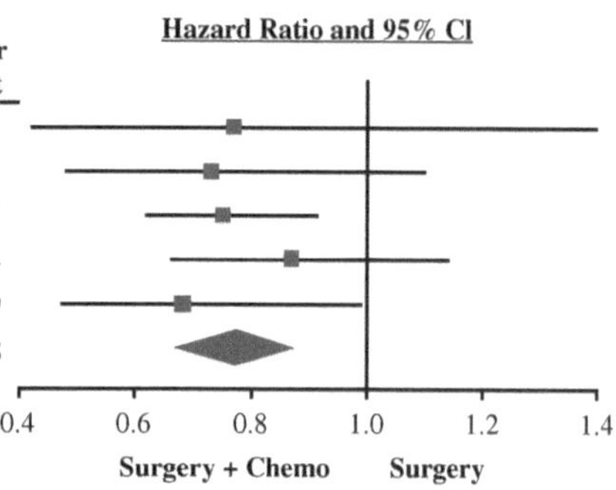

p <0.001

Test fot heterogeneity:
Q = 1.326 on 4 degrees of freedom (p= 0.857)
$i^2 = 0\%$

B

Study	Year	Hazard Ratio	Upper Limit	Lower Limit
Langer[21]	2002	0.78	0.46	1.31
Portier[21]	2006	0.66	0.45	0.96
Nordlinger[10]	2008	0.78	0.61	0.99
Adam[8]	2010	0.64	0.49	0.83
Fixed Effect		**0.71**	**0.61**	**0.83**

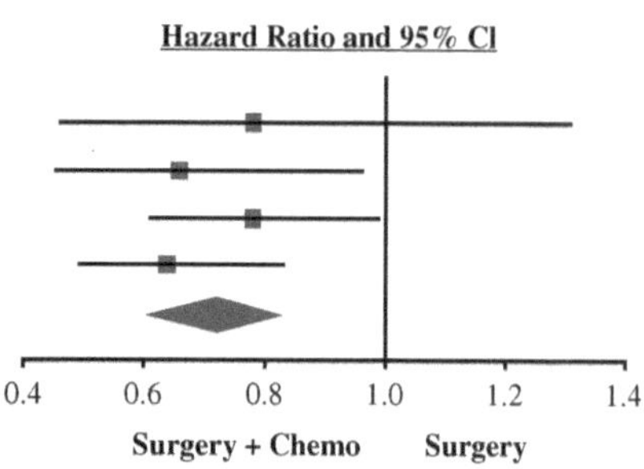

p <0.001

Test fot heterogeneity:
Q = 1.447 on 3 degrees of freedom (p= 0.695)
$i^2 = 0\%$

FIGURE 3.—Forest plots of studies comparing hazard ratios and fixed effects between surgery alone and surgery with additional chemotherapy for the treatment of patients with potentially resectable colorectal liver metastases (CRLM). a Forest plot comparing overall survival. b Forest plot comparing recurrence-free survival. (Reprinted from Araujo RLC, Gönen M, Herman P. Chemotherapy for patients with colorectal liver metastases who underwent curative resection improves long-term outcomes: systematic review and meta-analysis. *Ann Surg Oncol.* 2015;22:3070-3078, with permission from Society of Surgical Oncology.)

the literature for randomized controlled trials between 1990 and 2013 and observational comparative studies deemed to be of high quality based on the methodological index for nonrandomized studies. Of 673 reports, 83 were selected for further review, and of these, there were 3 randomized controlled trials and 1 observational study found to be appropriate for analysis. These studies included 2475 patients, 1451 of whom had surgery alone and 1024 who surgery and chemotherapy. The 3 randomized controlled trials consisted of 620 total patients. Two of the randomized studies evaluated 6 cycles of adjuvant chemotherapy, which was 5-fluorouracil (FU) based, and this included Langer et al[1] with 107 patients, and Portier et al[2] with 171 patients. The third trial by Nordlinger et al[3] included 364 patients who received 6 cycles of FOLFOX before and 6 cycles after surgery. The observational study included was that of Parks et al,[4] which included 792 patients receiving 5-FU-based chemotherapy. The final analysis consisted of these 4 trials clearly employing adjuvant chemotherapy (with some preoperative chemotherapy given in the Nordlinger trial[3]).

The findings of this study were that overall survival was improved by 23% when chemotherapy was given versus surgery alone, for a hazard ratio of 0.77 ($P < .001$). In terms of recurrence-free survival, there was a 29% improvement in patients receiving chemotherapy versus surgery alone, with a hazard ratio of 0.71 ($P < .001$; Fig 3). The authors conclude that the use of adjuvant chemotherapy in patients having hepatic resection for metastatic colorectal surgery is worthwhile to improve overall and recurrence-free survival. Limitations of this study were the small number of trials examined, the differences in regimens used, and the inclusion of an observational study. In the end, it is difficult to be confident that this question has been answered, but this study at least attempts to combine the larger studies (that may have been underpowered individually) to bring us closer to the truth.

J. R. Howe, MD

References

1. Langer, et al. *Proc Am Soc Clin Oncol.* 2002;21:149A.
2. Portier G, Elias D, Bouche O, et al. Multicenter randomized trial of adjuvant fluorouracil and folinic acid compared with surgery alone after resection of colorectal liver metastases: FFCD ACHBTH AURC 9002 trial. *J Clin Oncol.* 2006;24:4976-4982.
3. Nordlinger B, Sorbye H, Glimelius B, et al. Perioperative chemotherapy with FOLFOX4 and surgery versus surgery alone for resectable liver metastases from colorectal cancer (EORTC Intergroup trial 40983): a randomised controlled trial. *Lancet.* 2008;371:1007-1016.
4. Parks R, Gonen M, Kemeny N, et al. Adjuvant chemotherapy improves survival after resection of hepatic colorectal metastases: analysis of data from two continents. *J Am Coll Surg.* 2007;204:753-761.

Hepatocellular

Analysis of Recurrence Patterns After Anatomical or Non-anatomical Resection for Hepatocellular Carcinoma

Marubashi S, Gotoh K, Akita H, et al (Osaka Med Ctr for Cancer and Cardiovascular Diseases, Japan; et al)

Ann Surg Oncol 22:2243-2252, 2015

Background.—Recurrence patterns after hepatic resection has been poorly understood in view of tumor blood flow drainage (TBFD) area. Our goal was to clarify the recurrence patterns after anatomical versus nonanatomical hepatic resection for hepatocellular carcinoma (HCC).

Methods.—A total of 424 consecutive patients with HCC, who were treated by curative resection (R0) at our hospital from 2001 to 2012, were evaluated. Among these, we compared the outcomes of the anatomical resection group (AR group, $n = 243$) and the nonanatomical resection group (NR group, $n = 181$). We performed an analysis of the recurrence patterns of HCC based on the preoperative CT during hepatic arteriography in these 424 patients.

Results.—Preoperative liver function was better in the AR group than the NR group ($P < 0.001$), and tumor size was larger in the AR group than the NR group ($P < 0.001$). HCC recurrence was recorded in 145 patients (59.7 %) of the AR group and 102 patients (56.4 %) of the NR group with no significant differences between the two groups ($P = 0.590$). The incidences of extrahepatic and intrahepatic recurrence (solitary/multiple) were similar between the two groups. In addition, the rate of recurrences by local dissemination, either recurrences in the same subsegment in the NR group or recurrences in the TBFD area in the AR group, was sufficiently low (1.4 %) as to be considered negligible.

Conclusions.—The incidence and patterns of HCC recurrence were similar between the anatomical and nonanatomical resection. Recurrence by local dissemination may be considered to be negligible in both surgical methods (Fig 3).

▶ Hepatocellular cancer (HCC) is the second leading cause of cancer death internationally. Patients undergoing surgical resection for HCC have recurrence rates as high as 50% within the first 3 years after resection. It is thought that recurrence occurs through portal vein dissemination, from systemic circulating tumor cells that recolonize the liver or from de novo development of new tumors. If portal vein dissemination is one of the main mechanisms through which spread occurs, then anatomic resections may reduce recurrence compared with nonanatomic resections.

This study set out to look at patterns of HCC recurrence in patients at a single institution in Japan who had anatomic (AR) versus nonanatomic (NR) resection. They included 424 patients who had an R0 resection, which included 243 with AR and 181 with NR. In patients undergoing AR, they occluded the portal vein and hepatic artery, injected dye into the appropriate branch by ultrasound,

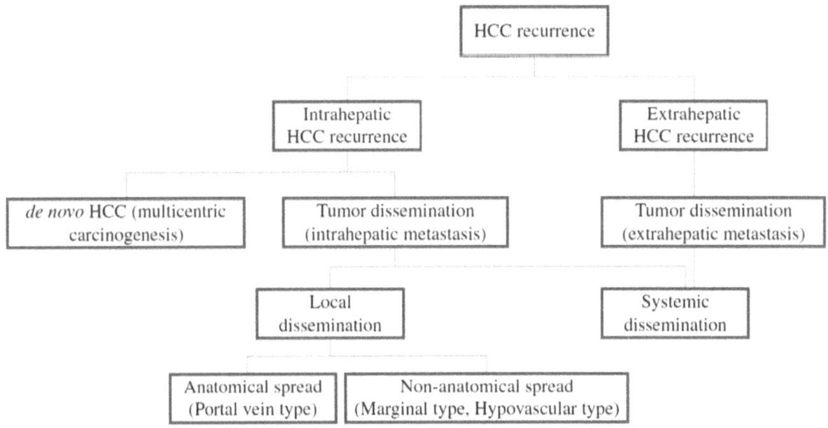

FIGURE 3.—Tree diagram of HCC recurrence. HCC recurrence is divided into intrahepatic and extrahepatic recurrence. Intrahepatic recurrence is divided into groups, as shown in the *diagram*, while extrahepatic recurrence always occurs as a result of systemic dissemination. (Reprinted from Marubashi S, Gotoh K, Akita H, et al. Analysis of recurrence patterns after anatomical or non-anatomical resection for hepatocellular carcinoma. *Ann Surg Oncol.* 2015;22:2243-2252, with permission from Society of Surgical Oncology.)

then performed parenchymal dissection along the line of demarcation. ARs consisted of 137 sectionectomies, 84 right or left lobectomies, 3 trisegmentectomies, and 19 subsegmentectomies. In the case of NRs, an attempt to obtain 5- to 10-mm margins was carried out. These patients were not randomized and were instead selected for the surgical procedure by the surgeons based on a variety of clinical and anatomic factors. The groups differed in that patients having NR generally were more likely to be hepatitis C—positive, have smaller tumors, smaller resected liver segments, shorter operative time, less blood loss, have well differentiated tumors, were less likely to have microvascular invasion, and were more likely to be stage 1. Postoperative morbidity was higher in patients undergoing AR, with an incidence of bile leak at 8.6% versus 1.7% in NR group, but patterns of other complications were similar. HCC recurrence was similar in both groups at 60% for the AR group versus 56% for the NR group, with a mean follow-up of just under 4 years. Multivariate analysis revealed that factors predicting for recurrence included preoperative AST, albumin, Des-γ-carboxy prothrombin marker, tumor size, lesion multiplicity, and blood loss. Whether a patient had AR or NR was not a risk factor for recurrence. Of these recurrences, the patterns were similar between the 2 groups. Distant metastases occurred in 10% of those undergoing AR versus 4% of those having NR, while solitary recurrence in the liver occurred in 25% of patients in each group, and multiple HCC recurrences occurred in 25 and 27% in the AR and NR groups, respectively. These differences were not statistically significant. Local tumor dissemination was seen in only 6 patients total (1.4%), with 1 case in the AR group and 5 cases in the NR group. The vast majority of recurrences were thought to be systemic or de novo development of HCC.

Limitations of the study are that it was not randomized and therefore the groups were not equal for all biological factors; the patterns of recurrence were determined by imaging; and it is generally difficult to determine whether recurrences originate de novo without genomic analysis. The main conclusions to draw from this study were that when performed with adequate surgical margins, the incidence of recurrence after NR is quite similar to that of AR, and therefore either surgical method could be used in these patients. The main patterns of recurrence seen were tumor dissemination with intrahepatic metastases or de novo HCCs, which might not be prevented by larger AR procedures.

J. R. Howe, MD

Antiviral Therapy Improves Postoperative Survival in Patients With Hepatocellular Carcinoma: A Randomized Controlled Trial

Huang G, Lau WY, Wang Z-G, et al (Natl Innovation Alliance for Hepatitis & Liver Cancer, Shanghai, China; et al)

Ann Surg 261:56-66, 2015

Objective.—A randomized controlled trial was conducted to find out whether antiviral therapy in patients with hepatitis B–related hepatocellular carcinoma (HCC) improves long-term survival after hepatic resection.

Background.—Despite advances in surgery and in multidisciplinary treatment, there is still no effective adjuvant treatment to prevent HCC recurrence after R0 resection for HCC. Whether antiviral therapy is useful in reducing postoperative HCC recurrence is unclear.

Methods.—Between May 2007 and April 2008, patients who received R0 hepatic resection for HBV-related HCC were randomly assigned to receive no treatment (the control group, n = 100) or antiviral therapy (adefovir 10 mg/d, the antiviral group, n = 100).

Results.—The baseline clinical, laboratory, and tumor characteristics of the 2 groups were comparable. The 1-, 3-, and 5-year recurrence-free survival rates for the antiviral group and the control group were 85.0%, 50.3%, 46.1% and 84.0%, 37.9%, 27.1%, respectively. The corresponding overall survival rates for the 2 groups were 96.0%, 77.6%, 63.1% and 94.0%, 67.4%, 41.5%, respectively. The recurrence-free survival and overall survival for the antiviral group were significantly better than the control group ($P = 0.026$, $P = 0.001$). After adjusting for the confounding prognostic factors in a Cox model, the relative risks of recurrence and death for antiviral treatment were 0.651 [95% confidence interval (CI): 0.451–0.938; $P = 0.021$] and 0.420 (95% CI: 0.271–0.651; $P < 0.001$). Antiviral therapy was an independent protective factor of late tumor recurrence (HR = 0.348, 95% CI: 0.177–0.687; $P = 0.002$) but not of early tumor recurrence [hazard ratio (HR) = 0.949, 95% CI: 0.617–1.459; $P = 0.810$].

Conclusions.—In patients with hepatitis B–related HCC, adefovir antiviral therapy reduced late HCC recurrence and significantly improved overall survival after R0 hepatic resection (Fig 3).

▶ Approximately 350 million people across the world have chronic hepatitis B infection, and more than half of hepatocellular carcinoma (HCC) cases are

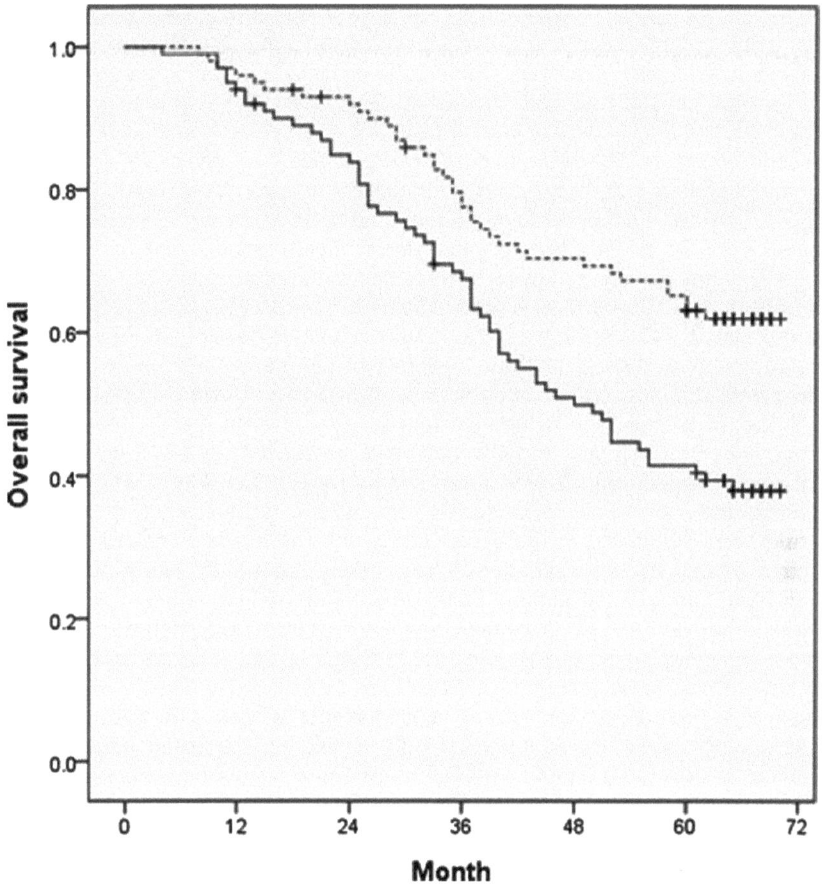

FIG 3.—Comparison of overall survivals between the 2 groups. Dotted line: the antiviral group (n = 100). Solid line: the control group (n = 100). Log-rank test: $P = 0.001$. (Reprinted from Huang G, Lau WY, Wang Z-G, et al. Antiviral therapy improves postoperative survival in patients with hepatocellular carcinoma. *Ann Surg*. 2015;261:56-66, with permission from Lippincott Williams & Wilkins.)

attributable to this virus. Effective vaccination is available for prevention, and in the past decade, multiple options for antiviral therapy have also become available. Besides interferon, the new promising agents are nucleoside/nucleotide analogues, which inhibit hepatitis B virus DNA polymerase activity and suppress replication. There are several agents available, including lamivudine, adefovir, telbivudine, and entecavir. Because hepatitis B replication has been shown to play an important role in the recurrence of HCC, one of the unanswered questions is whether treatment with antiviral medications after resection of HCC can improve survival or reduce recurrence rates.

This study from China randomized patients into antiviral treatment versus no treatment after resection of HCC. This study required that patients were positive for hepatitis B surface antigen, negative for hepatitis C or HIV, and that the hepatitis B viral DNA levels were greater than 2000 IU/mL. They also required that patients had Barcelona Clinic Liver Cancer Stage 0A or solitary tumors > 5 cm in size, with no evidence of hepatic metastasis or radiologic suggestion of invasion; patients also had to be Child-Pugh class A. Patients also were not previously treated for HCC or with antiviral therapy, and all had to have negative resection margins. The antiviral drug used was adefovir, given orally at 10 mg per day beginning at 4 to 7 days after surgery and continued throughout the study. One hundred patients were randomized to each arm with a medium follow-up of 60 months. Both groups were similar in terms of patient characteristics. Patients receiving antiviral therapy had a rate of undetectable HBV-DNA of 85% at 1 year and 93% at 5 years, versus 12% and 22%, respectively, for the control group. Fifteen patients treated with antivirals developed drug-resistant mutations. With respect to the end points of recurrence and overall survival, there were significant improvements seen in patients receiving antiviral therapy and control groups. The recurrence-free survival rates in the antiviral therapy group were 85% at 1 year and 46% at 5 years, versus 84% and 27% for the control group, respectively. Overall survival rates were 96% at 1 year and 63% at 5 years for the antiviral group, versus 94% and 41.5%, respectively (Fig 3). These results were significant at the 5-year end point. Multivariate analysis revealed factors leading to tumor recurrence were tumor size > 5 cm, surgical margins of < 1 cm, tumor encapsulation, presence of microsatellite nodules, and microportal tumor vein thrombus. Antiviral therapy was also associated with reduced tumor recurrence. For overall survival, the factors that were most important included these same factors plus albumin < 35 g/L and a high Ishak fibrosis score. The hazard rate for recurrence of patients treated with antivirals was 0.65, and for overall survival were 0.42, both highly significant. Interestingly, antiviral therapy did not reduce the risk of early tumor recurrence but did reduce the risk of late tumor recurrence. This excellent, randomized controlled study demonstrates the benefits of antiviral therapy in reducing tumor recurrence after resection of HCC in those patients infected with hepatitis B. The mechanism may be because active replication of hepatitis B virus may initiate HCC formation, and sustained high viral loads may impair immune responses. The authors believe that the benefit of antiviral therapy was not by a direct antitumor effect but rather by reducing chronic inflammation, thereby reducing the risk of developing new HCCs. The finding of the study is significant in that it will likely lead to the introduction of adjuvant treatment of these patients with oral nucleoside/nucleotide agents.

J. R. Howe, MD

HIPEC

A Simplified Preoperative Assessment Predicts Complete Cytoreduction and Outcomes in Patients with Low-Grade Mucinous Adenocarcinoma of the Appendix

Dineen SP, Royal RE, Hughes MS, et al (MD Anderson Cancer Ctr, Houston, TX; Natl Cancer Inst, Bethesda, MD; et al)

Ann Surg Oncol 22:3640-3646, 2015

Background.—Complete cytoreduction with hyperthermic intraperitoneal chemotherapy (CRS/HIPEC) has been shown to improve survival in patients with low-grade mucinous adenocarcinoma (LGMA). However, incomplete cytoreduction exposes patients to significant morbidity without a similar survival benefit. Preoperative assessment of the ability to achieve CRS is therefore a critical step in selecting patients for CRS/HIPEC.

Objective.—The aim of this study was to develop and validate a preoperative scoring system to accurately predict the ability to achieve complete cytoreduction in patients with LGMA of the appendix.

Methods.—A simplified preoperative assessment for appendix tumor (SPAAT) score was developed based on computed tomography scan findings thought to predict incomplete cytoreduction. We applied the SPAAT score to patients with LGMA to determine the ability of the score to predict complete cytoreduction. This scoring system was then applied to a separate cohort of patients from a different institution. Sensitivity and specificity were determined for the SPAAT score. Survival was calculated and correlated with the SPAAT score and the completeness of cytoreduction score.

Results.—A SPAAT score of <3 is a significant predictor of complete cytoreduction in the derivation cohort. In the validation cohort, 40 of 42 patients with a SPAAT score <3 achieved a complete cytoreduction, for a positive predictive value of 95.2 % and a negative predictive value of 100 %. Additionally, the SPAAT score was a significant predictor of disease-free survival.

Conclusions.—The SPAAT score is a useful tool in the preoperative assessment of patients with LGMA who are under consideration for cytoreductive surgery. Prospective analysis of this scoring system is warranted to appropriately select patients who will benefit from CRS/HIPEC (Table 1).

► Adenocarcinoma of the appendix is rare but can become a big problem if it perforates, leading to pseudomyxoma peritonei. If these lesions are low grade, they are amenable to cytoreduction with hyperthermic intraperitoneal chemotherapy. It has been shown that with this strategy, patients can have excellent 5-year survival, which may range from 30% to 75%. Predictors of poor survival are incomplete resection, high-grade lesions, and patient comorbidities. It is often difficult to determine preoperatively whether metastatic

TABLE 1.—SPAAT Score of 3 Demonstrates Best Results in Derivation and Validation Cohorts

Cutoff	Sensitivity (%)	Specificity (%)	PPV (%)	NPV (%)	Spearman
Derivation cohort ($n = 27$)					
SPAAT ≥ 2	100	36.4	69.6	100	0.503
SPAAT ≥ 3	100	100	100	100	1.0
SPAAT ≥ 4	92	100	100	50	0.678
Validation cohort ($n = 70$)					
SPAAT ≥ 2	62.5	93.3	92.6	65.1	0.568
SPAAT ≥ 3	100	93.3	95.2	100	0.943
SPAAT ≥ 4	100	70	81.6	100	0.756

NPV negative predictive value, *PPV* positive predictive value, *SPAAT* simplified preoperative assessment for appendix tumor

Reprinted from Dineen SP, Royal RE, Hughes MS, et al. A simplified preoperative assessment predicts complete cytoreduction and outcomes in patients with low-grade mucinous adenocarcinoma of the appendix. *Ann Surg Oncol.* 2015;22:3640-3646, with permission from The Author(s).

disease will be amenable to complete cytoreduction, which is important because these are morbid procedures with complication rates of 30% to 50%.

This article attempts to develop a preoperative method for determining which patients are most likely to have cytoreduction achieved. They call it the simplified preoperative assessment for appendix tumor (SPAAT), which relies on findings seen on CT scans. This is scored by looking at 5 areas on an abdominal CT with contrast, and scores can range from 0 to 7. One point is given for each if there is scalloping on the liver, spleen, pancreas, or portal vein. Three additional points are possible depending on the status of the small bowel and its mesentery. If the small bowel is floating in the mucinous ascites, this receives a score of 0; on the other extreme, if there is mesenteric foreshortening, tethering of the small bowel, and cauliflowering, then a score of 3 is awarded. On the basis of the 7-point scale, the authors reviewed data from 27 patients treated at 1 institution between 2008 and 2009 and assessed these patients for the SPAAT score. They then evaluated different cutoffs of the SPAAT score, and looked at sensitivity, specificity, and positive predictive value of these different scores for complete cytoreduction (Table 1). Twenty-three patients with a SPAAT score < 3 had complete cytoreduction and 4 patients with 3 or greater had incomplete cytoreduction, making the sensitivity, specificity, and positive predictive value 100% in this derivation cohort of 27 patients. They then looked at 70 patients treated at another institution as their validation cohort. Of these, 42 had a score of < 3 and 28 had a score of 3 or greater. Once again, a cutoff of 3 gave the best results with a sensitivity of 100%, specificity of 93%, and positive predictive value of 95%. As seen in other series, there was significantly improved overall and disease-free survival in patients who had complete cytoreduction versus incomplete cytoreduction. For patients with SPAAT score < 3 versus 3 or greater, disease-free survival was significantly improved, and there was a trend for improved overall survival. The complication rates were similar between groups, and all 3 mortalities were in patients who had a SPAAT score of > 3. Median follow-up was 52 months in this series. The authors conclude that this SPAAT score is useful for predicting whether patients will achieve a complete cytoreduction, and the big advantage is that it can be done using a preoperative CT scan rather than at exploration. Therefore, patients with significant comorbidities with a high SPAAT score can be saved the potential complications of surgery. However, having a SPAAT score >3 does not preclude attempted cytoreduction, and patients still may benefit from incomplete cytoreduction. An important limitation to this scoring system is that this study only included patients with excellent performance status and therefore may not be as generalizable to patients with more limited performance status, nor should it be used for patients who have high-grade appendiceal tumors.

J. R. Howe, MD

Extent of Colorectal Peritoneal Carcinomatosis: Attempt to Define a Threshold Above Which HIPEC Does Not Offer Survival Benefit: A Comparative Study

Goéré D, Souadka A, Faron M, et al (Gustave Roussy, Cancer Ctr, Villejuif Cedex, France)

Ann Surg Oncol 22:2958-2964, 2015

Background.—The main prognostic factors after complete cytoreductive surgery (CCRS) of colorectal peritoneal carcinomatosis (PC) followed by intraperitoneal chemotherapy (IPC) are completeness of the resection and extent of the disease. This study aimed to determine a threshold value above which CCRS plus IPC may not offer survival benefit compared with systemic chemotherapy.

Methods.—Between March 2000 and May 2010, 180 patients underwent surgery for PC from colorectal cancer with intended performance of CCRS plus IPC.

Results.—Among the 180 patients, CCRS plus IPC could be performed for 139 patients (curative group, 77 %), whereas it could not be performed for 41 patients (palliative group, 23 %). The two groups were comparable in terms of age, gender, primary tumor characteristics, and pre- and postoperative systemic chemotherapy. The mean peritoneal cancer index (PCI) was lower in the curative group (11 ± 7) than in the palliative group (23 ± 7) ($p < 0.0001$). After a median follow-up period of 60 months (range 47–74 months), the 3-year overall survival (OS) rate was 52 % [95 % confidence interval (CI) 43–61 %] in the curative group compared with 7 % (95 % CI 2–25 %) in the palliative group. Comparison of the survivals for each PCI (ranging from 5 to 36) shows that OS did not differ significantly between the two groups of patients when the PCI was higher than 17 (hazard ratio 0.64; range 0.38–1.09).

Conclusion.—This study confirmed the major prognostic impact of PC extent. When the PCI exceeds 17 in PC of colorectal origin, CCRS plus IPC does not seem to offer any survival benefit (Fig 2).

► Patients with peritoneal carcinomatosis from colorectal cancer uniformly had a poor prognosis until the advent of cytoreductive surgery and heated

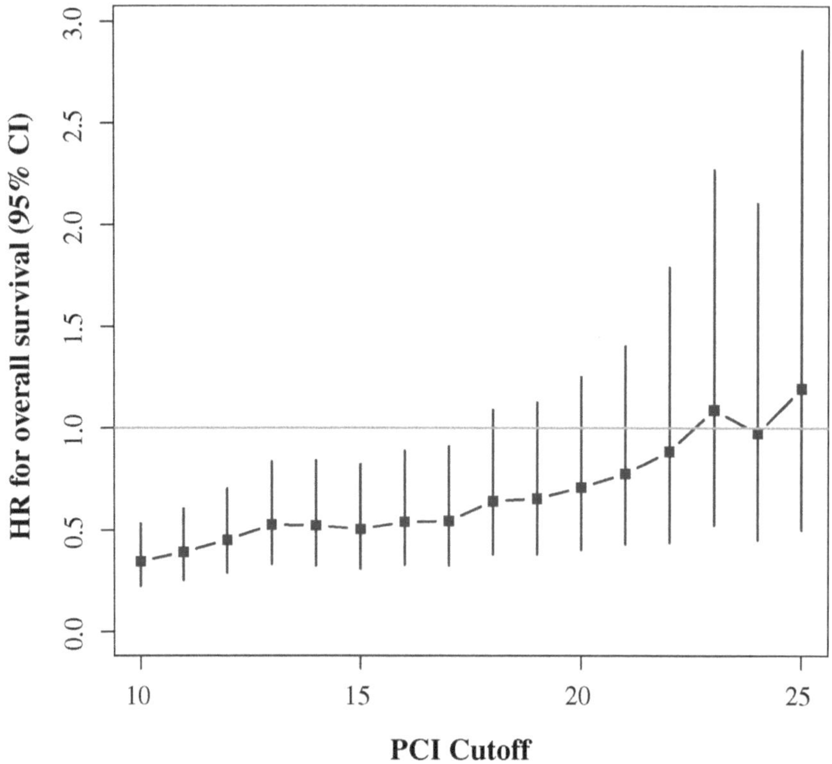

FIGURE 2.—Evolution of the hazard ratio (HR) for overall survival between the patients in the curative group and those in the palliative group according to each value of peritoneal carcinomatosis (PCI: 10 to 25). The overall survival rates did not differ significantly between the curative and palliative patients when the PCI was higher than 17 (HR 0.64; range 0.38–1.09). (Reprinted from Goéré D, Souadka A, Faron M, et al. Extent of colorectal peritoneal carcinomatosis: attempt to define a threshold above which HIPEC does not offer survival benefit: a comparative study. *Ann Surg Oncol.* 2015;22:2958-2964, with permission from Society of Surgical Oncology.)

intraperitoneal chemotherapy. This improved 5-year survival to 30% to 50%. However, it would help to identify factors to determine which patients are the most likely to benefit from this potentially morbid therapy. It has previously been reported that the completeness of cytoreduction and the extent of intraperitoneal carcinomatosis (PC) are major factors related to prognosis. The degree of peritoneal carcinomatosis is determined by the peritoneal carcinomatosis index, which divides the abdomen into 9 sectors and the small intestine into 4 regions (upper and lower jejunum, upper and lower ileum). The size of the lesions in each of these regions is determined on a scale of 0 to 3, with 0 being no microscopic disease, 1 $<$0.5 cm, 2 up to 5 cm of disease, and 3 $>$5 cm or confluent nodules. Therefore, the PC Index (PCI) score can range from 0 to 39. Previous studies have shown that PCI scores of higher than 16 to 20 have negative prognostic implications, although this number is not an absolute contraindication to cytoreductive surgery.

The objective of this study was to determine whether there was a threshold value at which cytoreductive surgery and hyperthermic intraperitoneal chemotherapy (HIPEC) did not provide any survival advantage versus postoperative systemic chemotherapy alone. This was a single-institutional study in which 180 patients with colorectal peritoneal carcinomatosis were evaluated over a 10-year period between 2000 and 2010, and eventually cytoreductive surgery and intraperitoneal chemotherapy were performed in 139; in 41 patients this could not be achieved, and they had palliative procedures only. These groups were then compared for factors that were different in patients who could have complete cytoreduction versus those could not. Significant differences between the 2 groups were that the mean PCI was 11 in the curative group versus 23 in the palliative group, the median length of stay was 23 days in the curative group versus 10 days in the palliative group, and the incidence of postoperative complications was 53% in the curative group versus 20% in the palliative group. Otherwise, there were no significant differences in nodal status, T stage, site of primary, and preoperative or postoperative chemotherapy administration. Sixty percent of patients had synchronous peritoneal carcinomatosis and 40% had metachronous, and these were not significantly different between the groups, nor was the presence of extraperitoneal metastasis (excluding ovarian metastasis). Most of these were located in the liver, and candidates were considered for resection when this disease was limited. Eight patients in the curative group died postoperatively, whereas 2 died postoperatively in the palliative group. Median follow-up was 60 months, and the 3-year overall survival was 52% in the curative group versus 7% in the palliative group. They then performed hazard ratios for different PCI cutoffs (Fig 2), and overall survival did not differ significantly between the curative and palliative groups when the PCI was found to be >17. Univariate analysis revealed that several factors were associated with overall survival, which included the PCI score, achievement of complete cytoreduction and receiving HIPEC, and age. On multivariate analysis, age fell out of this. The important findings of this study were that there may be a cutoff for patients who are candidates for cytoreduction in terms of the PCI. However, it is difficult to calculate the PCI preoperatively; CT scans underestimate this, and laparoscopy also underestimates the PCI. Therefore, this is not particularly helpful in preoperative decision making, but it is helpful in intraoperative decision making because of the high morbidity of these procedures. This study was limited in that it was a single-institution study with retrospective evaluation, but it still provides valuable selection criteria for patients who may undergo HIPEC.

J. R. Howe, MD

Peritoneal Surface Disease (PSD) from Appendiceal Cancer Treated with Cytoreductive Surgery (CRS) and Hyperthermic Intraperitoneal Chemotherapy (HIPEC): Overview of 481 Cases

Votanopoulos KI, Russell G, Randle RW, et al (Wake Forest Baptist Health, Winston-Salem, NC)

Ann Surg Oncol 22:1274-1279, 2015

Background.—Cytoreductive surgery (CRS) and hyperthermic intraperitoneal chemotherapy (HIPEC) used to treat peritoneal surface disease (PSD) from appendiceal cancer have shown variability in survival outcomes. The primary goal of this study was to determine predictors of surgical morbidity and overall survival. The secondary goal was to describe the impact of nodal status on survival after CRS/HIPEC for PSD from low-grade appendiceal (LGA) and high-grade appendiceal (HGA) primary lesions.

Methods.—A retrospective analysis of 1,069 procedures from a prospective database was performed. Patient characteristics, tumor grade, nodal status, performance status, resection status, morbidity, mortality, and survival were reviewed.

Results.—The study identified 481 CRS/HIPEC procedures: 317 (77.3 %) for LGA and 93 (22.7 %) for HGA lesions. The median followup period was 44.4 months, and the 30 day major morbidity and mortality rates were respectively 27.8 and 2.7 %. Major morbidity was jointly predicted by incomplete cytoreduction ($p = 0.0037$), involved nodes ($p < 0.0001$), and comorbidities ($p = 0.003$). Multivariate negative predictors of survival included positive nodal status ($p = 0.003$), incomplete cytoreduction ($p < 0.0001$), and preoperative chemotherapy ($p = 0.04$) in LGA patients and incomplete cytoreduction ($p = 0.0003$) and preoperative chemotherapy ($p = 0.0064$) in HGA patients. After complete cytoreduction, median survival was worse for patients with positive nodes than for those with negative nodes in LGA (85 months vs not reached [82 % alive at 90 months] $p = 0.002$) and HGA (30 vs 153 months $p < 0.0001$).

Conclusions.—Positive nodes are associated with decreased survival not only for HGA patients but also for LGA patients even after complete cytoreduction. Nodal status further stratifies histologic grade as a prognostic indicator of survival. Patients with nodenegative HGA primary lesions who receive a complete cytoreduction may experience survival comparable with that for LGA patients (Table 3).

▶ Appendiceal cancers are rare but, when they perforate, can lead to peritoneal carcinomatosis. Treatment of these patients have been problematic because this peritoneal disease does not often respond to systemic chemotherapy, and therefore surgeons have become increasingly aggressive by performing peritoneal debulking cytoreductive surgery (CRS) and hyperthermic intraperitoneal chemotherapy (HIPEC).

This was a very large, single-institution study from a center of excellence with HIPEC in which the authors retrospectively reviewed procedures they

TABLE 3.—Factors Predictive of Survival With Low-and High-Grade Appendiceal Primary Lesions (Uni-/Multivariate Analysis)

Variable	Lowgrade Appendiceal		Highgrade Appendiceal	
	Univariate p Value	Multivariate p Value	Univariate p Value	Multivariate p Value
Resection status	<0.001	<0.001 HR = 2.5 (R2a vs R0/1), 9 (R2b vs R0/1), 3.8 (R2c vs R0/1)	<0.001	<0.001 HR = 3.8 (R2a vs R0/1), 4.9 (R2b vs R0/1), 5.9 (R2c vs R0/1)
Lymph nodes	<0.001	0.003 HR = 3.6 P vs N	0.02	
Age	0.004		0.64	
Race	0.22		0.44	
Gender	0.19		0.79	
Albumin	0.002		0.99	
ECOG performance status	<0.001		0.82	
Repeat CRS-HIPEC	0.12		0.56	
No. of comorbidities	0.19		0.42	
Minor vs no morbidity	0.66		0.04	
Major vs no morbidity	0.18		<0.001	
No. of organs resected	<0.001		0.04	
Peritoneal carcinomatosis index	0.001		0.008	
Preoperative chemotherapy	0.003	0.05 HR = 2.2 Y vs N	0.02	0.006 HR = 2.5 Y vs N
Postoperative chemotherapy	0.88		<0.001	

HR hazard ratio, *ECOG* Eastern Cooperative Oncology Group, *CRS-HIPEC* cytoreductive surgery with hyperthermic intraperitoneal chemotherapy, *P* positive, *N* negative, *Y* yes, *N* no

Reprinted from Votanopoulos KI, Russell G, Randle RW, et al. Peritoneal surface disease (PSD) from appendiceal cancer treated with cytoreductive surgery (CRS) and hyperthermic intraperitoneal chemotherapy (HIPEC): overview of 481 cases. *Ann Surg Oncol.* 2015;22:1274-1279, Society of Surgical Oncology.

performed on patients with appendiceal cancer. The objectives were to determine factors that would predict for surgical morbidity, overall survival, and to also look at the impact of nodal status on overall survival. To do this, they retrospectively reviewed their database of patients over a 22-year period for those with primary tumors of the appendix, excluding patients with neuroendocrine features, unresectable primary lesions, and extra-abdominal disease. Patients were divided into low grade and high grade based on histology, with mucinous lesions being considered low grade, and signet ring cells as high grade. Patients were explored and CRS was performed followed by HIPEC, predominantly with mitomycin C, but some patients received oxaliplatin. Patients who had R0 or R1 resections were considered to have complete cytoreduction, and residual microscopic disease was subcategorized into R2A when there were lesions < 5 mm were left behind, R2B > 5 mm, and < 2 cm, and R2C > 2 cm. In their patients, 77% had low-grade lesions, 23% had high-grade lesions, and the median follow-up was 44.4 months. Concomitant colorectal resections were performed in 55% of patients; 44% had R0 or R1 disease, 28% had the R2A disease, 19% R2B disease, and 9% had R2C disease. The 30-day major morbidity rate was 28%, minor morbidity rate was 21%, and mean hospital stay was 9 days. Thirty-day mortality was 3%, and 90-day mortality was 6%. With respect to factors that predicted for morbidity, incomplete cytoreduction, medical comorbidities, and nodal involvement were all significantly associated on multivariate analysis. On multivariate analysis of survival, resection status (complete vs incomplete resection), lymph node involvement, and administration of preoperative chemotherapy were all significant (Table 3). Overall survival of patients with R0 or R1 cytoreduction was 175 months versus 73 months for patients with R2A resections. Another interesting finding was that node-negative high-grade patients did better than node-positive low-grade patients who had had complete cytoreduction. Furthermore, postchemotherapy did not seem to help low-grade patients, whereas it seemed to have some benefit in high-grade patients.

This is an important study because it represents a very large series of a rare tumor and gives us insight into prognostic factors for long-term survival. Clearly, complete cytoreduction, if it can be performed, leads to improved overall survival. Positive lymph nodes result in markedly reduced survival. Patients with high-grade primary lesions can still benefit from this procedure, and high-grade node-negative patients actually do better than patients who are node-positive with low-grade lesions. Finally, giving preoperative chemotherapy to these patients may not be beneficial. It may not reach significant levels penetrate in the peritoneal cavity and may reduce the functional status of patients. The limitations of this study were the potential for selection and referral bias, the fact that some patients had attempted cytoreduction elsewhere, and that patients not responding to chemotherapy were then referred for cytoreductive surgery. However, these retrospective data do help us to understand the expected survival and factors associated with morbidity in patients with these challenging tumors.

J. R. Howe, MD

Other

Comparison of Ivor-Lewis vs Sweet Esophagectomy for Esophageal Squamous Cell Carcinoma: A Randomized Clinical Trial

Li B, Xiang J, Zhang Y, et al (Fudan Univ Shanghai Cancer Ctr, China; et al)

JAMA Surg 150:292-298, 2015

Importance.—Sweet esophagectomy is performed widely in China, while the Ivor-Lewis procedure, with potential benefit of an extended lymphadenectomy, is limitedly conducted owing to concern for a higher risk for morbidity. Thus, the role of the Ivor-Lewis procedure for thoracic esophageal cancer needs further investigation.

Objective.—To determine whether Ivor-Lewis esophagectomy is associated with increased postoperative complications compared with the Sweet procedure.

Design, Setting, and Participants.—A randomized clinical trial was conducted from May 2010 to July 2012 at Fudan University Shanghai Cancer Center, Shanghai, China, of 300 patients with resectable squamous cell carcinoma in the middle and lower third of the thoracic esophagus. Intent-to-treat analysis was performed.

Interventions.—Patients were randomly assigned to receive either the Ivor-Lewis ($n = 150$) or Sweet ($n = 150$) esophagectomy.

Main Outcomes and Measures.—The primary outcome of this clinical trial was operative morbidity (any surgical or nonsurgical complications). Secondary outcomes included oncologic efficacy (number of lymph nodes resected and positive lymph nodes), postoperative mortality (30-day and in-hospital mortality), and patient discharge.

Results.—Resection without macroscopical residual (R0/R1) was achieved in 149 of 150 patients in each group. Although there was no significant difference between the 2 groups regarding the incidence of each single complication, a significantly higher morbidity rate was found in the Sweet group (62 of 150 [41.3%]) than in the Ivor-Lewis group (45 of 150 [30%]) ($P = .04$). More patients in the Sweet group (8 of 150 [5.3%]) received reoperations than in the Ivor-Lewis group (1 of 150 [0.7%]) ($P = .04$). The median hospital stay was 18 days in the Sweet group vs 16 days in the Ivor-Lewis group ($P = .002$). Postoperative mortality rates in the Ivor-Lewis (1 of 150) and Sweet (3 of 150) groups were 0.7% and 2.0%, respectively ($P = .25$). More lymph nodes were removed during Ivor-Lewis esophagectomy than during the Sweet procedure (22 vs 18, $P < .001$).

Conclusions and Relevance.—Early results of this study demonstrate that the Ivor-Lewis procedure can be performed with lower rates of postoperative complications and more lymph node retrieval. Ivor-Lewis and Sweet esophagectomies are both safe procedures with low operative mortalities.

Trial Registration.—clinicaltrials.gov Identifier: NCT01047111.

▶ There are multiple approaches for resection of esophageal cancer, including the transhiatal approach, which is popular in the United States; the Ivor-Lewis esophagectomy, performed with an upper midline and the right thoracotomy incision; and the Sweet esophagectomy through a left thoracic incision (with division of the diaphragm for mobilization of the stomach). Practice patterns are different in Asia, and this study compared 2 methods of esophagectomy using thoracic approaches at a single institution.

The authors randomized 300 patients with squamous cell carcinoma of the esophagus to arms, 1 receiving Ivor-Lewis and the other Sweet esophagectomy. Surgeons performing the procedures had each done at least 400 esophagectomies and were familiar with both approaches. The primary outcomes of this study to be evaluated were operative morbidity, oncologic efficacy, and postoperative mortality. Both groups were similar in terms of patient demographics and tumor stage. With respect to morbidity, this was higher in patients undergoing Sweet esophagectomy (41% of patients vs 30% in the Ivor-Lewis group), which was statistically significant. The most common complications were cardiac, pulmonary infection, chylothorax, and anastomotic leakage. There were significantly more reoperations in the Sweet group versus the Ivor-Lewis group (8 vs 1, respectively). Mortality was also higher in the Sweet group, with 3 deaths versus 1 in the Ivor-Lewis group, but this was not statistically significant (Table 3 in the original article). Operative time was significantly longer in the Ivor-Lewis group (by 28 minutes), but length of stay was reduced to 16 days in the Ivor-Lewis group versus 18 days for the Sweet. The total number of lymph nodes removed was significantly higher in the Ivor-Lewis group at 22, versus 18 in the Sweet group. Advantages of the Ivor-Lewis approach were that it allows for dissection of lymph nodes along both recurrent laryngeal nerves (which was not accessible in the Sweet procedure) and the hepatic artery and celiac axis (which is difficult through the transdiaphragmatic incision in the Sweet procedure). The authors conclude that, based on these results, that the Ivor-Lewis was superior to the Sweet procedure with respect to adequacy of lymphadenectomy, postoperative complications, and a lower reoperative rate. Longer term follow-up will be needed to determine whether there is a survival benefit, and this study did not look at quality-of-life issues.

J. R. Howe, MD

Progression and Management of Duodenal Neoplasia in Familial Adenomatous Polyposis: A Cohort Study

Serrano PE, Grant RC, Berk TC, et al (McMaster Univ, Hamilton, Ontario, Canada; Univ of Toronto, Ontario, Canada; Mount Sinai Hosp, Toronto, Ontario, Canada; et al)

Ann Surg 261:1138-1144, 2015

Objective.—To describe the natural history and outcomes of surveillance of duodenal neoplasia in familial adenomatous polyposis (FAP).

Background.—Duodenal cancer is the most common cause of death in FAP.

Methods.—Cohort study of patients prospectively enrolled in an upper endoscopic surveillance protocol from 1982 to 2012. The duodenum was assessed by side-viewing endoscopy and classified as stage 1 to 5 disease. Endoscopic and/or operative interventions were performed according to stage.

Results.—There were 218 patients in the protocol (98 with advanced stage). They had a median of 9 endoscopies (range: 2–25) over a median of 11 years (range: 1–26). Median age at diagnosis of stage 3 disease (adenoma: 2.1–10 mm) was 41 years and stage 4 disease (adenoma >10 mm) was 45 years. Median time from first esophagogastroduodenoscopy to stage 4 disease was 22.4 years. The risk of stage 4 disease was 34.3% [95% confidence interval (CI) 23.8–43.4] at 15 years. In multivariate analysis, sex, type of colorectal surgery, years since colorectal surgery, and stage were significantly associated with risk of progression to stage 4 disease. Five of 218 (2.3%) patients developed duodenal cancer at median age of 58 years (range: 51–65). The risk of developing duodenal cancer was 2.1% (95% CI: 0–5.2) at 15 years.

Conclusions.—Patients with advanced duodenal polyposis progress in the severity of disease (size and degree of dysplasia); however, the rate of progression to carcinoma is slow. Aggressive endoscopic and surgical intervention, especially in the presence of large polyps and high-grade dysplasia, appears to be effective in preventing cancer deaths in FAP (Table 1).

▶ Familial adenomatous polyposis (FAP) is an autosomal dominantly inherited condition in which patients develop hundreds of adenomatous polyps in the colon and inevitably develop colorectal cancer if colectomy is not performed. In patients undergoing colectomy, the most common cause of death has become duodenal polyps progressing to cancer or desmoid tumors. There have been few studies to evaluate the factors leading to duodenal polyps and cancers, and screening protocols to minimize this risk. This single institutional study looked at patients followed at 1 hospital over a 32-year period with FAP who followed an endoscopic protocol. Polyps were classified as stage 1 to 5, with 1 being a normal duodenum to 5 being adenocarcinoma, and stages

TABLE 1.—Staging and Management of Duodenal Polyposis in Familial Adenomatous Polyposis

Stage	Size, mm	Histologic Findings	Management
1	0	Normal	EGD every 5 yrs
2	1–2	Adenoma	EGD every 3 yrs
3*	2.1–10	Adenoma	EGD every 6 mo
4	>10	Adenoma	Endoscopic or surgical resection
5	Any	Adenocarcinoma	Radical surgery

EGD indicates esophagogastroduodenoscopy.

*The finding of high-grade dysplasia in this group changes the management to that of stage 4 disease. Radical surgery denotes pancreaticoduodenectomy when feasible.

2, 3, and 4 being classified by size (Table 1). Polypectomies were performed when possible, with argon beam coagulation or photodynamic therapy for smaller polyps or carpeting, and some patients underwent surgical management.

There were 218 patients in the study, all of whom had colorectal surgery at some point, with only a small fraction (16%) being screened by esophagogastroduodenoscopy (EGD) before colectomy. Three-quarters of patients had 5-year follow-up, and more than half had 10-year follow-up. Fifteen patients died in this cohort of 218 patients, 2 of duodenal cancer, 3 of pancreatic cancer, 2 desmoids, the others of various cancers, 1 of complications from endoscopic therapy. The 5 patients who refused follow-up were not included but ended up dying of duodenal cancer as well. Other metrics looked at this study were how many patients progressed to stage 4 polyps (> 10 mm in size), and the authors found that 66 of 167 patients who presented with stage 1, 2, or 3 polyps progressed to stage 4, with a median time from their first EGD to stage 4 being 22.4 years. Five patients developed adenocarcinoma out of 184 who initially had stage 1, 2, 3, or 4 polyps, with the overall risk being 2.1% at 15 years. This was a relatively low rate, and these duodenal cancers developed at a median of 15 years after the first endoscopy. Sixty percent of patients had endoscopic polypectomies beginning at a median age of 47.5 years, and 62% of procedures yielded polyps >10 mm in size. The complication rate of endoscopic management was 20%, including bleeding in 11%, and pancreatitis in 9% of cases, with 1 death due to severe pancreatitis and sepsis. Recurrence was common when polyps were removed piecemeal, as well as after snare polypectomy and ablation procedures. With respect to surgical management, 21 patients had surgical resection, which included 15 pancreaticoduodenectomies, 9 open polypectomies or ampullectomies, and 1 segmental resection. These procedures were performed for polyps that were >10 mm in size without high-grade dysplasia (28%), >10 mm with high-grade dysplasia (52%), or duodenal cancer (20%). In the 5 patients who developed duodenal cancer, 1 died of carcinomatosis, 1 was unresectable due to previous pancreatitis episodes, another of complications of desmoid tumor, and 2 were alive at last follow-up. Factors significant on multivariate analysis for progression to stage 4 polyps were time from colorectal surgery, and stage 1, 2, or 3 polyps at the first EGD, which increased the risk sequentially. There was no attempt at correlation of genotype with phenotype in this study. The major conclusion to be drawn from this is that with this surveillance program few patients progressed in duodenal carcinoma, and the length of time it took for this progression was quite long. Their recommendations for screening begin with EGD at 25 years of age, with follow-up EGD every 5 years for stage 1 polyps, every 3 years for stage 2 polyps, every 6 months for stage 3 polyps. Endoscopic or surgical resection is recommended in those with polyps >10 mm in size and surgical resection in those with adenocarcinoma (Table 1).

J. R. Howe, MD

Survival Benefit of Adjuvant Chemoradiotherapy in Patients With Ampulla of Vater Cancer: A Systematic Review and Meta-analysis

Kwon J, Kim BH, Kim K, et al (Seoul Natl Univ College of Medicine, Republic of Korea)

Ann Surg 262:47-52, 2015

Objective.—We conducted a systematic review and meta-analysis focusing on the impact of adjuvant radiotherapy (RT) on overall survival (OS) in ampulla of Vater (AoV) cancer.

Background.—The adjuvant treatment for AoV cancer is a subject of controversy without convincing evidence from randomized study.

Methods.—A comprehensive search was performed in the databases of EMBASE, PubMed,Web of Science, Cochrane Library, and Ovid from inception to July 2014. We included studies, which compared survival between patients with or without adjuvant RT after curative surgery solely for AoV cancer. Hazard ratio (HR) for OS was extracted, and a random-effects model was used for pooled analysis.

Results.—Ten retrospective studies including 3361 patients met all inclusion criteria and were included for the final meta-analysis. Adjuvant RT was delivered with concurrent chemotherapy, mostly 5-fluorouracil, in all institutional studies. Generally, adjuvant RT groups included more patients with locally advanced disease or lymph node metastasis than did the surgery alone groups. The pooled results demonstrated that adjuvant RT significantly reduced the risk of death (HR = 0.75; $P = 0.01$). Exploratory analyses showed that patients with lymph node metastasis (HR = 0.52; $P = 0.001$) and locally advanced disease (HR = 0.42; $P = 0.001$) may also have survival benefit from adjuvant RT. No clear evidence of publication bias was found.

Conclusions.—This is the first meta-analysis evaluating the role of adjuvant RT in AoV cancer. Our results suggest the potential for survival benefit of adjuvant chemoradiotherapy. Further studies, preferably randomized clinical trials, are needed to confirm our results (Fig 2).

▶ Carcinomas of the ampulla of Vater generally have a better prognosis than most pancreatic or bile duct cancers. The ESPAC-3 trial showed that adjuvant chemotherapy for periampullary cancers with either 5-FU or gemcitabine did not lead to improved survival; however, this included a variety of different tumor types. Tumors of the ampulla of Vater are fairly rare, accounting for only about 0.5% of gastrointestinal cancers, and therefore no randomized trial in this specific tumor type has been undertaken. This study set out to specifically examine whether radiation therapy was helpful in patients with resected ampullary cancers. Because there are no randomized trials, the authors of this article performed a meta-analysis of the available retrospective studies. They searched the English-language literature for papers on ampullary cancer where adjuvant therapy was given and selected articles in which there were both surgery alone and radiation therapy arms. Most patients receiving radiation

	Overall survival HR (95% CI)	Weight (%)
Willett[2]	0.79 (0.40-1.57)	7.4
Lee[3]	0.96 (0.22-4.18)	2.1
Sikora[4]	1.30 (0.87-1.93)	13.5
O'connell[5]	0.78 (0.63-0.97)	19.4
Krishnan[6]	1.02 (0.46-2.25)	6.0
Kim[7]	0.52 (0.26-1.07)	7.0
Showalter[9]	0.83 (0.34-2.04)	5.0
Narang[8]	0.41 (0.25-0.67)	11.1
Palta[10]	0.41 (0.22-0.76)	8.4
Miura[11]	0.88 (0.73-1.07)	20.1

Test for overall effect : 0.75 (0.60-0.94)
Heterogeneity : $I^2 = 55\%$ (P = 0.02)
Z = 2.46 (P = 0.01)

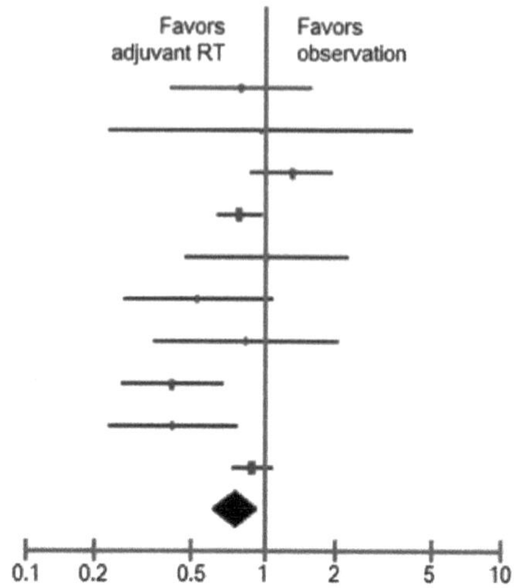

FIGURE 2.—Forest plot of HRs for OS from the included studies comparing adjuvant RT with observation. The pooled effects were calculated with a random-effects model. (Reprinted from Kwon J, Kim BH, Kim K, et al. Survival benefit of adjuvant chemoradiotherapy in patients with ampulla of vater cancer: a systematic review and meta-analysis. *Ann Surg*. 2015;262:47-52, with permission from Wolters Kluwer Health, Inc.)

also received sensitizing chemotherapy with either 5-fluorouracil or gemcitabine.

There were 10 studies that were included in the meta-analysis, 2 of which were population studies from the Surveillance, Epidemiology, and End Results (SEER) Program database and the other 8 were single institutional studies (6 from the United States, 1 from India, and 1 from Korea). There were a total of 3361 patients included in these 10 studies, which were all retrospective and thought to be relatively free of bias. The total number of patients in the surgery alone arm was 1418 and the adjuvant radiation therapy arm groups were 642. When these studies were pooled, it appeared that there was a survival benefit to radiation therapy, which reduced the risk of death with a hazard ratio of 0.75 (P = .01; Fig 2). When the 2 studies showing the highest effect from radiation therapy were removed, the hazard ratio still remained significantly decreased for patients receiving radiation at 0.86. It was clear from these studies that patients receiving radiation therapy generally had more locally advanced (T3-4) tumors and positive lymph nodes. On this basis, the expectation would be that these patients would do worse than patients having surgery alone due to the selection bias for more advanced tumors. When the 3 studies that detailed information on nodal metastases were compared, the improved survival for radiation therapy showed a hazard ratio of 0.52, and for T3-T4 tumors, the hazard ratio with radiation was 0.42. This study therefore showed that when pooling retrospective analyses radiation therapy seemed to improve the risk of death. Unfortunately, all these studies were retrospective, they all had their own potential for selection bias, and the majority of patients were contributed by a single, large SEER study (1287 of 2060 total patients). If anything, the selection bias seemed to favor patients with more advanced tumors getting radiation therapy, and therefore the effect of radiation therapy may be even greater than suggested in this meta-analysis. On the other hand, the addition of radiation therapy for pancreatic cancer has not convincingly shown a survival benefit, but tumors of the ampulla of Vater generally have a better prognosis, and perhaps these patients live longer so that a survival benefit is realized. It is unlikely that a randomized study will be done in patients with ampullary cancer because of their small numbers, and this meta-analysis is the best evidence that we have on the survival benefits of adjuvant radiation.

J. R. Howe, MD

Comparison of Perioperative Radiation Therapy and Surgery Versus Surgery Alone in 204 Patients With Primary Retroperitoneal Sarcoma: A Retrospective 2-Institution Study

Kelly KJ, Yoon SS, Kuk D, et al (Memorial Sloan Kettering Cancer Ctr, New York; et al)

Ann Surg 262:156-162, 2015

Objective.—To compare outcomes of patients with retroperitoneal or pelvic sarcoma treated with perioperative radiation therapy (RT) versus those treated without perioperative RT.

Background.—RT for retroperitoneal or pelvic sarcoma is controversial, and few studies have compared outcomes with and without RT.

Methods.—Prospectively maintained databases were reviewed to retrospectively compare patients with primary retroperitoneal or pelvic sarcoma treated during 2003–2011. Multivariate Cox regression models were used to assess associations with the primary endpoints: local recurrence-free survival (LRFS) and disease-specific survival.

Results.—At 1 institution, 172 patients were treated with surgery alone, whereas at another institution 32 patients were treated with surgery and perioperative proton beam RT or intensity-modulated RT with or without intraoperative RT. The groups were similar in age, tumor size, grade, and margin status (all $P > 0.08$). The RT group had a higher percentage of pelvic tumors ($P = 0.03$) and a different distribution of histologies ($P = 0.04$). Perioperative morbidity was higher in the RT group (44% vs 16% of patients; $P = 0.004$). After a median follow-up of 39 months, 5-year LRFS was 91% (95% confidence interval, 79%–100%) in the RT group and 65% (57%–74%) in the surgery-only group ($P = 0.02$). On multivariate analysis, RT was associated with better LRFS (hazard ratio, 0.26; $P = 0.03$). Five-year disease-specific survival was 93% (95% confidence interval, 82%–100%) in the RT group and 85% (78%–92%) in the surgery-only group ($P = 0.3$).

Conclusions.—The addition of advanced-modality RT to surgery for primary retroperitoneal or pelvic sarcoma was associated with improved LRFS, although this did not translate into significantly better disease-specific survival. This treatment strategy warrants further investigation in a randomized trial (Figs 1 and 3).

▶ Retroperitoneal sarcomas are challenging tumors to treat because by the time of diagnosis, they are often very large and generally make contact with important structures. Therefore, complete resection is difficult, and local recurrence is a major issue. Previous studies have shown that the addition of radiation therapy (RT) to surgical resection can improve local recurrence rates but not necessarily increase overall survival.

Previous studies RT in retroperitoneal sarcoma have been limited in size, so this one compared patients having surgery alone at 1 institution to those receiving surgery plus preoperative RT at another institution over the same time period. This included 172 surgical patients from Memorial Sloan-Kettering Cancer Center and 32 patients from the Massachusetts General Hospital who had surgical resection and RT. Of the latter group, 30 patients had preoperative

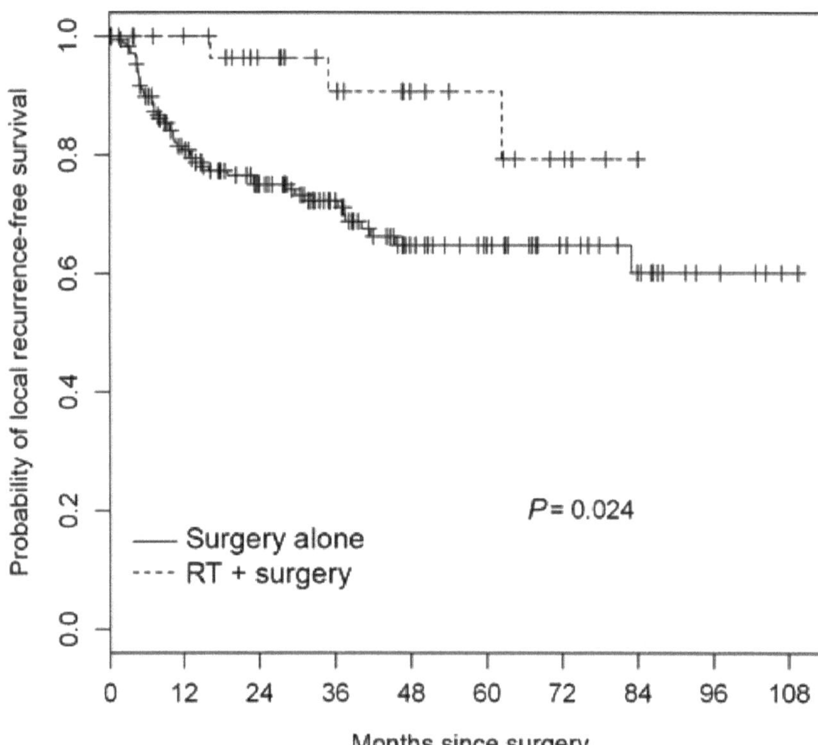

FIGURE 1.—Kaplan-Meier curve and log-rank analysis of local recurrence-free survival in patients with RPPS treated with perioperative RT versus those treated without perioperative RT at a median follow-up of 38.7 months. Perioperative RT was associated with a statistically significant increase in local recurrence-free survival. (Reprinted from Kelly KJ, Yoon SS, Kuk D, et al. Comparison of perioperative radiation therapy and surgery versus surgery alone in 204 patients with primary retroperitoneal sarcoma: a retrospective 2-institution study. *Ann Surg.* 2015;262:156-162, with permission from Wolters Kluwer Health, Inc.)

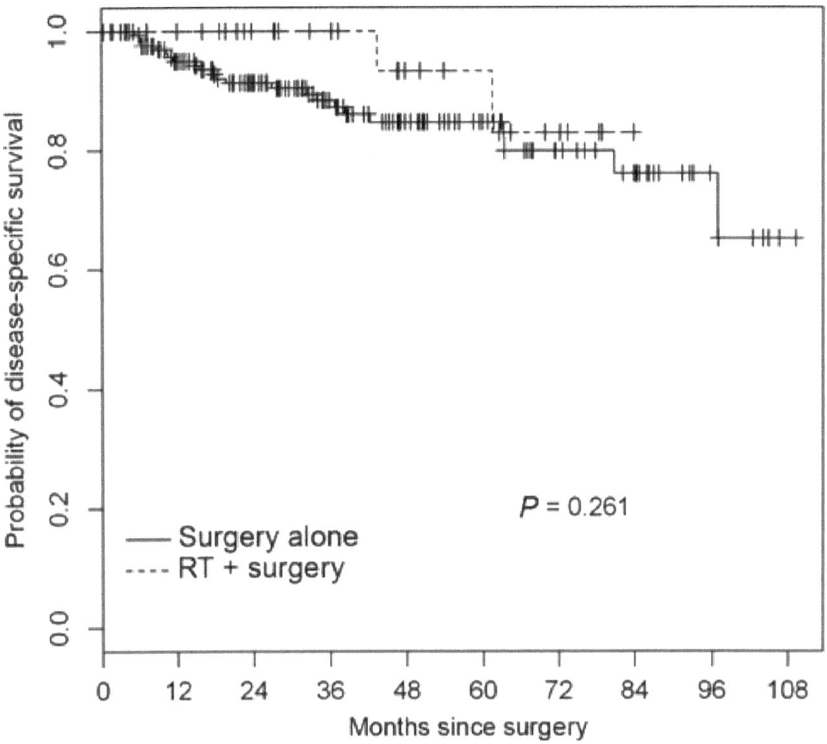

FIGURE 3.—Kaplan-Meier curve and log-rank analysis DSS in patients with RPPS treated with perioperative RT versus those treated without perioperative RT. There was not a statistically significant difference in DSS between the 2 treatment modalities. (Reprinted from Kelly KJ, Yoon SS, Kuk D, et al. Comparison of perioperative radiation therapy and surgery versus surgery alone in 204 patients with primary retroperitoneal sarcoma: a retrospective 2-institution study. *Ann Surg*. 2015;262:156-162, with permission from Wolters Kluwer Health, Inc.)

RT and 2 patients had postoperative RT; 19 had intensity-modulated RT (IMRT), 6 had proton beam, and 7 had both IMRT and proton beam. Intraoperative RT was also given in 15 patients. The median dose was 50 Gy for patients in the RT arm, including 10 Gy for those patients receiving intraoperative RT. Patients were only included in this study if they had an R0 or R1 resection; those with R2 resection or presenting with multifocal or recurrent disease were excluded. The significant findings from this study were that there was a statistically significant improved 5-year local recurrence-free survival in those receiving RT at a median follow-up of 38.7 months, which was 91% in the radiation therapy group versus 65% in the surgery only group (Fig 1). Multivariate analysis revealed that having RT, and well differentiated (vs dedifferentiated) liposarcoma were factors associated with improved local recurrence rates. Grade, size <18 cm, and R0 resection status were significant on univariate but not multivariate analysis. Within the 2 groups, there were a significantly higher percentage of patients with pelvic sarcomas in the RT/surgery group, with liposarcoma in the surgery alone group, and the operative times were higher and complication rates were greater in the RT/surgery group. There was no significant difference in 5-year disease-specific survival between the 2 groups, which was 93% in the RT/surgery group and 85% in the surgery group (Fig 3). On multivariate analysis, the only significant factor for improved disease-specific survival was decreased age. Complications seen in the study were mostly grade 1 or grade 2, and the overall rate of complications was 41% in the RT/surgery group versus 17% in the surgery only group. This study suggests that there is a significant advantage to delivering RT to patients with retroperitoneal sarcoma in those undergoing gross complete resection in terms of local recurrence, but no significant disease-specific survival advantage. This study suffered from being retrospective, with treatments being performed at 2 institutions, with patients who may have differed in surgical as well as pathologic factors. The answer to the important question of whether RT improves local recurrence rates and overall survival in resected retroperitoneal sarcoma awaits a randomized trial; however, this has been difficult to achieve in the past. The American College of Surgeons Oncology Group trial addressing this problem was never completed due to poor accrual, but there is a current trial ongoing in Europe (EORTC 62092-22092) that may answer this question in the future.

J. R. Howe, MD

Surgical Resection Provides an Overall Survival Benefit for Patients with Small Pancreatic Neuroendocrine Tumors

Sharpe SM, In H, Winchester DJ, et al (Univ of Chicago, IL; NorthShore Univ Health System, Evanston, IL)

J Gastrointest Surg 19:117-123, 2015

Background.—The optimal management of small (≤2 cm) pancreatic neuroendocrine tumors (PNETs) remains controversial. We evaluated these tumors in the National Cancer Data Base (NCDB) to determine if resection provides a survival advantage over observation.

Methods.—The NCDB was queried to identify patients with nonmetastatic PNETs ≤2 cm treated between 1998 and 2006. Kaplan-Meier survival estimates, stratified by grade and treatment type, evaluated the difference in 5-year overall survival (OS) between patients who underwent resection and observation. Multivariable Cox regression was used to determine the importance of resection in OS.

Results.—Three hundred eighty patients met inclusion criteria. Eighty-one percent underwent resection; 19% were observed. Five-year OS was 82.2% for patients who underwent surgery and 34.3% for those who were observed ($p < 0.0001$).When controlling for age, comorbidities, income, facility type, tumor size and location, grade, margin status, nodal status, surgical management, and nonsurgical therapy in the Cox model, observation [hazard ratio (HR) 2.80], poorly differentiated histology (HR 3.79), lymph node positivity (HR 2.01), and nonsurgical therapies (HR 2.23) were independently associated with an increase in risk of mortality ($p < 0.01$).

Conclusion.—Patients with localized PNETs ≤2 cm had an overall survival advantage with resection compared to observation, independent of age, comorbidities, tumor grade, and treatment with nonsurgical therapies (Fig 1).

▶ Pancreatic neuroendocrine tumors (PNETs) can have variable biological behavior, with some tumors being functional and making hormones while others are nonfunctional. Some are large, some are small, and some are poorly differentiated and display aggressive behavior. A dilemma for the clinician has been what to do with tumors < 2 cm in size. It is thought by many that these have a relatively indolent disease course and that the risk of operation on these tumors could potentially exceed the benefit. Relatively few studies have evaluated tumors < 2 cm in size, and these studies have had conflicting recommendations. This study is from the National Cancer Database (NCDB) where they selected patients for study who had < 2 cm, nonfunctional PNETS between 1998 and 2006. Patients with metastatic disease were not included. They found 380 patients meeting these criteria, of whom 309 (81.3%) had surgery and 71 (18.7%) were observed. Being a retrospective study, there was likely selection bias in the group of patients selected for observation over surgical resection. Comparison of the 2 groups revealed that the age was generally

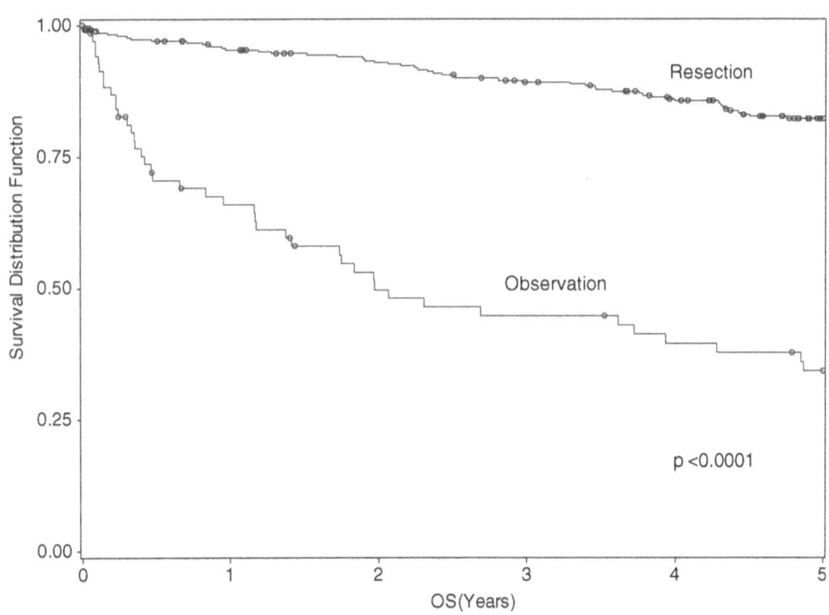

FIGURE 1.—Kaplan-Meier survival estimates comparing patients with PNETs ≤2 cm who underwent surgical resection or observation. (Reprinted from Sharpe SM, In H, Winchester DJ, et al, Surgical Resection provides an overall survival benefit for patients with small pancreatic neuroendocrine tumors. *J Gastrointest Surg.* 2015;19:117-123, with permission from The Society for Surgery of the Alimentary Tract.)

older in patients being observed, and there were more poorly differentiated tumors (14% vs 6.5%). There was a higher percentage of private insurance and of patients having operation in academic centers in patients undergoing resection. The number of tumors between 0 and 1 cm versus 1 and 2 cm was similar in each group. There was a significant difference in 5-year overall survival in the surgery (82%) relative to the observation group (34%; Fig 1). On multivariate analysis, significant factors for improved survival included surgical resection, negative lymph nodes, well or moderately differentiated tumors, and location in the body or tail. The hazard ratio for patients undergoing observation was 2.8 and for those with poorly differentiated tumors was 3.79. Interestingly, in patients with poorly differentiated tumors, the median survival was 2.4 years for those having surgery versus 0.4 years for those being observed. The authors suggest that the significant improvement of survival with surgery over observation suggests the significant benefit with surgery, and these results were not affected by the Charlson score, a measure of comorbidity. Previous studies have shown that 5% to 8% of tumors < 2 cm develop distant metastases, and the current study showed that the risk of nodal metastases was 29%, further reinforcing the recommendation. The results of this study should be interpreted with caution, however, because of its origin in a national database and their inherent limitations. This study looked at overall survival and not disease-specific survival, and the use of adjuvant treatments such as octreotide or other agents is not recorded. Furthermore, to be included in the database, patients need to have a tissue diagnosis of a PNET. This would have excluded the large number of patients found to have a small, enhancing mass consistent with PNET who were simply observed rather than having a biopsy performed; these numbers nationally could be quite high, and these patients could do very well, yet never be included in the observation group in the NCDB. This is an excellent question for a prospective, randomized trial; I hope this will be done someday to arrive at a definitive answer as to whether we should resect PNETs < 2 cm.

J. R. Howe, MD

11 Vascular Surgery

Aneurysm

Editor's Choice – Endovascular Aneurysm Repair Versus Open Repair for Patients with a Ruptured Abdominal Aortic Aneurysm: A Systematic Review and Meta-analysis of Short-term Survival

van Beek SC, Conijn AP, Koelemay MJ, et al (Academic Med Centre, Amsterdam, The Netherlands)

Eur J Vasc Endovasc Surg 47:593-602, 2014

Background.—There is clinical equipoise between open (OR) and endovascular aneurysm repair (EVAR) for the best treatment of ruptured abdominal aortic aneurysm (RAAA).

Objective.—The aim of the study was to perform a systematic review and meta-analysis to estimate the short-term (combined 30-day or in-hospital) survival after EVAR and OR for patients with RAAA. Data sources included Medline, Embase, and the World Health Organization International Clinical Trials Registry until 13 January 2014. All randomised controlled trials (RCTs), observational cohort studies, and administrative registries comparing OR and EVAR of at least 50 patients were included. Articles were full-length and in English.

Methods.—Standard PRISMA guidelines were followed. The methodological quality of RCTs was assessed with the Cochrane Collaboration's tool for assessing risk of bias. The quality of observational studies was assessed with a modified Cochrane Collaboration's tool for assessing risk of bias, the Newcastle-Ottawa Scale, and the Methodological Index for Non-Randomized Studies. The results of the RCTs, of the obersvational studies, and of the administrative registries were pooled separately and analysed with the use of a random effects model.

Results.—From a total of 3,769 articles, three RCTs, 21 observational studies, and eight administrative registries met the inclusion criteria. In the RCTs, the risk of bias was lowest and the pooled odds ratio for death after EVAR versus OR was 0.90 (95% CI 0.65-1.24). The majority of the observational studies had a high risk of bias and the pooled odds ratio for death was 0.44 (95% CI 0.37-0.53). The majority of the administrative registries had a high risk of bias and the pooled odds ratio for death was 0.54 (95% CI 0.47-0.62).

Conclusion.—Endovascular aneurysm repair is not inferior to open repair in patients with a ruptured abdominal aortic aneurysm. This supports the use of EVAR in suitable patients and OR as a reasonable alternative.

► The authors have performed an elegant randomized trial comparing endovascular (EVAR) and open surgical (OSR) aneurysm repair for patients with ruptured aortoiliac artery aneurysms. The study period spanned 5 years (2008-2013) and a total of 107 patients (EVAR, 51; OSR, 56) were enrolled. Notably, 524 patients underwent repair of ruptured aortoiliac aneurysms at the study institutions during the study period, inclusive of those enrolled in the study, with an estimated EVAR suitability rate of 33%. The study inclusion criteria required that the patients were hemodynamically stable (systolic blood pressure >80 mm Hg without vasopressor support), anatomically suitable for EVAR and the surgeon had to be facile with endovascular repair (defined as a minimum of 15 prior EVARS in symptomatic/asymptomatic patients). The authors reported that there were no differences between the 2 approaches in terms of 30-day mortality (18% vs 25%), 1-year mortality (30% vs 35%), and the perioperative major complication (45% vs 55%), although all favored the EVAR approach. There was a significant difference in the perioperative pulmonary complication rate, blood transfusion requirement, and intensive care length of stay (but not total length of stay) that favored EVAR, whereas the EVAR approach was also less costly. The study findings largely support the earlier Dutch AJAX[1] and IMPROVE[2] randomized trials that also failed to demonstrate a benefit from EVAR for the treatment of ruptured aneurysms, albeit somewhat counterintuitive for "endo-enthusiasts." It is important to note that the current trial was somewhat underpowered based on the authors' prestudy calculations that estimated 80 patients per treatment group based on a 20% mortality benefit for EVAR and a 40% mortality rate for OSR, and thus, it is conceivable that a difference actually exists (ie, type II error). This may be resolved by a meta-analysis of the results of the 3 randomized trials. The favorable mortality for the OSR likely reflects that fact that the patients were really the "best-case scenario" for either therapy considering the fact that they were hemodynamically stable and had anatomy suitable for an EVAR. Notably, the mean proximal neck and diameter in the EVAR group were 29.0 ± 22.8 and 23.8 ± 4.5 mm, respectively. The authors were somewhat circumspect in the interpretation of their data and concluded that "endovascular management of ruptured aneurysms (endoclamping as well as EVAR) must now be considered as major progress." I would contend that the data support and endovascular first approach for suitable, hemodynamically stable patients with ruptured aneurysms as has been adopted by most advanced centers. Furthermore, the data provide justification for the OSR if the endovascular approach is not available and reassurance that the mortality rates are comparable.

T. S. Huber, MD, PhD

References

1. Reimerink JJ, Hoornwg L, Vahl AC, et al. Amsterdam Aneurysm Trial Collaborators. Endovascular repair versus open repair of ruptured abdominal aortic aneurysms: a multicenter randomized controlled trial. *Ann Surg*. 2013;258:248-256.
2. IMPROVE Trial Investigators, Powell JT, Sweeting MJ, Thompson MM, et al. Endovascular or open repair strategy for ruptured abdominal aortic aneurysm; 30 day outcomes from IMPROVE randomized trial. *BMJ*. 2014;348:f7661.

Comparison of a Vascular Study Group of New England risk prediction model with established risk prediction models of in-hospital mortality after elective abdominal aortic aneurysm repair

Eslami MH, for the Vascular Study Group of New England (Boston Univ School of Medicine, MA; Boston School of Public Health, MA)

J Vasc Surg 62:1125-1133, 2015

Background.—A certain number of deaths may result from elective abdominal aortic aneurysm (AAA) repair due to inherent risks of operation; however, no agreement exists about which predictive model for in-hospital mortality is most accurate in predicting these events. This study developed a risk prediction model using Vascular Study Group of New England (VSGNE) data and compared it with established models.

Methods.—VSGNE data (2003-2013) were queried for patients undergoing elective AAA repair by open or endovascular techniques. Clinical variables and known predictors of mortality were included in a full prediction model. Backward elimination with $\alpha = .2$ was used to construct a parsimonious model. This VSGNE model was compared with established models—Medicare, Glasgow Aneurysm Score (GAS), and Vascular Governance North West (VGNW)—based on the scope of VSGNE data collection. Model fit was compared with the Vuong test. Model discrimination was compared in equally sized risk-group VSGNE terciles.

Results.—The overall mortality rate for 4431 elective AAA patients was 1.4%. The discriminating ability of the VSGNE model was high (C statistic = 0.822) and corrected slightly to 0.779 after internal validation. Vuong tests yielded significant overall fit difference favoring the VSGNE model over the Medicare (C statistic = 0.769), VGNW (C statistic = 0.767), and GAS (C statistic = 0.685) models. The VGNW and Medicare models performed better than GAS in predicting mortality among risk-group terciles.

Conclusions.—The VSGNE risk prediction model is best at forecasting mortality among this patient population. The Medicare and VGNW models showed good discrimination (Tables 3A and 3B).

▶ The authors have used data from the Vascular Study Group of New England (VSGNE), a regional group of the Vascular Quality Initiative (VQI), to develop a predictive model for mortality after abdominal aortic aneurysm repair (Tables 3A and 3B), both open and endovascular. Furthermore, they have compared their

TABLE 3A.—Point Scoring Proposed in this Model Based on the β-Estimates to Predict Risk of Mortality

Parameter	Points
Treatment	
EVAR	0
OAR (infrarenal)	2
OAR (suprarenal)	4
Aneurysm size, mm	
<65	0
≤65	2
Age, years	
≤75	0
>75	1
Gender	
Male	0
Female	1
Comorbidities	
Myocardial disease	1
Cerebrovascular disease	1
Chronic obstructive pulmonary disease	2
Laboratory value	
Creatinine, mg/dL	
<1.5	0
1.5 to <2	2
≥2	2

EVAR, Endovascular aneurysm repair; OAR, open aneurysm repair.
(Reprinted from Eslami MH; for the Vascular Study Group of New England. Comparison of a Vascular Study Group of New England risk prediction model with established risk prediction models of in-hospital mortality after elective abdominal aortic aneurysm repair. *J Vasc Surg.* 2015;62:1125-1133, with permission from Society for Vascular Surgery.)

TABLE 3B.—Proposed Risk Categories Based on the Model

Points	Probability of Mortality, %	Proposed Risk Designation
0	0.12	Low-risk group
1	0.20	
2	0.34	
3	0.59	
4	1.00	
5	1.71	Medium-risk group
6	2.91	
7	4.90	
8	8.14	High-risk group
9	13.2%	
10	20.75	
11	31.05	Prohibitive high-risk group
12	43.63	
13	57.10	
14	69.59	

(Reprinted from Eslami MH; for the Vascular Study Group of New England. Comparison of a Vascular Study Group of New England risk prediction model with established risk prediction models of in-hospital mortality after elective abdominal aortic aneurysm repair. *J Vasc Surg.* 2015;62:1125-1133, with permission from Society for Vascular Surgery.)

predictive model with several other available ones (Medicare, Glasgow Aneurysm Score, Vascular Governance North West) and found that their model was superior. This publication is timely given the increased emphasis on patient outcomes and overall quality that we have all experienced at our parent institutions and the dissemination of our outcomes to the public in terms of various scorecards and dashboards. I would readily concede that mortality may not be a good maker of overall quality, but my objections are irrelevant because it is a well-established metric. The individual components of the scoring system involve a combination of demographic, clinical, and anatomic variables that are readily available and part of the routine preoperative evaluation. Unfortunately, the definitions of the comorbidities were not detailed in the article but are fairly generic. They are available in the "help text" in the VSGNE and VQI data entry forms for the institutions that participate. It is interesting to see the impact of the various components of the predictive model, particularly the impact of a suprarenal clamp (odds ratio (OR) 6.72) and a creatinine >2.0 (OR 2.48). In our practice, we still do a lot of open aortic surgery for aneurysms, but it seems invariable that they involve a suprarenal clamp because the patients do not have suitable infrarenal neck for an endograft (or to place an infrarenal clamp). Some type of predictive model should likely be incorporated into all of our preoperative evaluation and planning processes. This is particularly important for elective aneurysm repairs because it is essentially a prophylactic operation with the operative decision based on the risk of repair, the rupture risk, patient preference, and life expectancy. The predicted mortality can help decide the most appropriate diameter threshold for repair (eg, 5.5 vs 6.0 cm) and further help articulate the anticipated risk to the patient. Furthermore, it may help identify potential strategies to reduce the inherent risk in terms of pushing the envelope or limits for endovascular repair for patients with a high predicted risk for open repair. These data should be interpreted with some caution because they await further external validation from another source, although the overall sample size is large (n = 4431) and likely robust. The model outperformed the others analyzed in the publication, but these were selected for comparison because they included similar components. There are likely other valid predictive models that could be used that include different input variables than those analyzed in the study.

T. S. Huber, MD, PhD

Endovascular strategy or open repair for ruptured abdominal aortic aneurysm: one-year outcomes from the IMPROVE randomized trial

IMPROVE Trial Investigators ()

Eur Heart J 36:2061-2069, 2015

Aims.—To report the longer term outcomes following either a strategy of endovascular repair first or open repair of ruptured abdominal aortic aneurysm, which are necessary for both patient and clinical decision-making.

Methods and Results.—This pragmatic multicentre (29 UK and 1 Canada) trial randomized 613 patients with a clinical diagnosis of ruptured aneurysm; 316 to an endovascular first strategy (if aortic morphology is suitable, open repair if not) and 297 to open repair. The principal 1-year outcome was mortality; secondary outcomes were re-interventions, hospital discharge, health-related quality-of-life (QoL) (EQ-5D), costs, Quality-Adjusted-Life-Years (QALYs), and cost-effectiveness [incremental net benefit (INB)]. At 1 year, all-cause mortality was 41.1% for the endovascular strategy group and 45.1% for the open repair group, odds ratio 0.85 [95% confidence interval (CI) 0.62, 1.17], $P = 0.325$, with similar re-intervention rates in each group. The endovascular strategy group and open repair groups had average total hospital stays of 17 and 26 days, respectively, $P < 0.001$. Patients surviving rupture had higher average EQ-5D utility scores in the endovascular strategy vs. open repair groups, mean differences 0.087 (95% CI 0.017, 0.158), 0.068 (95% CI −0.004, 0.140) at 3 and 12 months, respectively. There were indications that QALYs were higher and costs lower for the endovascular first strategy, combining to give an INB of £3877 (95% CI £253, £7408) or 4356 (95% CI 284, 8323).

Conclusion.—An endovascular first strategy for management of ruptured aneurysms does not offer a survival benefit over 1 year but offers patients faster discharge with better QoL and is cost-effective.

Clinical Trial Registration.—ISRCTN 48334791.

▶ The authors report the longer-term results of the IMPROVE Trial comparing a pragmatic strategy of endovascular versus open repair for patients with ruptured abdominal aortic aneurysms. Notably, the pragmatic study design was established to compare an endovascular-first strategy with an open-first strategy. Patients were randomly assigned at the time of the in-hospital clinical diagnosis but before a CT scan was obtained. Accordingly, a significant proportion of the patients in the endovascular-first strategy underwent open repair (35%-40%) because they were not anatomically endovascular candidates (criteria: neck diameter <32 mm, neck length >10 mm, neck angulation <60°) and there were patients randomly assigned in both groups that did not actually have ruptured aneurysms on CT. The initial report from the trial failed to demonstrate a 30-day mortality benefit for the endovascular strategy (endovascular aneurysm repair [EVAR], 35.7% vs open, 39.3%) although it was uncertain whether the equivocal findings persisted longer term. Consistent with the initial findings, the authors failed to find a mortality difference at 1 year (EVAR, 41.1% vs open, 45.1%). These findings were consistent throughout the various subgroups analyzed with the exception of women and those patients with a Hardman Index of greater than 2, which favored the endovascular approach. The authors did report that the endovascular-first approach was associated with a shorter length of hospital stay and discharge home (vs facility) during the index admission, better scores on the quality-of-life assessment tool (EQ-5D QoL), and a lower mean cost. These findings are reminiscent of those from the seminal open-versus-endovascular trials (EVAR-1, DREAM, OVER) for intact aneurysms that failed to demonstrate a long-term mortality benefit but favored the endovascular repairs for the softer outcome measures. I am not certain that these findings will truly impact clinical practice. I think that it is the general impression that an endovascular approach is favorable for both intact and ruptured aneurysms while being the preferred choice by both patients and providers. It is reassuring that the mortality rates, both at 30 days and 1 year, are comparable for the institutions that do not have programs that can provide endovascular repair around the clock and for the diminishing group of surgeons that do not feel comfortable with the approach.

T. S. Huber, MD, PhD

Rupture rates of untreated large abdominal aortic aneurysms in patients unfit for elective repair

Parkinson F, Ferguson S, Lewis P, et al (Royal Gwent Hosp, Newport, United Kingdom)

J Vasc Surg 61:1606-1612, 2015

Background.—Elective abdominal aortic aneurysm (AAA) surgery relies on balancing the risk of the intervention against the risk of the aneurysm causing death. Although much is known about intervention at 5.5 cm, little is known about the fate of the patient unfit for elective surgery at this threshold. Medical therapy and endovascular surgery have revolutionized management of aortic aneurysms in the last 20 years and are thought to have affected rupture rates.

Methods.—MEDLINE via PubMed, EMBASE, and the Cochrane Library Database were searched for studies reporting follow-up of untreated large AAA approach from inception to January 2014. Data were pooled using random-effects analysis with standardized mean differences and 95% confidence intervals (CIs) reported. The primary end points were rupture rates and all-cause mortality per year by AAA size.

Results.—The search strategy identified 1892 citations, of which 11 studies comprising 1514 patients experiencing 347 ruptured AAA were included. The overall incidence of ruptured AAA in patients with AAA >5.5 cm was 5.3% (95% CI, 3.1%-7.5%) per year. This represented cumulative yearly rupture rates of 3.5% (95% CI, −1.6% to 8.7%) in AAAs 5.5 to 6.0 cm, 4.1% (95% CI, −0.7% to 9.0%) in AAAs 6.1 to 7.0 cm, and 6.3% (95% CI, −1.8% to 14.3%) in AAAs >7.0 cm. There was no heterogeneity between studies ($I^2 = 0\%$). Only 32% of these patients were offered repair on rupturing an AAA, with a perioperative mortality of 58% (95% CI, 32%-83%). The risk of death from causes other than AAA was higher than the risk of death from rupture.

Conclusions.—Rupture rates of untreated AAA were lower than those currently quoted in the literature. Non-AAA-related mortality in this group of patients is high.

▶ The authors have performed a meta-analysis to define the rupture risk of large abdominal aortic aneurysms (AAA) in patients deemed "unfit" for elective repair. They performed an extensive review of the literature but were only able to identify 11 studies that fulfilled their study criteria, encompassing a total of 1514 patients. Notably, these studies included 6 prospective cohort studies, 3 retrospective studies, and 1 randomized trial. The studies were deemed high quality based on their Newcastle-Ottawa score, and the GRADE analysis showed a moderate strength of evidence. The authors reported that the diameter-specific annual rupture risks (5.5-6.0 cm, 3.5%; 6.1-7.0 cm, 4.1%; >7.0 cm, 6.3%) were lower than those traditionally reported with death from rupture accounting for less than half of the annual mortality rate (5.5-6.0 cm, 9.9%; 6.1-7.0 cm, 8.9%, >7.0 cm, 12.0%). These data are intriguing and suggest that the traditionally quoted rupture risks used to help determine the specific diameter threshold for elective repair may be too high. These data must be interpreted with some cause given the underlying quality of the studies, the lack of autopsies to confirm the actual cause of death (ie, ruptured aneurysm), and the inherent selection bias in terms of whether the findings in patients deemed "unfit" for repair are applicable to those deemed "fit" for repair. It is likely that the net effect of these limitations is such that the authors have underestimated the annual diameter-specific rupture risk. The concept of "unfit" for repair is somewhat surgeon-specific and is more of an overall qualitative impression rather than an objective or quantitative assessment. The definition of "unfit" has also likely evolved over the past few decades with the expansion of the endovascular therapies and the general overall improvement of medical and surgical care. Indeed, it is interesting that a significant percentage of "unfit" patients in the meta-analysis actually ultimately underwent elective repair. The authors also reported that 32% of the patients underwent emergent repair of their aneurysms (presumably for symptomatic, intact aneurysms or ruptures) and that the overall mortality rate was 58%, a number larger than traditionally quoted for the repair of ruptured aneurysms. This finding provides some guidance for providers when caring for that difficult cohort of patients who were deemed prohibitive risk for elective repair and present with a rupture. Overall, the data have several practical implications, and they can be used to reassure patients deemed "unfit" for repair that their annual rupture risk is likely lower than traditionally quoted although their annual mortality rate remains significant. They also suggest that these same patients can undergo repair in the event that they rupture with some expectation of survival. The data can also potentially be used to refine the diameter-specific threshold for repair for "fit" patients because they suggest that the rupture risks may not be as high as we have traditionally reported.

T. S. Huber, MD, PhD

Predictors and outcomes of endoleaks in the Veterans Affairs Open Versus Endovascular Repair (OVER) Trial of Abdominal Aortic Aneurysms

Lal BK, for the OVER Veterans Affairs Cooperative Study Group (Univ of Maryland School of Medicine, Baltimore; et al)

J Vasc Surg 62:1394-1404, 2015

Objective.—The Veterans Affairs Open Versus Endovascular Repair (OVER) Trial of Abdominal Aortic Aneurysms study was a randomized controlled trial comparing open vs endovascular repair (EVAR) in standard-risk patients with infrarenal aortic aneurysms. The analysis reported here identifies characteristics, risk factors, and long-term outcome of endoleaks in patients treated with EVAR in the OVER cohort.

Methods.—The OVER trial enrolled 881 patients, of whom 439 received successful EVAR. Logistic regression analysis was used to identify predictors for endoleaks and secondary interventions. Kaplan-Meier survival analysis, longitudinal plots, and generalized linear mixed models methods were used to describe time to endoleak detection, resolution, or death.

Results.—During a mean follow-up of 6.2 ± 2.4 years, 135 patients (30.5%) developed 187 endoleaks. Four patients with EVAR went on to rupture; these four patients did not all have an endoleak. Mortality between patients who did and did not develop endoleaks was not significantly different. The 187 endoleaks included 12% type I, 76% type II, 3% type III, 3% type IV, and 6% indeterminate. Patient demographics and vascular risk factors were not associated with endoleak development. The presence of endoleaks resulted in an increase in aneurysm diameter over time ($P < .0001$). Fifty-three percent of endoleaks resolved spontaneously, and 31.9% received secondary interventions. The initial aneurysm size independently predicted a need for secondary interventions ($P < .0003$). Delayed type II endoleaks (detected >1 year after EVAR) were associated with aneurysm enlargement compared with the early counterpart. There was no difference in aneurysm size or length of survival between type II and other types of endoleak.

Conclusions.—We present one of the most comprehensive and longest follow-up analyses of patients treated with aortic endografts. Endoleaks were common and negatively affected aneurysm diameter reduction. Delayed type II endoleaks were associated with late aneurysm diameter enlargement. Endoleaks and aneurysm diameter enlargement were not associated with excess mortality compared with those without these features.

▶ The authors have used the long-term data from the Open Versus Endovascular Repair (OVER) Trial to examine the durability of endovascular repair (EVAR) and the rate of endoleaks. Note that the seminal publication reported an early mortality advantage for endovascular repair, but it was lost after 2 years, similar to the EVAR 1 and DREAM trials. The current study focuses on the 439 patients that had a successful EVAR with their mean follow-up of 6.2 ± 2.4 years.

Importantly, the patients randomized in the trial fulfilled the instructions for use for the various devices deployed, although a variety were used in the trial. The follow-up included scheduled visits at 1, 6, and 12 months after repair and then yearly thereafter with CT scans and plain radiographs obtained at each visit. The authors found that 30.5% of the patients developed some type of endoleak with the majority being classified as type II (I, 12%; II, 76%; III, 3%; IV, 3%; indeterminate, 6%). The largest percentage of the endoleaks was detected within the first month although a sizable proportion was not detected until after 2 years (<1 month, 45%; 1 month to 2 years, 33%; >2 years 22%). Multivariate analysis failed to identify and patient- or aneurysm-specific characteristics that predicted the development of an endoleak and all types of endoleaks occurred in the 3 most commonly deployed devices. More than half of the endoleaks resolved spontaneously with 31.9% requiring some type of intervention. The presence of an endoleak attenuated the general decrease in aneurysm diameter, whereas patients with a type II endoleak identified after 1 year had a significant increase in aneurysm diameter compared with those detected early. Importantly, there was no difference in long-term mortality between the patients with an endoleak and those without one. There were 4 patients (0.9%) who ruptured their aneurysms after EVAR, although, interestingly, none had evidence of an endoleak. These data support the long-term safety of the EVAR approach in appropriately selected patients, but the significant incidence of endoleaks and ruptures underscore the importance of long-term surveillance and remediation. Unfortunately, the trial did not include guidelines for the management of the various endoleaks, and, thus, it is impossible to comment on the appropriate management of the various types, particularly the type II leaks that seem the most controversial.

Furthermore, it is important to temper the study findings that the presence of an endoleak is not associated with a decrease in mortality with the statement provided that they are managed similar to the OVER investigators.

T. S. Huber, MD, PhD

Debate: Whether evidence supports reducing the threshold diameter to 5 cm for elective interventions in women with abdominal aortic aneurysms

Vavra AK, Kibbe MR, Bown MJ, et al (Northwestern Univ, Chicago, IL; Univ of Leicester, UK; et al)

J Vasc Surg 60:1695-1702, 2014

Current practice guidelines recommend repair of asymptomatic abdominal aortic aneurysms once they reach the 5.5-cm-diameter threshold and are based on information from randomized controlled trials. However, because aneurysms are more common in men, women are underrepresented in these trials, and questions persist about whether this repair threshold should apply to them. In addition, women have smaller aortas to begin with and in most aneurysm cohorts are older, have more atherosclerotic risk factors, are less likely to be anatomic candidates for endovascular repair, and do poorer after emergency or elective repair of their aneurysm.

These are just some of the issues that our discussants address in determining whether the repair threshold should be at a smaller diameter for women.

▶ The authors present a thoughtful debate about the most appropriate diameter threshold for abdominal aortic aneurysm (AAA) repair (5.0 cm vs 5.5 cm) for intact aneurysms in women. The authors emphasize that the decision represents a balance between the rupture risk and the risk of repair. However, I would add that this complex decision should also include life expectancy and, perhaps most important, patient preference. The authors on both sides of the debate generally concede that women have constitutionally smaller aortic diameters, a higher risk of rupture risk per specific aneurysm diameter, a higher mortality for operative repair (both endovascular and open), are less likely to be endovascular candidates, and are older with a higher burden of comorbidities at the time of repair. The debate largely centers on the interpretation of the data regarding the gender-specific rupture risk per specific aneurysm diameter. The authors that advocated repair at the 5.0-cm threshold concede that the randomized trials comparing repair with expectant management (ie, UK Small Aneurysm Trial, ADAM, PIVOTAL, CEASAR) were underpowered to detect a difference in outcome based on gender. However, they contended that a follow-up report from the UK Small Aneurysm Trial along with other studies demonstrate that female gender is an independent risk factor for rupture with smaller aortic diameter a contributing factor. They go on to state that "a lack of data from large randomized controlled trials does not mean there are not convincing data to support a lower diameter threshold in female patients." The authors on the contrary side summarized the same data stating that "very little robust evidence is available regarding the diameter-specific rupture rates of small AAAs in women" emphasizing that the "lack of power, underline the need for actual evidence in this area." The authors on the contrary side go on to summarize the best available evidence (unpublished data analysis) and suggest that there is a survival benefit for surveillance in women with aneurysms between 5.0 and 5.5 cm. The question remains as to the ideal threshold for operative repair (or who wins the debate). In my own practice, I have offered repair (either open or endovascular depending on anatomy) to "good risk" women with 5.0-cm aneurysms. In addition to the arguments highlighted here, this approach is also justified by observations from small aneurysm trials indicating that aneurysms continue to grow and that the overwhelming majority of patients ultimately require repair. I would echo the American and European guidelines that state repair should be "considered" in women with AAAs between 5.0 and 5.4 cm.

T. S. Huber, MD, PhD

Open repair of asymptomatic popliteal artery aneurysm is associated with better outcomes than endovascular repair

Eslami MH, Rybin D, Doros G, et al (Boston Univ School of Medicine, MA; Boston School of Public Health, MA)

J Vasc Surg 61:663-669, 2015

Objective.—Open (OPAR) and endovascular (EPAR) repair are both used to treat popliteal artery aneurysm (PAA). We assessed outcomes of both modalities in the treatment of asymptomatic PAAs.

Methods.—Vascular Quality Initiative (VQI) databases (2010 to 2013) were queried for patients undergoing asymptomatic PAA repair using OPAR and EPAR. The groups were compared with respect to demographics, medical history, and procedural characteristics. Outcomes of interest were length of stay (LOS), major adverse limb events (MALE), MALE or perioperative death (MALE-POD), and loss of primary patency compared using Kaplan-Meier estimates. Proportional hazard Cox regression was used to compare the outcomes across the treatment groups. Multivariable regression with backward elimination procedure ($\alpha = .5$) was used to construct parsimonious models to predict MALE and MALE-POD. Gamma regression was used to compare LOS.

Results.—From 2010 to 2013, 390 patients with asymptomatic PAAs were identified (221 OPAR, 169 EPAR) and included in this study. Preoperative comorbidities were similar between the two groups, except for a higher rate of congestive heart failure (19.5% vs 11.8%, $P = .042$) and chronic obstructive pulmonary disease (19.5% vs 11.8%, $P = .042$) in the EPAR group. No in-hospital mortality was observed. LOS was significantly longer in the OPAR group (3.8 ± 2.5 vs 1.4 ± 1.9 days; $P < .001$). OPAR patients had a significantly higher MALE-free survival (95% vs 80%; $P < .001$) as was MALE-POD-free survival (93% vs 80%; $P < .001$) rates at 1 year after the procedure. OPAR was associated with lower hazard of MALE (hazard ratio [HR], 0.35; 95% confidence interval [CI], 0.15-0.86; $P < .05$), MALE-POD (HR, 0.28; 95% CI, 0.13-0.63; $P < .05$), and primary patency loss (HR, 0.25; 95% CI, 0.10-0.58; $P < .05$).

Conclusions.—This retrospective analysis suggests that OPAR is associated with better outcomes than EPAR. Ultimately, the ongoing, adequately powered Open versus Endovascular Popliteal Artery Aneurysm Repair (OVERPAR) trial will definitively compare these procedures.

▶ The authors report the largest experience with management of asymptomatic popliteal artery aneurysms and compare outcomes after open (OPAR, $n = 221$) and endovascular (EPAR, $n = 169$) repair. Data were obtained from the Vascular Quality Initiative, a national quality improvement effort sponsored by the Society for Vascular Surgery that encompasses more than 290 centers across the United States and Canada. The analysis was restricted to asymptomatic aneurysms in an attempt to reduce any bias due to the quality of the arterial outflow, thus allowing the most rigorous comparison of the 2 interventions. Notably, the mean ankle brachial indices in the 2 groups were almost 1 (OPAR: 1.10; EPAR: 0.99), suggesting that the infrageniculate outflow was not flow limiting. The authors reported that the choice of procedure affected the outcomes at 1 year and that the open approach was consistently associated with better outcome in terms of major adverse limb events (amputation + reintervention), major adverse limb events plus mortality, and patency. Admittedly, the patients in the EPAR group were older and had a higher incidence of both congestive heart failure and chronic obstructive pulmonary disease, although it was only the choice of procedure that was a significant predictor of outcome in the adjusted analysis. Not surprisingly, the length of stay was longer in the open group; there were no perioperative deaths in either group. These data seem to support the open approach and make a nice contribution to the literature. Indeed, the overall published experience with the open and endovascular approach for popliteal aneurysms is confusing with reports justifying each approach. The single randomized, controlled trial reported that the outcomes were comparable for patients with for normal infrageniculate runoff, although the sample size was small ($n = 30$).[1] Despite the support for the open approach, the report must be interpreted with some caution. There is an inherent selection bias in terms of the choice and appropriateness of the index procedure inherent in the retrospective study design. The longer term outcomes were limited primarily to the perioperative events and do not capture any complications after the index hospitalization. The terminal outcome measure was at 1 year, and thus, it is impossible to predict outcomes beyond that time point. A number of details that potentially affect outcome for both the open and endovascular approach, such as quality of conduit, type of popliteal stent, and quality of the runoff vessels, were not captured. Lastly, it is impossible to draw any conclusions about the utility of the approaches in patients with symptomatic aneurysms. The authors have launched a prospective study (OVERPAR—Open vs Endovascular Popliteal Artery Aneurysm Repair) through the Vascular Quality Initiative that should overcome many of these limitations and provide further guidance on the choice of procedures.

T. S. Huber, MD, PhD

Reference

1. Antonello M, Frigatti P, Battocchio P, et al. Open repair versus endovascular treatment for asymptomatic popliteal artery aneurysm: results of a prospective randomized study. *J Vasc Surg*. 2005;42:185-193.

Abdominal compartment syndrome associated with endovascular and open repair of ruptured abdominal aortic aneurysms

Rubenstein C, Bietz G, Davenport DL, et al (Hadassah Hebrew Univ, Jerusalem, Israel; Peripheral Vascular Associates, San Antonio, TX; Univ of Kentucky College of Medicine, Lexington)

J Vasc Surg 61:648-654, 2015

Background.—Abdominal compartment syndrome (ACS) is a known complication of ruptured abdominal aortic aneurysm (rAAA) repair and can occur with either endovascular (EVAR) or open repair. We hypothesize that the underlying mechanism for the development of ACS may differ for patients treated with EVAR or open operation.

Methods.—All patients who presented with rAAA at a tertiary care medical center between January 2005 and December 2010 were included in the study. Demographic factors, type of repair (open vs EVAR), development of ACS, intraoperative and postoperative fluid requirements, estimated blood loss, length of stay, and morbidity and mortality were recorded. Student *t*-test and Fisher exact test were performed. A *P* value <.05 was considered significant.

Results.—Seventy-three patients, 62 men and 11 women with an average age of 70.5 years, were treated for rAAA. Forty-four (60%) underwent open repair; 29 (40%) had EVAR. Overall mortality was 42% (31 of 73), with mortality being 31% (9 of 29) in EVAR and 48% (21 of 44) in open repair. ACS developed in 21 patients (29%), more frequently in open repair than in EVAR (15 of 44 [34%] vs 6 of 29 [21%]; *P* = NS). Mortality was higher in patients who developed ACS compared with those without ACS (13 of 21 [62%] vs 17 of 52 [33%]; *P* =.022). This finding was especially pronounced in the EVAR group, in which mortality in patients with ACS was 83% (5 of 6) compared with 17% (4 of 23) without ACS (*P* =.005). Intraoperative fluid requirements were significantly higher in EVAR patients who developed ACS compared with those without ACS, including packed red blood cells (5600 mL vs 1100 mL; *P* < .0001), total blood products (9300 mL vs 1500 mL; *P* < .001), crystalloid (11,200 mL vs 4500 mL; *P* < .001), and estimated blood loss (5000 mL vs 660 mL; *P* =.006). In patients treated with open repair, there were no significant differences in intraoperative fluid requirements between those who developed ACS and those without ACS. However, patients who developed ACS after open repair required significantly more crystalloid on the first and second postoperative days (first postoperative day, 8300 mL vs 5600 mL [*P* =.01]; second postoperative day, 6500 mL vs 3800 mL [*P* =.004]).

Conclusions.—This study demonstrates that the development of ACS after repair of rAAA is associated with increased mortality, especially in EVAR-treated patients. The higher intraoperative blood and blood product requirements associated with ACS in EVAR patients suggest that one potential cause of early ACS is continued hemorrhage from lumbar and inferior mesenteric vessels through the ruptured aneurysm sac. Hence, open ligation of such vessels should be considered in patients developing early ACS after EVAR for rAAA.

▶ The authors describe their experience with abdominal compartment syndrome (ACS) after ruptured abdominal aortic aneurysm repair, both the open and endovascular (EVAR) approach. They reported an incidence of 29% (open: 24%; EVAR: 21%), which is significantly higher than generally reported in the literature. Importantly, the mortality rate was remarkably higher in patients that developed ACS (62% vs 33%; *P* = .022) and was particularly noteworthy among the patients that developed ACS after EVAR (83%). These findings do not establish causality because it is unclear whether the increased mortality rate is really due to the ACS or whether patients that did poorly (and had a higher mortality rate) were more likely to develop ACS. These findings emphasize the point that ACS can develop after EVAR and should serve to raise the level of suspicion in the postoperative period, particularly among those patients who required aortic balloon control and those with massive blood and fluid requirements as detailed in the study. Unfortunately, the diagnostic criteria in the current study were somewhat vague (ie, increased airway pressure, oliguria, tense abdomen), and no definitive treatment recommendations were provided. We have found that bladder pressures can be helpful in equivocal cases given the nonspecific diagnostic criteria detailed. Furthermore, we have taken an aggressive approach using decompressive laparotomy and placement of a vacuum dressing in patients with suspected ACS in all settings (not just after repair of ruptured aneurysms). We often leave the abdomen open at the time of the index procedure after open ruptured aneurysm repair and have a low threshold for performing the decompressive laparotomy at the time of the index EVAR repair if there is any suspicion about the diagnosis of ACS. The authors hypothesized that the development of the ACS after EVAR was potentially related to the development of a type II endoleak from the inferior mesenteric or lumbar arteries. Although no definitive evidence was provided to support this hypothesis, it seems reasonable to explore the aneurysm sac and exclude any ongoing bleeding at the time of decompressive laparotomy.

T. S. Huber, MD, PhD

Early and delayed rupture after endovascular abdominal aortic aneurysm repair in a 10-year multicenter registry

Candell L, Tucker L-Y, Goodney P, et al (Univ of California, San Francisco, Oakland; Kaiser Permanente, Oakland; Dartmouth-Hitchcock Med Ctr, Lebanon; et al)

J Vasc Surg 60:1146-1153, 2014

Objective.—Rupture after abdominal endovascular aortic aneurysm repair (EVAR) is a function of graft maintenance of the seal and fixation. We describe our 10-year experience with rupture after EVAR.

Methods.—From 2000 to 2010, 1736 patients with abdominal aortic aneurysm (AAA) from 17 medical centers underwent EVAR in a large, regional integrated health care system. Preoperative demographic and clinical data of interest were collected and stored in our registry. We retrospectively identified patients with postoperative rupture, characterized as "early" and "delayed" rupture (≤30 days and >30 days after the initial EVAR, respectively), and identified predictors associated with delayed rupture.

Results.—The overall follow-up rate was 92%, and the median follow-up was 2.7 years (interquartile range, 1.2-4.4 years) in these 1736 EVAR patients. We identified 20 patients with ruptures; 70% were male, the mean age was 79 years, and mean AAA size at the initial EVAR was 6.3 cm. Six patients underwent initial EVAR for rupture (n = 2) or symptomatic presentation (n = 4). Of the 20 post-EVAR ruptures, 25% (five of 20) were early, all occurring within 2 days after the initial EVAR. Of these five patients, four had intraoperative adverse events leading directly to rupture, with one type I and one type III endoleak. Of the five early ruptures, four patients underwent endovascular repair and one received repair with open surgery, resulting in two perioperative deaths. Among the remaining 15 patients, the median time from initial EVAR to rupture was 31.1 months (interquartile range, 13.8-57.3 months). Most of these delayed ruptures (10 of 15) were preceded by AAA sac increases, including three patients with known endoleaks who underwent reintervention. At the time of delayed rupture, nine of 15 patients had new endoleaks. Among all 20 patients, six patients did not undergo repair (all delayed patients) and died, nine underwent repeated EVAR, and five had open repair. For patients who underwent repair for delayed rupture, mortality at 30 days and 1 year were 44.4% and 66.7%, respectively. Multivariable Cox regression analysis identified age 80 to 89 (hazard ratio, 3.3; 95% confidence interval, 1.1-9.4; $P = .03$), and symptomatic or ruptured initial indication for EVAR (hazard ratio, 7.4; 95% confidence interval, 2.2-24.8; $P < .01$) as significant predictors of delayed rupture.

Conclusions.—Rupture after EVAR is a rare but devastating event, and mortality after repair exceeds 60% at 1 year. Most delayed cases showed late AAA expansion, thereby implicating late loss of seal and increased endoleaks as the cause of rupture in these patients and mandating vigilant surveillance.

▶ The authors examined the incidence of ruptured aneurysms after endovascular aortic aneurysm repair (EVAR) using a prospective multi-institutional registry (Kaiser Permanente Northern California). Notably, the registry spanned 2000 to 2010, encompassed 17 medical centers and 1736 index EVAR procedures, and had an impressive follow-up rate of 92%. The authors reported only 20 ruptures (1.2%) among which 5 occurred within 30 days of the index procedure. However, the overall follow-up was somewhat limited (median 2.7 years), and it is likely that additional ruptures will occur with longer follow-up. The perioperative mortality (42.9%) and morbidity rates among those who underwent attempted repair were significant and not different between the early and delayed ruptures. Notably, these mortality rates are comparable to those commonly reported for de novo ruptured aneurysms, not supporting the concept that a prior EVAR is somehow protective in the event of a subsequent rupture. Analysis of the early ruptures suggested that there were technical difficulties at the time of the original procedure (eg, type 1 endoleak) and/or potential anatomic limitations, although the latter were not recorded in the registry. Analysis of the delayed ruptures found that 12 of 15 patients had evidence of an endoleak at the time of the rupture, but there was no evidence of endoleak before the rupture in 9 of 12 patients. There were 2 type II endoleaks among these, but the type II endoleaks were found to occur in combination with either a type I or III endoleak; there were no isolated type II endoleaks. Among the 3 delayed ruptures without a detectable endoleak, there was evidence of aneurysm growth in 2 cases. Multivariable analysis of the delayed ruptures identified advanced age and urgent/emergent indications for the index procedure, potentially suggesting a role for increased surveillance in these patients. Although not particularly earth shattering, the findings underscore several important principles and are noteworthy given the large "community" experience and excellent follow-up. Notably, aneurysms can rupture after EVAR, although the incidence is quite small. The associated mortality and morbidity rates are significant, and the majority is associated with type I or III endoleaks. Isolated type II endoleaks are likely relatively benign, particularly in the absence of continued aneurysm growth. Continued aneurysm growth despite the presence of an identifiable endoleak can lead to rupture. Ruptures after EVAR are not device-specific and can likely occur with all devices. The likelihood of rupture is increased after EVARs performed for urgent/emergent indications and outside the instructions for use. Lastly, long-term surveillance is mandatory. Admittedly, these results must be interpreted with some caution given the retrospective analysis of the ruptures, the lack of standardized surveillance and intervention protocol, and the lack of specific anatomic details.

T. S. Huber, MD, PhD

Long-Term Outcomes of Abdominal Aortic Aneurysm in the Medicare Population

Schermerhorn ML, Buck DB, O'Malley AJ, et al (Beth Israel Deaconess Med Ctr, Boston, MA; Geisel School of Medicine at Dartmouth, Lebanon, NH; et al)

N Engl J Med 373:328-338, 2015

Background.—Randomized trials and observational studies have shown that perioperative morbidity and mortality are lower with endovascular repair of abdominal aortic aneurysm than with open repair, but the survival benefit is not sustained. In addition, concerns have been raised about the long-term risk of aneurysm rupture or the need for reintervention after endovascular repair.

Methods.—We assessed perioperative and long-term survival, reinterventions, and complications after endovascular repair as compared with open repair of abdominal aortic aneurysm in propensity-score–matched cohorts of Medicare beneficiaries who underwent repair during the period from 2001 through 2008 and were followed through 2009.

Results.—We identified 39,966 matched pairs of patients who had undergone either open repair or endovascular repair. The overall perioperative mortality was 1.6% with endovascular repair versus 5.2% with open repair ($P < 0.001$). From 2001 through 2008, perioperative mortality decreased by 0.8 percentage points among patients who underwent endovascular repair ($P = 0.001$) and by 0.6 percentage points among patients who underwent open repair ($P = 0.01$). The rate of conversion from endovascular to open repair decreased from 2.2% in 2001 to 0.3% in 2008 ($P < 0.001$). The rate of survival was significantly higher after endovascular repair than after open repair through the first 3 years of follow-up, after which time the rates of survival were similar. Through 8 years of follow-up, interventions related to the management of the aneurysm or its complications were more common after endovascular repair, whereas interventions for complications related to laparotomy were more common after open repair. Aneurysm rupture occurred in 5.4% of patients after endovascular repair versus 1.4% of patients after open repair through 8 years of follow-up ($P < 0.001$). The rate of total reinterventions at 2 years after endovascular repair decreased over time (from 10.4% among patients who underwent procedures in 2001 to 9.1% among patients who underwent procedures in 2007).

Conclusions.—Endovascular repair, as compared with open repair, of abdominal aortic aneurysm was associated with a substantial early survival advantage that gradually decreased over time. The rate of late rupture was significantly higher after endovascular repair than after open repair. The outcomes of endovascular repair have been improving over time. (Funded by the National Institutes of Health.)

▶ The authors have used the Medicare database to compare the longer term outcomes after open and endovascular (EVAR) aneurysm repair for intact aneurysms among beneficiaries >67 years of age. Notably, the 67-year age cutoff was to facilitate a 2-year period of observation before the index repair that served as a baseline for demographic and clinical variables, including abdominal operations. The authors reported that the perioperative mortality rates were significantly lower after EVAR (1.6% vs 5.2%) but that survival was comparable after 3 years (Fig 1A in the original article). The early survival benefit resulted in an increase in the total amount of time that the EVAR patients were expected to survive with mean values of 12.7 and 7 days at 4 and 7 years, respectively, values that were statistically significant but not clinically relevant. The perioperative complication rates and length of stay (3.5 ± 5.3 vs 9.8 ± 8.9) were also significantly lower after EVAR, but the early readmission rates (10.7% vs 11.0%) were comparable. The rate of reinterventions was significantly greater among the EVAR group (18.8% vs 3.7%), although those related to laparotomy were greater in the open group (17.7% vs 8.2%). Most of these remedial abdominal operations were for abdominal wall hernia repair, although there readmissions for bowel obstructions over the 8-year follow-up period were also significantly greater in the open group (22.2% vs 17.3%) Somewhat surprisingly, the aneurysm rupture rate after EVAR was 5.4%. These findings are largely consistent with the randomized trials comparing open and EVAR but are particularly impressive given the large sample size and rigorous analysis using propensity-score-matched controls (n = 39 966 pairs). It was reassuring that the outcomes for both open and EVAR have improved, although it is likely that the improvements in our collective surgical technique and the devices themselves have been partially offset by expanded indications outside the indications for use for the various devices. These data could be used to justify either the EVAR or open approach. The perioperative advantages favor the EVAR approach, whereas the comparable long-term outcomes and aneurysm rupture rate in the EVAR group favor the open approach. Regardless of the data, most patients and providers have adopted an EVAR-first approach with the open approach largely relegated to patients who are not endovascular candidates. Importantly, the data can be used to reassure patients who are not candidates for EVAR that their long-term outcomes are comparable.

T. S. Huber, MD, PhD

Carotid

Effect of Patching on Reducing Restenosis in the Carotid Revascularization Endarterectomy Versus Stenting Trial

Malas M, Glebova NO, Hughes SE, et al (Johns Hopkins Univ, Baltimore, MD; Univ of Colorado Denver, Aurora; Rutgers Univ, Newark, NJ; et al)

Stroke 46:757-761, 2015

Background and Purpose.—The purpose is to determine whether patching during carotid endarterectomy (CEA) affects the perioperative and long-term risks of restenosis, stroke, death, and myocardial infarction as compared with primary closure.

Methods.—We identified all patients who were randomized and underwent CEA in Carotid Revascularization Endarterectomy versus Stenting Trial. CEA patients who received a patch were compared with patients who underwent CEA with primary closure without a patch. We compared periprocedural and 4-year event rates, 2-year restenosis rates, and rates of reoperation between the 2 groups. We further analyzed results by surgeon specialty.

Results.—There were 1151 patients who underwent CEA (753 [65%] with patch and 329 [29%] with primary closure). We excluded 44 patients who underwent eversion CEA and 25 patients missing CEA data (5%). Patch use differed by surgeon specialty: 89% of vascular surgeons, 6% of neurosurgeons, and 76% of thoracic surgeons patched. Comparing patients who received a patch versus those who did not, there was a significant reduction in the 2-year risk of restenosis, and this persisted after adjustment by surgeon specialty (hazard ratio, 0.35; 95% confidence interval, 0.16–0.74; $P = 0.006$). There were no significant differences in the rates of periprocedural stroke and death (hazard ratio, 1.58; 95% confidence interval, 0.33–7.58; $P = 0.57$), in immediate reoperation (hazard ratio, 0.6; 95% confidence interval, 0.16–2.27; $P = 0.45$), or in the 4-year risk of ipsilateral stroke (hazard ratio, 1.23; 95% confidence interval, 0.42–3.63; $P = 0.71$).

Conclusions.—Patch closure in CEA is associated with reduction in restenosis although it is not associated with improved clinical outcomes. Thus, more widespread use of patching should be considered to improve long-term durability.

Clinical Trial Registration.—URL: http://www.clinicaltrials.gov. Unique identifier: NCT00004732.

▶ The authors used data from the seminal Carotid Revascularization Endarterectomy versus Stenting Trial (CREST) to determine whether carotid endarterectomy (CEA) with patching (patch, 753; no patch, 329) was associated with lower perioperative and longer-term risk. Although the study was not specifically designed to examine the benefit of patching, the parent study design was rigorous and incorporated duplex ultrasound scans at prespecified intervals (baseline and 1, 6, 12, 24, and 48 months). The authors reported that patching resulted in a significant reduction in the risk of restenosis at 2 years, although there were no significant reductions in the perioperative adverse events or ipsilateral stroke at 4 years. Notably, restenosis was defined as a greater than 70% diameter-reducing stenosis with a peak systolic velocity of greater than 3.0 m/sec. Based on these findings, the authors concluded that "more widespread use of patching should be considered to improve long-term disability." Although I don't disagree with the authors' conclusion, as it supports my bias, the data could easily be used to support primary closure after CEA given the comparable outcomes in terms of perioperative events and ipsilateral stroke, remembering that CEA is a therapy designed to reduce the risk of ipsilateral stroke (not necessarily the risk of recurrent stenosis). The rates of restenosis at 2 years (patch, 3%; primary, 11%) are within the range of those traditionally reported. Unfortunately, the incidence of neurologic symptoms related to these restenotic lesions was not reported, although 2.9% of the patients in the overall cohort analyzed underwent reintervention. These early (< 2 years) restenotic lesions typically result from intimal hyperplasia and are rarely symptomatic in contrast to the index atherosclerotic lesions. Furthermore, it is unclear whether they are associated with a higher incidence of neurologic symptoms longer term. It was interesting that the rate of patching varied by the surgeon type with most vascular and thoracic surgeons using a patch repair (vascular, 89%; thoracic, 76%; neurosurgery, 6%). This likely reflects differences in training paradigms and bias within the specialties. Despite the quality of the CREST, the current report fails to answer the ongoing question about the necessity of patch closure after CEA. It has always been my opinion that CEA is the benchmark operation for cardiovascular surgeons and that each provider should adopt a consistent approach in terms of the conduct of the operation (eg, shunt vs no shunt, regional vs general anesthesia) and not waiver from that approach, provided that his or her outcomes are acceptable. In our practice, we use general anesthesia and bovine patch closure and routinely shunt. Fortunately, our results have been good and well below the national standards for symptomatic and asymptomatic lesions.

T. S. Huber, MD, PhD

Mechanism of Procedural Stroke Following Carotid Endarterectomy or Carotid Artery Stenting Within the International Carotid Stenting Study (ICSS) Randomised Trial

Huibers A, Calvet D, Kennedy F, et al (Univ College London, United Kingdom; et al)
Eur J Vasc Endovasc Surg 50:281-288, 2015

Objective.—To decrease the procedural risk of carotid revascularisation it is crucial to understand the mechanisms of procedural stroke. This study analysed the features of procedural strokes associated with carotid artery stenting (CAS) and carotid endarterectomy (CEA) within the International Carotid Stenting Study (ICSS) to identify the underlying pathophysiological mechanism.

Materials and methods.—Patients with recently symptomatic carotid stenosis (1,713) were randomly allocated to CAS or CEA. Procedural strokes were classified by type (ischaemic or haemorrhagic), time of onset (intraprocedural or after the procedure), side (ipsilateral or contralateral), severity (disabling or non-disabling), and patency of the treated artery. Only patients in whom the allocated treatment was initiated were included. The most likely pathophysiological mechanism was determined using the following classification system: (1) carotid-embolic, (2) haemodynamic, (3) thrombosis or occlusion of the revascularised carotid artery, (4) hyperperfusion, (5) cardio-embolic, (6) multiple, and (7) undetermined.

Results.—Procedural stroke occurred within 30 days of revascularisation in 85 patients (CAS 58 out of 791 and CEA 27 out of 819). Strokes were predominately ischaemic (77; 56 CAS and 21 CEA), after the procedure (57; 37 CAS and 20 CEA), ipsilateral to the treated artery (77; 52 CAS and 25 CEA), and non-disabling (47; 36 CAS and 11 CEA). Mechanisms of stroke were carotid-embolic (14; 10 CAS and 4 CEA), haemodynamic (20; 15 CAS and 5 CEA), thrombosis or occlusion of the carotid artery (15; 11 CAS and 4 CEA), hyperperfusion (9; 3 CAS and 6 CEA), cardioembolic (5; 2 CAS and 3 CEA) and multiple causes (3; 3 CAS). In 19 patients (14 CAS and 5 CEA) the cause of stroke remained undetermined.

Conclusion.—Although the mechanism of procedural stroke in both CAS and CEA is diverse, haemodynamic disturbance is an important mechanism. Careful attention to blood pressure control could lower the incidence of procedural stroke (Fig 2).

▶ The authors have retrospectively analyzed the data from the International Carotid Stenting (ICSS) Trial to determine the mechanism and timing of periprocedural stroke after carotid endarterectomy (CEA) and stenting (CAS) with the hope that the elucidation of the underlying mechanisms would suggest preventative strategies. Note that the ICSS was a randomized, controlled trial comparing the 2 modalities for patients with symptomatic carotid stenoses >50% and that the overall stroke risk 7.3% for CAS and 3.3% for CEA. The

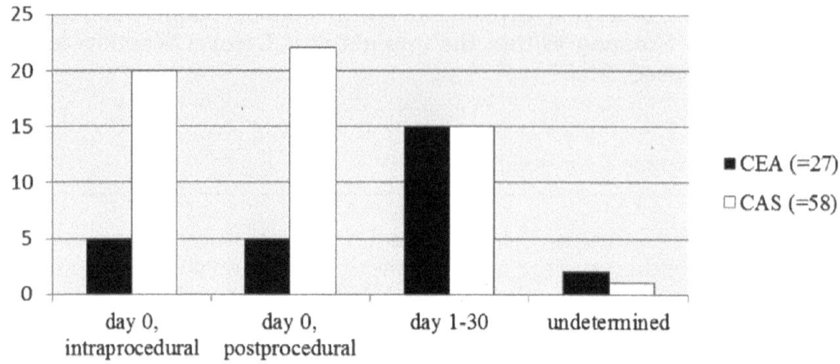

FIGURE 2.—Timing of strokes following CEA or CAS (CEA = carotid endarterectomy; CAS = carotid artery stenting). The difference in timings of event between CEA and CAS was statistically significant ($p = .014$, chi-square test). (Reprinted from Huibers A, Calvet D, Kennedy F, et al. Mechanism of procedural stroke following carotid endarterectomy or carotid artery stenting within the international carotid stenting study (ICSS) randomised trial. *Eur J Vasc Endovasc Surg.* 2015;50:281-288, with permission from Elsevier.)

authors found that the patterns of stroke varied by the treatment modality, with the majority of strokes in the CAS group being ischemic in nature, ipsilateral to the index lesion, nondisabling, and occurring on the day of the procedure (either intraprocedure or immediate postprocedure; Fig 2). In contrast, the majority of the strokes in the CEA group occurred between 1 and 30 days after the procedure and was more likely to be fatal or disabling. The majority of the strokes in the CEA group was also more likely to be ipsilateral to the index lesion and ischemic in nature, although a significantly larger percentage were hemorrhagic compared with the CAS group. The underlying responsible mechanisms also varied by the treatment modality with hemodynamic and hyperperfusion accounting for the leading causes in the CAS and CEA groups, respectively (CAS – hemodynamic > carotid-embolism > thrombus/occlusion > hyperperfusion = cardio-embolic = multiple causes; CEA – hyperperfusion > hemodynamic > carotid-embolic = thrombus/occlusion > cardiac = embolic = multiple causes). These data underscore the importance of perioperative blood pressure control, both hypo- and hypertension, and provide an avenue for quality improvement that may lead to better outcomes. These efforts may require good blood pressure control not only at the time of discharge, but throughout the prolonged postoperative period given the number of strokes that occurred within the 1- to 30-day period in both treatment groups. Indeed, the strokes related to hyperperfusion, the most common mechanism in the CEA group, frequently occur 1 to 5 days after the index procedure when the patients are at home. It was somewhat surprising that only a minority of the strokes resulted from thrombosis or occlusion of the carotid artery because this has been implicated as a major mechanism for strokes after CEA. In contrast, it was not surprising that technical difficulties were encountered during several of the CAS procedures that resulted in strokes, suggesting that it may be better to abort the procedure and that alternative approaches (eg, CEA, CAS with different approach) should be considered in this setting.

These data should be interpreted with some caution given the retrospective nature of the analysis and the inherent difficulties determining the actual cause of the strokes. Notably, the cause of stroke was unable to be determined in 23% of the cases. Furthermore, they are only relevant for symptomatic patients with > 50% stenosis, although they are likely applicable to asymptomatic patients with comparable lesions.

T. S. Huber, MD, PhD

National variation in preoperative imaging, carotid duplex ultrasound criteria, and threshold for surgery for asymptomatic carotid artery stenosis

Arous EJ, Simons JP, Flahive JM, et al (Univ of Massachusetts Med School, Worcester; et al)

J Vasc Surg 62:937-944, 2015

Objective.—Carotid endarterectomy (CEA) for asymptomatic carotid artery stenosis is among the most common procedures performed in the United States. However, consensus is lacking regarding optimal preoperative imaging, carotid duplex ultrasound criteria, and ultimately, the threshold for surgery. We sought to characterize national variation in preoperative imaging, carotid duplex ultrasound criteria, and threshold for surgery for asymptomatic CEA.

Methods.—The Society for Vascular Surgery Vascular Quality Initiative (VQI) database was used to identify all CEA procedures performed for asymptomatic carotid artery stenosis between 2003 and 2014. VQI currently captures 100% of CEA procedures performed at >300 centers by >2000 physicians nationwide. Three analyses were performed to quantify the variation in (1) preoperative imaging, (2) carotid duplex ultrasound criteria, and (3) threshold for surgery.

Results.—Of 35,695 CEA procedures in 33,488 patients, the study cohort was limited to 19,610 CEA procedures (55%) performed for asymptomatic disease. The preoperative imaging modality used before CEA varied widely, with 57% of patients receiving a single preoperative imaging study (duplex ultrasound imaging, 46%; computed tomography angiography, 7.5%; magnetic resonance angiography, 2.0%; cerebral angiography, 1.3%) and 43% of patients receiving multiple preoperative imaging studies. Of the 16,452 asymptomatic patients (89%) who underwent preoperative duplex ultrasound imaging, there was significant variability between centers in the degree of stenosis (50%-69%, 70%-79%, 80%-99%) designated for a given peak systolic velocity, end diastolic velocity, and internal carotid artery-to-common carotid artery ratio. Although 68% of CEA procedures in asymptomatic patients were performed for an 80% to 99% stenosis, 26% were performed for a 70% to 79% stenosis, and 4.1% were performed for a 50% to 69% stenosis. At the surgeon level, the range in the percentage of CEA procedures performed for a <80% asymptomatic carotid artery stenosis is from 0% to

100%. Similarly, at the center level, institutions range in the percentage of CEA procedures performed for a <80% asymptomatic carotid artery stenosis from 0% to 100%.

Conclusions.—Despite CEA being an extremely common procedure, there is widespread variation in the three primary determinants—preoperative imaging, carotid duplex ultrasound criteria, and threshold for surgery—of whether CEA is performed for asymptomatic carotid stenosis. Standardizing the approach to care for asymptomatic carotid artery stenosis will mitigate the significant downstream effects of this variation on health care costs.

▶ The authors have used data from the Vascular Quality Initiative (VQI) to examine the national practice variability for carotid endarterectomy (CEA) performed for asymptomatic stenoses (n = 19 610 CEA). Notably, 58% of the procedures in the database were performed for asymptomatic stenoses. The authors focused on the variability in preoperative imaging, criteria for the degree of stenosis, and operative thresholds for the degree of stenosis. They reported that the majority of patients underwent a single preoperative imaging study (usually duplex ultrasound) and underwent repair for stenoses > 80%, although there was a fair amount of variability in the criteria used to determine the actual degree of stenosis. These findings are reassuring and suggest that the vascular surgery community (or at least those surgeons that participate in the VQI) has an appropriate, conservative approach for CEA in asymptomatic patients. Admittedly, I find the data reassuring because they largely reflect my own bias and management strategy. The authors concluded that there was a "widespread variation in the three primary determinants—preoperative imaging, carotid duplex ultrasound criteria, and threshold for surgery," although I would contend that the national practice is probably more homogenous than they suspect or we are led to believe by their conclusions. Although only 57% of the patients had a single imaging study, I suspect that may of the other or second imaging studies were actually obtained by the nonvascular surgeon providers referring the patients (eg, family practice, neurology). It is quite common in our practice to have patients referred to clinic with several outside imaging studies. Regardless, we tend to obtain a duplex ultrasound in our own Intersocietal Accreditation Commission Vascular Testing–approved laboratory to confirm the degree of stenosis. Second, the thresholds for repair were pretty consistent with only 5% of patient undergoing CEA for a stenosis < 70%. We tend to use a threshold of > 80% as an indication for CEA in good risk, younger patients with reasonable life expectancy, but readily concede that the difference between a 70% to 79% and > 80% stenosis is fairly minimal and well within the indications for CEA as defined by the Asymptomatic Carotid Atherosclerosis Study. There was indeed a fair amount of variability in the criteria for determining the degree of carotid stenosis. However, I think that this stems from the facts that there are not any universally accepted criteria and that each institution really needs to validate its own criteria using its specific equipment. Overall, I was quite reassured by the study findings and think that the quality of care is likely appropriate based on the current literature, conceding that the indications for CEA in asymptomatic patients is a bit of a moving target that may change with the results of the current randomized trials in progress (ie, ACST-2, CREST-2).

T. S. Huber, MD, PhD

The value and economic analysis of routine postoperative carotid duplex ultrasound surveillance after carotid endarterectomy

AbuRahma AF, Srivastava M, AbuRahma Z, et al (West Virginia Univ, Charleston; et al)

J Vasc Surg 62:378-384, 2015

Background.—Several studies have reported on the role of postoperative duplex ultrasound surveillance after carotid endarterectomy (CEA) with varying results. Most of these studies had a small sample size or did not analyze costeffectiveness.

Methods.—We analyzed 489 of 501 CEA patients with patch closure. All patients had immediate postoperative duplex ultrasound examination and were routinely followed up both clinically and with duplex ultrasound at regular intervals of 1 month, 6 months, 12 months, and every 12 months thereafter. A Kaplan-Meier analysis was used to estimate the rate of ≥50% and ≥80% post-CEA restenosis over time and the time frame of progression from normal to ≥50% or ≥80% restenosis. The cost of post-CEA duplex surveillance was also estimated.

Results.—Overall, 489 patients with a mean age of 68.5 years were analyzed. Ten of these had residual postoperative ≥50% stenosis, and 37 did not undergo a second duplex ultrasound examination and therefore were not included in the final analysis. The mean follow-up was 20.4 months (range, 1-63 months), with a mean number of duplex ultrasound examinations of 3.6 (range, 1-7). Eleven of 397 patients (2.8%) with a normal finding on immediate postoperative duplex ultrasound vs 4 of 45 (8.9%) with mild stenosis on immediate postoperative duplex ultrasound progressed to ≥50% restenosis ($P = .055$). Overall, 15 patients (3.1%) had ≥50% restenosis, 9 with 50% to <80% and 4 with 80% to 99% (2 of these had carotid artery stenting reintervention), and 2 had late carotid occlusion. All of these were asymptomatic, except for one who had a transient ischemic attack. The mean time to ≥50% to <80% restenosis was 14.7 months vs 19.8 months for ≥80% restenosis after the CEA. Freedom from restenosis rates were 98%, 96%, 94%, 94%, and 94% for ≥50% restenosis and 99%, 98%, 97%, 97%, and 97% for ≥80% restenosis at 1 year, 2 years, 3 years, 4 years, and 5 years, respectively. Freedom from myocardial infarction, stroke, and deaths was not significantly different between patients with and without restenosis (100%, 93%, 83%, and 83% vs 94%, 91%, 86%, and 79% at 1 year, 2 years, 3 years, and 4 years, respectively; $P = .951$). The estimated charge of this surveillance was 3.6 × 489 (number of CEAs) × $800 (charge for carotid duplex ultrasound), which equals $1,408,320, to detect only four patients with ≥80% to 99% restenosis who may have been potential candidates for reintervention.

Conclusions.—This study shows that the value of routine postoperative duplex ultrasound surveillance after CEA with patch closure may be limited, particularly if the finding on immediate postoperative duplex ultrasound is normal or shows minimal disease.

▶ Dr AbuRahma and his colleagues have retrospectively analyzed the benefit of postoperative duplex ultrasound surveillance after carotid endarterectomy (CEA). Their protocol included duplex studies within the first 24 hours, then at 1 month and 12 months, and yearly thereafter. Notably, they had previously validated their duplex criteria for defining the degrees of stenosis (ie, > 50% and > 80%) after CEA and their noninvasive laboratory was accredited by the Intersocietal Commission for the Accreditation of Vascular Laboratories (ICAVL). The authors reported that 2% of the patients had an early or residual postoperative stenosis (> 50%), whereas 3.4% developed a late stenosis (> 50%) at an overall mean follow-up of 20.4 months. Notably, only 3 of 489 (0.6%) and 2 of 442 (0.4%) of the patients with early or late stenoses, respectively, underwent remedial intervention, and there was only 1 patient in the whole series who developed a neurological symptom attributed to the recurrent stenosis. The freedom from restenosis > 80% was estimated to be 93% at 4 years by the Kaplan-Meier method, and the corresponding freedom from the composite endpoint of stroke, myocardial infarction, and death at the same time point was 83%; the latter was not affected by the presence of restenosis. The estimated hospital changes and reimbursement for detecting the 4 patients with stenosis > 80% that would have been candidates for reintervention were $1 408 320 and $702,400, respectively. The report is particularly timely given the national emphasis on the "appropriateness" of care. The data clearly raise the question about the utility of postoperative duplex surveillance and emphasize the points that the practice is expensive while providing little yield or patient benefit. Unfortunately, the authors failed to make a real recommendation or draw any formal conclusions about the most appropriate surveillance protocol (if any protocol is worthwhile). In their discussion, they suggested that the immediate postoperative study is valuable and that a second study may be justified for patients with a normal postoperative study at 18 months, a time point that corresponds to the intimal hyperplastic response. It has been our practice to obtain an early postoperative study (< 6 weeks) to exclude any technical problems and then a repeat study at 1 year to exclude any recurrent stenosis. We have not obtained subsequent studies in patients with < 50% stenosis unless we are following their contralateral side. The current data must be interpreted with a mild amount of caution. They are reported from a center of excellence that has made an extensive contribution to the carotid literature. The mean follow-up is fairly short, and the outcomes were estimated by the Kaplan-Meier method. Furthermore, all of the patients in the series underwent a patch repair, and thus, the findings may not be applicable to patients who were not patched. Lastly, it is important to emphasize that the focus was on surveillance of the ipsilateral carotid after CEA and point out that there may be a role for duplex surveillance of the contralateral carotid system.

T. S. Huber, MD, PhD

Long-term outcomes after stenting versus endarterectomy for treatment of symptomatic carotid stenosis: the International Carotid Stenting Study (ICSS) randomised trial

Bonati LH, for the International Carotid Stenting Study investigators (Univ College London, UK; et al)

Lancet 385:529-538, 2015

Background.—Stenting is an alternative to endarterectomy for treatment of carotid artery stenosis, but long-term efficacy is uncertain. We report long-term data from the randomised International Carotid Stenting Study comparison of these treatments.

Methods.—Patients with symptomatic carotid stenosis were randomly assigned 1:1 to open treatment with stenting or endarterectomy at 50 centres worldwide. Randomisation was computer generated centrally and allocated by telephone call or fax. Major outcomes were assessed by an independent endpoint committee unaware of treatment assignment. The primary endpoint was fatal or disabling stroke in any territory after randomisation to the end of follow-up. Analysis was by intention to treat ([ITT] all patients) and per protocol from 31 days after treatment (all patients in whom assigned treatment was completed). Functional ability was rated with the modified Rankin scale. This study is registered, number ISRCTN25337470.

Findings.—1713 patients were assigned to stenting (n = 855) or endarterectomy (n = 858) and followed up for a median of 4·2 years (IQR 3·0–5·2, maximum 10·0). Three patients withdrew immediately and, therefore, the ITT population comprised 1710 patients. The number of fatal or disabling strokes (52 *vs* 49) and cumulative 5-year risk did not differ significantly between the stenting and endarterectomy groups (6·4% *vs* 6·5%; hazard ratio [HR] 1·06, 95% CI 0·72–1·57, $p = 0·77$). Any stroke was more frequent in the stenting group than in the endarterectomy group (119 *vs* 72 events; ITT population, 5-year cumulative risk 15·2% *vs* 9·4%, HR 1·71, 95% CI 1·28–2·30, $p < 0·001$; per-protocol population, 5-year cumulative risk 8·9% *vs* 5·8%, 1·53, 1·02–2·31, $p = 0·04$), but were mainly non-disabling strokes. The distribution of modified Rankin scale scores at 1 year, 5 years, or final follow-up did not differ significantly between treatment groups.

Interpretation.—Long-term functional outcome and risk of fatal or disabling stroke are similar for stenting and endarterectomy for symptomatic carotid stenosis.

▶ The study reports the seminal, long-term outcomes (median 4.2 years) from the International Carotid Stenting Study (ICSS) comparing carotid stenting

(CAS; n = 855) and carotid endarterectomy (CEA; n = 858) for symptomatic carotid stenosis (> 50% stenosis). The study reported that there was no difference in the incidence of fatal or disabling strokes between the groups (6.4% vs 6.5%, cumulative 5-year risk), the primary end point of the study. There was a higher incidence of any stroke (15.2% vs 9.4%, cumulative 5-year risk) and a higher incidence of the combined outcome of procedure-related stroke or procedure-related death or ipsilateral stroke (11.8% vs 7.2%, cumulative 5-year risk) in the CAS that was largely attributable to nondisabling strokes. Notably, the functional outcomes as assessed by the Rankin scores were not different between the groups. Furthermore, the incidence of recurrent stenosis (> 70%), as assessed by duplex ultrasound, were comparable between the groups (10.8% vs 8.6%) despite the fact that the criteria for stenosis were not corrected for the presence of a stent. These findings suggest that both CAS and CEA are effective, that sustained stroke prevents therapies for symptomatic carotid stenoses, and that the incidence of recurrent carotid stenosis is moderate. These findings are largely consistent with those from the other major randomized trials (ie, CREST, EVA-3, SPACE) in terms of the incidence of fatal or nondisabling strokes and the incidence of periprocedural strokes. Notably, the current study did not report an age-dependent difference in outcome, although it was not sufficiently powered to detect a difference. Previous meta-analyses of the CAS/CEA randomized trials have demonstrated a significant increase in the risk associated with stenting for patients > 70 years of age and a higher incidence of myocardial infarction, cranial nerve injury, and wound complications with CEA. These findings in toto seem to justify more widespread use of CAS for symptomatic patients < 70 years of age as an alternative to CEA.

T. S. Huber, MD, PhD

Acute Stroke After Carotid Endarterectomy: Time for a Paradigm Shift? Multicenter Experience With Emergent Carotid Artery Stenting With or Without Intracranial Tandem Occlusion Thrombectomy

Spiotta AM, Vargas J, Zuckerman S, et al (Univ of South Carolina, Charleston; Vanderbilt Univ, Nashville, TN; et al)

Neurosurgery 76:403-410, 2015

Background.—Stroke in the immediate postoperative period after carotid endarterectomy is a rare complication. Many centers have begun incorporating angiography before surgical re-exploration, which has the advantage of confirming carotid occlusion and treating tandem intracranial lesions if present.

Objective.—To determine the safety and efficacy of this strategy.

Methods.—A retrospective review was performed of all patients undergoing acute stenting of the carotid artery after carotid endarterectomy from November 2009 to June 2013 at 4 centers. Charts and angiographic images were reviewed. Eleven cases of carotid thrombosis within 72 hours of carotid endarterectomy and subsequent treatment strategies are summarized.

Results.—All patients had >50% carotid stenosis before carotid endarterectomy. One patient had intraoperative occlusion and dissection of the internal carotid artery, which was noted on intraoperative carotid duplex ultrasound. All patients underwent postoperative computed tomography or computed tomography perfusion scans with subsequent cerebral angiography and stent reconstruction within 11 hours of symptom onset. In all cases, carotid recanalization was successfully completed between 32 and 160 minutes from groin puncture. There were no procedural complications. Four patients had a tandem middle cerebral artery occlusion, 3 of whom underwent successful recanalization.

Conclusion.—Emergent endovascular evaluation in the setting of acute post–carotid endarterectomy thrombosis is a safe and timely treatment option, with the benefit of detecting and treating embolic intracranial lesions. Immediate angiography and intervention in this rare surgical complication show promising initial results.

▶ The authors have reported the collective outcome of patients undergoing carotid artery stenting (CAS) for acute stroke after carotid endarterectomy (CEA) and have advocated a "paradigm shift" in the treatment of this rare condition. Notably, the retrospective report identified 11 patients in 4 medical centers treated over a 3.5-year period. Unfortunately, neither the total number of CEAs performed nor the number of post-CEA strokes that occurred at the sites during the study period was reported, so it is difficult to define the actual incidence of the interventions. The authors performed CT and/or catheter-based arteriography as a diagnostic tool with the definitive treatment being CAS. This approach contrasts with the more traditional approach of routine neck exploration and balloon catheter thromboembolectomy. The authors justified their approach by their excellent technical result (ie, 100% recanalization) and the findings that several of the events resulted from lesions that would not have been amenable to open surgical treatment (carotid dissection = 1, tandem intracranial lesions = 4). Unfortunately, less than half (4 of 9) of the patients were asymptomatic at the time of follow-up, a rate consistent with the reports in the literature for the open surgical approach. I concur with the authors in that there has been a gradual evolution in the treatment of neurologic events after CEA given the advances in neuroimaging, the ability to treat intracranial lesions and the availability of hybrid open/endovascular suites in many major medical centers. However, I am not certain that I am ready to embrace a true "paradigm" shift and abandon the open surgical approach in favor of CAS given the limitations of the current study. Alternatively, I would contend that the open and endovascular techniques are complementary. It is important to remember that the treatment of the neurologic event should be the focus in this setting rather than the degree of carotid stenosis and/or the CEA itself. The neurologic events after CEA can result from thrombosis, emboli, and/or dissection. Accordingly, the responsible mechanism should be identified and definitive treatment (if possible) performed as expeditiously as possible with the specific approach dictated by the timing of the neurologic event relative to the procedure (eg, event in

OR, event in recovery room, event on floor) and the available resources (both imaging and personnel). CT and/or catheter-based arteriography can usually be obtained in a timely fashion and the results used to plan the definitive salvage procedure, either open or endovascular. In our own institution, we would favor an emergent catheter-based arteriogram in the hybrid suite for neurologic events that occur in the operating room or in the recovery room with the decision for open or endovascular treatment dictated by the findings. We favor open surgical thrombectomy for occluded internal carotid artery but would obtain a completion arteriogram to identify any additional intracranial lesions potentially amenable to endovascular treatment.

T. S. Huber, MD, PhD

Peripheral Arterial Occlusive Disease

Outcomes of completion imaging for lower extremity bypass in the Vascular Quality Initiative

Woo K, Palmer OP, Weaver FA, et al (Univ of Southern California, Los Angeles)
J Vasc Surg 62:412-416, 2015

Objective.—The objective of this study was to determine the association of intraoperative completion imaging (CI) for lower extremity vein bypass to a below-knee target with primary patency in the Vascular Quality Initiative.

Methods.—The Vascular Quality Initiative database was queried from January 2003 to October 2013 for lower extremity bypass (LEB) procedures that were elective, had an indication of occlusive disease, used a single-segment greater saphenous vein conduit, and had a below-knee target. LEBs with inflow arteries above the knee and below the knee were included. LEBs with concomitant endovascular procedures were excluded. CI was defined as completion angiography, completion duplex ultrasound, or both. The end points were primary patency at discharge and at 1 year. Multivariable analysis was performed controlling for patient demographics, comorbidities, bypass characteristics, and center.

Results.—Of 14,284 LEBs that were performed during the study period, 3147 satisfied the inclusion and exclusion criteria. Of 1457 (46%) that underwent CI, 287 (20%) underwent duplex ultrasound, 1116 (77%) underwent angiography, and 54 (3.7%) underwent both duplex ultrasound and angiography. There were more patients in the CI group with a history of smoking and a bypass graft crossing the knee. There was no difference in primary patency at discharge between the two groups (CI, 93.2% vs no CI, 93.8%; $P = .52$). Of the patients who underwent CI, the discharge primary patency was 95.1% for completion duplex ultrasound vs 92.8% for completion angiography ($P = .17$). On multivariable analysis, there was no significant association of CI with discharge primary patency ($P = .69$). The 1-year primary patency was 63% in the CI group vs 68% in the no CI group ($P = .051$). The 1-year primary patency was 60% for the duplex ultrasound group vs 65% for the angiography group

(P =.61). On multivariable analysis, there was no significant association of CI with 1-year primary patency (P =.69).

Conclusions.—In electively performed LEBs using single-segment saphenous vein to a below-knee target artery for occlusive disease, CI does not influence primary graft patency at discharge or at 1 year.

▶ The authors have used the Vascular Quality Initiative (VQI) database to retrospectively examine the utility of intraoperative completion imaging (CI; catheter-based arteriography or duplex ultrasound) after lower extremity bypass procedures. Notably, the procedures were limited to those performed electively using a single segment of saphenous vein with the bypass target below the knee. Admittedly, this is a fairly circumscribed patient population, justified by the authors to eliminate other confounding variables (eg, disadvantaged vein, simultaneous endovascular inflow procedure) that may not reflect a true association with the CI. The authors reported that the primary patency rates were comparable at discharge (CI 93% vs no CI 94%) and significantly greater at 1 year in the no CI group (CI 63% vs no CI 68%, P = .05), although there was no association with CI in terms of 1-year patency after correcting for the covariates. These data suggest that there may not be a benefit for completion imaging after lower extremity bypass, but they must be interpreted with some caution. First, there is likely a tremendous amount of selection bias in terms of the individual surgeons' use of completion imaging, and, unfortunately, the authors were not able to determine which surgeons used the CI routinely, selectively, or never. Second, the findings from the completion imaging and the ultimate impact on the conduct of the index operation and/or any remedial interventions were not available. Third, the procedures analyzed were fairly highly selected and represented only 22% (3147 of 14 284) of the lower extremity bypass procedures recorded in the VQI during the time course of the study, and, thus, the findings may not be applicable to other types of bypasses (eg, femoral-peroneal bypass with composite vein). Fourth, the findings may not be applicable to surgeons outside of the VQI. Although the VQI participants include academic centers, community centers, and nonacademic teaching hospitals, it is not clear that the results truly reflect real-world practice. Lastly, 1-year follow-up was available for only 59% of the procedures. I think that the authors' conclusions were very appropriate and justified, although I am not certain that they will change the opinion or bias of too many surgeons. The data suggest that the surgeons that elect not to do completion imaging in the study cohort likely have pretty good judgment that is justified by the comparable outcomes. I routinely do CI after all my lower extremity bypasses (and will continue to do so) because it "seems" like a good idea, but will readily concede that I rarely find something that mandates remediation during the index procedure.

T. S. Huber, MD, PhD

Endovascular Revascularization and Supervised Exercise for Peripheral Artery Disease and Intermittent Claudication: A Randomized Clinical Trial

Fakhry F, Spronk S, van der Laan L, et al (Erasmus Univ Med Ctr, Rotterdam, the Netherlands; Dutch Health Care Inspectorate, Utrecht, the Netherlands; Amphia Hosp, Breda, the Netherlands; et al)

JAMA 314:1936-1944, 2015

Importance.—Supervised exercise is recommended as a first-line treatment for intermittent claudication. Combination therapy of endovascular revascularization plus supervised exercise may be more promising but few data comparing the 2 therapies are available.

Objective.—To assess the effectiveness of endovascular revascularization plus supervised exercise for intermittent claudication compared with supervised exercise only.

Design, Setting, and Participants.—Randomized clinical trial of 212 patients allocated to either endovascular revascularization plus supervised exercise or supervised exercise only. Data were collected between May 17, 2010, and February 16, 2013, in the Netherlands at 10 sites. Patients were followed up for 12 months and the data were analyzed according to the intention-to-treat principle.

Interventions.—A combination of endovascular revascularization (selective stenting) plus supervised exercise (n = 106) or supervised exercise only (n = 106).

Main Outcomes and Measures.—The primary end point was the difference in maximum treadmill walking distance at 12 months between the groups. Secondary end points included treadmill pain-free walking distance, vascular quality of life (VascuQol) score (1 [worst outcome] to 7 [best outcome]), and 36-item Short-Form Health Survey (SF-36) domain scores for physical functioning, physical role functioning, bodily pain, and general health perceptions (0 [severe limitation] to 100 [no limitation]).

Results.—Endovascular revascularization plus supervised exercise (combination therapy) was associated with significantly greater improvement in maximum walking distance (from 264 m to 1501 m for an improvement of 1237 m) compared with the supervised exercise only group (from 285 m to 1240 m for improvement of 955 m) (mean difference between groups, 282 m; 99% CI, 60-505 m) and in pain-free walking distance (from 117 m to 1237 m for an improvement of 1120 m vs from 135 m to 847 m for improvement of 712 m, respectively) (mean difference, 408 m; 99% CI, 195-622 m). Similarly, the combination therapy group demonstrated significantly greater improvement in the disease-specific VascuQol score (1.34 [99% CI, 1.04-1.64] in the combination therapy group vs 0.73 [99% CI, 0.43-1.03] in the exercise group; mean difference, 0.62 [99% CI, 0.20-1.03]) and in the score for the SF-36 physical functioning (22.4 [99% CI, 16.3-28.5] vs 12.6 [99% CI, 6.3-18.9], respectively; mean difference, 9.8 [99% CI, 1.4-18.2]). No significant differences were found for the SF-36 domains of physical role functioning, bodily pain, and general health perceptions.

Conclusions and Relevance.—Among patients with intermittent claudication after 1 year of follow-up, a combination therapy of endovascular revascularization followed by supervised exercise resulted in significantly greater improvement in walking distances and health-related quality-of-life scores compared with supervised exercise only.

Trial Registration.—Netherlands Trail Registry Identifier: NTR2249.

▶ The authors report the results of a well-conducted randomized trial comparing endovascular revascularization alone with the combination of revascularization and a supervised exercise program for patients with moderate intermittent claudication. Notably, the inclusion criteria included a resting ankle brachial index of <.90, documented stenoses in the aortoiliac or femoropopliteal segment by noninvasive imaging, and a maximum walking distance between 100 and 500 m as assessed by a graded treadmill test. The study was designed to determine whether the combination therapy was better, although the authors conceded in their introduction that the first-line treatment for claudication (medical vs exercise vs revascularization) remains unresolved with endovascular revascularization being applied more frequently because of physician reimbursement, patient compliance, and the lack of funding for supervised exercise programs. The authors reported that the combination therapy was associated with a significant increase in the maximum walking distance at 12 months (difference 282 m), their primary outcome measure, although both strategies resulted in significant increases from baseline. These observed benefits for the primary outcome measure were consistent across almost all of the outcome measures with the combined therapy being superior to exercise (eg, pain-free walking distance, disease specific VascuQol score, Rating score), but exercising demonstrating an improvement from baseline. Further analysis of the data demonstrated some interesting findings. First, the ankle-brachial index (ABI) were significantly improved in the combination group although only minimally affected in the exercise group, underscoring the fact the underlying mechanism for improvement in the exercise group is not due to a marked increase in blood, at least as measured by the ABI. Second, 22% of the patients in the exercise group needed a remedial intervention for their claudication, but only 8% in the combination group required the same despite a restenosis rate of up to 32% in the latter group. Paradoxically, the freedom from intervention rate was significantly higher in the combination group. Third, the observed significant differences in the pain-free walking distance between the groups decreased with time (1 month, 566 m; 6 months, 409 m; 12 months, 282 m) suggesting that the exercise component of the therapy may take longer to achieve its maximal benefit and/or that the revascularization component may not be sustained. These data seem to justify the combined treatment and provide further support for the appropriate funding for supervised exercise program, something that is woefully lacking. However, they fail to provide any real guidance about the most appropriate first-line therapy for claudication, and it is worth emphasizing that endovascular revascularization is associated with significant cost and some adverse complications, albeit small. My recommended first-line therapy is exercise and I tell.

T. S. Huber, MD, PhD

Cilostazol and freedom from amputation after lower extremity revascularization

Neel JD, Kruse RL, Dombrovskiy VY, et al (Univ of Missouri School of Medicine, Columbia; Rutgers-Robert Wood Johnson Med School, New Brunswick, NY)

J Vasc Surg 61:960-964, 2015

Objective.—Cilostazol, an antiplatelet agent with vasodilating properties, has not been well evaluated in conjunction lower extremity revascularization (LER). We evaluated the association between cilostazol and limb salvage after endovascular or open surgery for LER.

Methods.—Patients aged ≥65 years undergoing LER were identified from 2007 to 2008 Medicare Provider Analysis and Review and Carrier files using International Classification of Diseases-9 Edition-Clinical Modification and Current Procedural Terminology-4 codes. Covariates included demographics, comorbidities, and disease severity. Use of cilostazol was identified using National Drug Codes and Part D files. Outcomes were compared using χ^2 and Kaplan-Meier analyses and Cox regression.

Results.—We identified 22,954 patients undergoing LER: 8128 (35.4%) with claudication, 3056 (13.3%) with rest pain, and 11,770 (51.3%) with ulceration/gangrene. Among them, 1999 patients (8.7%) used cilostazol before LER. More patients received endovascular (14,353) than open (8601) procedures. Cilostazol users had fewer amputations than nonusers at 30 days (7.8% vs 13.4%), 90 days (10.7% vs 18.0%), and 1 year (14.8% vs 24.0%; $P < .0001$ for all). Cox proportional hazards regression with adjustment for age, gender, race, comorbidities, type of procedure, and atherosclerosis severity showed noncilostazol users were more likely to undergo amputation ≤1 year after surgery (hazard ratio [HR], 1.15; 95% confidence interval [CI], 1.02-1.29; $P = .02$). Subgroup analyses using Cox proportional hazards models adjusted for age, gender, and comorbidities demonstrated significantly improved 1-year amputation-free survival for patients with renal failure (HR, 1.61; 95% CI, 1.28-2.02; $P < .001$) and diabetes (HR, 1.61; 95% CI, 1.36-1.92; $P < .001$) who were taking cilostazol.

Conclusions.—In patients undergoing LER, cilostazol use was associated with improved 1-year freedom from amputation. Patients with renal failure and diabetes also demonstrated a significant benefit from taking cilostazol. Further studies are needed to evaluate the benefits of cilostazol after LER.

▶ The authors have used the Medicare databases from 2007—2008 to examine the impact of cilostazol on limb salvage after lower extremity revascularization.

The analysis included both open and endovascular procedures performed for claudication and limb-threatening ischemia. They reported that the amputation rate was 15% higher (hazard ratio [HR] 1.15, 95% confidence interval [CI] 1.02–1.29) during the first year after revascularization among those who were not taking cilostazol at the time of the index procedure. Note that this beneficial effect was found after adjustment for age, gender, comorbidities, and indication for procedure (ie, claudication vs limb-threatening ischemia) using multivariable logistic regression. Among patients with diabetes and renal failure, the benefit of preoperative cilostazol was even greater after a similar adjustment (renal failure: HR 1.61, 95% CI 1.28–2.02; diabetes: HR 1.61, 95% CI 1.36–1.92). These data suggest that cilostazol should be part of the routine medical therapies for patients undergoing lower extremity intervention for their peripheral artery occlusive disease, similar to statins and antiplatelet agents. It is not clear that all patients with lower extremity occlusive disease should be on cilostazol, although this may be a reasonable extension of the data (and indications). Admittedly, the overall benefit was quite modest despite the impressive benefits identified in the subgroup analyses. Fortunately, the safety profile is quite good, and the medication seems to be relatively well tolerated. I suspect that the additional cost would be offset by the reduced number of amputations given their associated financial and psychosocial costs. The effects of cilostazol in terms of improving walking distances are presumed secondary to vasodilation and platelet inhibition, but the exact mechanism leading to limb preservation remains elusive. It is interesting to note that cilostazol has been reported to provide some benefit for patients with critical limb ischemia and it may reduce restenosis after balloon angioplasty.[1,2] The interpretation of the data are limited by the usual issues associated with administrative databases. Furthermore, I am concerned that the large number of interventions performed for claudication and the greater use of cilostazol among this cohort may be driving the improved limb salvage rates despite the statistical adjustments because the amputation rate at a year should be essentially zero for claudicants. Regardless of the limitations, I believe that the medication may have a role in the treatment of our patients, and I look forward to further reports examining its benefit in this setting.

T. S. Huber, MD, PhD

Reference

1. Soga Y, Iida O, Kawasaki D, et al. Impact of cilostazol on angiographic restenosis after balloon angioplasty for infrapopliteal artery disease in patients with critical limb ischemia. *Eur J Vasc Endovasc Surg.* 2012;44:577-581.
2. Shalhoub J, Davies AH, Franklin IJ. Cilostazol may improve outcome in critical limb ischemia. *Int Angiol.* 2009;28:363-366.

Access

Prospective multicenter study with a 1-year analysis of a new vascular graft used for early cannulation in patients undergoing hemodialysis

Glickman MH, Burgess J, Cull D, et al (Sentara Vascular Specialists, Norfolk, VA; Surgical Specialists of Charlotte, NC; Greenville Hosp System, SC; et al)

J Vasc Surg 62:434-441, 2015

Objective.—More than 85% of patients with end-stage renal disease start dialysis through a tunneled dialysis catheter (TDC) for long periods while their arteriovenous fistula or vascular access graft (arteriovenous graft [AVG]) matures. Because TDCs are associated with a high risk of complications, including death and infection, use of an AVG that can be cannulated safely immediately after implantation may reduce morbidity in these patients by allowing earlier TDC removal. We report a prospective multicenter study of a new early-cannulation AVG (Gore ACUSEAL Vascular Graft; W. L. Gore & Associates, Flagstaff, Ariz).

Methods.—Patients requiring creation of a prosthetic vascular access for hemodialysis were enrolled between July 2010 and February 2012 and observed for 12 months. Data were collected on the patients' baseline characteristics; location, position, loss of patency, and revisions of prior AVGs; dialysis sessions using the AVG; and major adverse events related to graft implantation or cannulation. Cumulative and primary unassisted graft patency rates were calculated. A subgroup analysis compared outcomes in patients in whom the AVG was first cannulated within 72 hours after implantation with outcomes in patients in whom the initial cannulation was performed >21 days postoperatively.

Results.—The population of this study was formed by 138 patients who received an ACUSEAL graft. During follow-up, 17 patients died and the AVG was abandoned in 27. The median value for follow-up was 360 days for all patients (variance 15,387). The overall mean time to initial cannulation was 15 days, with 54 grafts (40%) first cannulated within 72 hours after graft implantation and 33 grafts first cannulated >21 days afterward. The reason for late cannulation in some patients was dependent on the implanting surgeon's decision and the surgeon's personal experience with early cannulating grafts. The 1-year overall cumulative patency rate was 79% (95% confidence interval, 71%-85%); the primary unassisted patency rate was 35% (95% confidence interval, 27%-44%). Adverse events included 6 hematomas (two of which were related to cannulation and occurred 107 and 169 days, respectively, after AVG implantation), 15 graft infections, and 15 cases of steal syndrome requiring intervention. Patients in the early- and later-cannulation groups had similar characteristics and no significant differences in rates of cumulative or primary unassisted patency or adverse events.

Conclusions.—This study demonstrated that the new, early-cannulation AVG graft can be cannulated soon after implantation without a significant difference in patency and complication rates compared with rates associated with standard cannulation of expanded polytetrafluoroethylene grafts in the literature. This new AVG may allow early removal or avoidance of TDC use in patients undergoing hemodialysis, potentially reducing or eliminating the number of days of catheter-dependent dialysis, but further studies will be needed to demonstrate this potential.

▶ The authors report the results of a prospective evaluation (n = 138) of the ACUSEAL prosthetic arteriovenous hemodialysis access (AVG, Gore ACUSEAL Vascular Graft). The graft has a trilayer design comprising an inner layer of heparin-bonded ePTFE, a middle layer of an elastomeric membrane, and an outer layer of ePTFE. It was specifically designed to facilitate early cannulation, and the instructions for use, approved by the Food and Drug Administration, state that it can be cannulated for hemodialysis within 24 hours of implantation. The authors reported a primary and cumulative patency rate at 1 year of 35% and 79%, respectively, with an infectious and ischemic complication rate of 11% each. Notably, the authors reported that there were no differences in the patency or complication rates between the grafts that were cannulated within 72 hours postoperatively and those cannulated > 21 days in their subgroup analysis. These findings suggest that the AVG may indeed be suitable for early cannulation as concluded by the authors. An early cannulation graft has a tremendous amount of appeal and affords the potential to significantly reduce the duration of tunneled dialysis catheter use and the associated complications, including those related to both infection and central venous stenosis. Although most of the focus on tunneled catheter use has focused on the infectious complications, I would contend that the longer term central venous complications are equally nefarious and account for the expanding cohort of patients with complex access problems. There have been other attempts at early cannulation grafts, including one from the current study sponsor, but they have not been well adopted. It has been our impression that patients do not like being cannulated early after implantation because it just plain hurts to access the graft due to the surgical trauma from the incisions and tunnel. Although encouraging, the results must be interpreted with some caution due to several study limitations. First, the study was not a randomized trial, and the most important findings (ie, comparison of early vs late cannulation) were a result of a subgroup analysis. The decision to cannulate the graft early (< 72) or late (> 21 days) was based on the "surgeon's decision and the surgeon's personal experience" and includes a tremendous amount of selection bias. The study design was most unfortunate, and I would contend that the sponsor missed a nice opportunity to perform a quality randomized trial. Second, the outcomes are relatively short term, particularly given that one of the predecessor early cannulation grafts was associated with significant infectious complication rates. Lastly, the study was sponsored by the graft manufacturer itself. Despite these limitations, the concept of an early cannulation graft is exciting and may afford the opportunity to develop an effective catheter-free algorithm for patients presenting for hemodialysis access.

T. S. Huber, MD, PhD

A prospective randomized study of heparin-bonded graft (Propaten) versus standard graft in prosthetic arteriovenous access

Shemesh D, Goldin I, Hijazi J, et al (Shaare Zedek Med Ctr, Jerusalem, Israel)

J Vasc Surg 62:115-122, 2015

Objective.—Prosthetic grafts continue to be required for hemodialysis access when the options for native fistulas have been exhausted. The inferior long-term patency of grafts makes the possibility of preventing occlusion with heparin-bonded grafts an attractive alternative. We carried out a prospective randomized study to compare the patency of standard grafts with heparin-bonded grafts.

Methods.—Patients with end-stage renal failure requiring a prosthetic access were randomized to receive either a standard expanded polytetrafluorethylene (ePTFE) graft or a heparin-bonded ePTFE graft. Patients were enrolled from June 2007 until November 2011 and were followed up until July 2013, when the study concluded.

Results.—In this study, 160 patients were randomized and followed up for a median of 23.5 months. No patient was lost to follow-up. Primary patency was 35% and 14% for heparin-bonded grafts and 29% and 12% for standard ePTFE grafts at 6 and 12 months, respectively (P =.48). Assisted primary patency was 54%, 41%, and 27% for heparin-bonded grafts and 41%, 30%, and 23% for standard grafts at 12, 24, and 36 months, respectively (P =.12). Secondary patency was 83%, 83%, and 81% for heparin-bonded grafts and 81%, 73%, and 68% for standard grafts at 12, 24, and 36 months, respectively (P =.33). There were significantly fewer thromboses in heparin-bonded grafts during the first 5 months (P =.020). Of 80 standard grafts, 24 were eventually abandoned vs 17 heparin-bonded grafts (P =.188). Bleeding complications, infections, and intervention rates were similar in both groups.

Conclusions.—Heparin-bonded grafts demonstrated a trend to improved patency, but the difference was not statistically significant. Heparin-bonded grafts had a significantly lower early thrombosis rate that was sustained only for the first 5 months of follow-up.

▶ The authors report their results from a single-center, randomized controlled trial comparing heparin-bonded ePTFE (Propaten) with standard wall ePTFE grafts (AVGs) for patients (N = 160) undergoing prosthetic arteriovenous hemodialysis accesses. Notably, the majority of the patients in both groups underwent forearm AVGs (ie, brachial-basilic, brachial-cephalic) using 4- to 7-mm stretch grafts. The authors reported that there were no differences in primary, primary assisted, or secondary patency rates. Furthermore, they reported that there were no differences in the overall complication rates between the groups. The authors did "massage" their data a bit and identified some difference in terms of the time to the first thrombosis and the number of thromboses that favored the heparin-bonded grafts, although these were not the primary study end points. These data do not support the use of the heparin-bonded graft for hemodialysis access, particularly because it is more expensive (cost 18% more than standard wall graft at the authors' center). These findings are consistent with multiple other publications that have failed to demonstrate any real patency benefit for a specific nonautogenous AVG despite various modifications (eg, taper graft, material, anastomotic configuration). The reported primary patency rates at 12 months were dismal (heparin-bonded, 14%; standard, 12%), although the primary assisted (heparin-bonded, 54%, standard, 41%) and secondary rates (heparin-bonded, 83%; standard, 81%) were reasonable. This discrepancy in patency rates likely reflects the authors' aggressive approach to remediation of failing accesses. It does raise the question as to which patency measure is really the best one to assess the benefit of the heparin bound to the graft, likely the primary assisted patency as suggested by the authors. It is somewhat disheartening that the heparin-bonding did not provide a patency benefit. However, the mechanism of failure for most prosthetic arteriovenous accesses is intimal hyperplasia at the venous anastomosis, one that does not appear to be affected by the surface treatment of the graft with heparin.

T. S. Huber, MD, PhD

Venous

A Randomized Trial Comparing Treatments for Varicose Veins

Brittenden J, Cotton SC, Elders A, et al (Univ of Aberdeen, UK; et al)
N Engl J Med 371:1218-1227, 2014

Background.—Ultrasound-guided foam sclerotherapy and endovenous laser ablation are widely used alternatives to surgery for the treatment of varicose veins, but their comparative effectiveness and safety remain uncertain.

Methods.—In a randomized trial involving 798 participants with primary varicose veins at 11 centers in the United Kingdom, we compared the outcomes of foam, laser, and surgical treatments. Primary outcomes at 6 months were disease-specific quality of life and generic quality of life, as measured on several scales. Secondary outcomes included complications and measures of clinical success.

Results.—After adjustment for baseline scores and other covariates, the mean disease-specific quality of life was slightly worse after treatment with foam than after surgery ($P = 0.006$) but was similar in the laser and surgery groups. There were no significant differences between the surgery group and the foam or the laser group in measures of generic quality of life. The frequency of procedural complications was similar in the foam group (6%) and the surgery group (7%) but was lower in the laser group (1%) than in the surgery group ($P < 0.001$); the frequency of serious adverse events (approximately 3%) was similar among the groups. Measures of clinical success were similar among the groups, but successful ablation of the main trunks of the saphenous vein was less common in the foam group than in the surgery group ($P < 0.001$).

Conclusions.—Quality-of-life measures were generally similar among the study groups, with the exception of a slightly worse disease-specific quality of life in the foam group than in the surgery group. All treatments had similar clinical efficacy, but complications were less frequent after laser treatment and ablation rates were lower after foam treatment. (Funded by the Health Technology Assessment Programme of the National Institute for Health Research; Current Controlled Trials number, ISRCTN51995477.)

▶ The authors have performed an elegant randomized trial comparing 3 treatment modalities (ie, foam, laser, surgery) for symptomatic varicose veins. Importantly, the primary end point was quality of life at 6 months as determined using both disease-specific (ie, Aberdeen Varicose Vein Questionnaire) and generic (ie, EuroQoL Group 5-Dimension Self Report Questionnaire [EQ-5D], Medical Outcomes Study 36-Item Short-Form Health Survey [SF-36]) survey tools. They reported that disease-specific quality of life was somewhat worse in the foam group compared with the surgery group, although the difference was modest and likely not clinically relevant. There were no significant differences between the treatment groups for the EQ-5D or the SF-36 physical component scores, although the SF-36 mental component was slightly better in the laser group compared with foam. Analysis of the secondary end points suggested that the clinical success rates were roughly comparable at 6 months, although the success rate for ablating the saphenous vein was lower in the foam group. The major complication rates were also comparable (3%) between the groups, although the procedural-specific complication rates were lower in the laser group. The overall results suggest that the 3 treatment modalities are safe, effective, and relatively comparable. The small differences between the 3 groups may support an individual surgeon's bias; however, they do not seem sufficient to really justify changing techniques. The results must be interpreted with some caution given that the timeline for the primary end point was relatively short (ie, 6 months) and that it is conceivable there may be a difference in the quality of life or clinical success among the techniques after longer term follow-up. It is conceivable that the survey tools were not sufficiently sensitive to detect a difference among the techniques, although all 3 tools are fairly standard and have been widely validated. Furthermore, the radiofrequency ablation technique was not included in the study design, but the results in the literature have been comparable to the laser technique.

T. S. Huber, MD, PhD

Miscellaneous

Predictors of surgical site infection after hospital discharge in patients undergoing major vascular surgery

Wiseman JT, Fernandes-Taylor S, Barnes ML, et al (Univ of Wisconsin School of Medicine and Public Health, Madison)

J Vasc Surg 62:1023-1031, 2015

Objective.—Surgical site infection (SSI) is one of the most common postoperative complications after vascular reconstruction, producing significant morbidity and hospital readmission. In contrast to SSI that develops while patients are still hospitalized, little is known about the cohort of patients who develop SSI after discharge. In this study, we explore the factors that lead to postdischarge SSI, investigate the differences between risk factors for in-hospital vs postdischarge SSI, and develop a scoring system to identify patients who might benefit from postdischarge monitoring of their wounds.

Methods.—Patients who underwent major vascular surgery from 2005 to 2012 for aneurysm and lower extremity occlusive disease were identified from the American College of Surgeons National Surgical Quality Improvement Program Participant Use Files. Patients were categorized as having no SSI, in-hospital SSI, or SSI after hospital discharge. Predictors of postdischarge SSI were determined by multivariable logistic regression and internally validated by bootstrap resampling. Risk scores were assigned to all significant variables in the model. Summative risk scores were collapsed into quartile-based ordinal categories and defined as low, low/moderate, moderate/high, and high risk. Multivariable logistic regression was used to determine predictors of in-hospital SSI.

Results.—Of the 49,817 patients who underwent major vascular surgery, 4449 (8.9%) were diagnosed with SSI (2.1% in-hospital SSI; 6.9% postdischarge SSI). By multivariable analysis, factors significantly associated with increased odds of postdischarge SSI include female gender, obesity, diabetes, smoking, hypertension, coronary artery disease, critical limb ischemia, chronic obstructive pulmonary disease, dyspnea, neurologic disease, prolonged operative time >4 hours, American Society of Anesthesiology class 4 or 5, lower extremity revascularization or aortoiliac procedure, and groin anastomosis. The model exhibited moderate discrimination (bias-corrected C statistic, 0.691) and excellent internal calibration. The postdischarge SSI rate was 2.1% for low-risk patients, 5.1% for low/moderate-risk patients, 7.8% for moderate/high-risk patients, and 14% for high-risk patients. In a comparative analysis, comorbidities were the primary driver of postdischarge SSI, whereas in-hospital factors (operative time, emergency case status) and complications predicted in-hospital SSI.

Conclusions.—The majority of SSIs after major vascular surgery develop following hospital discharge. We have created a scoring system that can select a cohort of patients at high risk for SSI after discharge. These patients can be targeted for transitional care efforts focused on early detection and treatment with the goal of reducing morbidity and preventing readmission secondary to SSI (Fig 3, Table 3).

▶ The authors have used data from the American College of Surgeons National Surgical Quality Improvement Program (ACS NSQIP) to identify predictors of surgical site infections (SSIs) that occur after hospital discharge (postdischarge and < 30 days) in patients undergoing major, open vascular surgical procedures (abdominal aortic aneurysm repair, aortoiliac bypass, lower extremity revascularization). The analysis differs from the more common ones dealing with immediate, inpatient postoperative complications (including wound complications) and is timely given the current focus on readmission rates after major surgical procedures. Notably, wound complications account for the leading cause of preventable hospital readmissions after surgical procedures. The authors reported that the overall SSI rate for the procedures analyzed was 8.9% with 6.9% of these occurring after hospital discharge. The diagnosis was based on a composite measure from the data collected in NSQIP including predefined criteria for superficial SSI, deep SSI, organ space SSI, and wound dehiscence. The rates of the SSIs varied by the vascular surgical procedure with the highest rate reported for lower extremity revascularization (lower extremity revascularization, 11%; abdominal aortic aneurysm, 4.3%; aortoiliac, 8.5%). The predictors identified in their multivariate model (Table 3) were somewhat "predictable" to most vascular surgeons, and it no surprise that obese female patients undergoing a complex lower extremity revascularization for critical limb ischemia are at increased risk for wound complications. The authors' model (Fig 3 and Table 3) provides a nice benchmark for SSIs and can be used to identify patients at higher risk who may benefit from more intensive postdischarge surveillance than the typical "return to clinic visit in 2 weeks." These potential strategies include early postdischarge telephone communication, earlier clinic follow-up (ie, < 2 weeks), early primary care

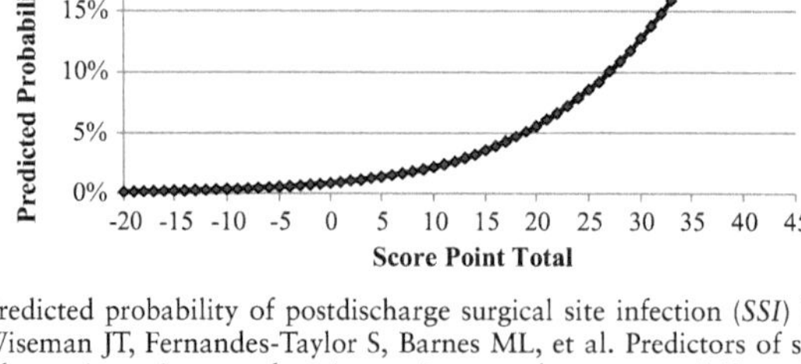

FIGURE 3.—Predicted probability of postdischarge surgical site infection (*SSI*) by total point score. (Reprinted from Wiseman JT, Fernandes-Taylor S, Barnes ML, et al. Predictors of surgical site infection after hospital discharge in patients undergoing major vascular surgery. *J Vasc Surg*. 2015;62:1023-1031, with permission from Society for Vascular Surgery.)

TABLE 3.—Risk Scores for 30-day Postdischarge Surgical Site Infection (SSI) Derived from the Multivariate Logistic Regression Final Model

Variables	Points
Lower extremity revascularization	12
Aortoiliac procedure	9
Obese	9
Operative time >6 hours	5
Female gender	4
Overweight	3
Operative time 4-6 hours	3
Insulin dependent DM	3
Non-insulin-dependent DM	2
Smoker	2
Hypertension	2
Critical limb ischemia	2
Dyspnea with moderate exertion	2
Groin anastomosis	2
ASA class 4 or 5	2
COPD	1
CAD	1
Neurologic disease	1
Age ≥65 years	−1
Black race	−2
Sepsis complication	−4
Renal complication	−6
Totally dependent functional status	−6
Prolonged LOS (≥14 days)	−9

The scores were generated as described in the Methods.

ASA, American Society of Anesthesiologists; CAD, coronary artery disease; COPD, chronic obstructive pulmonary disease; DM, diabetes mellitus; LOS, length of stay.

Reprinted from Wiseman JT, Fernandes-Taylor S, Barnes ML, et al. Predictors of surgical site infection after hospital discharge in patients undergoing major vascular surgery. *J Vasc Surg*. 2015;62:1023-1031, with permission from Society for Vascular Surgery.

follow-up for medical optimization, and/or "virtual" follow-up using telemedicine or Health Insurance Portability and Accountability Act—compliant imaging sharing tools. These strategies are based on the hope that early recognition will result in the initiation of wound care strategies (eg, debridement, antibiotics) that will prevent progression of the problem and avoid readmission, although this has not been clearly established. It was interesting that the predictors of the inpatient wound complications were somewhat different and largely associated with perioperative factors (eg, emergency case) in contrast to the postdischarge complications that were largely associated with patient comorbidities. The ultimate goal should be to reduce the overall incidence of SSIs, both inpatient and postdischarge, although it is somewhat sobering that not many of the identified predictors are modifiable in the preoperative period.

T. S. Huber, MD, PhD

Preoperative β-blockers do not improve cardiac outcomes after major elective vascular surgery and may be harmful

Scali S, Patel V, Neal D, et al (Univ of Florida, Gainesville; Harvard Med School, Boston, MA; et al)

J Vasc Surg 62:166-176, 2015

Objective.—Routine initiation β-blocker medications before vascular surgery is controversial due to conflicting data. The purpose of this analysis was to determine whether prophylactic use of β-blockers before major elective vascular surgery decreased postoperative cardiac events or mortality.

Methods.—The Society for Vascular Surgery Vascular Quality Initiative (SVS-VQI) data set was used to perform a retrospective cohort analysis of infrainguinal lower extremity bypass (LEB), aortofemoral bypass (AFB), and open abdominal aortic aneurysm (AAA) repair patients. Chronic (>30 days preoperatively) β-blocker patients were excluded, and comparisons were made between preoperative (0-30 day) and no β-blocker groups. Patients were risk stratified using a novel prediction tool derived specifically from the SVS-VQI data set. Propensity-matched pairs and interprocedural specific risk stratification comparisons were performed. End points included in-hospital major adverse cardiac events (MACEs), including myocardial infarction (MI; defined as new ST or T wave electrocardiographic changes, troponin elevation, or documentation by echocardiogram or other imaging modality), dysrhythmia, and congestive heart failure, and 30-day mortality.

Results.—The study analyzed 13,291 patients (LEB, 68% [n = 9047]; AFB, 11% [n = 1474]; and open AAA, 21% [n = 2770]); of these, 67.7% (n = 8999) were receiving β-blockers at time of their index procedure. Specifically, 13.2% (n = 1753) were identified to have been started on a preoperative β-blocker, 54.5% (n = 7426) were on chronic β-blockers, and 32.3% (n = 4286) were on no preoperative β-blockers. Among the three procedures, patients had significant demographic and comorbidity differences and thus were not combined. A 1:1 propensity-matched pairs analysis (1459 pairs) revealed higher rates of postoperative MI with preoperative β-blockers (preoperative β-blocker relative risk, 1.65; 95% confidence interval, 1.02-2.68; $P = .05$ vs no β-blocker), with no difference in dysrhythmia, congestive heart failure, or 30-day mortality. When stratified into low-risk, medium-risk, and high-risk groups within each procedure, all groups of preoperative β-blocker patients had no difference or higher rates of MACEs and 30-day mortality, with the exception of high-risk open AAA patients, who had a lower rate of MI (odds ratio, 0.35; 95% confidence interval, 011-0.87; $P = .04$).

Conclusions.—Exclusive of high-risk open AAA patients, preoperative β-blockers did not decrease rates of MACEs or mortality after LEB, AFB, or open AAA. Importantly, exposure to prophylactic preoperative β-blockers increased the rates of some adverse events in several subgroups. Given these data, the SVS-VQI cannot support routine initiation of preoperative β-blockers before major elective vascular surgery in most patients.

▶ The authors have attempted to examine the role of perioperative (< 30 days) beta blockade in patients undergoing high-risk, open vascular surgical procedures (lower extremity bypass, aortofemoral bypass, aneurysm repair) using the Society for Vascular Surgery Vascular Quality Initiative (VQI) database. The major outcome measures were perioperative mortality and major cardiovascular events (myocardial infarction, dysrhythmia, congestive heart failure) as defined in the database, although the authors also examined 1-year mortality. Although retrospective, a variety of sophisticated statistical analyses were implemented to truly dissect out any potential benefit (or harm) from the agents. The authors reported that perioperative beta blockade was associated with a higher incidence of postoperative myocardial infarction (2.9% vs 1.8%, relative risk 1.65, 95% confidence interval 1.02-2.68, $P = .05$) for the whole cohort using their propensity-matched pairs. Analysis of the procedure-specific outcomes demonstrated additional negative effects of perioperative beta blockade with a benefit in terms of postoperative myocardial infarction only demonstrated in the highest risk tertile of the patients undergoing open aneurysm repair. Notably, the mortality at 1 year was not significantly different among the matched pairs based on perioperative beta blockade, although, somewhat predictably, mortality increased among the higher risk tertiles. The analysis is particularly timely and relevant given the controversy surrounding the role of perioperative beta blockade, confounded by the concerns regarding the integrity of the data from the Dutch Echocardiographic Cardiac Risk Evaluation Applying Stress Echocardiography (DECREASE) family of trials that provided level 1 data supporting their benefit. The current data do not support the initiation beta-blockers in the perioperative period for the cohort of vascular surgery patients analyzed, those deemed the highest risk for major adverse cardiac events. The beta-blockers failed to demonstrate any real benefit with noted exception above and potentially caused harm, albeit the difference in terms of perioperative myocardial infarction may be more statistically significant than clinically relevant. Unfortunately, the data do not provide any guidance in terms of the management of patients that are already on beta-blockers (54.5% of the patients undergoing the index procedures in the VQI during the study period), although the national guidelines dictate they should be continued. The analysis is limited by its retrospective nature and the inherent selection bias in terms of the patients that were treated with beta-blockers, both acutely and chronically. The data could be used to justify a randomized trial for the initiation of perioperative beta-blockers in patients undergoing open aneurysm repair, although the enthusiasm is likely limited by the negative experience by the previous beta-blocker trials and the diminishing number of open repairs that has resulted from the evolution of the endovascular therapies.

T. S. Huber, MD, PhD

Office-based endovascular suite is safe for most procedures

Jain K, Munn J, Rummel MC, et al (Advanced Vascular Surgery, Kalamazoo, MI)

J Vasc Surg 59:186-191, 2014

Objective.—This study was conducted to identify the safety of endovascular procedures in the office endovascular suite and to assess patient satisfaction in this setting.

Methods.—Between May 22, 2007, and December 31, 2012, 2822 patients underwent 6458 percutaneous procedures in an office-based endovascular suite. Demographics of the patients, complications, hospital transfers, and 30-day mortality were documented in a prospective manner. Follow-up calls were made, and a satisfaction survey was conducted. Almost all dialysis procedures were done under local anesthesia and peripheral arterial procedures under conscious sedation. All patients, except those undergoing catheter removals, received hydrocodone and acetaminophen (5/325 mg), diazepam (5-10 mg), and one dose of an oral antibiotic preprocedure and three doses postprocedure. Patients who required conscious sedation received fentanyl and midazolam. Conscious sedation was used almost exclusively in patients having an arterial procedure. Measurements of blood urea nitrogen, creatinine, international normalized ratio, and partial thromboplastin time were performed before peripheral arteriograms. All other patients had no preoperative laboratory tests. Patients considered high risk (American Society of Anesthesiologists Physical Status Classification 4), those who could not tolerate the procedure with mild to moderate conscious sedation, patients with a previous bad experience, or patients who weighed >400 pounds were not candidates for office based procedures.

Results.—There were 54 total complications (0.8%): venous, 2.2%; aortogram without interventions, 1%; aortogram with interventions, 2.7%; fistulogram, 0.5%; catheters, 0.3%; and venous filter-related, 2%. Twenty-six patients required hospital transfer from the office. Ten patients needed an operative intervention because of a complication. No procedure-related deaths occurred. There were 18 deaths in a 30-day period. Of patients surveyed, 99% indicated that they would come back to the office for needed procedures.

Conclusions.—When appropriately screened, almost all peripheral interventions can be performed in the office with minimal complications. For dialysis patients, outpatient intervention has a very low complication rate and is the mainstay of treatment to keep the dialysis access patent. Venous insufficiency, when managed in the office setting, also has a low complication rate. Office-based procedural settings should be seriously considered for percutaneous interventions for arterial, venous, and dialysis-related procedures.

▶ The authors describe their extensive experience with office-based endovascular procedures ($N = 6458$) in an attempt to determine safety and patient satisfaction. Given the data presented, the approach appeared to be safe as reflected by the overall complication rate (0.8%), postprocedure hospital transfer rate (0.4%), and 30-day mortality. Notably, none of the deaths ($n = 18$) within 30 days of the procedure were specifically related to the procedure. The complication rate varied by the type of procedure with the arterial procedures associated with intervention (2.7%) and the venous procedures (2.2%) being the highest. The overwhelming majority (99%) of the patients stated that they were happy with the approach and would have another office-based procedure as necessary. Unfortunately, the efficacy of the procedures in terms of the longer-term outcomes was not presented in the analysis. Although I concur with the results of the article and the utility of the approach, the results must be interpreted with some minor caution. First, dialysis access–related procedures accounted for the largest percentage of the various procedures (42%). Although the patients with chronic kidney disease and end-stage renal disease often have multiple comorbidities, the access-related procedures tend to be more straightforward and, thus, less likely to result in complications and/or adverse outcomes. Notably, the authors stated that they performed relatively few peripheral arterial procedures within the early phase of their experience. Second, the patients were selected to do well in terms of the inclusion/exclusion criteria. Specifically, the exclusion criteria included obesity (>400 pounds), American Society of Anesthesiologists classification 4, previous contrast reaction, requirement for general anesthesia, and previous adverse experience with office-based procedures. Lastly, a variety of safeguards were implemented to reduce the incidence of adverse outcomes including Advanced Cardiac Life Support certification, limited sedation, preferential use of small diameter sheaths, ultrasound-guided access, closure devices, adequate inventory of covered stents, and the development of a protocol to manage emergencies. I readily concede that these "limitations" may just be good practice policies and recommend the article and overall clinical approach to individuals that are considering developing an office-based endovascular practice. Unfortunately, the widespread adoption of office-based endovascular procedures seems to be associated with an expansion of the indications given the associated additional reimbursement. It is not clear that moving these procedures from the hospital setting to the office actually reduces cost for the health care system. However, I think it is incumbent on all providers to maintain the same, rigorous indications for the procedures regardless of the remuneration and clinical setting.

T. S. Huber, MD, PhD

12 General Thoracic Surgery

Miscellaneous

The use of extracorporeal membrane oxygenation in blunt thoracic trauma: A study of the Extracorporeal Life Support Organization database

Jacobs JV, Hooft NM, Robinson BR, et al (St. Joseph's Hosp and Med Ctr, Phoenix, AZ; et al)

J Trauma Acute Care Surg 79:1049-1053, 2015

Background.—Reports documenting the use of extracorporeal membrane oxygenation (ECMO) after blunt thoracic trauma are scarce. We used a large, multicenter database to examine outcomes when ECMO was used in treating patients with blunt thoracic trauma.

Methods.—We performed a retrospective analysis of ECMO patients in the Extracorporeal Life Support Organization database between 1998 and 2014. The diagnostic code for blunt pulmonary contusion (861.21, DRG International Classification of Diseases—9th Rev.) was used to identify patients treated with ECMO after blunt thoracic trauma. Variations of pre-ECMO respiratory support were also evaluated. The primary outcome was survival to discharge; the secondary outcome was hemorrhagic complication associated with ECMO.

Results.—Eighty-five patients met inclusion criteria. The mean ± SEM age of the cohort was 28.9 ± 1.1 years; 71 (83.5%) were male. The mean ± SEM pre-ECMO Pao_2/FIO_2 ratio was 59.7 ± 3.5, and the mean ± SEM pre-ECMO length of ventilation was 94.7 ± 13.2 hours. Pre-ECMO support included inhaled nitric oxide (15 patients, 17.6%), high-frequency oscillation (10, 11.8%), and vasopressor agents (57, 67.1%). The mean ± SEM duration of ECMO was 207.4 ± 23.8 hours, and 63 patients (74.1%) were treated with venovenous ECMO. Thirty-two patients (37.6%) underwent invasive procedures before ECMO, and 12 patients (14.1%) underwent invasive procedures while on ECMO. Hemorrhagic complications occurred in 25 cases (29.4%), including 12 patients (14.1%) with surgical site bleeding and 16 (18.8%) with cannula site bleeding (6 patients had both). The rate of survival to discharge was

74.1%. Multivariate analysis showed that shorter duration of ECMO and the use of venovenous ECMO predicted survival.

Conclusion.—Outcomes after the use of ECMO in blunt thoracic trauma can be favorable. Some trauma patients are appropriate candidates for this therapy. Further study may discern which subpopulations of trauma patients will benefit most from ECMO.

Level of Evidence.—Therapeutic/care management study, level V.

▶ Many adult trauma patients develop respiratory failure after severe injury. Several factors contribute to respiratory failure, including pulmonary contusion, systemic inflammation, aspiration, pneumonia, and long bone fractures causing fat emboli. Some trauma patients will have pulmonary injury that progresses to severe adult acute respiratory distress syndrome (ARDS), which has an associated mortality rate of 40% to 60% despite many medical advances in its treatment. The use of extracorporeal membrane oxygenation (ECMO) in adult patients suffering ARDS has been historically been controversial. Recently, some studies have revealed some promising results in adults treated with ECMO, with survival rates as high as 63%. Although the debate continues about which patients will benefit from the use of ECMO, the ideal ECMO patient has a reversible disease process, minimal comorbidities, good baseline cardiopulmonary function, and contraindication to anticoagulation.

In some of these ways, trauma patients would be ideal patients in that they often have recoverable injuries and are typically young and healthy with good cardiopulmonary function baseline. One potential complication of ECMO in trauma patient population is the increased risk of hemorrhage during its use. However, this is less of an issue with the use of heparin-bonded systems and shorter length circuits permitting ECMO use with little to no anticoagulation use. Several reports have demonstrated that patients with traumatic intracranial hemorrhage and respiratory failure can be successfully managed on heparin-free ECMO without increasing the size of the hemorrhagic lesion. The use of ECMO in trauma patients has not been well characterized. No single center has a large, high-volume, trauma ECMO service, making it difficult to make broad generalization.

The authors undertook a large multicenter database review to evaluate the use of ECMO in patients with blunt thoracic trauma. They hypothesized that the use of ECMO after blunt thoracic trauma would produce favorable mortality outcomes with an acceptable risk of bleeding. They studied 90 patients treated with ECMO support who were identified in the extracorporeal registry during the study period. Survivors and nonsurvivors were compared in the cohort. By univariate analysis, there were no significant differences found between the survivors and the nonsurvivors when demographic, clinical, and physiologic data end points were evaluated. Survivors did trend toward a shorter duration of ECMO. Survivors also commonly had venovenous ECMO compared to venoarterial ECMO. Age, intracranial hemorrhage, injuries with a greater risk hemorrhage, PaO_2/FIO_2 ratio, and pre-ECMO duration of intubation did not significantly predict survival.

This report reminds us that even with the current medical therapy for ARDS with protective lung ventilation strategies may fall short in some cases, and there may be a role for ECMO. Although ECMO for blunt thoracic trauma may not be a panacea, it may represent a reasonable option to employ in young, otherwise healthy patients and in some cases may result in a survivable patient.

C. T. Klodell, Jr, MD

Lung Cancer Resection at Hospitals With High vs Low Mortality Rates

Grenda TR, Revels SL, Yin H, et al (Univ of Michigan, Ann Arbor; et al)

JAMA Surg 150:1034-1040, 2015

Importance.—Wide variations in mortality rates exist across hospitals following lung cancer resection; however, the factors underlying these differences remain unclear.

Objective.—To evaluate perioperative outcomes in patients who underwent lung cancer resection at hospitals with very high and very low mortality rates (high-mortality hospitals [HMHs] and low-mortality hospitals [LMHs]) to better understand the factors related to differences in mortality rates after lung cancer resection.

Design, Setting, and Participants.—In this retrospective cohort study, 1279 hospitals that were accredited by the Commission on Cancer were ranked on a composite measure of risk-adjusted mortality following major cancer resections performed from January 1, 2005, through December 31, 2006. We collected data from January 1, 2006, through December 31, 2007, on 645 lung resections in 18 LMHs and 25 HMHs. After adjusting for patient characteristics, we used hierarchical logistic regression to examine differences in the incidence of complications and "failure-to-rescue" rates (defined as death following a complication).

Main Outcomes and Measures.—Rates of adherence to processes of care, incidence of complications, and failure to rescue following complications.

Results.—Among 645 patients who received lung resections (441 in LMHs and 204 in HMHs), the overall unadjusted mortality rates were 1.6% (n = 7) vs 10.8% (n = 22; $P < .001$) for LMHs and HMHs, respectively. Following risk adjustment, the difference in mortality rates was attenuated (1.8% vs 8.1%; $P < .001$) but remained significant. Overall, complication rates were higher in HMHs (23.3% vs 15.6%; adjusted odds ratio [aOR], 1.79; 95% CI, 0.99-3.21), but this difference was not significant. The likelihood of any surgical (aOR, 0.73; 95% CI, 0.26-2.00) or cardiopulmonary (aOR, 1.23; 95% CI, 0.70-2.16) complications was similar between LMHs and HMHs. However, failure-to-rescue rates were significantly higher in HMHs (25.9% vs 8.7%; aOR, 6.55; 95% CI, 1.44-29.88).

Conclusions and Relevance.—Failure-to-rescue rates are higher at HMHs, which may explain the large differences between hospitals in mortality rates following lung cancer resection. This finding emphasizes the need for better understanding of the factors related to complications and their subsequent management.

▶ In this important study, the authors seek to identify factors that distinguish low-mortality hospitals from high-mortality hospitals, specifically in regard to major lung resections. After ranking the hospitals from lowest to highest mortality, 645 patients were identified from the low-mortality hospitals (441 patients) and high-mortality hospitals (204 patients). Adding to a growing body of evidence, they found that the distinguishing factor separating the 2 categories was the low-mortality hospital's ability to recognize a complication or problem as it was developing and implement an appropriate change to alter the clinical course. The term "failure to rescue" has been identified in previous studies reviewing other types of procedures as a significant difference distinguishing top-performing hospitals.

As the authors point out, the factors that lead to a "failure to rescue" are unclear and warrant further investigation. These data appear to support previous studies looking at outcomes associated with complex surgical procedures. Hospitals with higher volumes have demonstrated better outcomes and a lower mortality across a broad spectrum of surgical procedures. In the current study, as well as prior studies, the 2 groups demonstrated a similar number of complications. The significant difference between the groups arises in the process of recognizing and acting on the complications, resulting in either a positive or negative outcome. This likely reflects the ability of the hospital system to care for a certain group of patients (eg, postoperative thoracic cancer patients), rather than the ability of a single individual or surgeon. Standardized health care processes (eg, DVT prophylaxis, preoperative antibiotics, etc) was not shown to have a significant benefit between the 2 groups. By having a dedicated or consistent team of care providers, often working from a standardized protocol, however, it is plausible to anticipate problems will be identified in a more timely fashion and acted on in a successful manner. This appears to support the notion that complex or high-risk surgical procedures are best performed in centers where not necessarily the surgeon, but the entire care team, has a robust experience with the clinical disease process.

V. C. Daniel
C. T. Klodell, Jr, MD

Which Patients With ARDS Benefit From Lung Biopsy?

Palakshappa JA, Meyer NJ (Univ of Pennsylvania Perelman School of Medicine, Philadelphia)

Chest 148:1073-1082, 2015

A central tenet of caring for patients with ARDS is to treat the underlying cause, be it sepsis, pneumonia, or removal of an off ending toxin. Identifying the risk factor for ARDS has even been proposed as essential to diagnosing ARDS. Not infrequently, however, the precipitant for acute hypoxemic respiratory failure is unclear, and this raises the question of whether a histologic lung diagnosis would benefit the patient. In this review, we consider the historic role of pathology in establishing a diagnosis of ARDS and the published experience of surgical and transbronchial lung biopsy in patients with ARDS. We reflect on which pathologic diagnoses influence treatment and suggest a patient-centric approach to weigh the risks and benefits of a lung biopsy for critically ill patients who may have ARDS.

▶ Acute respiratory distress syndrome (ARDS) is recognized as an entity that can complicate various severe environmental insults. Often treating the underlying infection or inflammatory condition is considered the most important therapeutic goal. Unfortunately several conditions may mimic ARDS clinically and radiographically, yet have distinct treatments such as pulmonary alveolar proteinosis, acute eosinophilic pneumonia, or hypersensitivity or organizing pneumonia. These considerations may prompt a discussion of an aggressive strategy to obtain a precise diagnosis including open lung biopsy (OLB). However, this must be balanced with the fact that often the diagnostic yield of OLB may not be as high as desired. The real goal of an OLB is to provide the physician with additional diagnostic information and to guide targeted therapy and interventions. Additionally, the overall risk of performing OLB in these critically ill patients who are mechanically ventilated is not insignificant. In fact, in 1 study, the overall mortality for patients who underwent OLB was estimated to be 44%. Transbronchial lung biopsy may be an alternative for histologic lung sampling. However, in the early bronchoscopy literature mechanical ventilation was considered a contraindication although several case series have now been reported as to its safety and efficacy.

The question of whether to pursue OLB in a patient with a clinical syndrome of ARDS does not have a clear answer. The benefit of obtaining a potentially treatable diagnosis must be weighed carefully against the inherit risk of the invasive procedure in a mechanically ventilated patient and the risk of a result that does not affect therapy.

A few key principles can guide us. First, we should not perform a biopsy merely to prove that there is diffuse alveolar damage, because diffuse alveolar damage on pathology is neither specific nor sensitive for the diagnosis of ARDS. Second, we should consider a biopsy if there is a high clinic suspicion for a contributive result and the risk of the empirical therapy is too high, or when empirical therapy has already been implemented and has been proven to be unsuccessful. Third, we must remember that OLB does carry additional risks, but in general they are not disproportionate to the risk of the underlying illness. Patients with ARDS who undergo OLB have similar survival rates to those with ARDS who did not undergo biopsy recognizing that the biopsy was unlikely to have dramatically altered their outcome in an adverse fashion if no diagnostic material resulted in any therapeutic change. Finally, we must not perform the biopsies merely to satisfy the physician's curiosity or desire for certainty.

One other principle to consider is that our outcomes are closely scrutinized in this era, and we must be careful in our documentation if we are to undertake these high-risk procedures. Even though the index procedure is relatively low risk, the overall 30-day survival may be such that it draws the attention of regulatory boards and institutional quality metric reviews. In the end, we must make an individualized choice on a case-by-case basis to determine the best strategy.

C. T. Klodell, Jr, MD

Outcomes in Thoracic Surgical Management of Non-Small Cell Lung Cancer

Wyler von Ballmoos MC, Johnstone DW (Med College of Wisconsin, Milwaukee)

J Surg Oncol 110:539-542, 2014

Thoracic surgeons traditionally have measured their outcomes in terms of mortality, complication rates, recurrence patterns, and long-term survival for their cancer patients. These metrics of quality continue to be important today, but increasingly surgeons are under scrutiny for resource utilization, patient experience, and cost effectiveness. Intelligent decisions about resource use require knowledge of utility, disutility, and cost – information that is still limited and not easily implemented at the time treatment decisions are made. If we accept the proposition that lung cancer care requires a multidisciplinary team making best use of available resources to minimize unwarranted variation, maximize outcomes, and control costs, then three critical needs can be identified: consensus on goals, robust data, and alignment of incentives across disciplines.

▶ Non–small cell lung cancer is the most common malignancy in modern thoracic surgical practice. Surgical programs have long focused on standard outcome metrics to validate their thoracic oncology programs. However, surgeons are increasingly under scrutiny for resource utilization and cost-effectiveness. The value equation, which is the ratio of care quality to expense, has found its way into nearly every discussion about modern programs. Surgical programs now must pay as much attention to the cost of care as they do the quality of care they provide.

Quality indicators are generally divided into structural, process, and outcomes elements. Structural indicators comprise characteristics of the setting and organization of health care providers. This may include teaching versus nonteaching, cancer center designations, and so on. Compelling research has shown that high-volume lung cancer surgery centers have superior outcomes to lower volume sites, even with more complex case mixes. Early postoperative outcomes are better in lung cancer when surgery is performed by someone who is board certified in thoracic surgery and when performed at teaching hospitals. Interestingly, the individual surgeon volume does not appear to be as important a factor as the program volume, suggesting institutional experience and processes may be more important.

Process indicators are derived from clinical research, evidence-based treatment algorithms, and direct the flow of the care delivered. Process indicators focus on smoking cessation consultation for all patients undergoing resection, staging workup, pulmonary function testing, radiation dose limits, and so on.

Outcome indicators are easily understood and have traditionally been used to measure success. Simple end points such as survival and complication rates have been standard.

More recently, end points such as patient satisfaction and pain control have been added to the list. These end points must be given equal attention even though they do not contribute directly to long-term survival or cancer cure. National and regional lung cancer guidelines and care pathways have been developed and now form the foundations for most thoracic oncology programs. They are used for internal program quality assessments and to help with reimbursement. We must accept that lung cancer care requires a multidisciplinary team to make the best use of resources, minimize variation, and control costs. The team must come to consensus on goals, accumulate robust programmatic data, and eliminate financial constraints and silos.

Modern programs must learn to embrace these myriad metrics that will be used to judge our programs. We must scrutinize all these factors internally, while concurrently realizing that in the future, many of them may be publically reported.

C. T. Klodell, Jr, MD

Bronchoscopic lung volume reduction with endobronchial valves for patients with heterogeneous emphysema and intact interlobar fissures (the BeLieVeR-HIFi study): a randomised controlled trial

Davey C, Zoumot Z, Jordan S, et al (Imperial College London, United Kingdom)

Lancet 386:1066-1073, 2015

Background.—Lung volume reduction surgery improves survival in selected patients with emphysema, and has generated interest in bronchoscopic approaches that might achieve the same effect with less morbidity and mortality. Previous trials with endobronchial valves have yielded modest group benefits because when collateral ventilation is present it prevents lobar atelectasis.

Methods.—We did a single-centre, double-blind sham-controlled trial in patients with both heterogeneous emphysema and a target lobe with intact interlobar fissures on CT of the thorax. We enrolled stable outpatients with chronic obstructive pulmonary disease who had a forced expiratory volume in 1 s (FEV_1) of less than 50% predicted, significant hyperinflation (total lung capacity >100% and residual volume >150%), a restricted exercise capacity (6 min walking distance <450 m), and substantial breathlessness (MRC dyspnoea score ≥3). Participants were randomised (1:1) by computer-generated sequence to receive either valves placed to achieve unilateral lobar occlusion (bronchoscopic lung volume reduction) or a bronchoscopy with sham valve placement (control). Patients and researchers were masked to treatment allocation. The study was powered to detect a 15% improvement in the primary endpoint, the FEV_1 3 months after the procedure. Analysis was on an intention-to-treat basis. The trial is registered at controlled-trials.com, ISRCTN04761234.

Findings.—50 patients (62% male, FEV_1 [% predicted] mean 31·7% [SD 10·2]) were enrolled to receive valves (n = 25) or sham valve placement (control, n = 25) between March 1, 2012, and Sept 30, 2013. In the bronchoscopic lung volume reduction group, FEV_1 increased by a median 8·77% (IQR 2·27–35·85) versus 2·88% (0–8·51) in the control group (Mann-Whitney $p = 0{\cdot}0326$). There were two deaths in the bronchoscopic lung volume reduction group and one control patient was unable to attend for follow-up assessment because of a prolonged pneumothorax.

Interpretation.—Unilateral lobar occlusion with endobronchial valves in patients with heterogeneous emphysema and intact interlobar fissures produces significant improvements in lung function. There is a risk of significant complications and further trials are needed that compare valve placement with lung volume reduction surgery.

▶ This article introduces the concept of bronchoscopically placed endobronchial valves as a treatment option for severe chronic obstructive pulmonary disorder. In a limited number of patients, the authors were able to demonstrate a statistically significant benefit by using these endoscopically placed devices. What does not appear to be demonstrated, however, on either a scientific or intellectual level, is how this technique is superior to surgical lung volume reduction therapy. First, the valves are placed unilaterally, whereas in most instances of heterogenous emphysema, the pathology is present bilaterally. Bilateral surgical resection intellectually addresses this issue. Second, it appears that these endobronchial valves by definition create a shunt in that no ventilation or oxygenation occurs yet the lung remains perfused. Again, in the setting of LVRS this issue is addressed with resection of the affected lung. Further, lung volume reduction surgery can preferentially remove only those portions of the lung with severe emphysematous disease present. Placement of a valve within the segmental bronchus may have a deleterious effect on lung parenchyma, which is relatively spared by the pathology present. Finally, the earlier points could probably be overlooked if the procedure demonstrated a significantly improved safety profile. Unfortunately, in the 25 patients treated with the endobronchial valves, 2 patients died within a 90-day period. These mortalities occurred despite the operating physician having a considerable amount of experience performing this procedure. This suggests the placement of these valves requires a certain amount of experience for proficiency, and despite this, it remains a potentially challenging therapeutic intervention. The study suggests there is a distinct subset of patients that may benefit substantially from this intervention. Much more work, however, will be needed to help identify and stratify those patients who would most likely benefit (ie, identifying preprocedure the presence of collateral ventilation and subsequent device failure). And perhaps more important, a prospective trial needs to be performed to demonstrate any potential benefit endobronchial valves may have over the long-term effectiveness demonstrated by lung volume reduction surgery.

V. C. Daniel
C. T. Klodell, Jr, MD

Socioeconomic Risk Factors for Long-Term Mortality after Pulmonary Resection for Lung Cancer: An Analysis of More Than 90,000 Patients from the National Cancer Data Base

Khullar OV, Gillespie T, Nickleach DC, et al (Winship Cancer Inst, Atlanta, GA)
J Am Coll Surg 220:156-168, 2015

Background.—Several clinical variables, such as tumor stage and age, are well established factors associated with long-term survival after surgical resection of lung cancer. Our aim was to examine the impact of other clinical and demographic variables, controlling for known predictors of long-term survival, in order to investigate how outcomes varied according to important nonclinical factors.

Study Design.—The National Cancer Data Base, jointly supported by the Commission on Cancer of the American College of Surgeons and the American Cancer Society, was used to identify patients undergoing pulmonary resection for lung cancer and perform a retrospective cohort study. The cohort consisted of patients diagnosed with nonsmall cell lung cancer from 2003 to 2006, who underwent resection; overall survival data are available only for patients diagnosed through 2006. A Cox proportional hazards survival model was used to examine factors associated with risk of mortality.

Results.—A total of 92,929 patients were identified as diagnosed during the study period and undergoing surgical resection for lung cancer. On multivariable analysis, several socioeconomic factors such as lack of insurance, lower income, less education, and treatment at community centers vs academic or research programs predicted worse overall survival after controlling for disease characteristics known to be predictors of worse survival, such as tumor stage, histology, age, and extent of resection.

Conclusions.—Diminished long-term survival after pulmonary resection was associated with a number of socioeconomic factors. To date, this represents the largest database analysis of long-term mortality in patients undergoing surgical resection for lung cancer.

The disparities in survival outcomes reported here require further detailed investigation.

▶ Long-term survival after treatment for non—small cell lung cancer has previously been associated with several clinical factors. Established factors include tumor stage, lymph node metastases, distal metastases, histology tumor grade, sex, and age. Beyond tumor and patient care characteristics, treatment parameters, such as completeness of surgical resection, lobar versus sublobar resection, number of lymph nodes sampled, and the use of adjuvant and neoadjuvant chemoradiotherapy, have all been associated with survival. However, nonclinical demographic variables such as race, income, and insurance status have been analyzed in a variety of other cancers, such as breast, colon, and gastric cancers, and have been shown to have a significant impact on survival. Limited knowledge exists about how survival after surgical treatment of lung cancer varies according to important nonclinical factors. The authors performed a retrospective cohort study using the National Cancer Database to assess risk factors for overall mortality after pulmonary resection for non—small cell lung cancer only. They identified just about 93 000 patients over a 3-year period. The most common presentation of lung cancer was stage I (62.9%). The majority of patients underwent lobectomy (74.9%). Nearly 90% of patients had some form of lymph node surgery; however, 31% of patients had 3 or fewer lymph nodes examined. The mean number of lymph nodes examined was 7.8, and the mean tumor size was 3.42 cm.

Despite improvements in diagnosis, cancer care and operative care of non—small cell lung cancer, survival rates remain poor and have shown little improvement over time. Lung cancer continues to be the leading cause of cancer-related death in the United States. The authors sought to examine the socioeconomic risk factors that worsened survival after controlling the previously identified clinical risk factors. This study represents the largest retrospective database analysis of surgically resected non—small cell lung cancer to date examining survival as an end point. Controlling for the previously associated risk factors, they were able to more closely examine the impact of the nonclinical factors. Interestingly, similar to other cancers, demographic and socioeconomic characteristics were identified as being associated with worse survival. These included male sex, less education, lower income, government and no insurance, and treatment at no comprehensive community cancer programs. Consistent with other cancers that have been examined, being treated at an academic medical center with active research programs or being treated at a comprehensive community-based cancer center positively affected survival. However, as we focus on future efforts and interventions for these patients, it is important to recognize that these subgroups may be at higher risk for long-term survival issues. This may alter our philosophical approach to their treatment or allow for the development of strategies to mitigate this risk.

C. T. Klodell, Jr, MD

A Contralateral Esophagus-Sparing Technique to Limit Severe Esophagitis Associated With Concurrent High-Dose Radiation and Chemotherapy in Patients With Thoracic Malignancies

Al-Halabi H, Paetzold P, Sharp GC, et al (Harvard Med School, Boston, MA)
Int J Radiat Oncol Biol Phys 92:803-810, 2015

Purpose.—Severe (Radiation Therapy Oncology Group [RTOG] grade 3 or greater) esophagitis generally occurs in 15% to 25% of non–small cell lung cancer (NSCLC) patients undergoing concurrent chemotherapy and radiation therapy (CCRT), which may result in treatment breaks that compromise local tumor control and pose a barrier to dose escalation. Here, we report a novel contralateral esophagus-sparing technique (CEST) that uses intensity modulated radiation therapy (IMRT) to reduce the incidence of severe esophagitis.

Methods and Materials.—We reviewed consecutive patients with thoracic malignancies undergoing curative CCRT in whom CEST was used. The esophageal wall contralateral (CE) to the tumor was contoured as an avoidance structure, and IMRT was used to guide a rapid dose falloff gradient beyond the target volume in close proximity to the esophagus. Esophagitis was recorded based on the RTOG acute toxicity grading system.

Results.—We identified 20 consecutive patients treated with CCRT of at least 63 Gy in whom there was gross tumor within 1 cm of the esophagus. The median radiation dose was 70.2 Gy (range, 63-72.15 Gy). In all patients, ≥99% of the planning and internal target volumes was covered by ≥90% and 100% of prescription dose, respectively. Strikingly, no patient experienced grade ≥3 esophagitis (95% confidence limits, 0%-16%) despite the high total doses delivered. The median maximum dose, V45, and V55 of the CE were 60.7 Gy, 2.1 cc, and 0.4 cc, respectively, indicating effective esophagus cross-section sparing by CEST.

Conclusion.—We report a simple yet effective method to avoid exposing the entire esophagus cross-section to high doses. By using proposed CE dose constraints of V45 <2.5 cc and V55 <0.5 cc, CEST may improve the esophagus toxicity profile in thoracic cancer patients receiving CCRT even at doses above the standard 60- to 63-Gy levels. Prospective testing of CEST is warranted.

▶ In this article, the author adapts a proven successful technique of radiation delivery used in the treatment of prostate cancer and applies those same principles in a novel manner to the treatment of thoracic malignancies to ameliorate the esophageal side effects. Their results are impressive in terms of reduced esophageal toxicity. By definition, many thoracic malignancies treated with definitive chemoradiation therapy will likely result in a significant esophageal exposure to the radiation field, particularly in the common scenario of mediastinal N2 and N3 disease. By sparing the contralateral wall of the esophagus from the direct radiation field, they have demonstrated a dramatic reduction in the severity of esophageal toxicity while maintaining a continuous treatment regimen and delivering a maximal dose of radiation treatment. Although the sample size was fairly small, the results were impressive, with no Grade 3 toxicity noted. What is not known is the efficacy of the treatment provided, which the authors clearly acknowledge in their discussion. The next steps would be to perform the same process in a prospective fashion and examine disease-free and overall survival as well as evaluating toxicity. Certainly as a proof of concept, however, the group should be congratulated for demonstrating effectiveness at reducing a significant toxicity associated with this therapy.

V. C. Daniel
C. T. Klodell, Jr, MD

To drain or not to drain? Predictors of tube thoracostomy insertion and outcomes associated with drainage of traumatic hemothoraces

Wells BJ, Roberts DJ, Grondin S, et al (Univ of Calgary, Canada; et al)
Injury 46:1743-1748, 2015

Introduction.—Historical data suggests that many traumatic hemothoraces (HTX) can be managed expectantly without tube thoracostomy (TT) drainage. The purpose of this study was to identify predictors of TT, including whether the quantity of pleural blood predicted tube placement, and to evaluate outcomes associated with TT versus expected management (EM) of traumatic HTXs.

Patients and Methods.—A retrospective cohort study of all trauma patients with HTXs and an Injury Severity Score (ISS) ≥12 managed at a level I trauma centre between April 1, 2005 and December 31, 2012 was completed. Mixed-effects models with a subject-specific random intercept were used to identify independent risk factors for TT. Logistic and log-linear regression were used to compute odds ratios (ORs) for mortality and empyema and percent increases in length of hospital and intensive care unit stay between patients managed with TT versus EM, respectively.

Results.—A total of 635 patients with 749 HTXs were included in the study. Overall, 491 (66%) HTXs were drained while 258 (34%) were managed expectantly. Independent predictors of TT placement included concomitant ipsilateral flail chest [OR 3.03; 95% confidence interval (CI) 1.04–8.80; $p = 0.04$] or pneumothorax (OR 6.19; 95% CI 1.79–21.5; $p < 0.01$) and the size of the HTX (OR per 10 cc increase 1.12; 95% CI 1.04–1.21; $p < 0.01$). Although the adjusted odds of mortality were not significantly different between groups (OR 3.99; 95% CI 0.87–18.30; $p = 0.08$), TT was associated with a 47.14% (95% CI, 25.57–69.71%; $p < 0.01$) adjusted increase in hospital length of stay. Empyemas (n = 29) only occurred among TT patients.

Conclusions.—Expectant management of traumatic HTX was associated with a shorter length of hospital stay, no empyemas, and no increase in mortality. Although EM of smaller HTXs may be safe, these findings must be confirmed by a large multi-centre cohort study and randomized controlled trials before they are used to guide practice.

▶ Hemothoraces are common after thoracic trauma and are associated with significant morbidity and mortality. The incidence of hemothoraces has been increasing due to the near ubiquitous use of computed tomography and the adoption of top to bottom scanning of trauma patients. Although hemothoraces are effectively managed through tube thoracostomy drainage of the pleural space, this intervention is associated with numerous potential complications, including iatrogenic injury, retained hemothoraces, and empyema. The consensus guideline suggests that all hemothoraces should be considered for drainage regardless of size, as well as the relatively low complication profile of the chest tube insertion.

However, it is unclear whether chest tubes are being overutilized. With this in mind, the authors undertook this study to identify predictors of tube thoracostomy including whether the quantity of pleural blood predicted tube placement, and evaluate outcomes associated with thoracic tube drainage versus expected management of traumatic hemothoraces. The working hypothesis was that thoracic tube placement would have no association with clinically relevant outcomes but may predispose patients to an increased risk of empyema. For this study, the authors assessed 635 patients with a total of 749 hemothoraces over a 7-year period. Their univariant analysis demonstrated that their tube thoracostomy was predicted by penetrating trauma mechanism, hemodynamic instability, concomitant ipsilateral injury, tachypnea, and endotracheal intubation, as well as intensive care unit admission. Additionally, the tube thoracostomy patients had a median hemathorax volume that was more than 2 times that of the expectantly managed hemothorax patients. There were, however, 110 patients that were initially slotted for expectant management that required a tube thoracostomy in delayed fashion. This is independently predicated by an ipsilateral pulmonary contusion or hemothorax size with an odds ratio of 1.03 per 10 cc increase in hemothorax volume.

Among severely injured patients with traumatic hemothoraces that present to a level 1 trauma center over this 8-year period, the authors find that concomitant ipsilateral hemithoracic in flail chest as well hemothorax size were independent predictors of thoracic tube. Although there was no associated mortality benefit from chest tube placement in this retrospective cohort analysis, there was an increase in hospital length of stay.

However, it is important to recognize that this is retrospective study design and that the management of traumatic hemothorax was not standardized. Although it remains plausible that not all severely injured patients with traumatic hemothoraces require thoracostomy drainage, we must remain circumspect when generalizing to the overall trauma population. It is possible and reasonable to consider in the clinically stable patient with adequate monitoring, and the absence of significant concomitant thoracic injury, that small traumatic hemothoraces may be safe to manage expectantly. However, without more broad study, in a multicenter randomized fashion, caution should be exercised at this time when applying this in a generalized fashion.

C. T. Klodell, Jr, MD

Resection of Primary and Secondary Tumors of the Sternum: An Analysis of Prognostic Variables

Ahmad U, Yang H, Sima C, et al (Memorial Sloan Kettering Cancer Ctr; et al)
Ann Thorac Surg 100:215-222, 2015

Background.—We sought to determine the prognostic variables associated with overall survival (OS) and recurrence-free probability (RFP) in patients with primary and secondary sternal tumors treated with surgical resection.

Methods.—A retrospective analysis of patients who underwent resection of primary or secondary sternal tumors at 2 cancer institutes between 1995 and 2013 was performed. OS and RFP were estimated using the Kaplan-Meier method, and predictors of OS and RFP were analyzed using the Cox proportional hazards model.

Results.—Sternal resection was performed in 78 patients with curative (67 [86%]) or palliative (6 [8%]) intent. Seventy-three patients (94%) had malignant tumors, of which 28 (36%) were primary and 45 (57%) were secondary malignancies. Sternal resections were complete in 13 patients (17%) and partial in 65 (83%). There were no perioperative deaths, and grade III/IV complications were noted in 17 patients (22%). The 5-year OS was 80% for patients with primary malignant tumors, 73% for patients with nonbreast secondary malignant tumors, and 58% for patients with breast tumors ($p = 0.85$). In the overall cohort, R0 resection was associated with prolonged 5-year OS (84% vs 20%) on univariate ($p = 0.004$) and multivariate (adjusted hazard ratio, 3.37; $p = 0.029$) analysis. On subgroup analysis, R0 resection was associated with improved OS and RFP only for patients with primary malignant tumors.

Conclusions.—Sternal resection can achieve favorable OS for patients with primary and secondary sternal tumors. R0 resection is associated with improved 5-year OS and RFP in patients with primary malignant tumors. We did not detect a similar effect in patients with breast or nonbreast secondary tumors.

▶ Resection of tumor involving the sternum is a challenging procedure because it puts both hemithoraces at risk of instability and requires complex reconstruction. Sternal resections have been performed for primary and secondary sternal tumors, including breast cancer with both curative and palliative intent. For patients with primary sternal tumors, a 5-year overall survival rate of 49% to 92% with better prognosis is determined based on tumor grade and completeness of resection, which have been shown to associate with overall survival in multiple reports. Secondary sternal tumors compose a heterogeneous group that includes metastatic tumors that involve invasion of local tissues such as breast cancer. Breast cancer is the most widely studied secondary sternal tumor and has a 5-year overall survival rate of 20% to 60% depending on the study. Although any chest wall invasion portends a poor prognosis, it may be appropriate to consider sternal resection in highly selected patients, such as those with isolated bone recurrence no nodal involvement and an extended disease-free interval. The authors undertook this study to examine the critical outcomes and prognostic factors associated with overall survival and recurrence-free probability for patients with primary and secondary sternal tumors and breast cancers treated with sternectomy. They queried a prospectively maintained database at 2 cancer centers and retrospectively for these patients that were treated between 1995 and 2013. As expected, sternal resection was performed with low morbidity and mortality. Primary malignant sternal tumors portend favorable overall survival and recurrence-free probability after resection especially associated with an R0 resection. Overall survival for breast cancer was poorer than for primary or other secondary malignant tumors. Chondrosarcomas are the most common primary malignant sternal tumors.

This large series closely parallels our experience with sternal resection. We are fortunate to have a robust orthopedic oncology group and therefore perform a relatively high number of sternal resections for sarcoma. Our experience has been that with R0 resection and good reconstruction with methylmethacrylate and Marlex sandwich type reconstruction that good survival and sternal stability can be achieved. Similar to the author's conclusions, we should be extremely circumspect when evaluating patients, particularly with breast cancer metastatic to the sternum and directly invading the chest wall and sternum, for appropriateness of resection. In appropriately selected cases, good survival benefit can be obtained.

C. T. Klodell, Jr, MD

VATS versus intrapleural streptokinase: A prospective, randomized, controlled clinical trial for optimum treatment of post-traumatic Residual Hemothorax

Kumar S, Rathi V, Rattan A, et al (Guru Teg Bahadur Hosp, New Delhi, India; JPN Apex Trauma Ctr, New Delhi, India)
Injury 46:1749-1752, 2015

Background.—Post-traumatic residual haemothorax (RH) is common and carries significant morbidity. However, its optimal treatment is not clear.

Aim.—The aim of this study was to find the extent of this problem and the choice of treatment between VATS and intra-pleural streptokinase instillation (IPSI).

Material and Methods.—This RCT, conducted over 18 months period, included all patients of chest trauma between 18 and 70 years of age, admitted with haemothorax or haemopneumothorax requiring intercostal drain (ICD) insertion. 154 events of haemothorax/haemopneumothorax requiring ICD insertion were enrolled. RH was seen in 48 (31%) patients: 13 patients were excluded from RCT after refusal for treatment. Seventeen (49%) patients of remaining 35 RH cases were randomized to IPSI group and 18 (51%) patients were randomized to VATS group. The outcome parameters were resolution of RH and treatment related complications.

Results.—RH resolved equally well in VATS and IPSI group [13 patients (72%) versus 12 patients (71%), respectively; continuity-adjusted $p = 1$]. Morbidity wise no difference (p-value 0.529) was seen in the two groups.

Conclusion.—Post-traumatic RH is seen in 1/3rd patients and is equally well treated by VATS and IPSI.

▶ Posttraumatic hemothorax is a collection of blood in the pleural space and may be caused by blunt or penetrating trauma. In most cases, simple drainage by an intercostal chest tube placed under local anesthetic is both sufficient and an excellent resolution of the problem. However, complete resolution of the hemothorax does not always succeed, and retained intrapleural collections can be referred to as a residual hemothorax. The incidence of residual hemothorax has been reported variable between 5% and 30% and may organize, resulting in a loss of lung volume and empyema if left untreated. Most residual hemothoraces therefore need evacuation.

Historically, thoracotomy had been used, but it carries significant complications, such as morbidity and mortality. More recently, video-assisted thorascopic surgery (VATS) has been shown to be highly successful for treatment of these residual collections. Alternatively, some have used intrapleural streptokinase instillation, which has been advocated as an alternative in low-resource settings where the relatively costly and sophisticated techniques of VATS may not be available, feasible, or applicable. The authors report their experience in a randomized trial in which all patients that had residual hemothorax at 48 hours after chest drain placement were randomized to receive either intrapleural streptokinase or VATS. This resulted in 154 events in 146 patients of retained hemothoraces who were studied. As expected, the hospital stay was longer in the streptokinase group compared with the VATS group; however, overall the ability to clear the hemothorax of retained blood products was very similar.

Chest trauma is a common aspect of polytrauma. Untreated chest trauma is associated with high morbidity and mortality; however, most cases simple intervention such as oxygen therapy and intrapleural chest drainage reduce the morbidity and mortality. Broadly speaking, any residual pleural collection beyond 48 to 72 hours after chest tube insertion should be addressed. These retained hemothoraces can become a significant cause of morbidity and mortality, leading to pleural sepsis or lung entrapment. Previously published large multicenter trial by DeBose et al showed promising results for treatment of residual hemothoraces with VATS. However, many patients required 2 or more procedures and thoracotomy was ultimately required in 20%. Those authors reported a residual hemothorax of less than 900 cc to be an independent predictor of successful outcome with VATS.

Intrapleural streptokinase instillation is a good alternative for high-risk surgical patients. In the current study, no hemorrhagic complications were found after the installation of streptokinase.

This is one of the few studies that provide comparative data between intrapleural streptokinase instillation and VATS in the treatment of residual hemothorax. Moreover, none of the prior studies were randomized prospectively such as this trial.

Residual hemothorax continues to affect a substantial proportion of patients with chest trauma who require chest tube drainage and have retained blood products at the 48-hour postinjury time point. When feasible, VATS has clear advantage with shorter length of stay and improved diagnostic and therapeutic extensions but may not be appropriate for every patient. A reasonable second choice is intrapleural streptokinase installation, which has been proven to be well tolerated, reasonably available, acceptable, and economically advantageous compared with VATS in the treatment of residual hemothorax, especially in the situations where VATS is contraindicated or not available.

C. T. Klodell, Jr, MD

Pre- and Postoperative Management

Unexpected readmission after lung cancer surgery: A benign event?

Puri V, Patel AP, Crabtree TD, et al (Washington Univ School of Medicine, St Louis, MO)

J Thorac Cardiovasc Surg 150:1496-1505, 2015

Objective.—The study objective was to study the incidence, predictors, and implications of unanticipated early postoperative readmission after lung resection for non–small cell lung cancer.

Methods.—Patients undergoing surgery for clinical stage I to III non–small cell lung cancer were abstracted from the National Cancer Database. Regression models were fitted to identify predictors of 30-day readmission and to study the association of unplanned readmission with 30-day and long-term survival.

Results.—Between 1998 and 2010, 129,893 patients underwent resection for stage I to III non–small cell lung cancer. Of these, 5624 (4.3%) were unexpectedly readmitted within 30 days. In a multivariate regression model, increasing age, male gender, preoperative radiation, and pneumonectomy (odds ratio, 1.77; 95% confidence interval, 1.56-2.00) were associated with unexpected readmissions. Longer index hospitalization and higher Charlson comorbidity score were also predictive of readmission. The 30-day mortality for readmitted patients was higher (3.9% vs 2.8%), as was the 90-day mortality (7.0% vs 3.3%, both $P < .001$). In a multivariate Cox proportional hazards model of long-term survival, increasing age, higher Charlson comorbidity score, and higher pathologic stage (hazard ratio, for stage III 1.81; 95% confidence interval, 1.42-2.29) were associated with greater risk of mortality. Unplanned readmission was independently associated with a higher risk of long-term mortality (hazard ratio, 1.40; 95% confidence interval, 1.34-1.47). The median survival for readmitted patients was significantly shorter (38.7 vs 58.5 months, $P < .001$).

Conclusions.—Unplanned readmissions are not rare after resection for non–small cell lung cancer. Such events are associated with a greater

risk of short- and long-term mortality. With the renewed national focus on readmissions and potential financial disincentives, greater resource allocation is needed to identify patients at risk and develop measures to avoid the associated adverse outcomes.

▶ Hospital readmission is sentinel event after lung cancer surgery and is seen in at least 5% to 15% of patients. Readmission may be planned, for instance, to place intravenous devices such as ports for chemotherapy, or they may be unplanned as a direct consequence of the operation. Unexpected postoperative readmission are a major financial burden to the health care system, and now the Affordable Care Act incorporates a reduction including mandating public reporting of readmission rates with potential penalties for institutions with excessive readmission rates. Therefore, understanding and ameliorating unexpected postoperative readmissions after lung resections are medical and financial necessities for thoracic surgery programs.

Several patient and treatment related factors have been found to be associated with a higher risk of readmission. These include increasing age, male gender, lower socioeconomic status, and higher levels of comorbidity. More complex operations such as pneumonectomy and chest wall resection are also risk factors. Major postoperative complications and lack of social support also predict a greater likelihood of unplanned readmission. Recently publications have also shown a greater risk of 90-day mortality related to early readmission after lung surgery. The authors conducted a retrospective review of all patients that underwent resection for stage I to stage III non–small cell lung cancer from 1998 to 2010 from a national cancer database. They extracted 129 893 patients, yielding 5624 or 4.3% with unexpected readmission within 30 days of surgery. Readmitted patients were more likely to be older and to be male, had a lower socioeconomic status, and had a higher comorbidity score. Readmitted patients were also more likely to be from rural areas, to be treated in nonacademic institutions, and have a longer in-hospital index hospitalization (7.3 vs 9.0 days, $P < .001$).

The 30-day mortality for readmitted patients was also higher at 3.9% versus 2.8% for those that did not require readmission. Similarly, the 90-day mortality was 7% versus 3.3% for those that did not require readmission. The main finding of this study is that early readmission after lung resection for non–small cell lung cancer is seen in more than 4% of patients. Although patient factors such as age, gender, comorbidity, and extent of surgery determine the risk of readmission, the predictive ability of every model tried thus far has been at best modest. Higher rates of early mortality were seen in readmitted patients. Readmission is noted to be an independent risk factor for long-term mortality.

Most unanticipated readmissions after lung resection are due to pleural or pulmonary pathology or health care–associated infections. Postoperative readmissions after lung cancer surgery are generally associated with a greater risk of short-term mortality. Another important finding of this study is that readmitted patients had a shorter overall long-term survival. This study did suffer from the fact that it is a retrospective database study and reflects a broad range from different centers and situations. The findings may not be applicable to highly focused institutions with streamlined care for thoracic oncology patients. However, we can draw from this study that unplanned readmissions are not rare events after resection for lung cancer. Additionally it should be noted that such events should be associated with a higher risk of short- and long-term mortality. With such enhanced national focus on readmissions and the potential financial disincentives to treating institutions, greater resources should be allocated to identifying the patients at risk for readmission and developing strategies for mitigating these risks.

C. T. Klodell, Jr, MD

Open Lung Biopsy Among Critically Ill, Mechanically Ventilated Patients: A Metaanalysis

Wong AK, Walkey AJ (Boston Univ School of Medicine, MA)

Ann Am Thorac Soc 12:1226-1230, 2015

Rationale.—Open lung biopsy may be performed to guide therapy in mechanically ventilated patients with diagnostic uncertainty regarding etiology of pulmonary infiltrates. Current evidence for open lung biopsy in mechanically ventilated patients comes from single-center case series.

Objectives.—We performed a metaanalysis of case series to determine diagnoses, complications, and changes in therapy after lung biopsy in critically ill patients requiring mechanical ventilation.

Methods.—We searched Medline for case series of lung biopsies in critically ill patients requiring mechanical ventilation. We pooled results of individual case series using random effects metaanalysis models to obtain summary proportions.

Measurements and Main Results.—We identified 14 case series including a total of 512 mechanically ventilated patients with 530 histopathological diagnoses. The most common diagnoses were "fibrosis/pneumonitis" (n = 155, 25%; 95% confidence interval [CI], 14–37%) and infection (n = 113, 20%; 95% CI, 15–27%). Viruses were the most commonly identified infectious etiology identified on open lung biopsy, representing 50% of potential pathogens. Diffuse alveolar damage was present in a minority of specimens (n = 100, 16%; 95% CI, 8–25%). Therapeutic changes after lung biopsy occurred in 399 patients (78%; 95% CI, 64–81%). Procedure-related complications occurred in 29% of patients (95% CI, 25–33%), most commonly persistent air leak. Mortality among mechanically ventilated patients after diagnostic open lung biopsy was 54%.

Conclusions.—Among mechanically ventilated patients with respiratory failure of unclear etiology, lung biopsy yielded a wide range of diagnoses and was associated with a change in therapy in most patients.

▶ In this article, the authors continue to add to the growing evidence that open lung biopsy provides beneficial information for patients with respiratory failure.

In their meta-analysis of 14 single-center case series, they found that of 512 ventilated patients, 78% had a change in therapy based directly on the results of the open lung biopsy. The majority of these changes came about from new therapy being instituted or tailoring of current therapy to a more specific pathogen (79%). Therapy was discontinued on the basis of the biopsy in 10%. This meta-analysis further supports the concept that open lung biopsy for unidentified parenchymal lung disease consistently results in a change of management and should therefore be strongly considered in patients in whom no tissue diagnosis is available and current treatment strategies are not successful. Similar benefits have been demonstrated for open lung biopsy in the diagnosis and treatment of interstitial lung disease as well. Although our imaging through technology has become increasingly sophisticated and invaluable to current clinical practice, it cannot replace the pathology and culture results provided by a surgical specimen. Too often clinical decisions are based solely on the imaging provided, and yet, as this study demonstrates, the working diagnosis of acute respiratory distress syndrome was identified pathologically in only 16% of patient specimens. Our ability to make an accurate diagnosis simply from a chest x-ray or chest CT continues to fall short, and tissue confirmation remains an important guide for clinical therapy. What this study does not demonstrate is how this change in therapy altered the ultimate outcome for the patient. Despite the majority of patients having a change in overall therapy, the mortality of mechanically ventilated patients undergoing an open lung biopsy remains high at 54%. What percentage that number would have been in the absence of a tissue diagnosis will likely be impossible to determine. The timing of the open lung biopsies averaged 7.8 ± 4.3 days after initiation of mechanical ventilation. It raises the question of how overall mortality would be affected if diagnostic tissue was obtained in an earlier time frame after mechanical ventilation was initiated and more appropriate therapy could be started. Conversely, in the culture of increased outcomes scrutiny, there must be excellent documentation of the anticipated clinical course and outcome when survival may be relatively low even with the lung biopsy.

V. C. Daniel
C. T. Klodell, Jr, MD

Safety of Outpatient Chest Tube Management of Air Leaks After Pulmonary Resection

Royer AM, Smith JS, Miller A, et al (Univ of Tennessee College of Medicine, Chattanooga)
Am Surg 81:760-763, 2015

Prolonged air leaks are the most common postoperative complication following pulmonary resection, leading to increased hospital length of stay (LOS) and cost. This study assesses the safety of discharging patients home with a chest tube (CT) after pulmonary resection. A retrospective review was performed of a single surgeon's experience with pulmonary resections from January 2010 to January 2015. All patients discharged home with a CT were included. Discharge criteria included a persistent air leak controlled by water seal, resolution of medical conditions requiring hospitalization, and pain managed by oral analgesics. Patient demographics, type of resection, LOS, and 30-day morbidity and mortality data were analyzed. Comparisons were made with the Society of Thoracic Surgery database January 2011 to December 2013. Four hundred ninety-six patients underwent pulmonary resection. Sixty-five patients (13%) were discharged home postoperatively with a CT. Fifty-eight patients underwent a lobectomy, two patients a bilobectomy, and five patients had a wedge excision. Two patients were readmitted: One with a lower extremity deep venous thrombosis and the other with a nonlife threatening pulmonary embolus. Four patients developed superficial CT site infections that resolved after oral antibiotics. Patients discharged home with a CT following lobectomy had a shorter mean LOS compared to lobectomy patients (3.65 *vs* 6.2 days). Mean time to CT removal after discharge was 4.7 days (range 1-22 days) potentially saving 305 inpatient hospital days. Select patients can be discharged home with a CT with reduced postoperative LOS and without increase in major morbidity or mortality.

▶ Chest tubes are placed at the time of pulmonary resection for removal of fluid from the pleural cavity, as well as evacuation of pneumothorax associated with postresection air leaks. Chest tubes are removed once fluid drainage has slowed and there is no evidence of air leak. Prolonged air leaks are the most prevalent postoperative complication after pulmonary resection, leading to prolonged hospital stay and increased cost. Historically, prolonged air leak has been any leak lasting longer than 5 days. With the modern techniques of minimally invasive surgery, patients are frequently ready for discharge before that time point. Historically, various devices, such as Heimlich valves and portable mini chest tube bottles have been used for postoperative air leaks. The authors of this study began prospectively collecting data in 2010 on patients managed as an outpatient with their chest tube still in place. Interestingly, they defined prolonged air leak as any patient with an air leak present that is otherwise ready for discharge. Before discharge home, all patients were placed on a mini portable drain and watched for a minimum of 3 hours. In total, they studied 65 patients, which represented 13% of their lung resection patients who were discharged home postoperatively with a chest tube in place. Nearly all these patients were operated on with a minimally invasive approach. The outpatient management was almost universally successful with minimal morbidity.

Thoracic surgery has evolved over the past decade to where intensive care unit admissions are almost nonexistent and minimally invasive surgery is commonplace. However, there has been little progress in the management of prolonged air leaks, and this often translates to a prolonged length of stay and increased hospital costs.

In this important study, the authors document their experience after pulmonary resection in which patients were discharged home on an average of postoperative day 3.65 and managed with a portable drain. This represents an earlier discharge than the average in the STS National Database of 6.2 days. Additionally, the morbidity associated with the outpatient management was minimal. This article nicely confirms that patients can be safely discharged earlier from the hospital and managed as an outpatient until their chest tube can be safely removed.

With increasing hospital and quality metric pressures directed toward shortening length of stay while increasing or maintaining quality, this represents an additional or potential facet of care in which there is an opportunity to expedite the patient transition to home without compromising their quality of care.

C. T. Klodell, Jr, MD

Esophageal Cancer

Treatment of Diaphragmatic Hernia Occurring After Transhiatal Esophagectomy

Narayanan S, Sanders RL, Herlitz G, et al (Rutgers Robert Wood Johnson, New Brunswick, NJ; et al)

Ann Surg Oncol 22:3681-3686, 2015

Background.—Postesophagectomy diaphragmatic hernia (DH) is an uncommon problem but an important one to recognize and treat because of the risk of significant complications such as incarceration and strangulation. Diaphragmatic hernia appears to occur more frequently following transhiatal esophagectomy (THE) than after transthoracic procedures, likely because of the enlargement of the diaphragmatic hiatus required to perform THE.

Methods.—After 199 consecutive esophagectomies were performed at Rutgers Robert Wood Johnson University Hospital between January 2000 and June 2013, ten patients were identified with DH; all underwent diaphragmatic hernia repair (DHR). All patients who underwent esophagectomy during this time period were cataloged in a prospectively maintained database that was then retrospectively reviewed. All DH were repaired using a novel biologic plug mesh technique.

Results.—Ten esophagectomy patients developed DH; nine post-THE and one post-McKeown esophagectomy. One patient was excluded from analysis because of atypical presentation. Demographic data were similar between esophagectomy patients who developed DH and those who did not. Administration of neoadjuvant chemoradiation correlated with development of DH, but did not reach statistical significance. Complications directly related to DHR were few and mostly infectious, including empyema and pneumonia, and were more likely to occur in those who presented with acute obstruction. One patient presented with dysphagia post repair.

Conclusions.—Diaphragmatic hernia development post esophagectomy is an uncommon complication, but can have devastating results when there is bowel compromise. Repair by plugging the diaphragmatic hiatus

with a biologic mesh is a safe and effective method for closing the defect and results in few complications.

▶ Transhiatal esophagectomy is a common operative treatment for esophageal cancer. It has a lower short-term complication rate than esophagectomy with thoracotomy, and the 5-year survival rate is comparable. It can prevent complications associated with intrathoracic anastomosis, such as mediastinitis secondary to leak, and some studies demonstrate a significantly lower incidence of pulmonary complications. Diaphragmatic hernias are an uncommon but serious complication following esophagectomy and can occur both early and late in the perioperative period. Early complications are thought to occur because of the absence of adhesion formation in immediate postoperative period, and late diaphragmatic hernia likely occurs as a result of progressive dilatation of the diaphragmatic hiatus secondary to increased intra-abdominal pressure.

Postesophagectomy diaphragmatic hernias are important to recognize and treat because of the risk of serious complications such as respiratory distress, intestinal obstruction, strangulation, intrathoracic perforation, sepsis, and death.

The incidence, time course, sequelae, and risk of diaphragmatic hernias after transhiatal esophagectomy have not been fully elucidated. The authors review a single-institution experience with postesophagectomy diaphragmatic hernia to determine risk factors, time course and patient outcomes, and the results of a novel biologic mesh plug treatment. They reviewed 199 esophagectomies over a period of 13 years. They identified 9 patients that had diaphragmatic hiatus after transhiatal esophagectomy and analyzed it for risk factors predicting the occurrence.

A total of 173 patients with diaphragmatic hernia development after esophagectomy have been reported in the literature since 1987. The majority of these hernias have been described in case reports and small series, with only a few larger studies. Most hernias occurred in patients who underwent transhiatal esophagectomy because of the technical necessity of widening the esophageal diaphragmatic hiatus to mobilize the gastric conduit into the chest and safely perform the mediastinal dissection. However, at least 1 large study in the literature failed to find a difference in the incidence of transthoracic esophagectomy and transhiatal esophagectomy, with each being slightly under 1%. The group reported a personal incidence of diaphragmatic hernia development postesophagectomy of 0.5% in this particular study. Despite those reports, little is known of the time course of diaphragmatic hernia following esophagectomy or the risk factors. The authors of the current study find the 5% occurrence of diaphragmatic hernia occurrence, which is in the range reported in the general literature but higher than some that were reported. Time course to development was extremely variable. In the current report, the only identifiable risk factor associated with the development of diaphragmatic hernia that reached near statistical significance was in patients who received neoadjuvant chemoirradiation before esophagectomy. No patients in this series developed recurrent diaphragmatic after repair, which might be related to the use of the biological mesh as a plug rather than an attempt to directly repair the hernia defect. These authors report a somewhat novel approach using biologic mesh loosely sutured to 270 degrees of the hiatus with no attempt to repair the crural defect directly. They report leaving approximately 4 cm of space between hiatus and conduit. Additionally, although no routine assessment of swallowing was performed, only 1 patient complained of dysphagia and was discovered to have pyloric narrowing secondary to mesh placement that improved with endoscopic dilation. No other mesh complications such as erosion were reported.

In conclusion, the incidence of diaphragmatic hernia following esophagectomy is low but seems to be higher, perhaps, in patients who have undergone transhiatal esophagectomy because of the technical nuances of the procedure. Urgent repair of postoperative hernias containing abdominal viscera are important to prevent devastating complications. The author's technique of using a biological mesh plug without any attempt to reapproximate the crural defect directly may be effective in preventing recurrences without compromising the gastric conduit.

C. T. Klodell, Jr, MD

Intra-Operative Concerns

Esophageal Perforation and Acute Bacterial Mediastinitis: Other Causes of Chest Pain That Can Be Easily Missed

Cross MR, Greenwald MF, Dahhan A (Univ of Iowa, Iowa City)
Medicine (Baltimore) 94:e1232, 2015

Esophageal perforation is a rare condition that is commonly missed. Male gender and alcohol use are predisposing risk factors. Most of the cases are iatrogenic or traumatic; nonetheless, spontaneous cases are not uncommon. It typically occurs after vomiting or straining as the increased intra-abdominal pressure transmits into the esophagus and results in the tear. One of the main complications is acute bacterial mediastinitis from contamination with esophageal flora. This condition can be life-threatening because it is very frequently misdiagnosed and appropriate management is often delayed.

A 49-year-old man presented with worsening sudden-onset interscapular back pain that then changed to chest pain with odynophagia and was found to have fever and leukocytosis.

Chest computed tomography revealed signs of mediastinitis with possible esophageal perforation. He reported symptoms started 2 days ago after lifting of heavy objects. Empiric antimicrobial was begun with conservative management and avoidance of oral intake. Barium esophagram and esophagogastroduodenoscopy revealed no signs of perforation or inflammation. His symptoms resolved and he gradually resumed oral intake. Blood cultures grew Methicillin-sensitive *Staphylococcus aureus* and he was discharged on appropriate antibiotics for 4 weeks. He did well on follow-up 3 months after hospitalization.

The case highlights the importance of considering esophageal etiologies of chest pain.

▶ Esophageal perforation is a somewhat rare but potentially lethal disease process. Untreated bacterial mediastinitis is associated with a high mortality. This case report highlights a 49-year-old man who presents with a 2-day history of chest pain in the setting of a spontaneous esophageal perforation. This is identified by findings of mediastinitis on chest CT. In addition to the more common diagnoses that accompany chest pain (eg, acute coronary disease, aortic dissection, pneumothorax, esophageal spasm), the article highlights esophageal perforation as a potentially lethal process that can also present clinically in a similar fashion. The diagnosis can generally be inferred from the history and chest CT findings. Confirmation of the diagnosis may be made by barium esophagram or endoscopy. Prompt treatment includes nothing by mouth (NPO), broad-spectrum antibiotics (including anaerobes and antifungals), and often mediastinal drainage if necessary to control the infection.

Esophageal perforation is a challenging clinical problem to manage. Severe sepsis, acute respiratory distress syndrome, multisystem organ failure, and death are all potential sequelae of perforation, and classically the longer the delay in diagnosis, the poorer the outcome becomes. Furthermore, the management of esophageal perforations continues to evolve with no 1 method entirely successful for all presentations. Primary repair of the perforation, controlled fistulization (eg, via T-tube), exclusion, and mediastinal drainage, and more recently esophageal stent placement are all strategies used in the treatment of this process. However, no method will necessarily be appropriate for every perforation. The majority of perforations are iatrogenic and therefore may be recognized and acted on more promptly. Spontaneous esophageal perforation, typically in the form of postemetic esophageal rupture, may present in a more delayed fashion with associated greater morbidity and mortality. Early recognition and treatment, as highlighted in this article, is the key to achieving a potentially better outcome.

V. C. Daniel
C. T. Klodell, Jr, MD

Left upper lobectomy after coronary artery bypass grafting

Wei B, Broussard B, Bryant A, et al (Univ of Alabama at Birmingham Med Ctr)
J Thorac Cardiovasc Surg 150:531-535, 2015

Objective.—Left upper pulmonary lobectomy or segmentectomy after coronary artery bypass grafting (CABG) risks injury to the grafts. We reviewed our experience.

Methods.—This is a retrospective review of a prospective database from 1 surgeon, of patients who underwent left upper lobectomy after having previous CABG.

Results.—Between June 1998 and June 2014, a total of 2207 patients underwent lobectomy by 1 surgeon; 458 (21%) had a left upper lobectomy, and 28 (6.1%) had had a previous CABG. Twenty-seven patients (96.4%) had a left internal mammary artery (LIMA) used for the bypass. Twenty-six patients (96.2%) had significant adhesions between their lung and the bypass grafts. Of patients who had a LIMA graft, 25 (92.6%) had the left upper lobe completely dissected free from their grafts, whereas 2 patients (7.1%) had a sliver of their lung left on the grafts. No patient had a postoperative myocardial infarction, and 30-day and 90-day survival rates were both 100%. All patients had a curative resection, and all had complete thoracic lymphadenectomy.

Conclusions.—Left upper lobectomy after CABG, in patients with previous CABG and LIMA grafting, is safe. Usually the entire lung can be safely mobilized off the bypass grafts; if needed, a small sliver of lung can be left on the grafts. A curative resection is possible with minimal perioperative cardiac morbidity, and excellent 30- and 90-day mortality.

▶ Previous coronary bypass grafting can complicate lung surgery, related to the adhesion formation particularly at the location of bypass grafts. This may be predictably problematic when a pedicled left internal mammary artery has been strung across to the left anterior descending becomes adherent to the left upper lobe. Left upper lobectomy can then become somewhat treacherous because many patients may be dependent on the left internal mammary artery for coronary perfusion. The authors reviewed their single-center experience with a single surgeon over a 16-year period, during which time 28 patients with previous coronary artery bypass operations had left upper lobectomy. Nearly 90% of the patients underwent thoracotomy, as the original plan, and 3 patients had a robotic attempt with 2 of the 3 requiring conversion. In 93% of patients, the left upper lobe was able to be completely mobilized off the left internal mammary artery graft, and 2 (7.4%) had a thin wedge of lung left attached to it. In all cases, the planned resection was accomplished, and it was anticipated that the patients would have a good outcome.

Left upper lobectomy can certainly be difficult after coronary artery bypass grafting, especially when patients are graft-dependent and adhesions may be dense. This study reminds us that it is OK in extreme circumstances to leave a thin wedge of lung tissue adhered to the graft rather than risk damage to the graft. It also demonstrates again that resection can be safely performed, and reaffirms the findings of others in previous study looking at thoracoscopic lobectomy following coronary artery bypass grafting. I would strongly advocate for anyone considering an intrathoracic operation on someone with prior cardiac surgery to obtain the original operative report and review it carefully for any potential complications or pitfalls. Although this report focuses on left upper lobectomy, it reminds us that either hemithorax can be compromised after cardiac surgery. With the push toward arterial revascularization and more innovative ways of bypassing the vessels, it is not uncommon to find the right mammary artery with a pedicled graft as well. With the variability in the modern cardiovascular surgical techniques, including minimally invasive valve surgery, minimally invasive atrial fibrillation surgery, and creative strategies for coronary revascularization, the necessity of understanding the exact anatomy of mediastinum from previous operations before undertaking an intrathoracic procedure in either hemithorax cannot be overemphasized.

C. T. Klodell, Jr, MD

Analysis of Unexpected Conversion to Thoracotomy During Thoracoscopic Lobectomy in Lung Cancer

Byun CS, Lee S, Kim DJ, et al (Yonsei Univ Wonju College of Medicine, Republic of Korea; Yonsei Univ College of Medicine, Seoul, Republic of Korea)

Ann Thorac Surg 100:968-973, 2015

Background.—Since anatomical lung resection by video-assisted thoracoscopic surgery (VATS) was first introduced, VATS has played a major role in lung cancer. However, conversion to thoracotomy is a major concern because an unexpected thoracotomy increases the risk of potentially adverse outcomes. Therefore, we compared patients who were and were not converted to thoracotomy and identified the risk factors for thoracotomy conversion.

Methods.—Between January 2005 and December 2013, 69 of 1,110 VATS lobectomies for lung cancer required an unexpected conversion to thoracotomy. Each converted patient was individually matched to 3 randomly selected nonconverted patients based on date of operation, type of operation, and pathologic stage.

Results.—The most common cause of conversion was fibrocalcified lymph nodes, found in 28 patients (40.6%), followed by vascular injury in 20, tumor invasion or extension in 11, pleural adhesion in 5, incomplete interlobar fissure in 3, and failure of single-lung ventilation in 2. The differences in overall postoperative complications and in-hospital deaths were not significant; however, respiratory complications were significantly more common in the conversion group ($p = 0.012$). The independent risk factors for conversion were age 65 years and older, forced expiratory volume in 1 second of less than 1.8 L, and the presence of fibrocalcified lymph nodes on preoperative chest computed tomography.

Conclusions.—Unexpected conversion to thoracotomy during VATS lobectomy in lung cancer does not appear to increase overall surgical morbidity and mortality. However, with high-risk patients, the surgeon requires careful selection for VATS candidate. Also, if necessary, the decision to convert must be made promptly to reduce possible critical respiratory complications.

► The authors review their experience spanning 8 years of videoassisted thoracoscopic surgery (VATS) lobectomy for lung cancer to identify risk factors that may predict the risk of intraoperative conversion and what effect conversion may have on patient outcome. Not too surprisingly, their results did not demonstrate an increase in morbidity and mortality comparing thoracotomy versus VATS. Despite the limitations of their study design (retrospective review, randomly matched patient controls, low study power), their study probably reflects an accurate generalization that highlights the differences in VATS (or robotic-assisted) thoracic procedures and open procedures. Specifically, the trend toward higher respiratory complications (likely secondary to increased pain associated with a thoracotomy), increased blood loss (due to the larger thoracotomy incision as well as their second most common reason for conversion—uncontrolled bleeding at 29%), and longer intensive care unit and hospital stay are most likely reflective of the increased trauma and pain associated with a rib spreading technique.

Furthermore, the findings predictive of the need for thoracotomy also are not surprising. Dense fibrosis or calcification around the hilar vessels clearly presents a more technically challenging case surgically. In the event of uncontrolled bleeding, access through a larger incision will allow for control of intraoperative bleeding while it is definitively managed. Unexpected tumor extension, incomplete fissures, and dense pleural adhesions can all contribute to a difficult open procedure, much less thoracoscopic one. This work supports the concept that in cases in which an increased likelihood of operative conversion to thoracotomy exists based on the preoperative imaging (fibrocalcified nodes, tumor extension, lack of interlobar fissure), preoperative preparation may help with the postoperative recovery. Specifically, preoperative placement of an epidural catheter and expeditious conversion to thoracotomy if necessary may reduce operative time and potentially reduce the total blood loss associated with the procedure.

V. C. Daniel
C. T. Klodell, Jr, MD

Substernal goiter: when is a sternotomy required?

Nankee L, Chen H, Schneider DF, et al (Univ of Wisconsin, Madison)
J Surg Res 199:121-125, 2015

Background.—Sternotomy for substernal goiters (SSG) is associated with greater morbidity than a cervical approach to thyroidectomy. We sought to identify predictors for sternotomy as a surgical approach for the removal of SSG and analyzed the preoperative and postoperative characteristics of patients with SSG compared with those with large goiters contained entirely within the neck or a cervical goiter.

Methods.—A retrospective review of a surgical database was performed. We included patients with large (>100 g) thyroids or SSG, regardless of size. Between 1995 and 2013, 220 patients met these criteria. Comparisons were made between patients who had an SSG and patients who had a cervical goiter with particular focus on those who required sternotomy.

Results.—Of the 220 patients, 127 patients (58%) had SSG, of whom 7 (5.5%) required sternotomy. All patients who underwent sternotomy underwent preoperative computed tomography scanning and were more likely to have preoperative symptoms of chest pressure and voice complaints and have extension of the thyroid gland below the aortic arch. Sternotomy took an average of 2 hours longer than a cervical incision, was associated with significantly more blood loss (600 *versus* 190 mL, $P = 0.04$), and a longer length of stay (3.1 *versus* 1.8 d, $P = 0.03$) than cervical thyroidectomy.

Conclusions.—Sternotomy for SSG is rare. All patients necessitating sternotomy had extension below the aortic arch and were more likely to present complaining of chest pressure and voice issues.

▶ A retrosternal or substernal goiter is enlargement of the thyroid gland that extends into the mediastinum, posterior to the sternum. The prevalence is estimated in various studies to be between 2% and 19% among all patients with a goiter. Two of the most commonly accepted definitions are a goiter that is a descended below the plane of the thoracic inlet and a goiter with more than 50% of its mass lying below the thoracic inlet. Regardless of the definition, continued growth of a substernal goiter can lead to symptoms from compression of the great vessels, trachea, and esophagus. Medical management using exogenous thyroxin may reduce gland size slightly, but this is rarely sufficient. For this reason, surgical treatment is generally indicated for symptomatic patients, and many advocate for the removal of large retrosternal goiters before dangerous compression symptoms appear.

Most thyroidectomies can be performed safely through the cervical approach, but in some cases, a thoracic approach, such as a partial or total sternotomy, may be required. Accordingly, patients that are thought to have a more difficult operation, including perhaps more blood loss and more perioperative pain secondary to the sternotomy, have a longer length of stay. The authors performed retrospective review to try to identify pathologic, clinical, and radiologic factors associated with a thoracic approach being required. They include all patients who underwent total thyroidectomy that had large thyroids greater than 100 g or any mention of substernal component during their preoperative workup, regardless of the size of the gland. Over the period from 1995 to 2013, 3233 thyroidectomies were performed, and 220 had very large thyroids. Of those, 127 patients or 58% had substernal goiters, and a total of 7 or 5.5% required sternotomy. The authors found that the substernal goiter patients were older and presented with dysphagia or shortness of breath. Importantly, however, they had a higher incidence of voice issues and chest pressure compared with those who did not have substernal extension. Their operative course had more blood loss than those patients who did not have a sternotomy, and they had a longer length of stay. In nearly all cases, the preoperative evaluation predicted a high risk of sternotomy being required.

Although sternotomy is rarely required, for removal substernal goiter, it is somewhat predictive that the patients frequently have thyroid tissue below the level of the aortic arch, but not all patients with thyroid tissue below the level of the aortic arch require sternotomy. A CT scan is imperative for preoperative planning. Importantly, perioperative indicators such as blood loss and length of stay were higher for sternotomy patients, but this reflects the increased complexity of the surgical approach. Looking at long-term complications and outcomes, the patients who underwent sternotomy still had excellent long-term outcomes, and we should not fear the use sternotomy when appropriately selected patients present with substernal goiter.

C. T. Klodell, Jr, MD

Bilobectomy Versus Lobectomy for Non-Small Cell Lung Cancer: A Comparative Study of Outcomes, Long-Term Survival, and Quality of Life

Xie D, Deschamps C, Shen RK, et al (Mayo Clinic College of Medicine, Rochester, MN; et al)

Ann Thorac Surg 100:242-250, 2015

Background.—We aimed to compare long-term survival and quality of life (QOL) outcomes after bilobectomy and lobectomy for non-small cell lung cancer patients.

Methods.—A cohort of 951 consecutive patients was identified from a single treatment institution, of whom 128 underwent bilobectomy and 823, lobectomy. Propensity score matching (1:3) was applied to balance known confounders between the two surgical groups and resulted in 512 patients (matched cohort). Unmatched and matched analyses were performed to compare clinical outcomes between the two groups, including operative mortality rate, morbidity rate, long-term survival, overall QOL, and specific symptoms.

Results.—Operative mortality was higher in the bilobectomy group than in the lobectomy group (2.3% versus 0.5%, $p = 0.022$). Morbidity rates did not differ significantly between the two groups in either unmatched or matched cohort. In the unmatched analysis, the overall survival (OS [$p = 0.003$]) and disease-free survival (DFS [$p = 0.003$]) were significantly lower in the bilobectomy group; whereas in the matched analysis, no significant difference was found in either OS ($p = 0.473$) or DFS ($p = 0.387$). Using multivariate analysis, the operation type was not found to be a significant factor for either OS (hazard ratio 1.18; 95% confidence interval: 0.91 to 1.52; $p = 0.22$) or DFS (hazard ratio 1.22; 95% confidence interval: 0.95 to 1.58; $p = 0.13$). Patients who underwent bilobectomy appeared to have similar measures of QOL as lobectomy patients, except for coughing and dyspnea.

Conclusions.—Our findings indicate that patients with non-small cell lung cancer treated with bilobectomy had similar morbidity, OS, DFS, and overall QOL as patients treated with lobectomy, but had higher mortality by matched analysis.

▶ In this retrospective review of a prospectively collected database, the authors look at a host of patient parameters comparing lobectomy with bilobectomy. In their series of nearly 1000 patients, despite what one's initial impressions may suggest, their data found no significant difference in any of the variables examined in their propensity-matched prospective database except for mortality. After propensity score matching, the risk of mortality with bilobectomy was found to be higher than that of lobectomy, but lower than the reported mortality of 3% to 12% associated with pneumonectomy. This seems logical, that as the magnitude of anatomic resection increases in size and a larger portion of the lung is removed, the mortality would increase as well. Both their lobectomy and bilobectomy mortality numbers are well within the previously published ranges for these procedures. Perhaps the most striking finding was the lack of difference in morbidity, quality of life, and overall and disease-free survival. This confirms that centers such as this which use appropriate patient selection, dedicated thoracic surgery care teams, and consistently high thoracic case volumes can lead to consistently positive outcomes. As the authors have clearly demonstrated, the need for a bilobectomy is not an impediment to the patient receiving the optimal treatment for his or her lung cancer.

V. C. Daniel
C. T. Klodell, Jr, MD

Thoracic endometriosis: clinicopathologic updates and issues about 18 cases from a tertiary referring center

Ghigna M-R, Mercier O, Mussot S, et al (Marie Lannelongue Hosp, Le Plessis-Robinson, France)

Ann Diagn Pathol 19:320-325, 2015

Thoracic endometriosis is defined as the ectopic presence of endometrial glands and stroma in lung or pleura and constitutes an uncommon cause of spontaneous pneumothorax in nonsmoker women in childbearing age. From 2000 to 2014, 18 (7.3%) women of 246 had a histologically proven endometriosis-related pneumothorax. The examination of thoracic samples was performed on formalin-fixed, paraffin-embedded hematoxylin and eosin—stained slides. Immunohistochemistry was carried out on all samples. The pathologic findings included endometriosis foci appearing as a triad of endometrial glands, stroma, and hemosiderin-laden macrophages in 8 patients. In the remaining 10 patients, minute nests of endometrial stroma were recognized at histologic examination and immunohistochemistry. One patient displayed diaphragmatic endometriosis and pulmonary lymphangioleiomyomatosis. Thoracic endometriosis is an uncommon cause of recurrent pneumothorax necessitating histologic confirmation. The histologic diagnosis of endometriosis may be challenging on small pleural or lung biopsies because endometriosis mostly appears as minute nests of endometrial stromal cells. Here, we present our experience on thoracic endometriosis: considering frequent interpretation difficulties of biopsy samples, we propose a multidisciplinary diagnostic algorithm.

▶ Endometriosis is a disease characterized by ectopic dislocation of the endometrial components outside the uterine cavity. Ectopic endometrium can be found in abdominal scar, breast, lung, and the pleural cavity. Pelvic endometriosis constitutes most usual presentations of the disease and is characterized by abdominal pain, dysmenorrhea, and dyspareunia. The typical patient profile of thoracic endometriosis involves a woman of reproductive age with enduring symptoms of chest pain, cough, and dyspnea. Although most cases revealed themselves because of an occurrence of symptoms in association with menstrual cycle, some cases escape this standard, resulting in more difficult diagnosis. Over a 14-year period at the author's institution, a total of 1169 patients were treated for spontaneous pneumothorax, with 246 of those patients being women. The authors identified a 7.3% incidence or 18 patients, as having thoracic endometriosis. It is unclear whether this is only a small sampling and there are other cases that were missed, or if this accurately reflects the true incidence of the disease. Those patients presented with symptoms including chest pain, dyspnea, and cough. Pain was right-sided in all patients, and the chest x-rays showed pneumothorax in all cases.

Recurrent pneumothorax is a usual manifestation of thoracic endometriosis, because endometriosis implants normally involve the diaphragm and parietal pleural. The most popular and accepted theory is that this is a transdiaphragmatic crossing of air from the genital tract during menses. A more unusual manifestation of thoracic endometriosis is hemoptysis, which occurs with involvement of the bronchial tree. Thoracic endometriosis should be clinically expected in all woman of child-bearing age presenting with enduring respiratory symptoms that fluctuate with their menstrual cycle. Known risk factors associated with thoracic endometriosis include previous gynecologic surgery or primary or secondary infertility, and a history of pelvic endometriosis. Endometriosis is a common cause of recurrent pneumothorax, necessitating histologic confirmation for an adequate therapeutic management and long-term surveillance. Pleural or diaphragmatic endometriosis may be overlooked because of the scant and patchy distribution of the endometrial elements.

The clinical presentation of diaphragmatic anomalies, zones of perforation, or small brown nodules at the time of thoracoscopy for spontaneous pneumothorax should initiate a biopsy and pathologic examination to determine whether this is ectopic endometrial tissue. It is important in all cases of spontaneous pneumothorax undergoing thoracoscopy in women of child-bearing age to carefully inspect all visceral and parietal pleural surfaces, including the diaphragm.

C. T. Klodell, Jr, MD

Article Index

Chapter 1: General Considerations

Chapter 2: Trauma

Chapter 6: Surgical Infections

Chapter 7: Endocrine

Chapter 8: Nutrition

Chapter 9: Gastrointestinal

Chapter 10: Oncology

Chapter 11: Vascular Surgery

Chapter 12: General Thoracic Surgery

Author Index

A

B

C

D

E

F

G

H

M

N

O

P

R

S

T

U

V

W

X

Y

Z

FSC
www.fsc.org
MIX
Papier | Fördert
gute Waldnutzung
FSC® C083411

Kolibri 360 GmbH
Ferdinand-Jühlke-Straße 7
99095 Erfurt, Deutschland
produktsicherheit@kolibri360.de